Health
Services
Assistance

supporting nursing in acute care

3RD
Edition

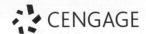

CENGAGE

Health Services Assistance: Supporting nursing in acute care
3rd Edition
Kathryn Austin

Portfolio manager: Sophie Kaliniecki
Senior content developer: Kylie Scott
Senior project editor: Nathan Katz
Cover designer: Mariana Maccarini
Text designer: Rina Gargano (Alba Design)
Permissions/Photo researcher: Liz McShane
Editor: Paul Smitz
Proofreader: James Anderson
Indexer: Max McMaster
Art direction: Mariana Maccarini
Cover: Courtesy Adobe Stock/Monkey Business
Typeset by KnowledgeWorks Global Ltd.

Any URLs contained in this publication were checked for currency during the production process. Note, however, that the publisher cannot vouch for the ongoing currency of URLs.

This third edition published in 2024

Part/Chapter-opening images courtesy iStock.com/ShotShare; iStock.com/sudok1.

Notice to the Reader
Publisher does not warrant or guarantee any of the products described herein or perform any independent analysis in connection with any of the product information contained herein. Publisher does not assume, and expressly disclaims, any obligation to obtain and include information other than that provided to it by the manufacturer. The reader is expressly warned to consider and adopt all safety precautions that might be indicated by the activities described herein and to avoid all potential hazards.

By following the instructions contained herein, the reader willingly assumes all risks in connection with such instructions. The publisher makes no representations or warranties of any kind, including but not limited to, the warranties of fitness for particular purpose or merchantability, nor are any such representations implied with respect to the material set forth herein, and the publisher takes no responsibility with respect to such material. The publisher shall not be liable for any special, consequential, or exemplary damages resulting, in whole or part, from the readers' use of, or reliance upon, this material.

For product information and technology assistance,
in Australia call **1300 790 853**;
in New Zealand call **0800 449 725**

For permission to use material from this text or product, please email
aust.permissions@cengage.com

National Library of Australia Cataloguing-in-Publication Data
ISBN: 9780170464116
A catalogue record for this book is available from the National Library of Australia.

Cengage Learning Australia
Level 5, 80 Dorcas Street
Southbank VIC 3006 Australia

Cengage Learning New Zealand
Unit 4B Rosedale Office Park
331 Rosedale Road, Albany, North Shore 0632, NZ

For learning solutions, visit **cengage.com.au**

Printed in Malaysia Papercraft
1 2 3 4 5 6 7 27 26 25 24 23

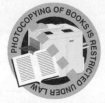

Brief Contents

Contents

Guide to the text

As you read this text you will find a number of features in every chapter to enhance your study of Health Services Assistance and help you understand how the theory is applied in the real world.

PART-OPENING FEATURES

Part openers introduce each of the chapters within the part and give an overview of how they relate to each other.

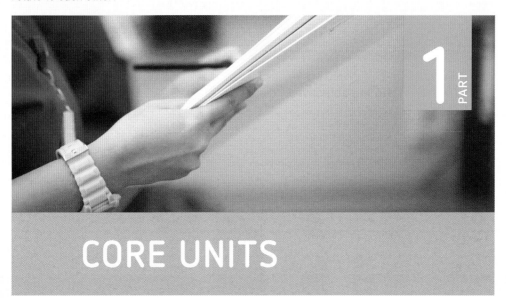

CORE UNITS

As a health services assistant, you will work in acute and subacute settings as part of a healthcare team, assisting nurses to provide client care. An understanding of foundational concepts support and facilitate the provision of the highest standards of client care in these environments. These concepts are demonstrated throughout the initial chapters of this text, which reflect the core units from the national qualification.

As part of this healthcare team and under duty of care, you have ethical and legal responsibilities to carry out your work in a way that ensures each individual's health and safety is protected.

Chapters 1 and 2 provide an overview of specific workplace risks, hazards and associated safety practices. Also included are strategies to maintain personal protection and prevent the transmission of infections from person to person. It is important for you to build on your acquired knowledge of and skills in health, safety and infection control to maintain a safe work environment.

An essential part of providing care is to recognise and understand the anatomy and physiology of body systems and to communicate and use appropriate terminology associated with care. Chapters 3, 4 and 5 provide you with knowledge of the healthy functioning of the human body and practical aspects of disease management. Appropriate use of medical terminology and communication techniques for the workplace are described so that you can function as an effective team member who contributes to meeting the basic human needs and ongoing care for individuals.

Chapters 6 and 7 apply this knowledge further with cultural care using a client-centred approach and prioritising work so that you can meet organisational goals and objectives and use lifelong learning to improve your workplace practices.

CHAPTER-OPENING FEATURES

Identify the key concepts you will engage with through the **learning objectives** at the start of each chapter.

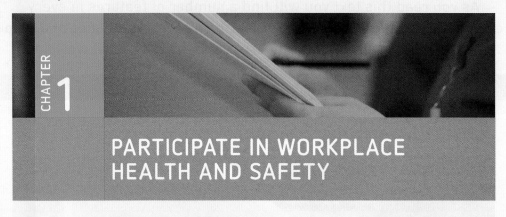

CHAPTER 1

PARTICIPATE IN WORKPLACE HEALTH AND SAFETY

Learning objectives

By the end of this chapter, you should be able to:

1   follow safe work practices
2   implement safe work practices
3   contribute to safe practices in the workplace
4   reflect on your own safe work practices.

Introduction

This chapter highlights the requirements for you, as a health services assistant (HSA), to participate in work health and safety (WHS) processes in the workplace. This is essential to ensure your own health and safety at work, as well as that of others who may be

FEATURES WITHIN CHAPTERS

Each chapter opens with **Industry Insights** from a Health Services Assistant perspective, contextualising key concepts from the chapter in workplace examples.

INDUSTRY INSIGHTS

Safety huddles and WHS

My first day in the new wa[rd] safety and quality issues f[...] and implement controls t[...] was identified: a bariatric[...] who needed assistance to[...] manual handling and per[...]

In implementing cont[...] and training needs, inclu[...]

- provision of a bariatri[...] their use

◄ REFLECTING ON THE INDUSTRY INSIGHT

1   After our safety huddle meeting, we identified additional hazards in the ward. Which of the following is *not* a hazard in a healthcare environment?
    a   Presence of bodily fluids from an infected wound.
    b   Used sharps left unattended in the equipment room.
    c   Performing a risk assessment on a patient.
    d   Violent or aggressive behaviour from a new admission.

2   Our bariatric patient required a transfer to a wheelchair and one of the staff involved felt a pain in her back after the procedure. An incident report was completed. Which of the following does the report always need to include?
    a   Person's occupation.
    b   Where and when the incident occurred.

After you have worked through the chapter, revisit this section at the end of the chapter in the **Reflecting on the Industry Insight** to apply your knowledge with several multiple choice questions.

FEATURES WITHIN CHAPTERS

Engage actively and personally with the material by completing the practical activities in the **Activity** boxes. These help you to assess your own knowledge, beliefs, traits and attitudes.

Codes of practice

An approved code of practice is a practical guide to achieving the standards of health, safety and welfare required under the WHS Act and the WHS regulations. Search for the code of practice for *hazardous manual tasks* on Safe Work Australia's website (**https://www.safeworkaustralia.gov.au**) and answer the following questions:

1 What is a hazardous manual task?

2 What are the characteristics of hazardous manual tasks?

3 Who has WHS duties in relation to hazardous manual tasks?

4 Identify any other codes of practice from this website that are relevant to your work as an HSA.

Analyse practical applications of concepts through the **Scenario** box, with questions for reflection or discussion.

Following procedures for identifying hazards

Hillary, an HSA who worked in a small rural hospital, was concerned about the lack of manual handling equipment for use in the ward. She was worried that incorrect procedures might result in injuries to staff or patients. Hillary reported this to the RN who acknowledged her concerns and invited her to the WHS meeting, where Hillary presented the issue.

The committee conducted an open discussion about potential solutions, including the temporary hire of manual handling equipment until a thorough assessment of the types of patients and their needs was completed. Two months later, the hospital purchased an electronic hoist and three forearm support frames and cleared out an unused office for equipment storage. By following the correct procedures, Hillary and the HSC members ensured that the WHS concerns for patients and staff were acknowledged.

1 Risk control measures use the hierarchy of risk control. What level of control was used in this example?

2 What procedures would you follow if you identified a potential hazard in the ward during your work experience?

Important **Key terms** are marked in bold in the text and defined in the margin when they are used in the text for the first time. A full list of key terms is also available in the **glossary**, which can be found at the back of the book.

Emergency response

Your response to an emergency should be according to the policies and procedures of your organisation, which is outlined in the emergency action plan. As an HSA, you should be fully aware of your role in terms of:

* identifying an emergency situation
* how an emergency should be reported
* how to follow all organisational procedures in response to the emergency.

A response to an emergency may include activating an alarm or an evacuation, which is likely to include assisting patients from the wards. It is paramount that you obey all directions from designated personnel as demonstrated in your training on emergencies or as outlined in the emergency action plan. A response in the case of fire might be to:

* remove people
* alert fire brigade and nearby staff
* confine fire and smoke – close windows and doors if possible
* extinguish or control fire without taking risks.

In the case of a fire, it is important to remember to stay close to the ground. Patients in immediate danger should be removed first, with ambulatory patients accompanied or directed to

Emergency action plan
A plan that outlines an organisation's policies and procedures in response to an emergency situation.

END-OF-CHAPTER FEATURES

At the end of each chapter you will find several tools to help you to review, practise and extend your knowledge of the key learning objectives.

Review your understanding of the key chapter topics with the **Summary**.

SUMMARY

The entire healthcare team, as well as patients and others, has a responsibility to maintain work health and safety (WHS). The awareness of risks through hazard identification and management ensures that the workplace remains a safe environment. This chapter outlined the importance of participating in WHS processes as an HSA working in acute care. It emphasised the importance of identifying existing and potential hazards and undertaking elimination or minimisation measures to promote work health and safety.

The new **Apply your knowledge** feature encourages you to integrate the concepts discussed in the chapter and apply them to a real-world situation.

APPLY YOUR KNOWLEDGE

Emergency response

Whilst I was giving a bed bath to Mrs Frazier with the assistance of the registered nurse (RN), Mrs Frazier started to complain of chest pain. In no time she became pale and unconscious with no evidence of pulse or breathing.

The RN asked me to press the emergency button and we lowered the back of the bed to

Mrs Frazier was transferred to the high-dependency cardiac unit for further monitoring and I cleaned up the ward area after the team had left.

3   Look up Chapter 2, 'Comply with infection prevention and control policies and procedures', and identify the appropriate actions to take when disposing of contaminated waste.

Test your knowledge and consolidate your learning through the **Self-check questions** and the **Questions for discussion**.

SELF-CHECK QUESTIONS

1   Describe the WHS responsibilities for the employer and employee.
2   How can hazards be identified in the workplace?
3   What is the purpose of completing a risk assessment matrix?
4   Describe the control levels in the hierarchy of risk control.
5   What are examples of emergency alarms used in health care?

QUESTIONS FOR DISCUSSION

1   Discuss the purpose of the WHS Act.
2   Visit the Safe Work Australia website (http://www.safeworkaustralia.gov.au) and discuss how Safe Work Australia improves work health and safety and workers' compensation across Australia.
3   Discuss how you can contribute to the minimisation of risks in the workplace.
4   Discuss and give examples of how engineering controls can reduce risks in the healthcare environment.

Take your study further with research and group work in the **Extension activity**.

EXTENSION ACTIVITY

Work health and safety inspection

Identifying hazards is the first step in the risk management process. During your workplace experience, team up with a colleague to undertake a WHS inspection of the ward and complete the following activities:

1   Conduct the WHS audit using the checklist in Figure 1.14. (This checklist has been produced as a guide to decide whether a healthcare facility complies with WHS legislation.)
2   In groups, identify the hazards found and develop strategies to minimise or eliminate the risks that they pose.

Guide to the online resources

MINDTAP

Premium online teaching and learning tools are available on the *MindTap* platform – the personalised eLearning solution.

MindTap is a flexible and easy-to-use platform that helps build student confidence and gives you a clear picture of their progress. We partner with you to ease the transition to digital – we're with you every step of the way.

The *Cengage Mobile App* puts your course directly into students' hands with course materials available on their smartphone or tablet. Students can read on the go, complete practice quizzes or participate in interactive real-time activities.

MindTap for Austin's *Health Services Assistance* 3rd edition is full of innovative resources to support critical thinking, and help your students move from memorisation to mastery! Includes:

- Austin's *Health Services Assistance* 3rd edition eBook
- Polling questions, activities, worksheets and case studies.

MindTap is a premium purchasable eLearning tool. Contact your Cengage learning consultant to find out how *MindTap* can transform your course.

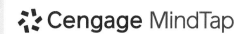

INSTRUCTOR RESOURCES PACK

Premium resources that provide additional instructor support are available for this text, including:

SOLUTIONS MANUAL

The **Solutions Manual** provides answers to every question in the text.

POWERPOINT™ PRESENTATIONS

Cengage **PowerPoint slides** are a convenient way to add more depth to your lectures, covering additional content and offering a selection of engaging features aligned with the textbook.

COGNERO® TEST BANK

A bank of questions has been developed in conjunction with the text for creating quizzes, tests and exams for your students. Create multiple test versions in an instant and deliver tests from your LMS, your classroom, or wherever you want using Cognero. Cognero test generator is a flexible online system that allows you to import, edit, and manipulate content from the text's test bank or elsewhere, including your own favourite test questions.

CASE STUDIES

Analyse in-depth **Case studies** that present issues in context, encouraging students to integrate the concepts discussed in the chapter and apply them to the workplace.

COMPETENCY-BASED ACTIVITY SHEETS

Chapter worksheets mapped to units of competency for instructors.

ARTWORK FROM THE TEXT

Add the digital files of graphs, pictures and flow charts into your learning management system, use them in student handouts, or copy them into your lecture presentations.

MAPPING GRID

This **Detailed Mapping Grid** aligns the content of this book to the elements of core and elective units of competency from HLT33115 – Certificate III in Health Services Assistance.

The Instructor Resource Pack is included for institutional adoptions of this text when certain conditions are met. The pack is available to purchase for course-level adoptions of the text or as a standalone resource. Contact your Cengage learning consultant for more information.

FOR THE STUDENT

MINDTAP

MindTap is the next-level online learning tool that helps you get better grades!

MindTap gives you the resources you need to study – all in one place and available when you need them. In the *MindTap Reader*, you can make notes, highlight text and even find a definition directly from the page.

If your instructor has chosen *MindTap* for your subject this semester, log in to *MindTap* to:
- Get better grades
- Save time and get organised
- Connect with your instructor and peers
- Study when and where you want, online and mobile
- Complete assessment tasks as set by your instructor.

When your instructor creates a course using *MindTap*, they will let you know your course link so you can access the content. Please purchase *MindTap* only when directed by your instructor. Course length is set by your instructor.

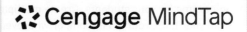

Preface

Increasing demand and an ageing population continue to shape the changing context for the health workforce in Australia. This has resulted in the need for health services assistants who can provide a high standard of personal and clinical care for patients, as well as the retention of highly skilled and experienced enrolled and registered nurses for more complex needs. This wide skill mix will result in high-quality care for every patient and the efficient use of healthcare services.

This text supports the beginning learner by describing the knowledge and skills required to work towards a Certificate III in Health Services Assistance (Assisting in Nursing Work in Acute Care). This nationally recognised qualification reflects the role of a variety of workers who use a range of factual, technical and procedural knowledge to provide assistance to health professional staff for the care of patients.

Health services assistants work under the delegation and supervision of registered nursing staff, and each chapter in the text identifies the scope of practice and range of activities that can be undertaken. The skills and knowledge required for the effective delivery of care, with examples, are detailed throughout the text, with the capacity for the learner to self-assess, and to use knowledge learnt through the 'Apply your knowledge' feature at the end of each chapter. Discussion and extension activities also provide opportunities for students to increase their knowledge.

Foundation knowledge and skills are developed throughout the initial chapters, which reflect the core units from the national qualification. These include work health and safety (WHS), infection control, anatomy and physiology, cultural care, communication and prioritising work. This underpinning knowledge can then be applied to gain a greater understanding of the specialist acute care elective specialisation chapters that follow. These discuss transporting and moving patients, nursing and using equipment in an acute care environment, and behaviours of concern. Additional chapters identify nursing care for people with dementia-specific, mental health and palliative care needs, as well as how to provide a high standard of client service. This highlights the ever-expanding role of the health services assistant. The final chapter on assisting with an allied health program is new to this edition and presents information for health services and allied health assistants on providing basic assistance to allied health professionals in a health or community context. This includes following treatment plans for therapeutic interventions and/or conducting programs under supervision.

Using this text will enable students to meet high standards of patient-focused care and provide teachers and facilitators with tools to support students throughout their learning journey.

About the author

Kathryn Austin DipAppSc Nursing, CIV TAE, GradDip VET, MEd, MBA has been driving the strategic and operational delivery of health programs in the Vocational Education and Training (VET) Sector as a Manager, Head Teacher and Facilitator for over 25 years. Other roles have included capability development with a focus on leadership and culture and how they can impact on effective workplace teams.

Kathryn is a principled advocate for health and community services and has presented at conferences on the changing needs of the healthcare sector and current vocational education and training issues. She is a professional member of the nursing and midwifery council and currently works in a compliance capacity for nursing and midwifery accreditation. She is committed to improving educational standards and promoting a culture of performance awareness to enhance the quality of education programs in the higher education and VET sectors.

Acknowledgements

The author and Cengage Learning would like to thank Geoff Arnott for his contribution to the first edition of this text, and the following reviewers for their incisive and helpful feedback:

- Melissa Slattery – Equals International
- Jodie Watkins – South Regional TAFE Albany
- Catherine Wallace – TAFE NSW
- Susan Boulter – TAFE NSW
- Catherine Fox – BRACE SkillsPlus
- Rosemary Henderson – Phillips Institute
- Lynelle Jenkinson – TAFE NSW
- Simone Best – ACU.

Cengage acknowledges Susie Gray for the contribution of Chapter 2 on infection control for the first edition.

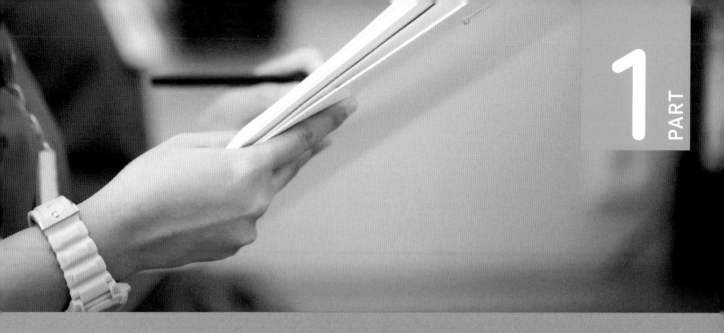

CORE UNITS

As a health services assistant, you will work in acute and subacute settings as part of a healthcare team, assisting nurses to provide client care. An understanding of foundational concepts support and facilitate the provision of the highest standards of client care in these environments. These concepts are demonstrated throughout the initial chapters of this text, which reflect the core units from the national qualification.

As part of this healthcare team and under duty of care, you have ethical and legal responsibilities to carry out your work in a way that ensures each individual's health and safety is protected.

Chapters 1 and 2 provide an overview of specific workplace risks, hazards and associated safety practices. Also included are strategies to maintain personal protection and prevent the transmission of infections from person to person. It is important for you to build on your acquired knowledge of and skills in health, safety and infection control to maintain a safe work environment.

An essential part of providing care is to recognise and understand the anatomy and physiology of body systems and to communicate and use appropriate terminology associated with care. Chapters 3, 4 and 5 provide you with knowledge of the healthy functioning of the human body and practical aspects of disease management. Appropriate use of medical terminology and communication techniques for the workplace are described so that you can function as an effective team member who contributes to meeting the basic human needs and ongoing care for individuals.

Chapters 6 and 7 apply this knowledge further with cultural care using a client-centred approach and prioritising work so that you can meet organisational goals and objectives and use lifelong learning to improve your workplace practices.

PARTICIPATE IN WORKPLACE HEALTH AND SAFETY

Learning objectives

By the end of this chapter, you should be able to:

1 follow safe work practices
2 implement safe work practices
3 contribute to safe practices in the workplace
4 reflect on your own safe work practices.

Introduction

This chapter highlights the requirements for you, as a health services assistant (HSA), to participate in work health and safety (WHS) processes in the workplace. This is essential to ensure your own health and safety at work, as well as that of others who may be affected by your actions. Your duty of care involves identifying workplace hazards and using risk management processes to eliminate or minimise the risk in order to maintain workplace safety.

This chapter will outline the WHS legislation in Australia, including the identification of hazards and risk control, how to safely conduct work in an acute care setting, and the importance of participating in consultative activities. The last part of the chapter considers the importance of reflecting on your own safe work practices so that continuous improvements can be made.

Following safe work practices is essential for all workers in healthcare settings. Awareness of hazards, risks and controls, and emergency procedures, as well as your own levels of stress, can ensure that the workplace is safe for both you and the individuals in your care.

INDUSTRY INSIGHTS 💬

Safety huddles and WHS

My first day in the new ward involved a safety huddle. This was a meeting to discuss safety and quality issues for both staff and patients to identify hazards, assess risks and implement controls to eliminate or minimise the risks. A hazardous situation was identified: a bariatric patient on our ward who weighed 180 kilograms and who needed assistance to mobilise. This posed a risk for all of us when undertaking manual handling and personal care tasks.

In implementing controls to minimise risks, we identified appropriate resources and training needs, including:

- provision of a bariatric bed, wheelchair, commode and chair, with instruction on their use
- ergonomics and manual handling training, including appropriate posture and consideration of bed height when undertaking activities at the bedside
- an appropriately sized blood pressure (BP) cuff when taking clinical measurements
- use of bariatric scales when taking weight
- use of the Waterlow or Braden pressure ulcer assessment tool
- an increase in the number of staff for manual handling and personal care tasks; for example, holding the skin folds when washing the patient, and assistance when rolling the patient for pressure area care
- psychological care, including maintaining patient dignity and respect when delivering care.

We recorded the strategies in the patient notes so that all the staff on each shift were aware and could access and use the resources. We were also informed that we must complete an incident report form if we suffered any injuries when performing tasks on this or any other patient. Our manager identified that some of us needed further training but ensured that we would be supervised in the meantime so that we could perform our duties safely.

Hazard
Anything that has the potential to harm the health or safety of a person.

Risk
The possibility that a hazard will actually cause harm.

Waterlow or Braden pressure ulcer assessment tool
A screening tool that provides predictive information about the risk of developing a pressure sore.

1 FOLLOW SAFE WORK PRACTICES

It is the responsibility of all workers to familiarise themselves with Australian WHS legislation, as well as their organisation's policies and procedures. These policies and procedures aim to inform workers about their responsibilities, reporting procedures, recording requirements and emergency procedures. As an HSA, it is your role to contribute to safety in the workplace by identifying any existing or potential workplace hazards, follow the organisation's risk assessment and management processes, and ensure that you are aware of emergency plans and procedures.

Follow workplace policies and procedures for safe work practices

The *Work Health and Safety Act 2011* (the WHS Act) provides the framework for the protection of the health, safety and welfare of workers at work as well as others affected by the work undertaken at the workplace.

Under the WHS Act, it is required that all workplaces follow safe work practices and that certain Australian Standards are maintained for all workers. Section 3 of the WHS Act describes the purpose of the Act, which is to:

Australian Standards
Documents setting out specifications, procedures and guidelines for Australia.

- protect the health and safety of workers and other people by eliminating or minimising risks arising from work or workplaces
- ensure fair and effective representation, consultation and cooperation to address and resolve health and safety issues in the workplace
- encourage unions and employer organisations to take a constructive role in improving WHS practices
- assist businesses and workers to achieve a healthier and safer working environment
- provide information, education and training on WHS
- provide effective compliance and enforcement measures
- deliver continuous improvement and progressively higher standards of WHS … 'health' includes psychological health as well as physical health.

Source: Safe Work Australia, 2016

The WHS Act provides the overall framework, while each state and territory has a WHS organisation with the power to enforce and regulate legislation related to WHS in the workplace. Safe Work Australia is a national body that is responsible for leading the development of policy to improve WHS and workers' compensation arrangements across Australia.

WHS responsibilities

The WHS Act and state and territory legislation covers:

Person conducting a business or undertaking (PCBU)
Individuals, businesses or organisations that are conducting business.

- person conducting a business or undertaking (PCBU) – individuals, businesses or organisations that are conducting business
- workers – anyone who performs paid work in any capacity for an employer, business or organisation is considered a worker; however, the term can also include unpaid workers such as volunteers or work experience students
- other people at a workplace – this includes patients and their visitors in acute care settings. PCBUs (employers) and workers (employees) both have WHS rights and responsibilities.

Employers must:

- properly orientate, train and supervise staff to ensure safe work practices are understood and followed by all employees
- consult with all employees about decisions that will affect safety in the workplace

Personal protective equipment (PPE)
Clothing and equipment designed to be a barrier between the worker and the hazard.

- provide suitable personal protective equipment (PPE) to make sure workers can do their job safely and train workers on how to use PPE correctly
- regularly check WHS systems and procedures to make sure that workers are adequately protected from workplace hazards
- provide adequate facilities for the welfare of employees, which covers everything from providing suitable toilet facilities to conducting risk assessments on premises and procedures

- be aware of their legal obligations under WHS legislation.
  Employees must:
- work safely to protect themselves and others from injury and follow all WHS instructions, such as:
  - wear all PPE provided
  - follow safe work procedures
  - not interfere with or misuse anything provided by the employer (equipment, signs etc.) that is used to keep the workplace safe
  - not behave in a way that puts themselves or others at risk
  - respond to a reasonable request to provide assistance or first aid to an injured person at work
- report any WHS issues, including hazards, injuries, illnesses and near misses.

Near miss
An accident that is just barely avoided; for example, almost receiving a needlestick injury.

Codes of practice

An approved code of practice is a practical guide to achieving the standards of health, safety and welfare required under the WHS Act and the WHS regulations. Search for the code of practice for *hazardous manual tasks* on Safe Work Australia's website (**https://www.safeworkaustralia.gov.au**) and answer the following questions:

1 What is a hazardous manual task?

2 What are the characteristics of hazardous manual tasks?

3 Who has WHS duties in relation to hazardous manual tasks?

4 Identify any other codes of practice from this website that are relevant to your work as an HSA.

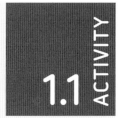
1.1 ACTIVITY

Identify, report and record existing and potential hazards in the workplace

A hazard can be defined as 'anything that has the potential to cause injury, illness or damage to your health' (Worksafe Tasmania, 2022). Hazards exist in acute care, and it is your responsibility to identify existing and potential hazards in your work area and to take actions to control the risk. A risk arises when it is possible that a hazard will actually cause harm. The level of risk will depend on factors such as how often the job is done, the number of workers involved and how serious any injuries that result could be. Risk management (see Figure 1.1) refers to the process of identifying, assessing, controlling and reviewing risks, so that strategies or changes can be made to work practices.

Risk management
The culture, processes and structures that are directed towards realising potential opportunities while managing adverse effects.

Hazard identification

According to Safe Work Australia (2020), traumatic joint/ligament and muscle/tendon injury accounted for 39 per cent of all injuries claimed in 2018–19. This highlights the importance of identifying hazards before they cause harm – the first step in the risk management process. The NSW WHS Regulations 2017 requires workers to identify hazards that can affect anyone at a workplace. Hazards in acute care settings include:

- physical – manual tasks, noise and radiation
- chemical – acids, heavy metals and dusts

FIGURE 1.1 Risk management process

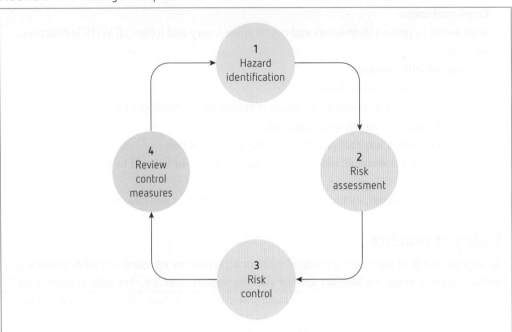

- biological – microorganisms, including bacteria and viruses
- mechanical/electrical – slips, trips and falls
- psychosocial – fatigue, stress and violence.
  Methods that can be used to identify hazards in your workplace include:
- consulting workers about any health and safety problems they have encountered in doing their work
- inspecting the workplace and observing how work tasks are performed
- WHS audits or workplace inspections
- review of incident/accident and near-miss reports.

New or emerging hazards

New hazards may sometimes emerge in the setting where you work. Examples of new or emerging hazards include:
- presence of bodily fluids from an infected wound
- excessive noise from new building works adjacent to the health facility
- evidence of worker fatigue or burnout
- violent or aggressive behaviour from a new admission.
  Remaining alert is the best way of identifying new or emerging hazards. If you do identify a new or emerging hazard, you are required to report it to your supervisor.

Risk assessment

Risk assessment

Analysis of the potential risks that may be involved in an activity.

Risk assessment is necessary to prevent accidents and to maintain workplace safety. It involves an analysis of the hazard in terms of the likelihood of it creating a workplace injury or illness. Risk assessments are very important because they form an essential part of a good safety management plan. They help to:
- create awareness of hazards and risks
- identify who may be at risk

- determine if existing control measures are adequate or if more should be done
- prevent injuries or illnesses when done at the design or planning stage
- prioritise hazards and control measures.

As an HSA, risk assessment involves looking at your workplace to identify those things, situations, processes and so on that may cause harm and reporting them to your supervisors. Formal assessments should be done by a competent team of individuals who have a good working knowledge of the workplace. Staff who should always be involved include supervisors and workers who work with the process under review because they are the most familiar with the operation.

A risk assessment matrix (see Figure 1.2) is used to determine the level of risk based on the assessment of likelihood and consequence. For example, a frequently used, slippery bathroom floor could be assessed as very likely to result in a major injury.

FIGURE 1.2 Risk assessment matrix

			Potential Consequences				
			L6	L5	L4	L3	L2
			Minor injuries or discomfort. No medical treatment or measureable physical effects	Injuries or illness requiring medical treatment. Temporary impairment	Injuries or illness requiring hospital admission	Injury or illness resulting in permanent impairment	Fatality
			Not Significant	Minor	Moderate	Major	Severe
Likelihood	Expected to occur regularly under normal circumstances	Almost Certain	Medium	High	Very High	Very High	Very High
	Expected to occur at some time	Likely	Medium	High	High	Very High	Very High
	May occur at some time	Possible	Low	Medium	High	High	Very High
	Not likely to occur in normal circumstances	Unlikely	Low	Low	Medium	Medium	High
	Could happen, but probably never will	Rare	Low	Low	Low	Low	Medium

Risk control

After identifying and assessing the risk, strategies for managing it must be developed in consultation with the healthcare team. Section 17 of the WHS Act requires risks to be eliminated; however, if this is not reasonably practicable, the risks must be minimised.

The control of risk should be based on a consideration of the work environment factors that may pose a threat to safety. The process for minimising or controlling risk is known as the **hierarchy of control**. The levels of controls are as follows (also see Figure 1.3 for examples of controls in practice):

- Level 1 controls:
  - Eliminate hazards.

Hierarchy of control

A step-by-step approach to eliminating or reducing risks, with a ranking of risk controls from the highest level of protection through to the lowest and least reliable protection.

FIGURE 1.3 Hierarchy of controls in practice

Level	Control	Example of control in practice
1	**Elimination** Remove the hazard completely	Where a healthcare facility has chosen not to purchase latex gloves to eliminate the risk of employees developing allergies/allergic reactions to latex materials
2	**Substitution** Replace the hazard with another process	Replacing flooring with a more slip-resistant surface to avoid slips or falls
2	**Isolate** Separate the hazard from people	Storing chemicals in an appropriate cabinet
2	**Engineering controls** Removing or isolating a hazard through technology	Using a ceiling-mounted system to transfer a person from bed to bathroom to take the load for the healthcare worker
3	**Administrative controls** Policies aimed at limiting exposure to a hazard, including guidelines, policies and procedures	Staff members working in pairs when providing care in high-risk psychiatric areas so as to discourage any threatening situations
3	**Personal protective equipment** Clothing and equipment designed to be a barrier between workers and the hazard	Using gowns, gloves, and masks and eye shields when caring for people with infective/viral respiratory disorders, such as sudden acute respiratory syndrome (SARS) This can also include earmuffs to help protect from noise

- Level 2 controls:
  - Substitute the hazard
  - Isolate the hazard
  - Use engineering controls.
- Level 3 controls:
  - Use administrative controls
  - Use PPE.

PPE is used when all other control measures are considered unsuitable. PPE requires training for use, implementation of maintenance programs and supervision to ensure it is used correctly.

All people should be familiar with the hazard control measures used in their workplace and refer to the hierarchy of control framework to assess that the appropriate WHS measures are being taken.

Residual risk

Residual risk

The risk of loss or harm remaining even after all controls have been implemented.

A residual risk is a risk that remains even after all controls have been implemented. It is not possible to eliminate or completely control all hazards, so part of a risk analysis is knowing that a level of risk may be considered acceptable if it is unlikely to occur; or if it does occur, it will have minimum impact.

Risk assessment and control

Respond to the following regarding risk assessment:

1   Undertake a risk assessment of the ward or facility during your workplace experience.
2   Identify hazards and complete a risk assessment matrix to determine their likelihood and consequences.
3   Using the hierarchy of control, identify how these risks could be minimised.

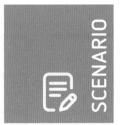

Review control measures

The fourth step in managing hazards is, in consultation with staff, monitoring and reviewing the changes made to control the hazard to ensure they have been effective and have not introduced additional hazards. This hazard reporting is essential for successful hazard management. Implementing the use of hazard report forms will encourage staff to identify and report hazards so that controls can be implemented before an injury occurs.

ADL Support Services Pty Ltd

Manual handling was identified as the most common cause of claims made to Safe Work Australia for ADL Support Services Pty Ltd, which runs a number of small private hospitals in north-western Victoria and southern New South Wales. It was already aware that manual handling was responsible for 58 per cent of all the injuries, but the company percentage was closer to 70 per cent with recorded back injuries by nurses, HSAs and its kitchen staff at all locations.

ADL decided to employ a consultancy firm to investigate causes and to come up with solutions based around hazard identification, risk assessment and control of risk at the various sites. As a part of its investigation, the consultancy firm studied available data, interviewed staff, made observations and wrote recommendations. The final report outlined the findings and emphasised the implementation of hierarchy of risk control measures, with recommendations based around substitution, engineering and administrative controls in relation to the risks.

The recommendations included:

- all beds to be of adjustable height and to be hydraulic
- heavy kitchen equipment to be substituted with lighter alternatives, and movement in and out of the kitchen to occur with the assistance of wheeled trolleys
- all staff to be provided with induction and ongoing training in safe manual handling techniques and use of equipment
- overhead hoists to be installed in all rooms including bathrooms and toilets
- all patients to be assessed during admission for required manual handling
- a plan to be established to reduce or eliminate manual handling by augmenting with suitable equipment.

1   What risk assessment tools and manual handling devices does your workplace use to identify and manage the risks associated with manual handling?
2   Why was it important for the consultancy firm to interview staff as part of the investigation?

Follow workplace emergency procedures

An *emergency situation* is any abnormal or sudden event that requires immediate action. It often occurs without warning and has the potential to cause injury, illness or death, as well as major disruption and damage to property. You should identify and report an emergency situation according to your organisational procedures. Simulation training should also be provided involving an emergency response or an actual evacuation drill.

It is also important to be aware of the location of emergency exits and the planned assembly points where everyone is to meet in the event of an evacuation. Evacuation maps will be displayed throughout your workplace with signs and symbols indicating the nearest exit and the assembly point for the building. Emergency procedure information must be kept in an accessible and obvious location in the workplace. It is important that you know where the information regarding emergency procedures is kept and the action to take in such instances. See the example of an evacuation plan in Figure 1.4.

FIGURE 1.4 An example of a typical evacuation plan

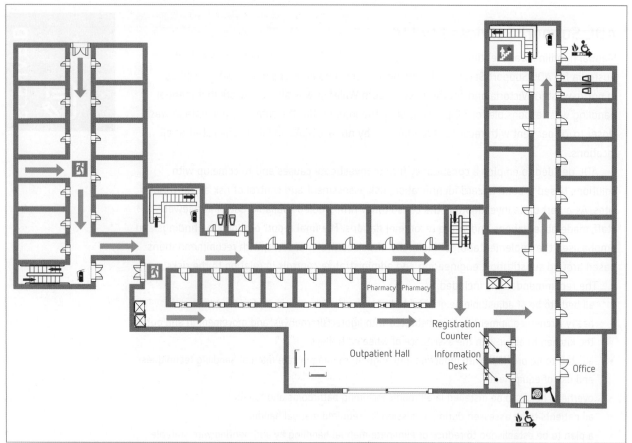

Pharmacy Pharmacy

Registration
Counter

Outpatient Hall

Information
Desk

Office

Source: Reproduced with permission from Wondershare and Edrawsoft.

Hospitals and healthcare facilities use a nationally recognised set of codes to prepare, plan, respond and recover from internal and external emergencies. Figure 1.5 identifies the hospital emergency codes which are based upon Australian Standard (AS) 4083 – 2010 Planning for emergencies – healthcare facilities:

FIGURE 1.5 Emergency codes

Fire or smoke	Code red
Evacuation	Code orange
Bomb threat	Code purple
Personal threat	Code black
Internal emergency	Code yellow
External emergency	Code brown
Medical emergency	Code blue

Examples of these emergency codes include:

- events requiring evacuation, such as fires, bomb threats or hazardous substances
- personal threats, such as intruders and disturbed/aggressive individuals
- internal emergencies, such as loss of power or water supply
- external emergencies and natural disasters, such as flood and storm
- critical medical emergencies, such as cardiac arrest.

You should identify emergency codes and alarms in your workplace and respond to them appropriately. Emergency signals and alarms may include:

- duress alarms
- machinery malfunction alarms
- fire alarms
- evacuation alarms or announcements
- beepers on mobile phones.

Emergency response

Your response to an emergency should be according to the policies and procedures of your organisation, which is outlined in the emergency action plan. As an HSA, you should be fully aware of your role in terms of:

- identifying an emergency situation
- how an emergency should be reported
- how to follow all organisational procedures in response to the emergency.

A response to an emergency may include activating an alarm or an evacuation, which is likely to include assisting patients from the wards. It is paramount that you obey all directions from designated personnel as demonstrated in your training on emergencies or as outlined in the emergency action plan. A response in the case of fire might be to:

- remove people
- alert fire brigade and nearby staff
- confine fire and smoke – close windows and doors if possible
- extinguish or control fire without taking risks.

In the case of a fire, it is important to remember to stay close to the ground. Patients in immediate danger should be removed first, with ambulatory patients accompanied or directed to an evacuation area. Non-ambulatory patients should be moved using wheelchairs or stretchers, when available, to the evacuation area.

Emergency action plan

A plan that outlines an organisation's policies and procedures in response to an emergency situation.

You may also be involved in a debriefing of the emergency response after the emergency has occurred. This is to assess the effectiveness of the emergency action plan in terms of continuous improvement, and determines:

- what occurred – the nature of the emergency in terms of what, how and when events occurred and who was involved
- how the emergency action plan worked – evaluation of operational effectiveness
- any recommended changes – proposed amendments to the emergency action plan.

ACTIVITY 1.3

Emergency action plans

Locate the emergency action plan in your workplace or classroom area to determine where the:

- evacuation area is located
- nearest emergency exit is.
Refer to emergency procedure guidelines in your workplace to answer the following questions:

1   What are the instructions to remove frail and immobile individuals in the event of a fire?
2   What is the procedure for answering the phone if there is a bomb threat?
3   What is the reporting procedure for a medical emergency such as a cardiac arrest?
4   What is the procedure for a Code Black – personal threat (armed or unarmed persons threatening injury to themselves or others)?

2   IMPLEMENT SAFE WORK PRACTICES

Implementing safe work practices means following all work procedures and instructions and reporting incidents and injuries to a designated person in your organisation. It also includes undertaking any required WHS housekeeping tasks in your work area. To ensure that you incorporate safe practices in your role, HSAs are required to know the meanings of safety signage and the location of policies and procedures, as well as their scope of practice when undertaking tasks.

Identify and implement WHS procedures and work instructions

Procedures and work instructions may be provided verbally, in writing and visually by WHS signage, symbols and other pictorial presentations. Each organisation will have a variety of policies and procedures in place; for example:

- storage and handling of chemicals
- manual handling risk assessments
- falls risk assessments
- incident reporting
- workplace violence
- standard and additional precautions
- emergency procedures
- smoking policies.

Identify safety signage

Safety signs in the workplace each convey a specific message regarding hazards and safety to those who view them. The messages include the location of safety and fire protection equipment, mandatory signs for safety equipment, hazards and emergency signals. The Australian Standard 1319–1994 Safety Signs for the Occupational Environment regulates the design and use of safety signs, which are identified by colour and shape. The common signs used in health care can be seen in Figure 1.6.

FIGURE 1.6 Safety signage

SIGN	PURPOSE	EXAMPLE
Prohibition signs	Indicates something that you must not do	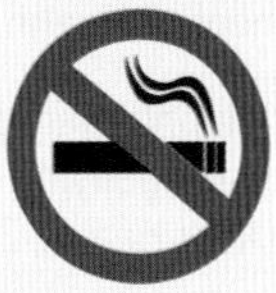
Mandatory signs	Indicates that you must wear special safety equipment, or specific processes that need to be undertaken to ensure employee safety	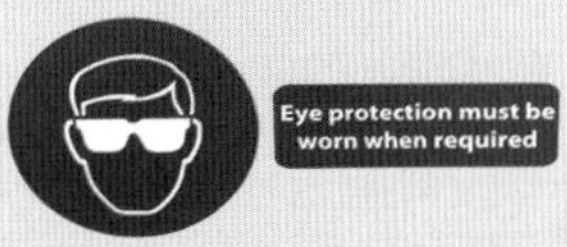
Hazard warning signs	Warns of a danger or risk to your health	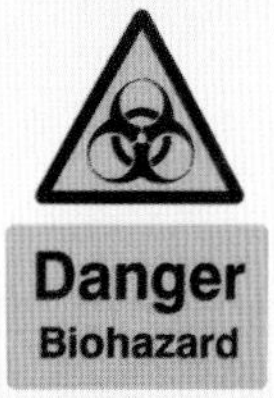
Emergency information signs	Shows the location of emergency safety equipment or emergency exits	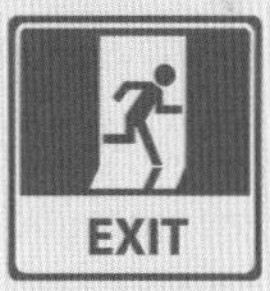
Fire signs	Indicates the location of fire alarms and firefighting facilities	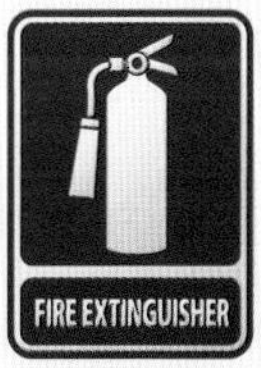
Danger hazard signs	Warns of a particular hazard or hazardous condition that could be life threatening	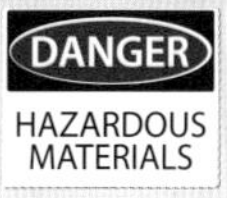

Sources from top: iStock.com/arcady_31; Alamy Stock Photo/Art Directors & TRIP; iStock.com/Gannet77; iStock.com/PSNJua; iStock.com/MyFortis; Shutterstock.com/Stephen Marques

Implement procedures

In order to implement WHS policies and procedures, it is the responsibility of an organisation to provide employees with the appropriate equipment, skills and knowledge to support safe work practices. This includes the distribution of policy documents to staff, including a **policy directive**, guidelines, information bulletins and procedure manuals. State or territory public health organisations have electronic databases for policy and procedure documents and smaller healthcare providers may have paper-based forms. Some examples of real policies and guidelines used across Australia can be seen in Figure 1.7.

FIGURE 1.7 Examples of policies and guidelines

POLICY/GUIDELINE	PURPOSE
COVID-19 vaccination – Australian COVID-19 Vaccination Policy (Australian Government, Department of Health, 2021)	This Australian COVID-19 Vaccination Policy outlines the approach to providing COVID-19 vaccines in Australia
Prevention and management of workplace bullying in NSW Health (NSW Health, 2018)	Assists managers to fulfil their obligations to eliminate or minimise the risk of bullying and manage complaints relating to bullying; and provides staff with information on their rights and obligations when they make a complaint
Workplace Aggression and Violence Policy (WA Health, 2021)	Outlines the minimum requirements and responsibilities of WA health system entities in providing a safe workplace where employees are not subject to aggression and violence
Hand hygiene clinical guideline (SA Health, 2020)	Outlines the specific hand hygiene practices required to minimise the risk of patients, visitors and staff acquiring a healthcare associated infection. The policy states when and how staff must perform hand hygiene

ACTIVITY 1.4

Hazardous chemicals in the workplace

Use relevant WHS regulations, policies and procedures to answer the following questions:

1   How should hazardous chemicals be labelled in the workplace?
2   How should hazardous chemicals be stored in the workplace?
3   What precautions should be used to minimise the risk of exposure to hazardous chemicals in the workplace?
4   How are hazardous chemicals disposed of in the workplace?

Identify and report incidents and injuries

An incident is any event that has caused, or has the potential to cause, injury, ill health or damage. In an acute care setting, an incident report must be completed if there is an error in treatment, a possible breach of duty of care or a sharps incident. A 'near miss' incident, where no injury occurred, is also a cause for completing an incident report.

Following an incident, it may be necessary to take immediate action to minimise further injury or damage occurring. This may include providing immediate care to the individual involved, making the area safe and removing or isolating the equipment/items. You must report all incidents and injuries to the registered nurse (RN), supervisor or manager and complete a report of the incident as soon as possible – but it must be within 24 hours of the incident or near miss occurring (see Figure 1.8).

FIGURE 1.8 Incident report form

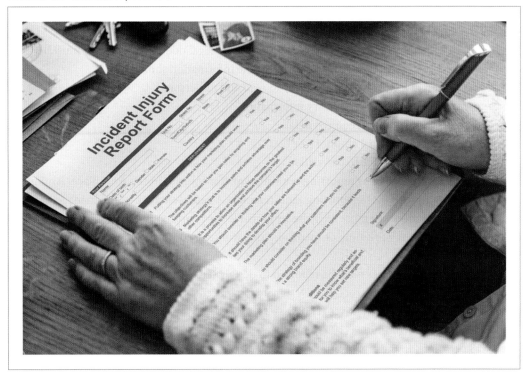

In many large organisations, an incident notification may be made electronically, with the notifier completing a number of mandatory fields when reporting an incident. These intranet-based incident record systems, known as electronic incident management system (IMS) (see Figure 1.9), use standardised processes for the collection, classification and notification of clinical incidents, WHS incidents and consumer feedback. Data collected gives information on the types, frequency and severity of clinical incidents so that continuous improvements can be made.

FIGURE 1.9 Electronic incident management system

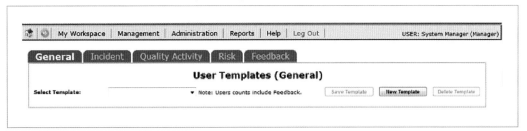

Source: https://my.riskman.net.au/Training/VHIMS/Administration%20Guides/VHIMS%20User%20Templates%20Guide.pdf

Incident reports vary in their format but always need to include:
- date, time and place
- name and address of person/people involved
- witnesses to the incident
- where and when the incident occurred

- the tasks or work that was being performed
- description of incident, injury or symptoms
- any treatment provided.

It must be remembered that incident report forms are legal documents, so they must be completed accurately, thoroughly and objectively. The information should be:

- *clear* – written in legible writing and easy to read and understand
- *concise* – includes only the necessary information
- *complete* – includes all the required detail
- *objective* – free of personal emotions or bias
- *correct* – accurate and able to be verified.

Each state in Australia has reporting requirements for injuries in the workplace. An injury register is an example of these reporting requirements. A representative of the management team of an organisation will most likely be responsible for coordinating the injury register. If an injury results in lost work time or medical costs, workers' compensation claim forms must be completed.

All incidents and injuries must be reported to designated management personnel in line with workplace procedures and instructions. Designated management personnel may include:

- health and safety representatives (HSRs)
- health and safety committee (HSC) members
- WHS personnel in the organisation.

ACTIVITY 1.5

Incident reporting

Identify the immediate actions that should be taken for each of the following incidents:

1. An HSA slipped and fell due to water on the floor in the hallway.
2. A patient's skin was very red and inflamed after dressing tape was removed.
3. Information about a patient was entered in the wrong patient's progress notes.
4. The strap on the stand-up lifter broke while a person was being moved.
5. An HSA caused a skin tear on the leg of an elderly patient when helping to reposition them.
6. An HSA was hit on the face by a confused patient.

In the interest of continuous improvement, an incident report is completed to enable a review of the incident, its cause and how to prevent its recurrence. It is important to remember that the contents of these reports are confidential and that copies of all incident reports need to be kept secure. If a person is being transferred to another hospital or to a medical centre, the report needs to be taken with them.

Maintain safe housekeeping practices in your work area

WHS housekeeping in your work area should be undertaken in line with workplace procedures and instructions. WHS housekeeping includes maintaining a clear, clean and tidy work area to improve health and safety. Prevention of accident, injury and illness in the workplace involves a commitment from all workers and includes:

- maintaining equipment and notifying a supervisor if any equipment is not working properly

- ensuring equipment is:
  - kept clean, as per guidelines
  - stored in the correct area as soon as possible after use
- keeping walkways, exits and traffic areas clear
- using a spills kit to clean up spills
- participating in WHS training
- observing safety signs and knowing what they mean, including signs for:
  - dangerous goods classifications
  - emergency equipment
  - PPE
  - specific hazards, such as sharps or radiation.

Before using equipment with a patient or co-worker, the equipment must be checked first to make sure that it is in good working order. This is called a pre-start check. Any unsafe equipment that cannot be effectively repaired should be withdrawn from use. Knowing that equipment is unsafe but is still being used could be a clear breach of duty of care. Equipment that is either not working or not working properly should be recorded and reported promptly to the designated person in your organisation. A pre-start check may also identify unnecessary clutter and potential tripping hazards in the wards, corridors and public spaces.

All equipment, including items used to transport people and mobility aids, must be in safe working order and undergo the required maintenance and safety checks. It is your responsibility to report equipment faults or defects so that a person can be transported safely (see Chapter 9, 'Transport individuals', for more on transporting individuals).

Infection prevention and control

Safe housekeeping practices aimed at avoiding infections in your work area should also be maintained (for more information, see Chapter 2, 'Comply with infection prevention and control policies and procedures'). Undertaking standard and additional precautions will prevent the spread of infection and as such it is important that all PPE fits correctly. Infection risks should be identified and reported according to your workplace procedures.

WHS housekeeping

Identify your WHS responsibilities in relation to the following scenarios:

1 You are being taught the clinical skill of urinalysis, which may involve contact with body fluids, and there are no gloves available in your size.

2 You are working in a hospital ward and the cleaner has mopped the floor but has left visible vomitus.

3 You are performing a shallow wound dressing and notice that there are blood stains on your gown.

4 You have been asked to work in the orthopaedic ward but you are unfamiliar with how to use the ceiling-mounted hoist.

ACTIVITY 1.6

3 CONTRIBUTE TO SAFE PRACTICES IN THE WORKPLACE

Contributing to safe work procedures in your workplace includes raising WHS issues and participating in WHS meetings, inspections and consultative activities. Workers can make a valuable contribution to workplace health and safety by supporting each other and questioning unsafe practices. As a member of a multidisciplinary team, an HSA should also provide input into the implementation of controls aimed at maintaining a safe environment for their co-workers and the individuals in their care.

Raise WHS issues according to organisational policies and procedures

When an employee needs to raise a WHS issue, they can refer to organisational policies and procedures to find out how to proceed. The issue may be resolved through management action, discussion with the group or person involved or referral to an HSC or HSR. It is the responsibility of this representative or committee to follow up any further action required to resolve the issue. If there is no committee or representative, a supervisor is responsible for dealing with the safety issue that has been identified.

An employer cannot dismiss an employee or change their work function or role to their detriment simply because they have raised safety issues or are part of an HSC. Grievances that cannot be resolved can be referred to each state or territory governing body for an inspector to investigate and assist in the resolution. All issues and grievances should be recorded, along with each step taken in the resolution process.

An employer, through its officers, has a duty under the WHS Act to consult with workers at all levels. Managers should promote and foster open lines of communication and consultation with workers by engaging with workers and by being visible and open to feedback and ideas.

There are significant penalties for disobeying WHS legislation and three categories of offences according to the WHS Act (Australian Government, 2011, Section 31–33):

- Category 1: Reckless conduct – the person is reckless as to the risk to an individual of death or serious injury or illness.
- Category 2: Failure to comply with a health and safety duty – and the failure exposes an individual to a risk of death or serious injury or illness.
- Category 3: Failure to comply with health and safety duty.

WHS policies and procedures should be continuously developed and monitored with consideration of any issues that have been raised. Appropriate WHS programs should then be developed in consultation with all levels of the organisation.

Grievance
A complaint because an event is believed to be incorrect or unfair.

ACTIVITY 1.7

WHS issues

Outline how an HSA is able to contribute to safe work practices in an acute care setting when the following factors are present:

1. There is the potential for aggression from clients.
2. The workload involves many manual handling tasks.
3. There is high potential for stress while working with acutely ill patients.
4. The patient has an infectious disease and there is high risk of it spreading.

Participate in WHS meetings, inspections and consultative activities and contribute to safe workplace policies and procedures

Consultation with employees/HSRs is a requirement of all the state and territory WHS legislation. Employee participation and consultation is crucial to achieve a successful and effective WHS program because:

- people are more likely to change if they are involved in the process
- common goals can be identified when people work together
- participation can provide a more fulfilling role for employees
- employees have detailed knowledge of any hazards in their work and often have ideas about how problems can be solved.

There are a number of opportunities to participate in WHS in your workplace (see also Figure 1.10), including:

- induction and orientation for new staff, which can provide an opportunity to ask questions about WHS issues
- staff meeting and debriefing sessions, which can raise existing and new issues that have an impact on WHS
- formal and informal meetings convened by the HSRs in work areas, which discuss specific issues and concerns
- regular HSC meetings as required under WHS legislation
- inspections and audits of the workplace environment to check for WHS adherence and for workplace hazards
- discussions about alterations to patient care plans and other documentation that have implications for WHS involvement.

FIGURE 1.10 Suggestions for WHS participation

SUGGESTION	WHS IMPLEMENTATION
Identifying a hazard	Robyn, the HSA, noticed that a patient's bed was no longer able to be raised. She reported it immediately and it was fixed as a matter of urgency
Clarifying understanding of WHS policies and procedures	The two new HSAs said to the nurse unit manager that they found it difficult to understand the incident forms. An in-service session was organised to ensure that all nursing staff understood and could use the form
Active involvement in training	Judy, an HSA with over five years' experience, completed her fire warden course and her required emergency evacuation training
Identifying unsafe equipment	Gerry reported that the walk belts being used in the ward were worn and frayed. New walk belts were purchased for use in the ward
Identifying potential for aggression and violence	Cathy reported that her patient Carl was becoming very short-tempered and aggressive towards her. She reported his behaviour to the RN who arranged a medical consultation
Communicating changes in support plans based on WHS concerns	Darryl reported that a patient was unable to assist with her transfer from bed to wheelchair and it was suggested that the stand-up lifter be used. This was noted in the patient's nursing care plan
Participating in HSCs and becoming an HSR	Clare agreed to become the HSR for the aged-care facility where she worked

Your active participation in WHS issues may result in a number of changes in the workplace, which could include changes in the:

- quality of support being provided to patients
- equipment being used
- workplace layout
- work organisation, involving policies, protocols and procedures
- job descriptions
- training and staff development.

Your work area should have an HSR who is a member of the HSC. The HSR has the power to investigate WHS issues that are raised in your work area and to carry out inspections. They also have access to all accident records.

The role of the elected HSR is crucial in terms of supporting others in working safely. This can be done through the establishment of support groups to encourage the effective development of individual and group competencies in WHS. A support group can be formed with terms of reference for involvement on issues in their work area; they can also contribute to ideas on improving health and safety.

SCENARIO

Following procedures for identifying hazards

Hillary, an HSA who worked in a small rural hospital, was concerned about the lack of manual handling equipment for use in the ward. She was worried that incorrect procedures might result in injuries to staff or patients. Hillary reported this to the RN who acknowledged her concerns and invited her to the WHS meeting, where Hillary presented the issue.

The committee conducted an open discussion about potential solutions, including the temporary hire of manual handling equipment until a thorough assessment of the types of patients and their needs was completed. Two months later, the hospital purchased an electronic hoist and three forearm support frames and cleared out an unused office for equipment storage. By following the correct procedures, Hillary and the HSC members ensured that the WHS concerns for patients and staff were acknowledged.

1 Risk control measures use the hierarchy of risk control. What level of control was used in this example?

2 What procedures would you follow if you identified a potential hazard in the ward during your work experience?

4 REFLECT ON YOUR OWN SAFE WORK PRACTICES

Safe work practices ensure that accidents or injuries are reduced. By complying with WHS legislation, you are protected from many workplace hazards. However, the nature of healthcare work can cause physical and psychological stress for workers. You need to reflect on your own stress levels and report any concerns as per workplace procedures, and you should participate in debriefings to address any individual needs.

Identify ways to maintain currency of safe work practices for systems, equipment and processes

Maintaining currency in safe work practices for systems, equipment and processes ensures that work undertaken is relevant, safe and complies with legislative requirements. Organisations regularly review their systems, equipment and processes through their HSCs, including the review of risk management processes, incident reporting or near-miss reporting. Safety data sheets (SDS), previously called material safety data sheets (MSDS), provide information on hazardous chemicals and how they can affect the health and safety of people. SDSs must be kept in the workplace where they are easily accessible to all staff. Information on the SDS includes:

- the identity of the chemical
- health and physicochemical hazards
- safe handling and storage procedures
- emergency procedures
- disposal considerations.

Your responsibilities as an employee include being aware of hazardous materials, reading and applying all updates on improvements in safe work practices, and participating in all formal and informal briefings. The updated information may be provided verbally, by hard copy or electronically and you should ensure that you are able to access all sources of information.

Maintaining currency may be provided by training sessions where information is covered on a range of WHS areas, including:

- legislative compliance
- regulations
- industry standards
- codes of practice
- organisational policy and procedures
- hazard identification and control.

Training sessions should occur as a part of an induction, and updates should be given regularly.

Inductions

A general induction provides an overview of the general safety obligations, policies and procedures of your organisation (see Figure 1.11). A specific induction identifies specific hazards and risks relevant to the employee's position or location and instructs the employee in the safe system of work for the completion of tasks or in the use of equipment or materials. An example may be an induction for workers to a radiology department where specific policies and procedures regarding safety are relevant.

FIGURE 1.11 General hospital ward induction activities

INDUCTION TOPIC
Emergency procedure guide
Fire evacuation plan
Fire stairs / doors
Fire extinguishers
Emergency alarm
Emergency evacuation area
Location of manual handling equipment
Location of resuscitation trolley
Hazard management register and hazard reporting procedure
Incident reporting procedure
Duress or panic alarms (if applicable)

Existing employees who have transferred from another department or location, employees who have returned to work after a period out of the workforce, and students should also undertake work health and safety induction training.

Work health and safety induction
An overview of the general WHS obligations, policies and procedures of your organisation.

Regular updates

Regular updates to WHS training ensure that employees' skills are kept up to date. Updates to training can include notification of any changes to WHS legislation and employee/employer obligations or information about new or changed procedures or risks. It can also include demonstrations on how to use new equipment. Updates may include information on:

* fire safety
* manual handling
* violence prevention and management
* sharps injuries
* hand hygiene
* basic life support.

WHS training is organised by management but should be based on consultation with the HSC and the elected HSRs. It is important that the committee and the representatives explain the benefits of the training to co-workers in their work area.

Reflect on own levels of stress and fatigue

Stress is the body's way of responding to a threat or perceived threat. It requires you to make a physical or emotional adjustment to your behaviour in order to manage the situation. Prolonged stress is damaging to the body and can lead to physical and emotional exhaustion. This, in turn, can result in accidents and injuries in the workplace. Stress and fatigue can be caused by a range of factors, including:

* shift work
* irregular work hours

- time pressures
- staff shortages
- dealing with behaviours of concern
- emotional trauma when caring for palliative patients
- exposure to infectious diseases or sharps.

Identifying your levels of stress and fatigue ensures that you can work safely and for long periods. It is your responsibility to report heightened stress or fatigue to your supervisors so that you do not cause harm to yourself or others. The physical and psychological signs of stress are listed in Figure 1.12.

FIGURE 1.12 Physical and psychological signs of stress

PHYSICAL	PSYCHOLOGICAL
Eating more or less	Depression and anxiety
Chest pain, rapid heartbeat	Procrastinating or neglecting responsibilities
Skin conditions, such as eczema	Inability to concentrate
Loss of sex drive	Constant worrying
Nausea, dizziness	Feeling overwhelmed
Diarrhoea or constipation	Moodiness, irritability or anger
Sleeping too much or too little	Loneliness and isolation
Frequent colds or flu	Using alcohol, cigarettes or drugs to relax

Managing your stress levels may be helped by:
- talking to others about your emotions, including co-workers and supervisors
- seeking professional support through counselling
- undertaking regular physical exercise
- staying positive about your role
- maintaining a balanced diet
- limiting alcohol and other drugs
- getting adequate sleep
- breathing exercises, meditation or yoga
- relaxing by doing things you like or developing new interests
- reflecting on your experiences.

Reflection

Reflection will help you to analyse and evaluate your stress levels, and this in turn will help you to learn new coping strategies. This is consistent with the Gibbs' reflective cycle model (see Figure 1.13), which can be used by healthcare workers in the acute setting. It considers:
- what happened
- how you felt about the event/s
- what was good and bad about the event/s
- how you make sense of the event/s
- on reflection, if there was anything you could have done differently
- what you would do if the events arose again.

FIGURE 1.13 Gibbs' reflective cycle

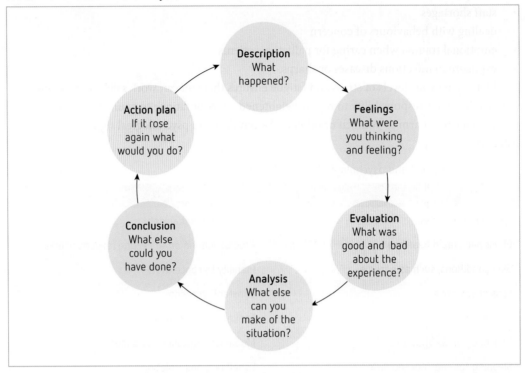

Source: Adapted from Gibbs, G. (1988). *Learning by doing: A guide to teaching and learning methods.*
Oxford: Oxford Brooks University.

ACTIVITY

1.8

Application of Gibbs' reflective cycle

1   Identify an event in your workplace that created personal stress.

2   Apply Gibbs' reflective cycle by describing:
    a   how you felt about the event
    b   what was good and bad about it
    c   how you made sense of it.

3   On reflection, is there anything you could have done differently?

4   If the event happened again, what would you do to help reduce your stress levels and to improve your work?

SUMMARY

The entire healthcare team, as well as patients and others, has a responsibility to maintain work health and safety (WHS). The awareness of risks through hazard identification and management ensures that the workplace remains a safe environment. This chapter outlined the importance of participating in WHS processes as an HSA working in acute care. It emphasised the importance of identifying existing and potential hazards and undertaking elimination or minimisation measures to promote work health and safety.

Particular aspects included an emphasis on WHS procedures and work instructions for your area and how to report to designated people. Identification and reporting of incidents and making sure that the work area remains clean and clear ensure that safe housekeeping practices are maintained.

The last part of the chapter emphasised that WHS is everyone's responsibility and that contributing in meetings, inspections and consultative activities is important. Additionally, by reflecting on your own safe work practices, you are able to recognise stress or fatigue, and take actions to minimise this risk and to maintain personal safety.

APPLY YOUR KNOWLEDGE

Emergency response

Whilst I was giving a bed bath to Mrs Frazier with the assistance of the registered nurse (RN), Mrs Frazier started to complain of chest pain. In no time she became pale and unconscious with no evidence of pulse or breathing.

The RN asked me to press the emergency button and we lowered the back of the bed to lie Mrs Frazier flat. The registered nurse and I commenced CPR until the arrest team arrived with the emergency trolley.

1   What is your responsibility as an HSA regarding responding to an emergency?

The arrest team took over the CPR and my role was to assist in any tasks as delegated by the RN during this episode. I removed the other patient from the room so that she would not become upset. I came back and was asked to get an additional IV pole from the storeroom. Mrs Frazier was defibrillated and given life-saving medications and she recovered from the cardiac arrest.

2   What potential hazards would need to be moved from the immediate area to ensure it was clear for the emergency team?

Mrs Frazier was transferred to the high-dependency cardiac unit for further monitoring and I cleaned up the ward area after the team had left.

3   Look up Chapter 2, 'Comply with infection prevention and control policies and procedures', and identify the appropriate actions to take when disposing of contaminated waste.

I found the whole scene quite distressing as Mrs Frazier reminded me of my elderly neighbour. We all attended a debrief session afterwards and the team encouraged me to let them know if I needed additional support.

4   Why is it important for the HSA to reflect on their own levels of stress after this emergency response?

5   Why is it important to have regular updates on emergency procedures?

6   How did the HSA demonstrate an understanding of the scope of their role as well as the WHS responsibilities as an employee during this emergency response?

◄ REFLECTING ON THE INDUSTRY INSIGHT ➕

1   After our safety huddle meeting, we identified additional hazards in the ward. Which of the following is *not* a hazard in a healthcare environment?
    a   Presence of bodily fluids from an infected wound.
    b   Used sharps left unattended in the equipment room.
    c   Performing a risk assessment on a patient.
    d   Violent or aggressive behaviour from a new admission.

2   Our bariatric patient required a transfer to a wheelchair and one of the staff involved felt a pain in her back after the procedure. An incident report was completed. Which of the following does the report always need to include?
    a   Person's occupation.
    b   Where and when the incident occurred.
    c   Diagnosis of injury.
    d   Name of the nursing unit manage (NUM) in the ward.

3   Being in a new ward can be stressful and tiring. Which of the following can help reduce fatigue at work?
    a   Drinking lots of strong, hot coffee.
    b   Avoiding too many late nights or excessive alcohol use.
    c   Taking long breaks and a larger patient load.
    d   Standing or bending over for long periods of time.

SELF-CHECK QUESTIONS

1   Describe the WHS responsibilities for the employer and employee.
2   How can hazards be identified in the workplace?
3   What is the purpose of completing a risk assessment matrix?
4   Describe the control levels in the hierarchy of risk control.
5   What are examples of emergency alarms used in health care?
6   List four examples of safety signage used in acute care facilities.
7   What is an example of a near miss and how is this different from an incident?
8   What is the purpose of safety data sheets (SDSs)?
9   Identify the physical and psychological effects of stress on your body.
10 What are your definitions of the following key words and terms that have been used in this chapter?

KEY WORD OR TERM	YOUR DEFINITION
PCBU	
Hazard	
Residual risk	

KEY WORD OR TERM	YOUR DEFINITION
Risk assessment	
Australian Standards	
Policy directive	
Grievance	
Work health and safety induction	

QUESTIONS FOR DISCUSSION

1 Discuss the purpose of the WHS Act.
2 Visit the Safe Work Australia website (**http://www.safeworkaustralia.gov.au**) and discuss how Safe Work Australia improves work health and safety and workers' compensation across Australia.
3 Discuss how you can contribute to the minimisation of risks in the workplace.
4 Discuss and give examples of how engineering controls can reduce risks in the healthcare environment.
5 Discuss the ways in which an HSA could maintain their currency of safe work practices in a healthcare setting.

EXTENSION ACTIVITY

Work health and safety inspection

Identifying hazards is the first step in the risk management process. During your workplace experience, team up with a colleague to undertake a WHS inspection of the ward and complete the following activities:

1 Conduct the WHS audit using the checklist in Figure 1.14. (This checklist has been produced as a guide to decide whether a healthcare facility complies with WHS legislation.)
2 In groups, identify the hazards found and develop strategies to minimise or eliminate the risks that they pose.

FIGURE 1.14 WHS audit checklist

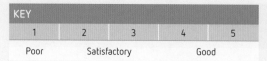

KEY				
1	2	3	4	5
Poor	Satisfactory		Good	

EQUIPMENT		1	2	3	4	5
Beds	Height adjustable					
	Fitted with brakes					
	Bedsides fitted with bedrails					
	Accommodates all lifting machines					
Office areas	The office chairs are adjustable					
	There is sufficient leg room for the worker					
	There is adequate space to work in					
	If the chair has castors, is it on carpet?					
	Shelving for manuals and folders					
Screen-based equipment	Variation from keyboard duties					
	Screens have sufficient contrast					
	Screens have minimal glare					
Workstation is adjustable to meet individual needs	Monitor					
	Desk					
	Keyboard					
	Sufficient room to work in					
Waste disposal & correct bins available	Appropriate colour-coded bags being used					
	General – paper etc.					
	Sharps					
	Food					
	Other: infected/cytotoxic/glass (circle which)					
Hazardous substances	A material safety data sheet for each chemical used (including cleaning agent)					
	Containment materials available for spills					
	Flammable agents in a flameproof cupboard					
	Storage of minimal quantities in the workplace					
	Ventilation with extraction available at source					
Personal protective equipment	Available					
	Used correctly					
	Suitable					

EQUIPMENT		1	2	3	4	5
Physical hazards	Are cleaning signs used appropriately?					
	Are all exits clear?					
Environment	The area has a suitable temperature. If not, circle one of the following: too hot / too cold					
	Taps are drip-free when turned off					
Wet areas	Non-slip surface					
	Water contained within the area					
Medical emergency – staff know	Where equipment is stored					
	Medications					
	Resuscitation equipment					
	Suction					
Lifting machine/ equipment	Brakes fitted					
	Wheels in good order					
	Slings in good condition					
	Correct slings available					

REFERENCES

Australian Government (2011). *Work Health and Safety Act 2011*. Retrieved 13 March 2017 from https://www.comlaw.gov.au/Details/C2011A00137

Australian Government (2021). Australian COVID-19 vaccination policy. Retrieved 2 April 2022 from https://www.health.gov.au/sites/default/files/documents/2020/12/covid-19-vaccination-australian-covid-19-vaccination-policy.pdf

Government of Western Australia Department of Health (2021). Workplace aggression and violence policy. Retrieved 2 April 2022 from https://ww2.health.wa.gov.au/~/media/Corp/Policy-Frameworks/Employment/Workplace-Aggression-and-Violence-Policy/Workplace-Aggression-and-Violence-Policy.pdf

New South Wales Government (1998). *Workplace Injury Management and Workers Compensation Act 1998* (NSW). Retrieved from https://www.legislation.nsw.gov.au/#/view/act/1998/86/whole

New South Wales Government (2011). Occupational Health and Safety Regulation 2001. Retrieved from https://www.legislation.nsw.gov.au/inforce/dae6f0b4-221e-4e28-bf73-8ae956eef3d8/2001-648.pdf

New South Wales Government (2018). Prevention and management of workplace bullying in NSW Health. Retrieved 19 January 2018 from https://www1.health.nsw.gov.au/pds/ActivePDSDocuments/PD2018_016.pdf

Safe Work Australia (2016). Guide to the *Model Work Health and Safety Act*. Retrieved from https://www.safeworkaustralia.gov.au/system/files/documents/1702/guide-to-the-whs-act-at-21-march-2016.pdf

Safe Work Australia (2020). Work-related injury and disease – Key WHS statistics Australia 2020. Retrieved 2 April 2022 from https://www.safeworkaustralia.gov.au/sites/default/files/2020-11/Key%20Work%20Health%20and%20Safety%20Stats%202020.pdf

South Australia Health (2020). Hand hygiene clinical guidelines. Retrieved 2 April 2022 from https://www.sahealth.sa.gov.au/wps/wcm/connect/765d5d0046d2cefe9be0fb2e504170d4/Guideline_Hand+Hygiene+Policy_v1.2_Oct2015.pdf?MOD=AJPERES

Worksafe Tasmania (2022). 4 steps to manage hazards and risk. Retrieved 2 April 2022 from https://worksafe.tas.gov.au/topics/Health-and-Safety/managing-safety/getting-your-safety-systems-right/4-steps-to-manage-hazards-and-risk

APPLY BASIC PRINCIPLES AND PRACTICES OF INFECTION PREVENTION AND CONTROL

Learning objectives

By the end of this chapter, you should be able to:

1   identify the role of infection prevention and control in the work setting
2   follow standard and transmission-based precautions for infection prevention and control in the work setting
3   respond to potential and actual exposure to infection risks within scope of own role.

Introduction

This chapter describes the skills and knowledge required to apply basic infection prevention and control principles in work settings, including implementing standard and transmission-based precautions and responding to risks. All healthcare workers (inclusive of health services assistants), regardless of their experience level, are required to understand applicable measures to control and manage the spread of infection.

Infection is commonly described as the damage to tissue or cells by invading microorganisms. The suggestion to separate patients with infections from others is documented in a hospital handbook published in 1877. Likewise, the importance of hand washing was noted in the mid-1800s in Vienna when the incidence of death due to infection after childbirth declined significantly following the introduction of simple hand washing techniques (WHO, 2009a, p. 9).

This chapter will give you an understanding of how infection might spread, the measures used to prevent infection, and how healthcare workers can control the spread of infection.

Infection
Damage to tissue or cells by invading microorganisms.

Microorganism
Any living microscopic entity, including bacteria and viruses.

1   IDENTIFY THE ROLE OF INFECTION PREVENTION AND CONTROL IN THE WORK SETTING

Infection prevention and control practices reduce the risk of transmission of infections between healthcare workers, patients and others. Utilising standards and guidelines provide healthcare workers valuable information on the preventative measures to minimise the risk of transmissions of infections. An understanding of hazards and microorganisms with their ability to transmit infections is also paramount in order to implement risk control measures to reduce the spread of infection. This prevention and control approach requires communication, cooperation and coordination between the health provider and their staff, patients and consumers.

Identify standards and guidelines relevant to own role and work setting

The National Safety and Quality Health Service (NSQHS) Standard number three, Preventing and Controlling Healthcare-Associated Infection, aims to prevent patients acquiring preventable healthcare associated infections and to effectively manage infections when they occur using evidence-based strategies (ACSQHC, 2017).

The standards allow healthcare providers a framework to develop protocols specific to their area of work that all healthcare workers can use. This can be used alongside the *Australian guidelines for the prevention and control of infection in healthcare* (2019) to ensure that the principles of infection prevention and control are applied to a wide range of healthcare settings. Employees must then follow their healthcare protocols and procedures and take suitable action to protect themselves and others in the workplace to ensure that infection control is an integral part of their care of the patient.

Identify infection risks and hazards

To understand infection control and its risks, it is important to understand the microorganisms, or germs, that cause infections. A microorganism is any living microscopic entity, which includes bacteria and viruses. The human body always has microorganisms, known as *flora*, living on the skin's surface or in the respiratory or gastrointestinal tracts without causing infection. These microorganisms are called *resident (normal) flora* because they are always present. *Transient flora* are temporary and easily transferred when touching surfaces; however, they are easily controlled with effective hand washing techniques.

Simply stated, it is usually when normal flora are transferred to a foreign site in the body that the potential for infection occurs. When microorganisms produce disease, they are called pathogens.

There are five types of pathogenic microorganisms:

- Bacteria – single-celled microorganisms found in all environments and which are not always harmful or pathogenic. Common bacterial infections include urinary tract infections, diarrhoea and outer ear infections. Some bacteria that are capable of causing serious disease are becoming resistant to most commonly available antibiotics. MRSA (Methicillin-resistant *Staphylococcus aureus*) is an infection caused by a strain of bacteria that is resistant to certain antibiotics, including penicillin. VRE (Vancomycin-resistant Enterococcus) is another bacterium commonly found in the gut and resistant to the antibiotic vancomycin.
- Viruses – microorganisms that live within cells, where they multiply and get nourishment by attacking the DNA within the host cell. Examples include the common cold, chicken pox and HIV, and more recently COVID-19.
- Fungi – usually single-celled and not always pathogenic; they are considered part of the body's normal flora. Fungi can cause disease in individuals who are immunologically impaired. Common sites of infection are the skin, nails and mucous membranes. Examples of fungal infections include tinea and ringworm.
- Protozoa – parasitic microorganisms usually found in polluted water that obtain nourishment from decaying organic matter. Infections such as gastroenteritis are spread by ingestion of affected food and water.
- Rickettsiae – microorganisms that can only survive within living tissue. They are spread by lice, fleas and ticks, causing infections such as typhus.

For an infection to spread, certain conditions must be met. This process is known as the chain of infection (CDC, 2016) and can be identified by six steps (see Figure 2.1):

1 **Infectious agent** – e.g., virus, bacteria, fungi
2 **Reservoir or source** – e.g., human (blood and bodily fluids), animal, environment (food, water, soil, waste)
3 **Portal of exit**, which is the path for the microorganism to escape – e.g., sneezing, bleeding, faeces

Pathogens
Microorganisms that produces disease.

Bacteria
Microorganisms capable of causing disease and infection.

Viruses
Microorganisms that multiply only within the living cells of a host. Examples include the common cold, chicken pox and HIV.

Fungi
Yeasts or moulds that may cause infections in the hair, nails, skin and mucous membranes.

Protozoa
Single-celled parasites causing infections such as gastroenteritis after ingestion of infected food or water.

Parasites
Microorganisms that survive and thrive on others while contributing nothing to the host cell. Protozoa and helminths are types of parasites.

Rickettsiae
Microorganisms that can only survive within living tissue and are spread by lice, fleas and ticks, causing infections such as typhus.

FIGURE 2.1 The chain of infection

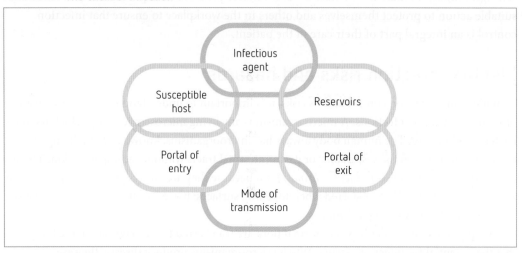

4 **Mode of transmission**, which is how the microorganism is transmitted to others – includes the following:
  – *Direct contact* – through touch, when physical contact transfers pathogenic microorganisms from an infected source to a susceptible host. An important example of this is infection via needlestick injury.
  – *Indirect contact* – when the pathogenic microorganism is transferred via an object when an infected source touches it (e.g., a tap) and a susceptible host then touches the same object. This can also include vectors (e.g., animal, insect, parasite).
  – *Droplet transmission* – the pathogenic microorganism is transmitted in saliva/mucus after being expelled from the source via coughing, sneezing or talking. The droplets are unable to travel more than a metre or so and therefore close proximity is required for transmission.
  – *Airborne transmission* – from coughing, sneezing or talking. The pathogenic microorganism is so small it is able to linger like an aerosol in the air for long periods, allowing it to attach to dust or other droplets for transfer. The space between the source and host can be great.
  Some diseases, such as varicella (chicken pox), can have more than one route of transmission and require several precautionary methods.

5 **Portal of entry**, which is where the microorganism enters the host

6 **Susceptible host**, or the person who is susceptible to the infectious agent. Those who are most susceptible to infection are those:
  – with lowered immune status
  – with wounds or devices, such as catheters or tubes
  – with multiple medical conditions (co-morbidities)
  – who are very young or aged.

If any of the links are broken, then the infection will not occur. Infection control principles are aimed at breaking one or more links in this chain.

Modes of transmission

Match the following terms with their correct definition by placing the correct number next to the description in column two:

ACTIVITY 2.1

TRANSMISSION MODE	DEFINITION
1 Direct contact	The microorganism is transferred via an object after the infected source touches it (e.g., a tap) and then the susceptible host touches the same object
2 Indirect contact	The microorganism is transmitted in saliva or mucus after being expelled from the source via coughing, sneezing or talking
3 Airborne	The microorganism is so small it lingers in the air like an aerosol, allowing it to attach to dust or other droplets for transfer
4 Droplet	Physical contact transfers microorganisms from an infected source to a susceptible host; such as via needlestick injury

Hazards

A hazard is anything that has the potential to harm. The risk of infection spreading from hazards in the healthcare setting is an area requiring constant attention because this can escalate quickly if allowed. Hazards include, but are not limited to, needlestick injuries, assisting patients with activities of daily living (ADLs), and exposure to blood and bodily fluids from catheters, cannulas, transfusions and airways.

Activities of daily living (ADLs)

A set of activities necessary for normal self-care. The activities are feeding, bathing, dressing, toileting, mobility and continence.

Identifying infection hazards

A hazard is anything that has the potential to harm.

1   Identify tasks that could be potential hazards.

2   List how those hazards could be minimised and what PPE you would require for protection.

ACTIVITY 2.2

Healthcare workers' roles and responsibility in infection prevention and control

Healthcare workers have a responsibility to their employer, patients and self to act responsibly to assist in the prevention and control of infection. The ongoing effort to minimise cross-infection by identifying infection risks and hazards and using control measures can only be successful if all team members accept their responsibility in this vital campaign.

Simple and easy day-to-day activities are to:

* know and understand the organisation's infection prevention and control policies and procedures
* ensure all provided equipment is used appropriately and at all times to prevent and control the spread of infection
* attend all training sessions provided by the employer

- attend to and report hazards, such as spills, immediately
- immediately report any hazardous behaviours, such as staff members not wearing gloves, because this may cause infection to spread
- not attend work when unwell to avoid placing other staff and patients at risk
- ensure all immunisations are current
- attend to your personal care and cleanliness
- avoid wearing jewellery or false/acrylic nails in the workplace because they have the potential to cause skin tears or bruising on patients and provide areas for germs to get trapped during hand washing
- ensure you wear a clean and well-laundered work uniform or clothing
- wear PPE as required and when provided
- ensure all equipment is cleaned thoroughly and as soon as practicable after use to avoid cross-infection via instruments.

Control measures to minimise risk

A risk is the possibility that an identified hazard will actually cause somebody harm. Effective risk management involves identification of hazards and assessment of the perceived risk before implementing a plan to minimise or eliminate the risk. Logical risk management will include consulting with all staff who should be involved in the hazard identification, risk assessment and risk control processes. Staff should nominate a representative to be involved in the consultation process and who can act as a resource when required (refer to the section 'Identify, report and record existing and potential hazards in the workplace' in Chapter 1).

Assess risks

Risk assessment is the process of gauging the danger associated with an identified hazard so the nature of the risk can be understood. This includes identifying the harm that may result from the hazard, the severity of that harm and the likelihood harm will occur. All healthcare workers should be able to critically assess infection risks within their working environment and adequately manage the issue to ensure correct control procedures are implemented. A healthcare worker, regardless of their role, should never assume a potential infection risk is not their problem. While the implementation of policies is the responsibility of management, the collective team of healthcare workers contributes to the identification of potential and actual risks, and the implementation of the decided guidelines and policies.

Communicating to management when a potential risk is identified is an important part of the assessment process. The risk management flowchart created by the NHMRC (2010) and shown in Figure 2.2 highlights the importance of communication, consultation, monitoring and review.

Generically, any risk assessment should cover the following points *before* evaluating how the identified hazard might *cause* harm:

1   identify the hazard and any factors that may be *contributing* to the risk
2   *assess* any available information that is relevant to the particular hazard
3   identify the *severity* of any potential harm by perceiving the types of injuries or damage that might result from the hazard.

As the level of risk increases, so will the likelihood and severity of harm. In order to assess the risk involved in any task, you should consider the risk of harm to yourself or the patient, and if the identified risk can be avoided or eliminated.

FIGURE 2.2 Risk management flowchart

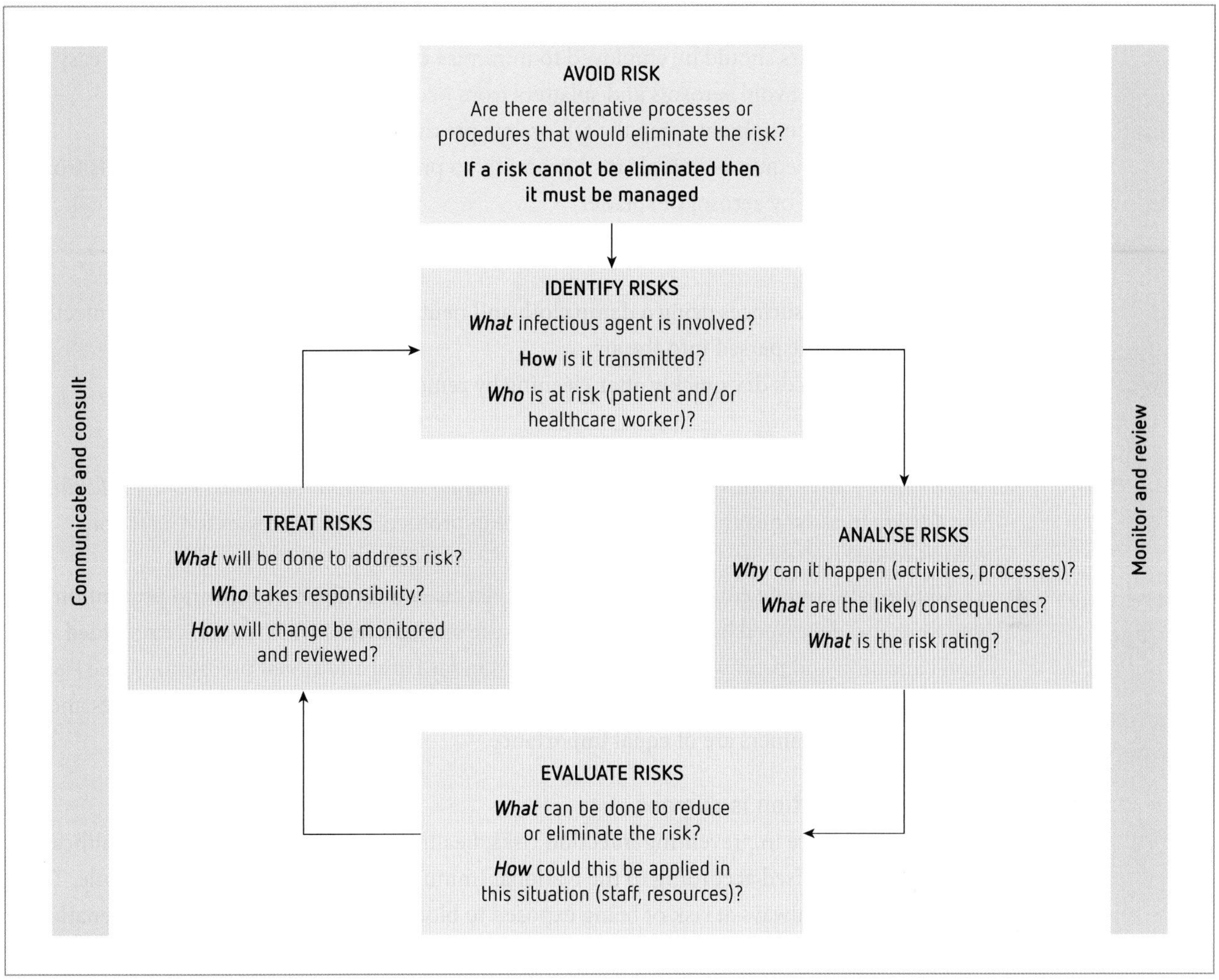

AVOID RISK

Are there alternative processes or procedures that would eliminate the risk?

If a risk cannot be eliminated then it must be managed

IDENTIFY RISKS

What infectious agent is involved?

How is it transmitted?

Who is at risk (patient and/or healthcare worker)?

TREAT RISKS

What will be done to address risk?

Who takes responsibility?

How will change be monitored and reviewed?

ANALYSE RISKS

Why can it happen (activities, processes)?

What are the likely consequences?

What is the risk rating?

EVALUATE RISKS

What can be done to reduce or eliminate the risk?

How could this be applied in this situation (staff, resources)?

Communicate and consult

Monitor and review

Source: Based on material provided by the National Health and Medical Research Council
© Commonwealth of Australia 2015, released under CC BY 3.0 AU licence

Minimise risk

Once infection control guidelines are implemented in a healthcare facility, your role in identifying, reporting and managing risks does not end. Not all risks are foreseeable or able to be eliminated, meaning the need for continuing vigilance by all healthcare workers is essential.

The most effective risk management comes from:

- ongoing recognition and implementation of best practice guidelines
- displaying appropriate signs for staff and visitors
- ensuring necessary equipment is available and in working order
- ensuring staff have appropriate vaccination status
- provision of ongoing education for staff.

One of the most effective ways to engage staff in ongoing education is to upskill several healthcare workers to act as 'champions' or 'go to' people.

Minimise risk of contamination via aerosols and splatter

Within any healthcare setting, contamination via aerosols and splatter should be anticipated, and workplace behaviours should be employed to minimise the potential. The following are easy and suitable methods to avoid aerosols and splatters from occurring:

*   when washing equipment, keep the tap on low pressure to reduce water splash
*   ensure reusable equipment is cleaned promptly to prevent potential infectious agents from being dispersed by aerosol or splatter
*   avoid using spray bottles to clean surfaces and apply cleaning agents directly to a cleaning cloth
*   maintain clean surfaces using a damp cloth and neutral detergent so that dust and infectious agents are not dispersed into the air
*   ensure all surfaces dry quickly after cleaning by removing any excess water.

Use appropriate signs

The NHMRC (2019) published *Australian guidelines for the prevention and control of infection in healthcare* to assist healthcare facilities to develop protocols and processes for infection prevention and control appropriate to their specific situation.

Additionally, online education modules, standardised infection controls, and prevention signs were also developed by the NHMRC to ensure staff, patients and visitors are provided with visual education and prompting on the need for standard and additional precautions (see Figure 2.3 and Figure 2.8, respectively). Usage of signs identifying clean and contaminated zones and different waste containers are of equal importance.

Ensure immunisation is current

As a control measure in preventing infection risks, healthcare facilities insist that all healthcare workers are immunised according to the National Immunisation Program (NIP) Schedule. This is because staff are always at risk of being exposed to blood-borne pathogens, such as hepatitis B and C, human immunodeficiency syndrome (HIV), diphtheria, pertussis, tetanus and measles. COVID-19 and flu vaccinations are also required in many healthcare environments.

ACTIVITY 2.3

Immunisations

Visit the 'National Immunisation Program Schedule' page at **https://www.health.gov.au/health-topics/immunisation/when-to-get-vaccinated/national-immunisation-program-schedule** to learn more about the National Immunisation Program (NIP) Schedule.

1   What categories of people are eligible for the free flu (influenza) vaccines each year?

2   What vaccination is recommended for those 70 years and over?

Communicate and record identified risks and risk management strategies

Healthcare facilities are required to have a collaborative approach to infection control, and this is achieved by listening to staff and ensuring clear policies and procedures are available for staff to follow. Facility management is also expected to provide appropriate initiation to new staff, with ongoing updates and refreshers throughout their employment.

Once a plan of action is in place to eliminate or control the risk, the need for documentation and record maintenance becomes a priority to ensure that the plan of action is, and continues to be, effective. Thorough and concise documentation enables accurate recording of infection control data. This not only ensures improved processes and procedures, with the aim of reducing risks in the future, but also allows tracking of historical data and supports the efforts made to control the risk. Subsequent risk assessments can be completed quickly when historical data is maintained. This is because a clear demonstration of previous decision-making practices shows how controls were intended to be implemented and if they were successful.

2 FOLLOW STANDARD AND TRANSMISSION-BASED PRECAUTIONS FOR INFECTION PREVENTION AND CONTROL IN THE WORK SETTING

In the health- and community-care setting, the risk of infection will always be a concern. Careful planning of care can significantly reduce risks. This includes implementing personal hygiene practices including handwashing and using appropriate personal protective equipment (PPE). Healthcare workers must also assess the environment and use additional precautions if required to ensure they protect themselves and their patients from hazards and the risk of infection.

In order to ensure their infection control guidelines are effective, healthcare facilities collect data under surveillance programs promoted by the NHMRC. These programs establish baseline data on the prevalence and type of infections, identify where the spread or chain of infection is most likely, and suggest appropriate infection control measures to limit spread.

Implement personal hygiene practices in the work setting

Personal hygiene practices include standard precautions, which are the basic practices used for all patients – regardless of whether a known infection exists – because they minimise the chance of spreading an infection. Adherence to standard precautions is essential in reducing and controlling the spread of infectious agents from healthcare workers to patients; in minimising risks associated with the handling of blood, all body fluids and mucous membranes; and in the management of hospital/facility-acquired infections. Hospital-acquired infection is a term used to describe an infection acquired in the healthcare facility that the patient was free of, and not incubating, at the time of admission.

It is the responsibility of every healthcare worker to employ standard precautions to protect their patients, visitors and themselves. Standard precautions (NHMRC, 2010, p. 21), as shown in Figure 2.3, include:

- following respiratory hygiene and cough etiquette
- performing hand hygiene before and after tending to a patient
- using personal protective equipment (PPE) when necessary, such as gloves, masks, gowns or aprons
- routine environmental cleaning, including surface cleaning and safe management of blood and body fluid spills
- safe handling and disposal of sharps
- ensuring shared patient equipment is clean and reprocessed
- using aseptic non-touch technique
- appropriate handling of linen and waste.

Standard precautions
Basic level of infection control that reduces the spread of possible infection.

Hospital-acquired infection
Also called nosocomial infections. An infection acquired in the healthcare facility by a patient who did not have it on admission.

FIGURE 2.3 Standard precautions

 Perform hand hygiene before and after every patient contact

 Clean and reprocess shared patient equipment

 Use personal protective equipment when risk of body fluid exposure

 Follow respiratory hygiene and cough etiquette

 Use and dispose of sharps safely

 Use aseptic technique

 Perform routine environmental cleaning

 Handle and dispose of waste and used linen safely

Source: Australian Commission on Safety and Quality in Health Care. Sydney: ACSQHC. Reproduced with permission. https://safetyandquality.gov.au/wp-content/uploads/2012/02/Approach-3-Standard-Precautions-Photo-PDF-693KB.pdf

Respiratory hygiene and cough etiquette

Personal hygiene practices, which include respiratory hygiene and cough etiquette should be as habitual for healthcare workers as the need for washing hands between attending to patients. Simple measures, such as covering the mouth and nose when coughing and sneezing, will prevent the dispersal of infected respiratory secretions into the air where others can inhale them. Using tissues and disposing of them immediately after use and before washing your hands also minimises the risk of infection spread.

The National Health and Medical Research Council (NHMRC, 2010, p. 90) stresses the need for all individuals to practise correct respiratory hygiene and cough etiquette by following these guidelines:

- cover the mouth and nose with a tissue when coughing, sneezing or blowing the nose
- always use tissues and dispose of them immediately in the waste after use
- if tissues are not available, sneeze or cough into the inner elbow instead of the hands
- always practise correct hand hygiene after coughing, sneezing or blowing the nose
- do not touch the eyes, nose or any mucous membranes with contaminated hands.

It is your responsibility to assist patients to contain their respiratory secretions if they are unable to do so effectively on their own. This also includes affording them the opportunity to clean their hands by offering a wet and dry washcloth for hand hygiene.

Practice hand hygiene in accordance with national standards and guidelines

In every infection control policy, hand hygiene is considered the cornerstone for preventing transmission of infection. Hands must be washed *correctly* before and after patient contact; after handling blood, any body fluids and contaminated items; and after gloves are removed. Correct hand hygiene protects the patient from microorganisms the healthcare worker may be carrying, protects the healthcare worker from microorganisms the patient may be harbouring, and ensures microorganisms are not transmitted during contact.

Routine hand wash

Hand washing is only effective if it is completed correctly. There are different types of hand washing depending on the situation. The routine hand wash is used by everyone in everyday life and includes hand washing in situations such as after going to the bathroom, before touching food or after patting a dog. In the healthcare setting, this includes washing hands before and after patient contact, between tasks and after removing gloves. Hand Hygiene Australia (HHA, 2013) identifies the five essential moments of hand hygiene as before and after touching a patient, before and after a procedure (including body fluid exposure risk) and after touching a patient's surroundings. Figure 2.4 illustrates the five moments of hand hygiene.

> **Routine hand wash**
> Lasts between 40 and 60 seconds and is used to remove visible soil and transient microorganisms.

The World Health Organization (WHO, 2009b, p. 3) suggests a routine hand wash should incorporate the following practices:

FIGURE 2.4 The five moments of hand hygiene

1 Before touching a patient

2 Before a procedure

3 After a procedure or body fluid exposure risk

4 After touching a patient

5 After touching a patient's surroundings

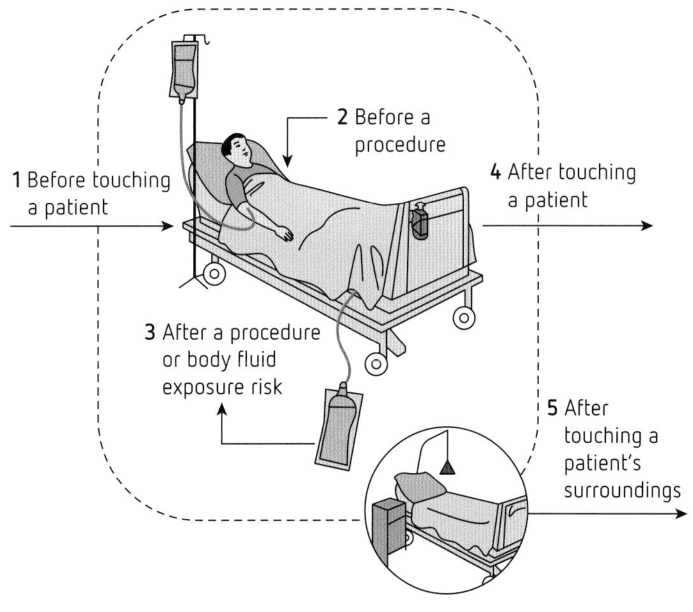

Source: Adapted from 'My 5 Moments for Hand Hygiene' in English, 2022. WHO is not responsible for the content or accuracy of this adaptation, https://www.who.int/campaigns/world-hand-hygiene-day, accessed December 2022

1   Wet hands with water and apply enough soap to cover all hand surfaces
2   Rub hands palm to palm, then right palm over left dorsum with fingers interlaced
3   Palm to palm with fingers interlaced followed by backs of fingers to opposing palms with fingers interlocked
4   Rotational rubbing of left thumb clasped in right palm, and vice versa
5   Rotational rubbing back and forth with clasped fingers of right hand in left palm, and vice versa
6   Rinse hands with water with palms facing down
7   Dry thoroughly with a single-use towel
8   Turn the tap off with the towel.
    This procedure is demonstrated in Figure 2.5.

Clinical and surgical hand wash

Clinical hand wash

A longer routine hand wash that takes a minimum of 60 seconds and is used by healthcare workers before commencing a dressing or procedure on a resident or patient, or before opening sterile equipment.

A clinical hand wash is used by healthcare workers before commencing a dressing or procedure on a patient, or before opening sterile equipment. Washing should last a minimum of 60 seconds and incorporate all the practices identified in the routine hand wash. This is different again from a surgical hand wash, which is recommended by the WHO to take between two and five minutes and is completed prior to surgery or an invasive procedure. The technique is consistent with the routine hand wash but also includes cleaning under the nails with a nail stick and extending beyond the hands to the elbows (WHO, 2009a).

Every healthcare facility employs a set of infection control guidelines with the expectation that all staff and visitors will comply with them. While universal guidelines exist, it is essential staff also adhere to the guidelines of their workplace.

Surgical hand wash

Completed prior to surgery or an invasive procedure, and takes between two to five minutes. The hands and forearms are scrubbed as well as areas under nails.

Hand rubs and gels

Alcohol-based hand rubs and gels are suitable for use on clean hands when the task involves minimal patient contact. Although recognised as a way of improving hand hygiene, the use of hand rubs and gels is not a substitute for washing soiled hands. The most effective hand rubs or gels for reducing the spread of microorganisms are those that contain 60 to 80 per cent alcohol content. Figure 2.6 shows the correct way to use hand rub.

Hand care procedures

It is essential to maintain the integrity of your skin because microorganisms can enter the body through breaks in the skin, such as cuts and scratches. Broken skin should be dressed with a waterproof dressing and changed as required. Fingernails should be kept short and clean, and jewellery should be kept to a minimum to avoid the risk of harm to patients, and to limit areas where microorganisms can be trapped during hand washing.

ACTIVITY 2.4

Hand washing

Consider everyday tasks that require hand hygiene and list how many times in a day you estimate you should be washing your hands.

1   Complete a list for a day at home and a day at your healthcare facility.
2   What precautions should you take if your skin becomes inflamed from handwashing?

FIGURE 2.5 How to hand wash

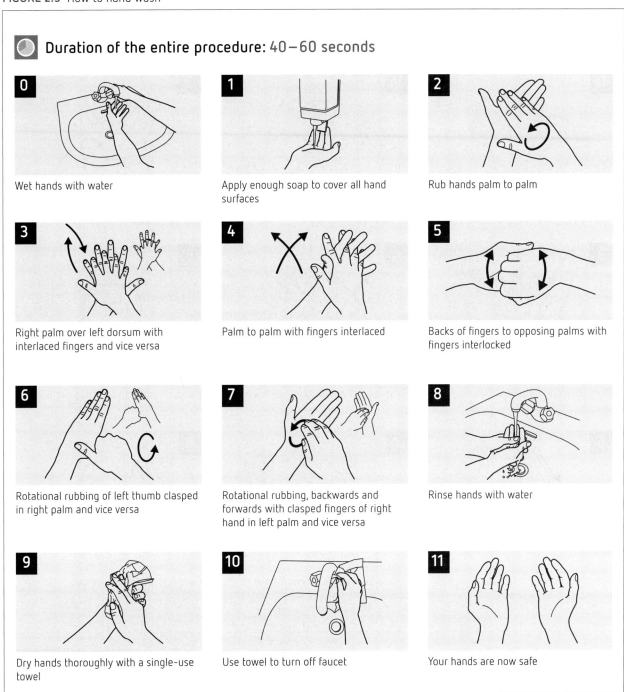

Duration of the entire procedure: 40–60 seconds

0 Wet hands with water

1 Apply enough soap to cover all hand surfaces

2 Rub hands palm to palm

3 Right palm over left dorsum with interlaced fingers and vice versa

4 Palm to palm with fingers interlaced

5 Backs of fingers to opposing palms with fingers interlocked

6 Rotational rubbing of left thumb clasped in right palm and vice versa

7 Rotational rubbing, backwards and forwards with clasped fingers of right hand in left palm and vice versa

8 Rinse hands with water

9 Dry hands thoroughly with a single-use towel

10 Use towel to turn off faucet

11 Your hands are now safe

Source: Reproduced from 'How to Handwash' , 2022. https://www.who.int/campaigns/world-hand-hygiene-day, accessed December 2022

FIGURE 2.6 How to use hand rub or gel

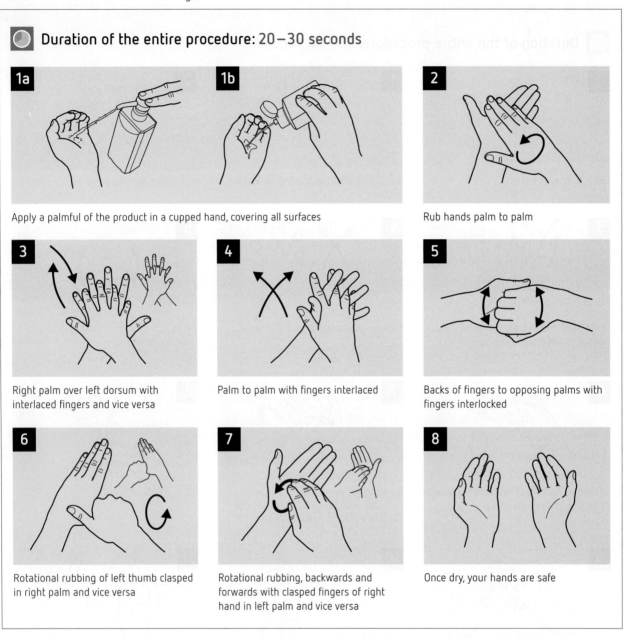

Duration of the entire procedure: 20–30 seconds

1a Apply a palmful of the product in a cupped hand, covering all surfaces

1b

2 Rub hands palm to palm

3 Right palm over left dorsum with interlaced fingers and vice versa

4 Palm to palm with fingers interlaced

5 Backs of fingers to opposing palms with fingers interlocked

6 Rotational rubbing of left thumb clasped in right palm and vice versa

7 Rotational rubbing, backwards and forwards with clasped fingers of right hand in left palm and vice versa

8 Once dry, your hands are safe

Source: Reproduced from 'How to Handrub' in English, 2022. https://www.who.int/campaigns/world-hand-hygiene-day, accessed December 2022

Use PPE according to current national standards and guidelines

Personal protective equipment – commonly called PPE – should always be available for use by healthcare workers. It includes gowns, gloves, masks and goggles, and should be used when there is a risk of exposure to blood or body fluids, the chance of a splash or spray of body fluid, or direct contact with mucous membranes and/or broken skin. Its usage is to protect both the person undergoing treatment and the healthcare worker by acting as a physical barrier to prevent the spread of microorganisms. PPE must not be worn outside the area it is required for, as this will increase the risk of cross-infection to other patients, visitors and staff. The *Work Health and Safety Act 2011* dictates not only the need for employers to provide PPE but also the need for healthcare workers to use the equipment safely and at the correct times. In order to determine the need for PPE, healthcare workers should continually assess the risk of the procedure about to be performed. To determine the risk, the following should be considered:

*   Does the person have a known infection?
*   If so, what is the likely route of transmission: droplet, airborne, or direct or indirect contact?
*   What type of procedure is being performed and how invasive is it?
*   Which type of PPE is best suited to the situation?

Gowns

Gowns may be cloth or waterproof, sterile or non-sterile, and may also be plastic. Sterile gowns are used in the surgical setting in conjunction with sterile gloves and masks to create a sterile field. Generally, the use of non-sterile gowns is appropriate when a splash or contact with body fluids is anticipated. If cloth gowns are used in these situations, it is suggested a plastic apron be worn under the outer gown for protection. Plastic aprons and fluid-resistant gowns must be considered single-use only and be discarded appropriately after use. A healthcare worker's uniform is not considered suitable PPE.

Gloves

Clean, non-sterile gloves are available in different sizes (small, medium, large and extra-large) throughout healthcare facilities. They must be used in any situation where there is the potential for the healthcare worker to be exposed to blood or body fluids, or if the healthcare worker has broken skin on their hands or around their nails. Everyday tasks where gloves should be used include, but are not limited to, showering a patient; emptying a pan, urinal or indwelling catheter (IDC) bag; applying pressure to a bleeding or weeping wound; and cleaning dentures. Gloves are considered single-use items and must be changed between patients, and between tasks on the same person. It is essential that you remove your gloves as soon as the procedure is complete and undertake hand washing immediately after removing them. If the healthcare worker or patient has a latex allergy, latex-free gloves must be used because allergic reactions can range from contact eczema to anaphylaxis. It may also be necessary to ensure that other equipment used in the person's care is free of latex.

Masks and eye protection

Masks, eye protection and face shields must meet the relevant Australian Standards to be considered adequate to protect the membranes of the mouth, nose and eyes from splashes or sprays of blood or other bodily fluids. They also serve to protect the patient from pathogenic microorganisms found in or on the healthcare worker.

Eyewear should be close fitting and provide protection at the sides. Single-use items should be discarded once the procedure is complete, otherwise they must be cleaned according to the manufacturer's instructions.

Masks should also be worn according to the manufacturer's instructions and once in place should not be touched until removed and discarded after completion of the procedure.

P2/N95 particulate-filtering facepiece masks should be fit-tested before use to ensure they form a tight seal around the face. NSW Health recommends that P2 masks should be removed and disposed of after about four hours of continuous use, or when they become moist. This is because the seal will not be as effective. After use, drop the mask into a contaminated waste bin and wash hands and arms thoroughly in soapy water, or use alcohol hand rub (NSW Health, 2020). The person who carries out the fit test should be appropriately trained, qualified and experienced, and the procedure should be undertaken in accordance with Australian Standards and manufacturer's guidelines.

Masks and face shields should not be pulled down and worn loosely around your neck, ready for reuse. Masks and face shields are considered single-use items.

Figure 2.7 highlights the sequence for donning and removing PPE.

Footwear

In all facilities, appropriate footwear is considered to be an enclosed and fastened shoe with a non-slip sole and closed-in toe. This type of shoe prevents the risk of injury from sharp items that may be on the floor or dropped, trips and bumps, and transmission of pathogenic microorganisms either from or to exposed feet.

Minimising the risk of cross-infection

Christopher, aged 27, lacerated his thigh while jumping over a wire fence at the local soccer field. He presented to the hospital two days later with an infected wound. Swabs were taken from the wound exudate and sent to pathology for testing. The sample was cultured and grew Methicillin-resistant *Staphylococcus aureus* (MRSA). The sample was also tested against different antibiotics for resistance or sensitivity and this indicated that the sample was sensitive to the antibiotic Vancomycin.

Christopher was admitted for wound drainage and cleansing. He was placed in a private room to prevent the spread of MRSA to other patients and intravenous antibiotics were commenced. Signage indicating the need for contact precautions and the use of appropriate personal protective equipment (PPE) was placed outside his room and staff used dedicated patient-care equipment (e.g. blood pressure cuffs, stethoscopes) and single-use disposable items (e.g. single-patient digital thermometer). All staff attending Christopher wore protective clothing (aprons and gloves) when they had physical contact with him and disposed of waste in the contaminated waste bins. His visitors were required to wash their hands thoroughly before and after seeing him. Christopher responded well to the antibiotic therapy and was discharged three days later on oral antibiotics and scheduled for a follow-up at the clinic.

1   How did Christopher's wound swab culture determine sensitivity to Vancomycin?
2   Why was Christopher placed in a private room?
3   What type of container is best used for Christopher's waste?

Culture
Growing microorganisms in a nutrient medium.

Environmental cleaning and management of waste

Most healthcare facilities have their own housekeeping staff; however, cleaning is everybody's business because housekeeping staff are not responsible for the routine cleaning of specific equipment such as nebulisers, blood pressure cuffs and any non-disposable items. Routine cleaning procedures are an essential part of infection control and should be adhered to as per

FIGURE 2.7 Donning and removing PPE

Sequence for donning PPE	Sequence for removing PPE
Step 1. Hand hygiene • Perform hand hygiene before putting on personal protective equipment 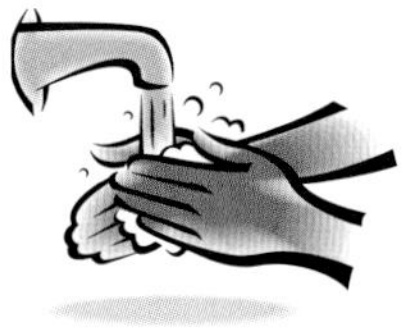	**Step 1. Gloves** • Grasp outside of glove with opposite gloved hand; peel off • Hold removed glove in gloved hand • Slide fingers of ungloved hand under remaining glove at wrist • Peel glove off over first glove • Discard gloves in waste 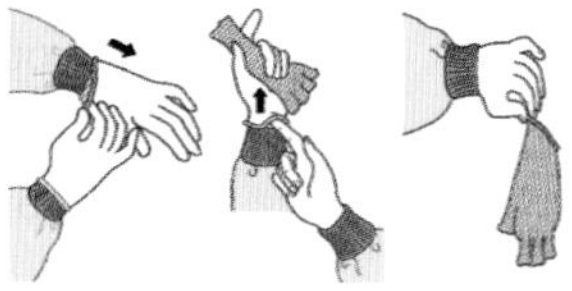
Step 2. Gown/apron • Fully cover torso from neck to knee, arms to end of wrist, and wrap around the back • Fasten in back at neck and waist 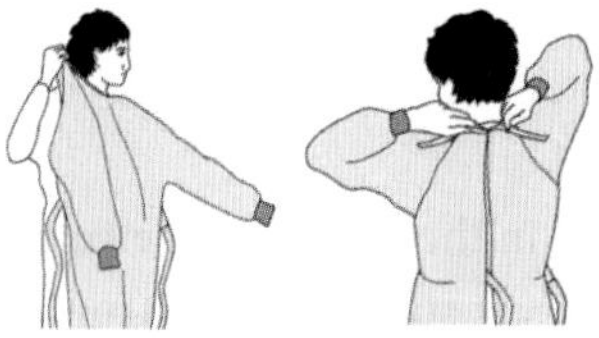	**Step 2. Hand hygiene** • Perform hand hygiene following removal of gloves • The use of a water-free skin cleanser is appropriate 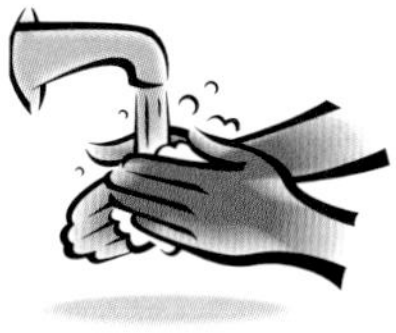
Step 3. Mask or respirator • Secure ties or elastic bands at middle of head and neck • Fit flexible band to nose bridge • Fit snug to face and below chin • Fit check mask/respirator 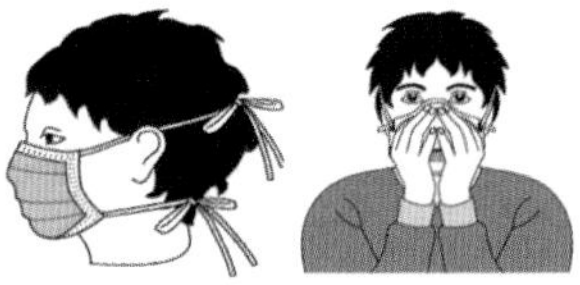	**Step 3. Protective eyewear** • To remove, handle by head band or earpieces • Place reusable eyewear in designated receptacle for cleaning or discard disposable eyewear into waste container for disposal 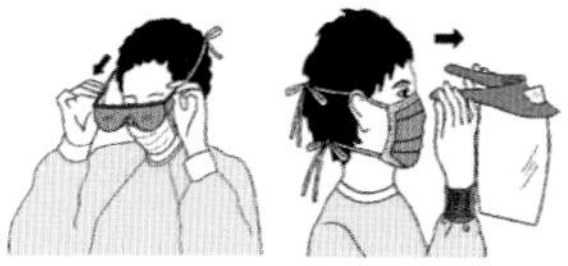
Step 4. Protective eyewear • Place goggles or face shield over face and eyes and adjust to fit 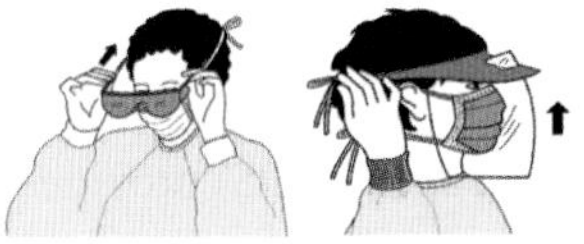	**Step 4. Gown** • Unfasten ties • Pull away from neck or shoulders, touching inside of gown only • Turn gown inside out • Fold or roll slowly into a bundle and discard into designated waste container 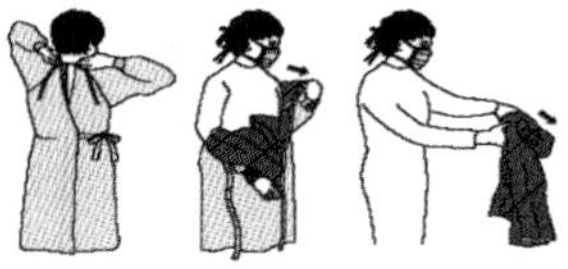
Step 5. Gloves • Extend to cover wrist of gown 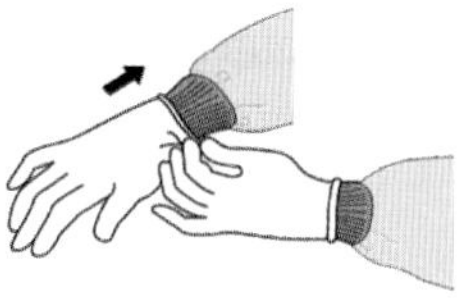	**Step 5. Mask or respirator** • Remove by touching tapes or ties only • Discard in designated waste container 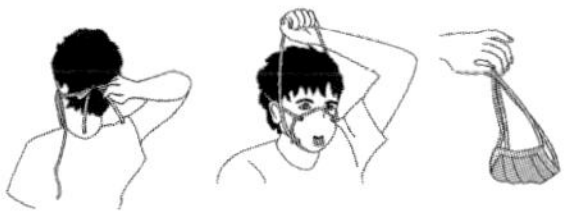
	Step 6. Hand hygiene • Perform hand hygiene following removal of all PPE 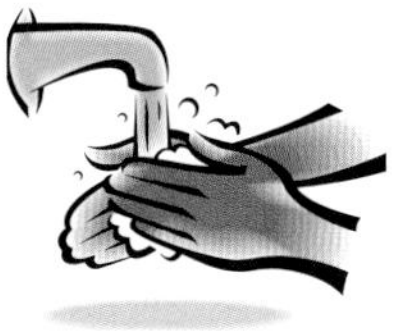

Source: Centers for Disease Control and Prevention (2016). Sequence for donning PPE. Retrieved 4 May 2019 from https://www.cdc.gov/HAI/prevent/ppe.html Siegel JD, Rhinehart E, Jackson M, Chiarello L, and the Healthcare Infection Control Practices Advisory Committee, 2007 Guideline for Isolation Precautions: Preventing Transmission of Infectious Agents in Healthcare Settings, June 2007 http://www.cdc.gov/ncidod/dhqp/pdf/isolation2007.pdf

the facility's policy. Routine cleaning is generally conducted daily or if there is an immediate and specific need. Dust, dirt from shoes, dead skin cells and other microbes on the floor or equipment surfaces act as potential sources of infection. Elderly patients in a compromised state of health become susceptible hosts for pathogenic microorganisms, and it is therefore important that cleaning schedules are adhered to and completed thoroughly, especially in areas of direct care.

Vacuuming carpeted areas, mopping linoleum floors and damp wiping surfaces with a clean cloth, warm water and detergent should be completed as routine daily practice to promote a reduction in contaminated surfaces. Any damp dusting should be followed by drying the surface, and any surface used for multiple functions, such as the bedside table or over-bed trolley, should be cleaned before and after each use. It is also important to inspect all surfaces for tears, rips or cracks because any disintegration or impairment creates a breeding ground for microorganisms and compromises the effectiveness of infection control measures. Any furniture or equipment found to be in disrepair should be reported through the correct channels relevant to facility policies for maintenance or replacement.

Three types of cleaning are identified in the healthcare setting: *cleansing*, *disinfection* and *sterilising*. While it is suitable to **cleanse** most surfaces or instruments with warm water and mild detergent, there are occasions when stronger agents are used. **Disinfection** is the removal or elimination of pathogenic microorganisms (except **spores**) with the use of chemical solutions. Use of a hospital-grade disinfectant is effective against most pathogens and must be approved by the Therapeutic Goods Administration. All surface soiling must be removed before disinfection can effectively occur. Chemical disinfectants must be diluted according to the labelled specifications and should never be mixed. Equipment requiring sterilising must also be cleaned of all visible biological matter such as organic tissue and blood before being sterilised by steam, chemicals or gamma irradiation. **Sterilisation** is the complete removal of and destruction of all microorganisms, including spores, from equipment. Where reusable equipment, instruments and devices are used, appropriate cleaning, disinfection and sterilisation ensures the risk to the patient is minimised. All cleaning products must be logged to ensure safe and correct handling and storage processes. A safety data sheet (SDS) provides relevant information about hazardous substances including regulations on storage, correct usage and emergency protocols if used inappropriately. It is the responsibility of any healthcare worker using these products to ensure the SDS is accurately completed and maintained, and all equipment remains in safe working order.

Cleaning for the health workforce during COVID-19

Clean and disinfect frequently touched surfaces, equipment and anything that has been exposed to respiratory droplets. Always adhere to hand washing principles and wear gloves and PPE to minimise your risk of getting coronavirus.

Respond to situations where transmission-based precautions or enhanced cleaning is required

Additional precautions, sometimes called transmission-based precautions (see Figure 2.8), are used when a known or suspected infection exists, and when it is identified that the use of standard precautions alone may not be sufficient to prevent the transmission of infection. They

Cleansing
The cleaning of surfaces or instruments with warm water and mild detergent.

Disinfection
The removal or elimination of pathogenic microorganisms (except spores) with the use of chemical solutions.

Spores
Cells produced by bacteria and fungi that can develop into new bacteria or fungi.

Sterilisation
The complete removal and destruction of all microorganisms (including spores) from equipment by either steam, chemicals or gamma irradiation.

Additional precautions
Also called transmission-based precautions. Special infection control measures used when standard precautions alone may not be sufficient to prevent the transmission of infection.

FIGURE 2.8 Additional precautions – used in addition to standard precautions

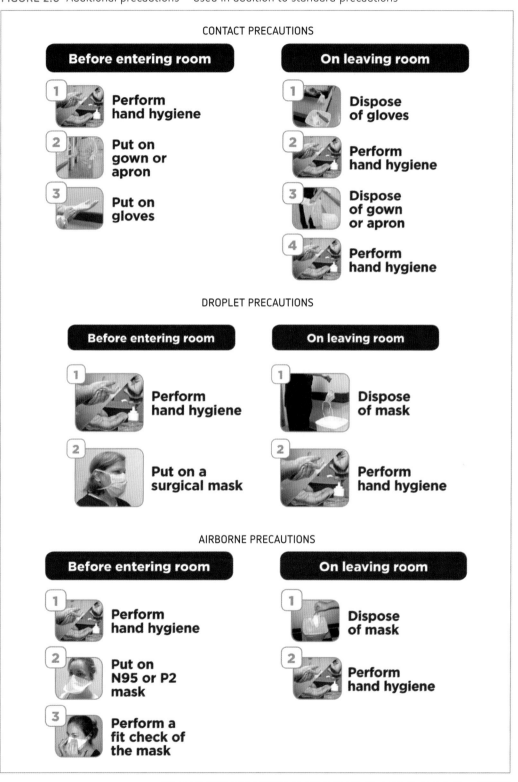

Source: Australian Commission on Safety and Quality in Health Care. Sydney: ACSQHC; NSW Clinical Excellence Commission 2012. Reproduced with permission. https://www.safetyandquality.gov.au/wp-content/uploads/2012/02/Portrait-NSW-Standardised-Infection-Control-and-Prevention-Signs.pdf

are therefore *used in addition to, not instead of, standard precautions* because they are intended to prevent transmission of a specific infectious disease. This may also include additional PPE depending on the mode of transmission. Other measures are also implemented in conjunction with additional surface cleaning of the patient areas, including isolation and **barrier nursing**, patient-dedicated equipment, **lamina flow environments** and specific respiratory protective masks. For example, all healthcare workers providing direct patient care for individuals with suspected or confirmed COVID-19 should have access to P2/N95 respirators that filter at least 95 per cent of airborne particles.

It is also considered appropriate to keep patients with the same infection within a confined area, tended by the same group of healthcare workers, and to restrict their movement.

ACTIVITY 2.5

Spread of infection

1 Create a list of common infections you are aware of, then consider how they are spread (i.e., their mode of transmission).

2 What standard and additional precautions can you use to limit their spread?

3 What are the specific precautions used to prevent the spread of infection of COVID-19?

Barrier nursing
Local isolation of a patient with an infectious disease to prevent the spread of the disease. The 'barrier' takes the form of gowns, caps, overshoes, gloves and masks that are donned by staff and visitors before approaching the patient and discarded before returning to the normal environment.

Lamina flow environment
An environment that minimises the amount of dust and particles in the air by filtering and exhausting the air in one direction only.

3 RESPOND TO POTENTIAL AND ACTUAL EXPOSURE TO INFECTION RISKS WITHIN SCOPE OF OWN ROLE

As a Health Services Assistant, it is important to identify risks, respond and communicate any breaches so that appropriate actions can be taken. Minimising contamination, appropriate cleaning following exposure to blood and bodily fluids, appropriate handling of linen and contaminated waste and cleaning spills will reduce the risk of exposure to infection. The final response is to provide accurate documentation to record and evaluate the risk to ensure that continuous improvements can be made to protect the staff, patients and public from infection risks. The level of documentation may vary according to local policies and guidelines.

Identify, respond to and communicate potential or actual breaches in infection control

Every healthcare provider has guidelines, policies and procedures for varying circumstances to protect patients, visitors and staff from the risk of infection or harm. A guideline directs people on how to do something and is usually formulated from evidence gathered through trials and research and from expert advice. As a result of the guideline, a policy is adopted to ensure everyone follows the same protocols. Adherence to facility guidelines for infection control, needlestick injuries, exposure to blood or bodily fluids when attending to personal care of the patient, or blood-borne pathogen infections such as MRSA, Hepatitis are all good examples of protecting patients, visitors and staff from risk.

Communication of infection control breaches involves incident reporting and documentation and it is up to the health services assistants to adhere to these reporting requirements as part of their scope of practice.

Assess risk and take appropriate action in accordance with industry and organisational guidelines

Regardless of the effort and importance placed by facilities on minimising and managing risk, the nature of a healthcare worker's role will always expose them to ongoing hazards requiring attention. Unfortunately, some guidelines are only able to be formulated and implemented after an event or accident has shown the need. However, recognising and assessing the potential risk from sharps injuries or blood borne viruses is the first step in the control of them. The health care worker should ensure that there are clear written instructions and systems in place for the management of these risks to make sure that staff and patients are safe.

Needlestick injuries

In the healthcare environment, a needlestick injury occurs when an uncapped needle penetrates the skin of a healthcare worker. If the needle has not been used it is considered 'clean'; and while the broken skin is cause for concern, the risk of infection is low. If the needlestick injury occurs after use, it is of greater concern and is considered 'dirty'. In this circumstance the wound should be immediately cleaned and facility protocol observed.

Needlestick injuries are not uncommon, and because of this many facilities employ policies for the administration of injections. Such policies will include a 'no recap' rule and will mandate sharps containers be available at the bedside to ensure sharps are disposed of immediately after use. Retractable needles are also becoming popular because they further reduce the risk of needlestick injury.

Activities of daily living

Many ADLs involve exposure to body fluids and are therefore a potential infection risk, particularly assisting with showering, cleaning teeth or dentures, and assisting with toileting or changing incontinence devices. Exposure to blood and bloodborne pathogens can occur when undertaking wound care. These include Hepatitis B and C, Human immunodeficiency virus (HIV) and multi resistant staphylococcus aureus (MRSA). You should use PPE and ensure any broken skin on your body is covered with a waterproof dressing. Assisting with ADLs is further complicated if the person is restricted to bed, aggressive or cognitively impaired. This will need consideration from a work health and safety perspective (refer to the section 'Identify, report and record existing and potential hazards in the workplace' in Chapter 1).

Control measures to minimise contamination of people, materials and equipment

Using control measure to limit contamination is an essential step in infection control. Although healthcare facilities differ from each other in many ways, they still share similarities in design, including the use of a centralised nurses' station where medical records, phones and computers are kept, and the separation of clean and dirty utility rooms. These areas are nominated as either *contaminated* or *clean* zones to ensure that cross-contamination does not occur.

Identify clean and contaminated zones

Contaminated and clean zones should be clearly marked so that all staff are aware and can limit crossover between the areas. Healthcare workers should ensure their workflow is from clean to contaminated zones and care should be taken to avoid contaminated items re-entering the clean area. High-risk areas for cross-contamination are areas touched or frequented by multiple people, and include floors, door handles, walking frames and other frequently used mobility aids, call bells, hand and bed rails, and light switches.

Clean zones

A clean zone is an area specifically designated for non-contaminated, sterile or disinfected items only, such as a client's room, treatment room, equipment and storage areas, administration areas and a kitchen. Medical records, materials and equipment is also stored in a designated clean area. It is important to remember that these areas must be kept free from contamination. Therefore, control measures of removing contaminated items such as PPE and ensuring correct hand hygiene is undertaken before entering these areas is important. Safety measures, such as wearing freshly laundered scrubs in the operating theatre suite or hairnets by staff in the kitchen area, can also limit the risk of cross-infection.

Contaminated zones

A contaminated zone is an area designated for cleaning and processing dirty equipment or an area that has become contaminated during a procedure, such as the bathroom and toilet, laundry room and dirty utility room. Signs will be available to remind staff to remove contaminated gloves and gowns before leaving a designated contaminated area. Dirty utility rooms, also known as sluice rooms, are found on all wards and are used for emptying, cleaning and decontaminating of bedpans, urinals and measuring jugs, and the measurement and testing of body fluids such as urine. Sinks in these rooms should be deep enough so that splashes are minimised with taps that are non-touch or that can be turned on and off with the elbow are effective control measures to minimise risk. These rooms should be located near patient rooms so that cross-contamination of the clean and contaminated zones is minimised, and transportation time and distance of contaminated material is reduced.

Handle, transport and process linen appropriately

Linen, including sheets, towels, gowns and bed clothes, are reservoirs for body fluids. Control measures to limit contamination include changing linen regularly and if soiled must be contained in an appropriately identified impervious bag for transportation to the laundry or for disposal as per facility guidelines. These measures can prevent contamination of clean linen and prevent transfer of microorganisms to other patients. An apron and gloves should be worn to prevent contaminated linen coming into contact with your uniform, and the linen should be placed immediately in the appropriate lined skip and removed from the area in a timely manner.

Transporting clean linen to the bedside should be done on a trolley to prevent the linen being held close to your uniform, which may have become dirty.

Dispose of contaminated waste

Not all waste in the clinical setting should be considered infectious and it is therefore important to segregate waste at the point of generation, using appropriately colour-coded and labelled containers. General waste includes domestic waste, recyclable waste such as cardboard boxes, and uncontaminated linen. Clinical waste is anything that has the potential to cause or spread disease. This type of high-risk waste is disposed of in sharps containers or colour-coded bins with appropriate labelling. Examples of high-risk waste labelling are outlined in Figure 2.9.

The WHO (2018) estimates that 85 per cent of all healthcare waste is general and non-hazardous, and the remaining 15 per cent is considered infectious, toxic or radioactive. The categories that the WHO groups all healthcare waste under are as follows:

- infectious waste – may be contaminated with blood and/or other body fluids, be waste from laboratory work such as an autopsy, or be from a patient in an isolation room
- pathological waste – human tissue, organs or fluids
- sharps – including needles, scalpels and blades
- chemical waste – solvents, chemicals, mercury and battery fluid
- pharmaceutical waste – out-of-date, unused or contaminated drugs
- genotoxic or cytotoxic waste – materials, equipment and residue that are contaminated by cytotoxic drugs. These drugs are commonly administered to people with cancer
- radioactive waste – the by-products of radioactive drugs used in various treatments
- general waste – does not cause any concern as a biological, chemical, radioactive or physical hazard.

FIGURE 2.9 Examples of labelling for high-risk waste containers

 International biohazard symbol visible on clinical waste

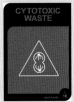 Cytotoxic waste symbol

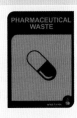 Pharmaceutical/anatomical waste symbol. Usually shown with the international biohazard symbol

 Radioactive symbol

 Recycle symbol

Sources from top: Shutterstock.com/strawberrytiger; Sustainability Victoria; Sustainability Victoria; Shutterstock.com/LadyM Studio; Shutterstock.com/kiberstalker

General waste

Domestic and recyclable waste, which does not cause any concern as a biological, chemical, radioactive or physical hazard.

Clinical waste

Any waste that has the potential to cause or spread disease.

Infectious waste

Waste contaminated with blood and/or other body fluids.

Pathological waste

Waste that includes human tissue, organs or fluids.

Sharp

Any equipment that contains a needle, scalpel or blade.

Chemical waste

Waste that is made from harmful chemicals such as solvents and mercury.

Pharmaceutical waste

Unused, expired or leftover medication that is no longer needed.

Genotoxic or cytotoxic waste

Includes cytotoxic drugs (e.g., used in chemotherapy).

Every healthcare worker has a responsibility to understand the risks and hazard identification associated with waste management. The person responsible for generating the waste is responsible for the correct handling, transport and disposal of the waste. If all waste is disposed of correctly, the risk of cross-infection and the cost involved are both minimised significantly.

Control measures include storing all clinical waste in well-lit and ventilated areas with clear signage and waste must not be accessible to the public. There is a variety of state and territory legislation governing the storage and disposal of waste in Australia. Examples include:

- *Protection of the Environment Operations Act 1997* – NSW
- *Environment Protection Act* (1994 Queensland; 1993 South Australia; 1970 Victoria; 1997 ACT; 1986 Western Australia).

Transporting specimens

Preparing specimens for collection and transport is important in order to protect couriers from risk. Control measures include leak-resistant bags with separate compartments for the request form and specimen. These are essential during transit because leaking specimens may not be accepted or processed by the pathology company.

<table>
<tr><td>ACTIVITY
2.6</td><td>

Breaking the chain of infection

The spread of infection was discussed earlier in this chapter. In order to effectively manage infection control, there needs to be a break in the spread or chain either at the source of infection, the mode of transmission or the susceptible host.

1. List some necessary processes you would use as a healthcare worker to promote infection control and prevention.
2. What conditions would make a person a susceptible host to infection?

</td></tr>
</table>

Follow process for management of spills and exposure to blood or body fluids

Needlestick injuries, attending to blood transfusions, accessing cannulas, removing surgical drapes, emptying catheters and handling other incontinence aids, changing dressings, and transferring urine and faeces in a bedpan or urinal to the dirty utility room are all examples of everyday tasks where you or an RN could be exposed to infection risks associated with blood and bodily fluids.

The following protocols are used by most facilities for care following exposure to body fluids.

Immediately after exposure to blood or body fluids, it is recommended that the exposed person undertake the following steps as soon as possible:

- wash wounds and skin sites that have been in contact with blood or body fluids with soap and water
- apply a sterile dressing as necessary, and apply pressure through the dressing if bleeding is still occurring
- if injured, do not squeeze or rub the injury site

- if blood gets on the skin, irrespective of whether there are cuts or abrasions, wash well with soap and water
- irrigate mucous membranes and eyes (remove contact lenses) with water or normal saline
    - if eyes are contaminated, rinse while they are open, gently but thoroughly (for at least 30 seconds) with water or normal saline
    - if blood or body fluids get in the mouth, spit them out and then rinse the mouth with water several times
- if clothing is contaminated, remove clothing and shower if necessary.

When water is not available, use of non-water cleanser or antiseptic should replace the use of soap and water for washing cuts or punctures of the skin or intact skin. The application of strong solutions (e.g. bleach or iodine) to wounds or skin sites is not recommended.

For human bites, the clinical evaluation should include the possibility that both the person bitten and the person who inflicted the bite were exposed to a blood-borne virus.

The exposed person should inform an appropriate person (e.g. supervisor or manager) as soon as possible after the exposure so assessment and follow-up can be undertaken in a timely manner. After reporting the incident, the worker should be released from duty so that an immediate risk assessment can be performed.

Remove spills

Blood and body fluid spills are unintentional and unexpected, but you should always be aware of correct procedural policy to deal with the situation without alarming or offending the person, who may be either very ill or embarrassed, and/or their visitors. This will include cleaning promptly and according to facility guidelines, and ensuring appropriate PPE is used. The majority of facilities have spill kits available, and it is essential that you know the location where they are kept.

Regardless of the size of a spill, a safety sign should be placed immediately at the site to alert others to the spill while cleaning is arranged and in progress. This is discussed further in the upcoming section 'Use appropriate signs'. It is essential that healthcare workers use PPE, including gloves, apron, mask and face shield. Visible fluid should be soaked up using disposable cloths or paper towels, which should then be immediately placed in the contaminated waste bag. The affected area should be washed with hot soapy water, and if only a small spill, should then be left to dry. Larger spills are usually greater than 10 centimetres in diameter and may need to be wiped with bleach (sodium hypochlorite) as per the facility's guidelines.

PPE should be removed and disposed of at the spill site and hand hygiene performed. The manager on duty must be informed and all appropriate documentation completed. This is usually an incident form; however, if bleach or other chemicals were used in the cleaning process it may be necessary to log the usage.

The safety sign must not be removed until the area is completely dry and safe to walk on.

Document and report incidents

All incidents must be reported and investigated. These include injuries or near miss incidents relating to infection control. Action 1.11 of the National Safety and Quality Health Service Standards describes the health service organisations' requirement to have organisation-wide incident management and investigation systems in place. This includes:

* supporting the workforce to recognise and report incidents
* supporting patients, carers and families to communicate concerns or incidents
* involving the workforce and consumers in the review of incidents
* providing timely feedback on the analysis of incidents to the governing body, the workforce and consumers
* using the information from the analysis of incidents to improve safety and quality
* incorporating risks identified in the analysis of incidents into the risk management system
* Regularly reviewing and acting to improve the effectiveness of the incident management and investigation systems.

Source: Adapted from https://www.safetyandquality.gov.au/standards/nsqhs-standards, Action 1.11, p.8.

Documentation can be paper-based or electronic and should include all information about the incident, actions taken, outcomes and changes made if necessary (refer to the section 'Identify and report incidents and injuries' in Chapter 1).

SUMMARY

Infection control may seem complex in all its areas of use; however, when you analyse your work environment and follow simple guidelines with a 'common sense' approach, the prevention of the spread of microorganisms becomes quite logical and methodical.

This chapter has identified that the pathogenic microorganisms responsible for causing infection require a susceptible host to infect and an entry site. If you maintain vigilance with hygiene practices and alert co-workers to potential risks, such as patients with broken skin or worrying infectious symptoms, the chain of infection required for the pathogenic microorganism to reproduce can be interrupted.

Maintaining clean zones, adhering to cleaning schedules, following facility procedures and protocols (guidelines) and using PPE correctly are all proven ways to maintain efficient working environments free of infection and risk.

Universally, every infection control group, association, council or organisation identifies correct hand washing techniques as being the single most effective infection control measure that can be used by healthcare workers and the general public to prevent the spread of potential pathogens. When used in conjunction with other standard and additional precautions, and safe work practices, as described in this chapter, you can effectively provide safe care to each individual.

APPLY YOUR KNOWLEDGE

Standard and additional precautions

Infection control measures are important in the prevention and mitigation of viral infections within health and aged care facilities.

Les, aged 87, was a resident of Poplars Aged Care Facility. For 24 hours he had been experiencing abdominal pain, lethargy, headache, diarrhoea and vomiting. Faecal samples were taken and the next day the samples confirmed that Les had norovirus gastroenteritis. This is a highly contagious viral infection that can easily be spread from person to person through touching a contaminated object or having direct contact with the person.

As the HSA working at Poplars, I was required to adhere to standard and additional precautions when caring for Les and to collect a faecal specimen for pathology testing.

1   What are the most important standard precautions to be practised when looking after Les?

2   How would the faecal specimen and form be prepared for collection?

3   How are contaminated linen items processed?

Les was managed by rest and oral rehydration solutions as well as being encouraged to drink plenty of fluids. Our role was to wear PPE when entering Les's room to reduce the likelihood of exposure to infectious vomitus or faecal material, especially if there was a risk of splashes to the face when Les was vomiting.

4   How should a vomitus spill be cleaned from the floor?

5   What are the important considerations when wearing masks and eye protection?

6   The management at Poplars decided to include information on infection control protocols for viruses for all new staff. Refer to Chapter 1, 'Participate in workplace health and safety', and describe the importance of specific inductions for new staff.

7   How did the HSA demonstrate an understanding of the scope of their role with infection control protocols during this case?

Les took a week to recover and lost 1.5 kilograms during his illness. He was educated in correct hand washing techniques to help prevent future infections. We continued with standard and additional precautions for two weeks after Les's recovery to ensure that transmission of the virus was reduced.

◄ REFLECTING ON THE INDUSTRY INSIGHT 💬 ➕

1 What alternative hand hygiene measures are used when hands are not visibly soiled?
   a No measures are required.
   b Alcohol-based hand rub.
   c Wiping hands on a paper towel.
   d No touch technique.

2 How can cross-contamination be minimised when attending to a patient's activities of daily living (ADLs)?
   a Do not assist the patient with ADLs.
   b Wear the same gloves when attending to all ADLs.
   c Complete all similar procedures on all patients before moving to the next procedure.
   d Ensure you wash hands and clean spills after each procedure.

3 When assisting a client with ADLs that expose you to bodily fluids, what precautions need to be taken?
   a Hand rub before and after the procedure.
   b Wear gloves and dispose of them afterwards.
   c Wear gloves and perform hand hygiene after the procedure.
   d No special precautions need to be taken.

SELF-CHECK QUESTIONS

1 Identify the five types of pathogenic microorganisms and explain why it is important to understand their differences.
2 Identify and explain each of the six steps in the chain of infection.
3 Explain the difference between standard and additional precautions.
4 Outline the five moments of hand hygiene.
5 What is PPE and when should each type be used?
6 Describe some simple measures that limit the spread of infection by droplet transmission, and thereby show your understanding of correct respiratory hygiene and cough etiquette.
7 Three types of cleaning are identified in the healthcare setting. List and explain their differences.
8 Why is it important to separate waste and dispose of each type appropriately?
9 How can the healthcare worker minimise contamination via aerosols and splatter?
10 What are your definitions of the following key words and terms that have been used in this chapter?

KEY WORD OR TERM	YOUR DEFINITION
Barrier nursing	
Spores	
Cytotoxic waste	
Blood-borne pathogen	
Pathology	
Safety data sheet	
Pharmaceutical waste	
Immunisation	

QUESTIONS FOR DISCUSSION

1   In this chapter you have learnt that correct hand washing techniques have been universally identified as the single most effective infection control measure a healthcare worker can undertake. Identify the different types of hand wash and provide an example of when each would be appropriate to use.

2   Discuss how the National Safety and Quality Health Service (NSQHS) Standard number three, Preventing and Controlling Healthcare-Associated Infection, uses evidence-based systems to prevent and control healthcare-associated infections.

3   Discuss the importance of mandatory COVID-19 vaccinations and boosters for the residential aged care workforce. Refer to the Australian Department of Health at **https://www.health.gov.au/ initiatives-and-programs/covid-19-vaccines/information-for-aged-care-providers-workers-and-residents-about-covid-19-vaccines/residential-aged-care-workers**

4   List and describe six of the types of waste identified by the World Health Organization (WHO, 2015) in its fact sheet 'Health-care waste'.

5   Outline the steps identified in the South Australian Department of Health's (2020) *Preventing and responding to work related exposure to infectious disease policy guideline* for care immediately following exposure to blood or body fluids.

EXTENSION ACTIVITY

Hand hygiene practice

In this chapter, you learnt that correct hand hygiene protects clients from microorganisms that healthcare workers may be carrying, protects healthcare workers from microorganisms the patients may be harbouring, and ensures microorganisms are not transmitted via contact during treatment.

1   In groups of three or four, practise hand washing techniques and critique each other.

2   Record the areas that your group decides are less effectively cleaned than others.

3   Share your discussion and critiquing with the other groups and listen to their feedback.

4   Glo Germ™ gel (for hands) and powder (for bench tops) contain harmless simulated germs that can be illuminated with ultraviolet light to test the effectiveness of your cleaning practices. In the same group, use the gel and powder to test how well your cleaning methods actually work:

   a   For the hand wash: rub the gel into your hands like a hand cream, then wash your hands as you normally would. Use the ultraviolet light to illuminate the germs left behind to identify the areas missed during your hand wash.

   b   For the bench-top clean: dust the powder onto the bench top, then clean the area as you normally would. Use the ultraviolet light to illuminate the germs left behind to identify the areas missed during your bench-top clean.

   c   Discuss why these particular illuminated areas are easy to miss during hand washing and surface cleaning.

REFERENCES

Australian Commission on Safety and Quality in Health Care (ACSQHC) (2017). National Safety and Quality Health Service Standard. Retrieved 4 May 2019 from https://www.nationalstandards.safetyandquality. gov.au/3.-preventing-and-controlling-healthcare-associated-infection

Australian Government (2011). *Work Health and Safety Act 2011*. Retrieved 13 March 2017 from https:// www.comlaw.gov.au/Details/C2011A00137

Centers for Disease Control and Prevention (CDC) (2016). How infections spread. Retrieved 7 May 2022 from https://www.cdc.gov/infectioncontrol/spread/index.html

Government of South Australia (2017). *Preventing and responding to work related exposure to infectious disease policy guideline*. Retrieved 14 October 2022 from https://www. sahealth.sa.gov.au/wps/wcm/connect/3903950041184cfd8d32df1afc50ebfc/Guideline_ Preventing+and+Responding+to+Work+Related+Exposure+to+Infectious+Disease_ Guideline_11.05.2017.pdf?MOD=AJPERES&CACHEID=ROOTWORKSPACE-3903950041184cfd8d32df1afc50ebfc-ocRiBKD

Hand Hygiene Australia (HHA) (2013). The National Hand Hygiene Initiative. Retrieved 15 March 2017 from http://www.hha.org.au/home.aspx

National Health and Medical Research Council (NHMRC) (2010). *Australian guidelines for the prevention and control of infection in healthcare*. Retrieved 17 October 2019 from https://www.nhmrc.gov.au/ sites/default/files/documents/attachments/19269%20NHMRC%20-%20Infection%20Control%20 Guidelines-accessible.pdf

National Health and Medical Research Council (NHMRC) (2019). *Australian guidelines for the prevention and control of infection in healthcare*. Retrieved 4 October 2019 from https://www.nhmrc.gov.au/about-us/publications/australian-guidelines-prevention-and-control-infection-healthcare-2019

NSW Health (2020). P2 mask. Retrieved 7 May 2022 from https://www.health.nsw.gov.au/environment/factsheets/Pages/face-mask.aspx

World Health Organization (WHO) (2009a). *Guidelines on hand hygiene in healthcare*. Retrieved 15 March 2017 from http://whqlibdoc.who.int/publications/2009/9789241597906_eng.pdf

World Health Organization (WHO) (2009b). Hand hygiene: Why, how & when? Retrieved 17 October 2019 from https://www.who.int/gpsc/5may/Hand_Hygiene_Why_How_and_When_Brochure.pdf

World Health Organization (WHO) (2015). Health-care waste. Factsheet number 253. Retrieved 15 March 2017 from http://www.who.int/mediacentre/factsheets/fs253/en/

World Health Organization (WHO) (2018). Health-care waste. Retrieved 17 October 2019 from https://www.who.int/news-room/fact-sheets/detail/health-care-waste

RECOGNISE HEALTHY BODY SYSTEMS

Learning objectives

By the end of this chapter, you should be able to:

1   work with information about the human body
2   recognise and promote ways to support healthy functioning of the body.

Introduction

This chapter describes the skills and knowledge required to work with basic information about the human body and to recognise and promote ways to maintain healthy functioning of body systems. An understanding of basic anatomy, physiology and healthy functioning will allow you to recognise body systems and their importance to good health, as well as the consequences in terms of disease when they do not function as expected.

By using and interpreting information about the human body and its healthy functioning, you will be able to contribute to the multidisciplinary team in care planning that supports the needs of the person being cared for. This chapter provides a broad overview and will enhance your quality of work activities by enabling you to effectively share information about the human body with your healthcare team.

INDUSTRY INSIGHTS 💬

Understanding anatomy and physiology

It wasn't until I started my first placement in the neurological ward that I realised the importance of understanding anatomy and physiology. Our patient, Mr Ford, had a closed head injury after falling off a second-floor balcony. I had learnt that anatomically, the skull is the hard casing that holds the brain tightly together so that it doesn't move and get damaged during everyday activities. After Mr Ford's injury, the bleeding between his brain and skull (epidural haematoma) caused an increase in pressure in his head. This interfered with the brain's ability to carry out all of its important functions, and so I understood why Mr Ford's symptoms included headache, confusion and dizziness, and why neurological observations to monitor pupil size, level of consciousness and motor function were needed to monitor his condition. Mr Ford required neurosurgery to drill a hole in his skull and suction the haematoma. This released the pressure inside his head (intracranial pressure) and Mr Ford recovered well.

I realised that an understanding of how the body works physiologically allows you to think more critically and to understand what happens when it is ill or injured, and what can be done about it. I aim to increase my knowledge of anatomy and physiology and use it to reflect on the reasoning behind the abnormal signs and symptoms of my patients in the future.

> ◆ Haematoma
> A collection of blood outside of blood vessels.

1 WORK WITH INFORMATION ABOUT THE HUMAN BODY

As a health services assistant (HSA) working in an acute care environment, it is important for you to have basic knowledge of the normal structure, function and location of the major body systems and to use correct medical terminology. This knowledge of normal functioning will enable you to identify abnormal functioning when it occurs. Additionally, an awareness of the relationships between major components of each body system and other structures emphasises that the wellbeing of a person is dependent on not just individual parts of the body, but also the body as a whole. This holistic approach allows you to identify the overall health of the person, including factors that support healthy functioning, and assists in determining their needs. This section will explore the normal structure and functioning of the human body for each body system as well as identifying factors that contribute to healthy functioning.

Describe the structure and function of the major body systems, and review factors that contribute to the maintenance of a healthy body

Anatomy describes how the body is structured, while *physiology* describes how the body functions. The basic structure and functions of the body systems and associated components are outlined in the following sections, along with body system changes that can occur and factors to maintain healthy functioning. These systems include:

* cells, tissues and organs
* cardiovascular system
* respiratory system
* musculoskeletal system
* endocrine system
* nervous system
* special senses – smell, taste, vision, equilibrium and hearing
* gastrointestinal system
* urinary system
* reproductive system
* integumentary system
* lymphatic and immune system.

Directional terms and body cavities

Each part of the human body has a role in supporting the body's overall healthy functioning. To accurately describe the human body, it is important to have knowledge of anatomical positions that describe directions and cavities. These directional terms allow you to report and record the location of an injury or symptom, and to clearly identify structures to avoid confusion.

The standard anatomical position for the body is upright, looking forward, with upper extremities at the sides and palms facing forward. Figure 3.1 outlines anatomical directions with examples to emphasise how this terminology can be used in a healthcare setting.

FIGURE 3.1(a) Anatomical directions with examples

TERM	DIRECTION	EXAMPLE
Superior	Towards the upper part of the body	The superior vena cava is above the heart
Inferior	Towards the lower part of the body	The inferior vena cava is below the heart
Medial	Towards the midline of the body	The medial ligament is towards the inner aspect of the knee
Lateral	Away from the midline of the body	The radius is lateral to the ulna
Proximal	Close to the origin of the body part	The proximal end of the tibia is at the knee
Distal	Further from the origin of the body part	The distal end of the tibia is at the foot
Superficial	At the body surface	The superficial layer of the skin is at the body's surface
Deep	More internal body	Deep wounds can affect internal structures

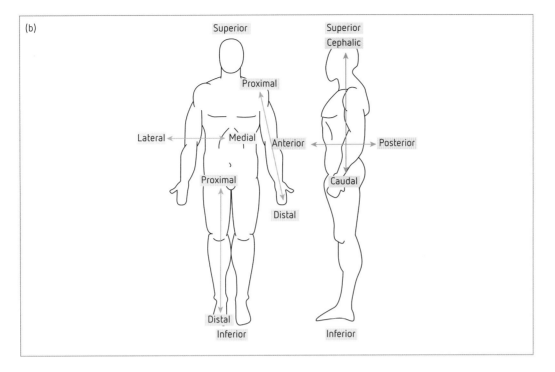

(b)

Body cavities are areas in the body that contain its internal organs. The cranial and spinal cavities are found in the dorsal cavity, while the thoracic and abdominopelvic cavities are found in the ventral cavity. Figure 3.2 illustrates the main body cavities. Smaller cavities are also found within the cranial cavity; these are the nasal, orbital and oral cavities.

Body cavities
Spaces inside the body that hold and protect internal organs.

FIGURE 3.2 The main body cavities

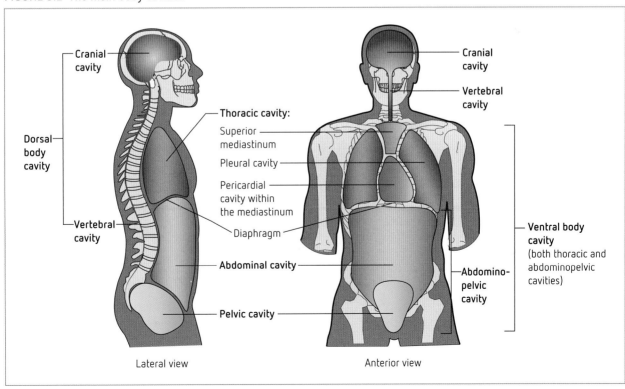

Lateral view

Anterior view

Cells, tissues and organs

The human body is a complex organism, with its simplest form being the *atom* – the microscopic building block of matter. Atoms combine to form *molecules,* which in turn combine to form cells. Cells vary in size, shape and function, with groups of similar cells combining to form tissues. A combination of two or more tissue types forms an organ, with each organ performing a specific function in the body. Organs combine to form the 11 organ systems that make up the human body (see Figure 3.3).

FIGURE 3.3 Structural organisation of the body from atom to organ system

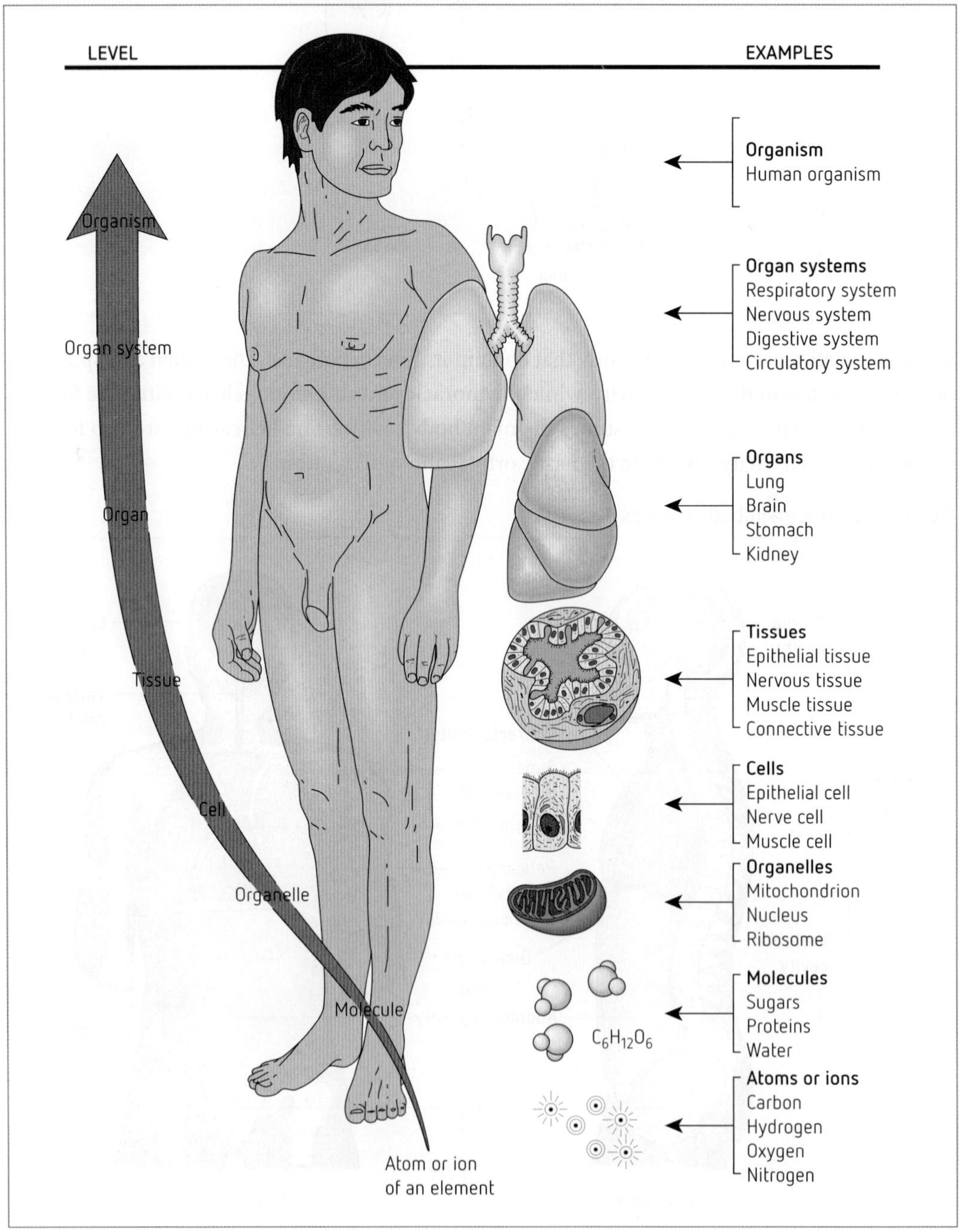

LEVEL

EXAMPLES

Organism
Organism
Human organism

Organ system
Organ systems
Respiratory system
Nervous system
Digestive system
Circulatory system

Organ
Organs
Lung
Brain
Stomach
Kidney

Tissue
Tissues
Epithelial tissue
Nervous tissue
Muscle tissue
Connective tissue

Cell
Cells
Epithelial cell
Nerve cell
Muscle cell

Organelle
Organelles
Mitochondrion
Nucleus
Ribosome

Molecule
Molecules
Sugars
Proteins
Water

$C_6H_{12}O_6$

Atom or ion
of an element
Atoms or ions
Carbon
Hydrogen
Oxygen
Nitrogen

Source: From Beck, *Theory and Practice of Therapeutic Massage,* 5E, p. 74. © 2011 Cengage

Cells

The fundamental unit of life is the cell. Humans have hundreds of different cells with common components called **organelles** or 'little organs' that perform various functions within the cell. The fluid inside each cell (intracellular fluid) is referred to as *cytoplasm*, and it is held inside the cell by the *plasma membrane*. This semipermeable membrane filters waste and allows nutrients to enter and leave the cell. Figure 3.4 outlines the basic structure of a cell.

The control centre of the cell is the nucleus, which contains genetic material or deoxyribonucleic acid (DNA). This genetic material directs the production of proteins that make the entire body function. Other organelles within the cell include the *endoplasmic reticulum*, a series of canals that connects the nucleus to the cytoplasm; the *Golgi apparatus*, which distributes the proteins and other products within and outside of the cell; and *lysosomes*, which clean up the waste products within the cell. The energy required for all these processes is supplied by organelles known as mitochondria.

Cells differ in function and size from long *nerve cells* (i.e., neurons) that gather information, to spherical *fat cells* that store nutrients. *Epithelial cells* cover body organs and have a honeycomb appearance, while *muscle cells*, which are long and have the ability to contract, allow movement of body parts. Some cells fight disease (i.e., macrophages) and others reproduce. The long *sperm cell* has a tail to allow it to swim to the *egg cell* for fertilisation.

> **Organelles**
> A number of organised or specialised structures within a living cell.

Tissues

Tissues also vary in size, shape and function. The four types of tissues (see Figure 3.5) that combine to form the organs and systems of the body are listed in Figure 3.6, with examples of each.

FIGURE 3.4 Cell structure

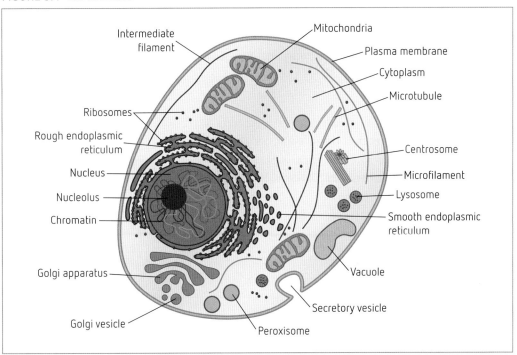

Source: Shutterstock.com/Vladimir Ischuk

FIGURE 3.5 The four types of tissues

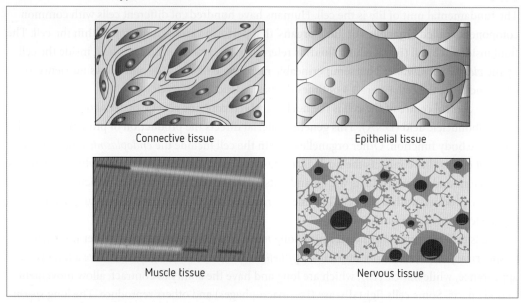

FIGURE 3.6 Tissue types and functions

TISSUE TYPE	FUNCTION	LOCATION
Connective	Supports the body and connects other tissues	Tendons, bones, blood, fat
Epithelial	Protects the outer body and lines internal organs. Its structure allows for secretion, absorption and filtration	Skin, sweat glands, alveoli
Muscle	Involved in voluntary and involuntary movements. It is classified as skeletal, cardiac or smooth muscle tissue	Skeletal muscles, heart, bladder
Nervous	Sends and receives electrochemical impulses from one part of the body to another	Neurons

ACTIVITY 3.1

Organs

List the organs found in each of the following body systems.

BODY SYSTEM	ORGANS
Cardiovascular	
Respiratory	
Musculoskeletal	
Endocrine	
Nervous	
Special senses	
Digestive	
Urinary	
Reproductive	
Integumentary	
Lymphatic and immune	

Cardiovascular system

The cardiovascular system comprises the heart and blood vessels (see Figure 3.7). The heart pumps blood through pathways called blood vessels to supply essential substances and nutrients, such as glucose, oxygen and hormones, to our cells. The blood vessels also carry waste away from those cells, which is then flushed out of the body in urine, faeces and sweat, as well as carbon dioxide via the lungs.

The heart lies in the thoracic cavity and is enclosed by a sac of serous membrane called the *pericardium*. The layers of the heart are the:

* *epicardium* – the outer layer
* *myocardium* – the middle muscle layer
* *endocardium* – the smooth inner layer.

The heart has two upper chambers, the left and right atria, which receive blood from the veins of the body. This blood then fills the two lower chambers, the left and right ventricles, which contract to pump blood out of the heart and into circulation around the body. Heart valves allow blood to flow in one direction only.

The heart functions as a double pump to circulate oxygenated and deoxygenated blood throughout the body. The pulmonary circulation takes deoxygenated blood from the right side of the heart to the lungs and back to the left side of the heart. The systemic circulation takes the

Cardiovascular system
Refers to the heart, blood vessels and blood.

FIGURE 3.7 Internal anatomy of the heart

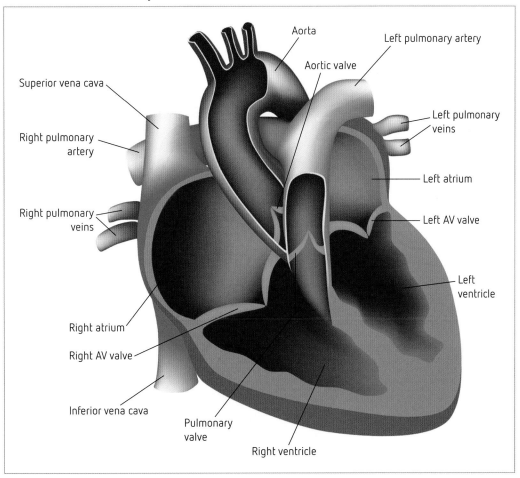

Source: Shutterstock.com / Alila Medical Media

oxygenated blood from the left side of the heart to the tissues and organs of the body and back to the right side of the heart.

The networks of vessels (see Figure 3.8) that transport blood around the body include:

- **Arteries** – thick-walled blood vessels that take oxygenated blood away from the heart. They divide into smaller *arterioles*. The largest artery in the body is the aorta.
- **Veins** – thin-walled blood vessels that return deoxygenated blood back to the heart. They divide into smaller *venules*. Many veins contain valves to ensure blood flows in one direction only. The largest veins in the body are the superior and inferior vena cava.
- **Capillaries** – small vessels that join arterioles and venules. Nutrients and oxygen are passed through capillaries into the cells of the body and waste products such as carbon dioxide are removed.

FIGURE 3.8 The network of blood vessels

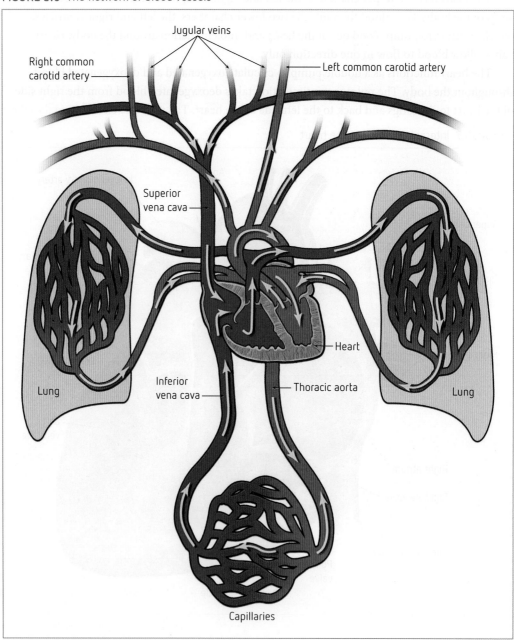

Source: Alamy.com/Nucleus Medical Media Inc.

Physiology

As the heart beats, the blood flows around the body. One complete heartbeat makes up a cardiac cycle, which consists of ventricular contraction (systole) that sends out blood to the systemic circulation and ventricular relaxation (diastole), which allows the ventricles to fill with blood again. A unique electrical conduction system causes the heart to beat and starts at the sinoatrial node (pacemaker) in the right atrium. The electrical impulse travels to the ventricles and causes the heart to contract. A disruption in this conduction can cause an arrhythmia (irregular beat).

Arrhythmia

An irregular heartbeat, ordinarily associated with a fluttering in the chest.

Body system changes and factors contributing to healthy functioning

As people get older, they may develop an abnormal build-up of fat, cholesterol and other substances in the inner lining of their arteries. This development is called atherosclerosis, and when the blood supply to the heart is affected it can cause the heart to overwork resulting in hypertension, *cardiac failure*, *angina* or heart attack. Signs of cardiac or coronary artery disease include:

* shortness of breath following activity
* pain, numbness, weakness or coldness in legs or arms
* pain in the chest, neck, jaw, throat or left arm
* irregular heartbeat, or slower or faster heartbeat
* light-headedness
* dizziness.

Atherosclerosis

Hardening and narrowing of the arteries caused by cholesterol, fat and other substances lining the arteries.

Common tests used to determine cardiac disorders include:

* coronary angiography to investigate blockages or narrowing of arteries
* blood tests to measure cholesterol, triglyceride and cardiac enzyme levels
* blood pressure monitoring to detect hypertension
* electrocardiogram to detect abnormal heart rhythms
* echocardiogram to monitor how the heart and valves are functioning
* stress tests to show how your heart works during exercise.

Maintaining healthy functioning of the cardiovascular system includes:

* avoiding smoking
* moderating alcohol intake
* eating foods which lower cholesterol
* controlling high blood pressure
* remaining at a healthy weight through regular exercise and a balanced diet.

Blood components

3.2 ACTIVITY

Blood transports nutrients, oxygen, wastes and hormones to all parts of the body so that vital functions can be performed. Address the following questions / tasks related to blood components:

1 Complete the following table by identifying the medical term and function of the blood cells listed.

BLOOD CELL	MEDICAL TERM	FUNCTION
Plasma		
White blood cells		
Red blood cells		
Platelets		

2   How much blood is contained within an average adult body?

3   What is haemoglobin?

4   What are the four different blood types? Which of these is the universal donor and which is the universal recipient?

Respiratory system

The human body requires oxygen for cell functioning and must eliminate the waste product carbon dioxide. This occurs through the respiratory system, which comprises the upper respiratory tract that purifies, humidifies and warms incoming air, and the lower respiratory tract, which is the site of gas exchange (see Figure 3.9).

Respiratory system

The organs involved in breathing with the exchange of oxygen and carbon dioxide.

Organs and functions of the upper respiratory tract

Air is drawn in through the nose into the nasal cavity where the nasal mucosa traps incoming bacteria and other debris. Air then passes to the pharynx (throat) and larynx (voice box), which

FIGURE 3.9 The respiratory system organs

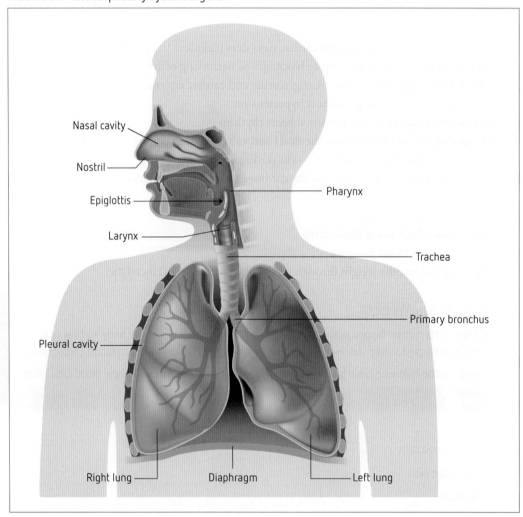

Source: Shutterstock.com / Alila Medical Media

has vocal cords that allow the formation of speech. The epiglottis protects the opening of the larynx and when we swallow it forms a lid at the opening of the larynx to protect from inhalation of food into the lungs. The rigid trachea (windpipe) is reinforced with c-shaped rings of *hyaline cartilage* to keep its shape open. The upper respiratory tract is where the air is warmed and moistened before it reaches the lungs.

Organs and functions of the lower respiratory tract

The trachea splits into two bronchi that lead to each lung. The right lung has three lobes and the left lung has two lobes. The smaller subdivisions of the main bronchi within the lungs are called *bronchioles*, which divide further to form *alveoli*.

Physiology

During inhalation, the accessory muscles of respiration enlarge the chest cavity. The diaphragm lowers and the intercostal muscles push upwards. Air is then drawn into the lungs due to the reduced pressure. During exhalation, the diaphragm contracts and the intercostal muscles relax to force air out of the lungs, through the trachea and out the nose and mouth (see Figure 3.10). These processes supply the body with oxygen and dispose of carbon dioxide, and occur through the following routes:

- *external respiration* – oxygen and carbon dioxide are exchanged between the alveoli and the pulmonary capillaries
- *internal respiration* – oxygen and carbon dioxide are exchanged between the blood and cells inside the body.

Body system changes and factors contributing to healthy functioning

Chronic asthma, especially in young people, is a major illness – the Australian Bureau of Statistics (2018) estimated 2.7 million Australians had asthma in 2017–18. Asthma symptoms are wheezing, breathlessness and chest tightness. Older people are also subject to a number of lung disorders such as COPD (chronic obstructive pulmonary disease) causing mild or severe shortness of breath. COPD includes emphysema and chronic bronchitis, which are common in older

Asthma

A type of chronic airways disease with symptoms of wheezing, breathlessness and chest tightness.

COPD (chronic obstructive pulmonary disease)

A disease with symptoms of mild or severe shortness of breath. COPD includes emphysema and chronic bronchitis.

FIGURE 3.10 The diaphragm and intercostals moving during inspiration and expiration

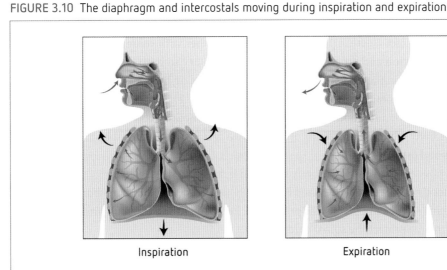

Inspiration

Expiration

people who have smoked during their lives. Other disorders include lung cancer and pneumonia. Signs of respiratory disorders include:

- cough – with or without sputum or coughing up blood
- dyspnoea – difficulty breathing
- cyanosis – bluish colour of the lips and fingertips
- shortness of breath
- noisy breathing.

    Common tests used to determine respiratory disorders include:
- auscultation to listen for abnormal lung sounds with a stethoscope
- chest X-ray to take images to detect lung consolidation or abnormalities
- arterial blood gas tests to determine the amount of oxygen in the blood
- pulmonary function tests to measure lung capacity and airway resistance (spirometry).

    Maintaining healthy functioning of the respiratory system includes:
- avoiding smoking
- avoiding triggers that can exacerbate asthma (air pollution, chemicals, physical exertion)
- avoiding people with colds and flu-like symptoms
- flu and COVID-19 vaccinations.

ACTIVITY 3.3

Health risks of smoking

Quitting smoking reduces the risk of developing smoking-related diseases and improves your health in multiple ways. Research the health risks of smoking and/or visit the Quit website (http://www.quit.org.au) to answer the following questions:

1   What are the health risks of smoking?

2   What are the health benefits of quitting?

3   What effects can smoking have during pregnancy?

4   Why is it important to stop smoking before surgery?

Musculoskeletal system

Musculoskeletal system
The bones, joints, cartilage, ligaments and connective tissue that support the body and help you move.

Erythrocytes
Red blood cells.

Tendons
Connective tissue that connects muscle to bone.

Cartilage
Tough connective tissue that lines joints and gives structure to the nose, ears, larynx and other parts of the body.

The musculoskeletal system includes the bones, joints, cartilage, ligaments and connective tissue that support the body (see Figure 3.11). The bones work together with voluntary skeletal muscles to maintain body position and produce movements. Involuntary smooth muscles operate automatically to maintain the necessary functions of life including breathing and digestion, and cardiac muscle maintains our heartbeat.

The 206 bones in the adult body perform the following functions:
- support the body – bones and groups of bones provide a framework for the attachment of soft tissues and organs
- store minerals – 99 per cent of the body's calcium is stored in the skeleton
- produce blood cells – erythrocytes (red blood cells) are produced in the red bone marrow
- protect organs – for example, the ribs protect the heart and lungs, the skull protects the brain and the vertebrae protect the spinal cord
- provide movement – tendons attach muscle to bone.

Bones consist of compact tissue on the external surface and spongy tissue inside, and they grow and develop through a process called *ossification*. Cartilage is a connective tissue that also provides support but is softer and more flexible than bone. It can be found in the nose, the flap of the ears and in movable joints.

FIGURE 3.11 The musculoskeletal system

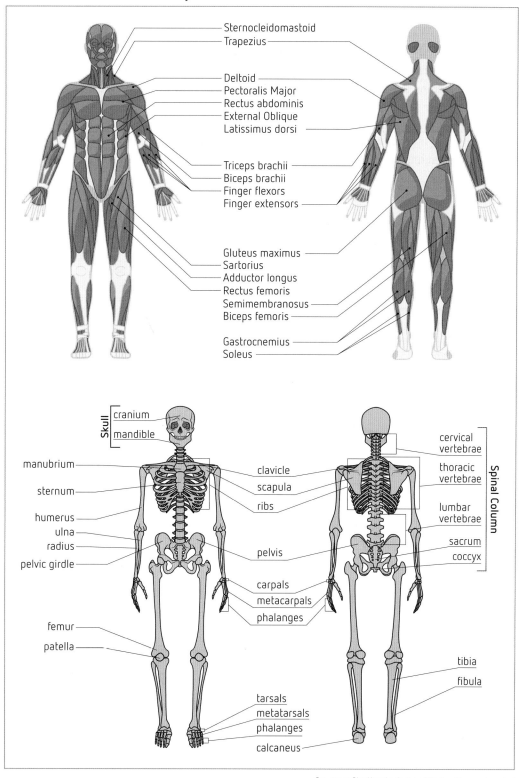

Sources: Shutterstock.com/NastyaSigne, elenabsl

Joints

Where two or more bones meet to allow for movement.

Synovial fluid

Thick liquid located between joints to provide lubrication.

Ligaments

Fibrous connective tissue that connects bones to other bones.

Joints occur where two or more bones meet, and can be classified as either:

- *fibrous* – immovable, such as the bones of the skull
- *cartilaginous* – slightly movable, such as the bones of the vertebrae
- *synovial* – freely movable, such as the bones of the knee.

Figure 3.12 identifies the different types of synovial joints found in the body. Synovial fluid provides lubrication in these joints and ligaments support the bones around the joints.

Physiology

As we move, our muscles contract and shorten, with most skeletal muscles working in pairs. For example, bending the elbow results in bicep contraction and tricep relaxation. These muscles

FIGURE 3.12 Different types of synovial joints

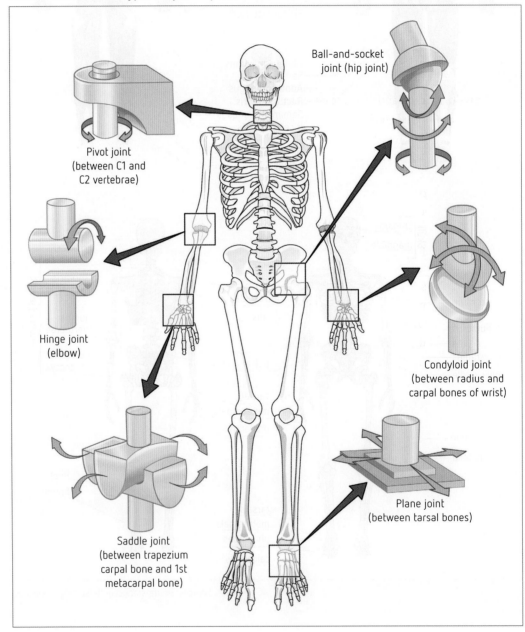

Source: OpenStax College via Wikicommons released under a CC BY 3.0 licence

are then supported by a network of connective tissue and tendons that anchor them to bones for strength and support. The movement of these muscles is a result of nervous stimulation. The response can be voluntary or involuntary, and an imbalance in the transmission of nerve impulses can cause uncoordinated or decreased musculoskeletal responses. This is seen in spinal cord injuries.

Body system changes and factors contributing to healthy functioning

As people age, joint tissues become less resilient to wear and tear and start to degenerate. This makes people susceptible to musculoskeletal diseases such as *osteoarthritis* and *osteoporosis*, as well as severe back pain. Other possible issues include *rheumatoid arthritis*, an autoimmune disease that causes chronic inflammation of joints, and muscular overuse, which can cause sprains, strains and tendonitis. Signs of musculoskeletal disorders include:

* pain or swelling in joints
* loss of mobility in joints
* deformity in joints.

Common tests used to determine musculoskeletal disorders include:

* X-rays to identify and evaluate bone density and structure
* bone scans to evaluate bone mineral density and degree of osteoporosis
* arthroscopy to examine, diagnose and repair a joint.

Maintaining healthy functioning of the musculoskeletal system includes:

* remaining at a healthy weight through regular exercise and a balanced diet
* avoiding overuse or straining of muscles
* avoiding poor posture and a sedentary lifestyle
* ensuring that dietary intake includes vitamin D and calcium
* undertaking passive exercises and active exercises.

Passive exercises (see Figure 3.13) are used to prevent stiffness and regain range of motion in muscles in persons who have difficulty doing independent exercise. They are also known as passive range of motion (ROM) exercises. Someone helps you move your muscles and joints through their full range of motion. **Active exercises** (see Figure 3.14) are patient initiated and help strengthen the muscles through increased movement.

Passive exercise

Exercise performed with the assistance of a person who moves your muscles and joints through their range of motion.

Active exercise

Using your own muscle power to move muscles and joints in the body.

FIGURE 3.13 Passive exercise

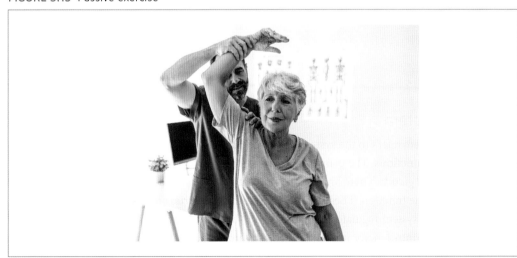

Source: iStock.com/ljubaphoto

FIGURE 3.14 Active exercise

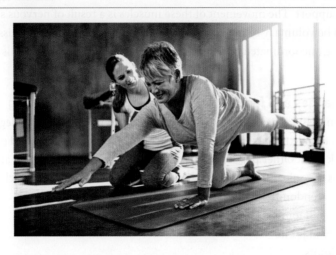

Source: iStock.com/PeopleImages

ACTIVITY 3.4

Body movements and exercises

The muscles in our body produce movement and provide posture and stability in joints. Complete the table below by describing the most common types of movements listed.

MOVEMENT	DESCRIPTION
Flexion	
Extension	
Rotation	
Abduction	
Adduction	
Circumduction	
Supination	
Pronation	
Inversion	
Eversion	

Endocrine system

The system of glands and organs that secretes hormones into the bloodstream to regulate bodily functions.

Endocrine system

The **endocrine system** refers to the system of glands that secretes chemicals into the bloodstream to regulate bodily functions. The primary glands are the *pituitary*, *pineal*, *thyroid*, *parathyroid*, *thymus* and *adrenal glands*. There are also organs that belong to other body systems but have a secondary endocrine function. These include the *pancreas*, *ovaries* and *testes* (see Figure 3.15).

The endocrine system regulates the human body by releasing chemical messengers called hormones, which control major processes such as reproduction, growth and development, fluid balance and metabolism.

FIGURE 3.15 The endocrine system

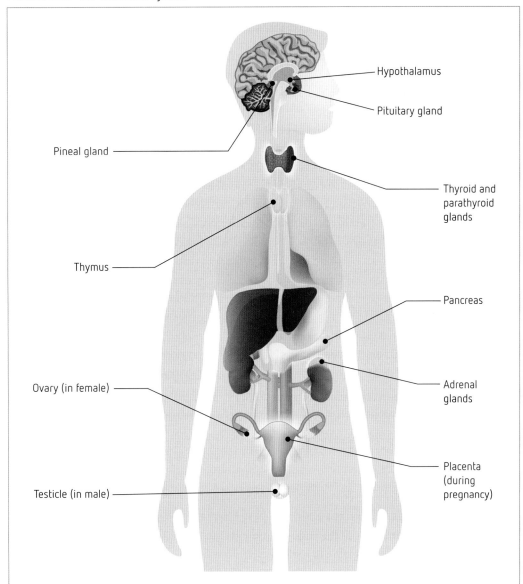

Hypothalamus

Pituitary gland

Pineal gland

Thyroid and parathyroid glands

Thymus

Pancreas

Ovary (in female)

Adrenal glands

Testicle (in male)

Placenta (during pregnancy)

Source: Shutterstock.com/Designua

Figure 3.16 outlines the major endocrine glands, their functions and the hormones they release.

Physiology

Hormones maintain homeostasis, which is the tendency of the internal environment of the body to maintain a balance or equilibrium. This is important because an imbalance in the body's internal environment can cause body system disorders or death. In most cases, the release of a hormone from its associated gland occurs via the gland's activation and inhibition, which is regulated by *negative feedback* mechanisms. This means that a decrease in homeostatic levels of hormones and their effects triggers more release of that hormone and vice versa. For example, pancreatic islets cells release glucagon in response to low blood sugar levels, but when blood sugar levels are within normal range, the glucagon release is inhibited.

Homeostasis

The ability of a system to maintain its internal equilibrium.

FIGURE 3.16 The major endocrine glands, their functions and the hormones released

GLAND	FUNCTION	MAJOR HORMONES
Anterior pituitary	Stimulates growth and development	Growth hormone
	Stimulates milk production	Prolactin
	Stimulates production of oestrogen, sperm and progesterone	Follicle stimulating hormone (FSH) and luteinising hormone (LH)
	Stimulates thyroid to release hormones	Thyroid stimulating hormone (TSH)
	Stimulates adrenal gland to release hormones	Adrenocorticotrophic hormone (ACTH)
Posterior pituitary	Contraction of uterus and lactation	Oxytocin
	Water regulation in the kidneys	Antidiuretic hormone (ADH)
Pineal	Circadian rhythm	Melatonin
Thyroid	Regulates metabolic rate	Thyroxin
	Decreases calcium levels in blood	Calcitonin
Parathyroid	Controls calcium/phosphate levels	Parathyroid
Thymus	Plays a role in immunity	Thymosin
Adrenals	Regulates electrolytes	Aldosterone
	Aids carbohydrate, protein and fat metabolism	Cortisol
	Influences secondary sex characteristics in males	Sex steroids
	Prepares body for 'fight–flight'	Epinephrine
Pancreatic islets	Glycogen breakdown to increase blood glucose level (BGL)	Glucagon
	Glucose storage to decrease BGL	Insulin
Ovaries	Development of female sexual characteristics	Oestrogen
		Progesterone
Testes	Development of male sexual characteristics	Testosterone

Body system changes and factors contributing to healthy functioning

As our body ages, the efficiency of the endocrine glands can decrease. This is seen in females during menopause where the decline in reproductive hormones causes atrophy of the reproductive organs, inability to bear children and the possibility of osteoporosis. The decline in thyroid hormone can cause hypothyroidism. The ability to resist stress and infection is also diminished for all people, and there may be a decline in insulin production, causing diabetes. Signs and symptoms of diabetes can include:

- excessive thirst (polydipsia)
- excessive urination (polyuria)
- fatigue and weight loss
- slow-healing sores
- numb or tingling feet.

Common tests used to determine endocrine disorders include:

- blood glucose monitoring to detect glucose levels
- urine tests to check abnormalities in hormone levels
- blood tests to check electrolyte and hormone levels.

Maintaining healthy functioning of the endocrine system includes:

Menopause

The period in a woman's life (typically between the ages of 45 and 50) when menstruation ceases.

Hypothyroidism

Where the thyroid gland is underactive and fails to secrete enough hormones into the bloodstream.

- remaining at a healthy weight through regular exercise and a balanced diet
- avoiding smoking
- having regular health check-ups.

Diabetes

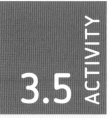

Research the causes and types of diabetes and answer the following questions:

1   How can diabetes affect other functions of the body?
2   What is the difference between type 1 and type 2 diabetes and what are the treatment options for each?
3   What are the complications of diabetes?
4   Practise your clinical skills by taking a blood glucose level (BGL).

Nervous system

The nervous system controls and coordinates all voluntary and involuntary activities of the body through functional units known as neurons. The structure of the nervous system comprises the:

- central nervous system – brain and spinal cord
- peripheral nervous system – cranial and spinal nerves.

Central nervous system

The largest part of the brain is the cerebrum, which controls thought, language, reasoning, perception and voluntary movement. The cerebrum has two hemispheres and four lobes (temporal, frontal, parietal and occipital), with each lobe having responsibility for various functions such as hearing, speech, pain and vision. The cerebellum lies beneath the cerebrum and coordinates muscle activity and balance, and the brain stem merges with the spinal cord at the base of the brain to relay messages to other parts of the body (see Figure 3.17). The brain stem consists of the *midbrain*, *pons* and *medulla oblongata*, which regulate the body's vital activities such as breathing, heart rate and blood pressure. The spinal cord carries motor and sensory messages to and from the brain.

The skull and vertebral column protect the central nervous system, with further protection provided by the meninges – connective tissue that surrounds the central nervous system. The meninges have a tough outer layer (dura mater), a middle layer (arachnoid mater) and an innermost layer (pia mater). Cerebrospinal fluid is found in the space between the arachnoid and pia mata (subarachnoid space) and provides nourishment and a watery cushioning around the brain and cord.

Peripheral nervous system

There are 12 pairs of cranial nerves and 31 pairs of spinal nerves. The *sensory (afferent) nerves* carry impulses to the brain and spinal cord, and the *motor (efferent) nerves* carry impulses away from the brain and spinal cord to muscles, organs and tissues. *Mixed nerves* transmit impulses in both directions.

Physiology

The nervous system functions to sense change, interpret information and respond through muscular contractions or glandular secretions. The central nervous system receives inputs from the sensory division and responds via the motor division. The nerve fibres (neurons) transfer these messages by the use of chemicals that carry the information from one nerve cell to the next.

Nervous system

Receives and interprets stimuli (via neurons) to control and coordinate activities in the body.

Cerebrum

The part of the brain that controls thought, language, reasoning, perception and voluntary movement.

Cerebellum

The part of the brain that lies beneath the cerebrum and coordinates muscle activity and balance.

Brain stem

Merges with the spinal cord at the base of the brain to relay messages to other parts of the body.

Spinal cord

Carries motor and sensory messages to and from the brain.

FIGURE 3.17 Anatomy of the human brain

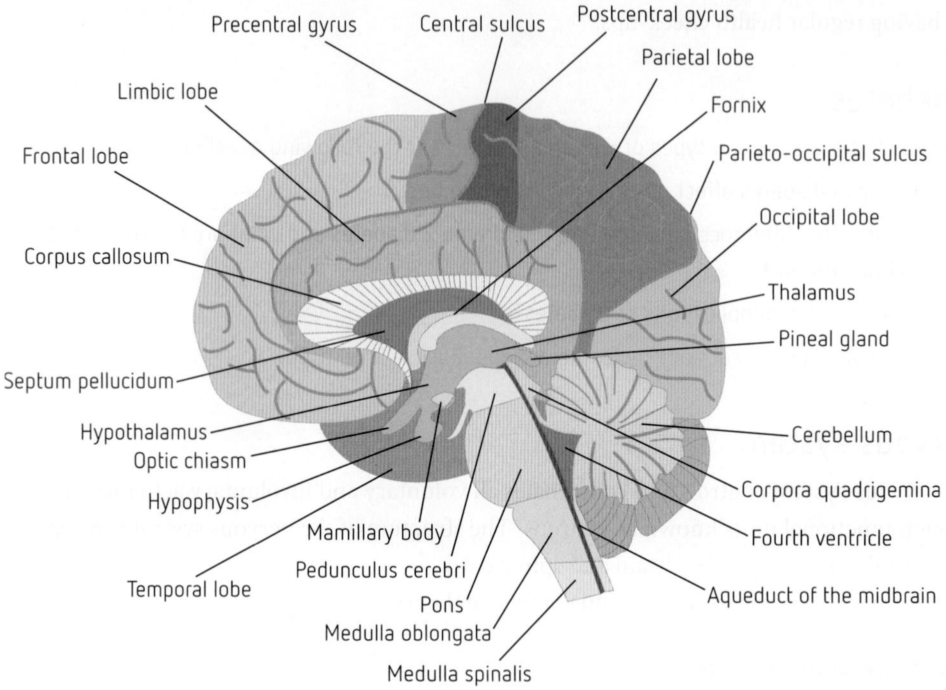

Source: Shutterstock.com/BigMouse

Somatic nervous system

Carries motor and sensory information to skin, sense organs and skeletal muscles.

Autonomic nervous system

Automatic or involuntary responses of the nervous system, as in the actions of smooth muscles, cardiac muscles and glands.

The voluntary or **somatic nervous system** initiates motor responses consciously or voluntarily to control skeletal muscles, whereas the **autonomic nervous system** initiates automatic or involuntary responses; for example, the actions of smooth muscles, cardiac muscles and glands. These actions can be either inhibiting (*parasympathetic* effects) or stimulating (*sympathetic* effects) as shown in Figure 3.18. An example can be seen when we walk into a brightly lit room. Our nervous system senses the change, interprets and responds by initiating muscular actions in the eye to constrict the pupil and limit the amount of light entering the eye. This response is automatic, rapid and involuntary.

Body system changes and factors contributing to healthy functioning

Disorders of the nervous system can affect either the brain or the spinal cord, and can be due to trauma, infection, autoimmune disorders, tissue degeneration, strokes or tumours. Examples of nervous system disorders include Alzheimer's disease and other forms of dementia, multiple sclerosis, Parkinson's disease and meningitis. Strokes can occur due to a blockage or bleed in the brain. The signs of stroke are:

- severe headache
- nausea and vomiting
- visual disturbances
- motor deficits
- loss of consciousness
- facial droop
- difficulty speaking
- confusion.

FIGURE 3.18 The organisation of the nervous system

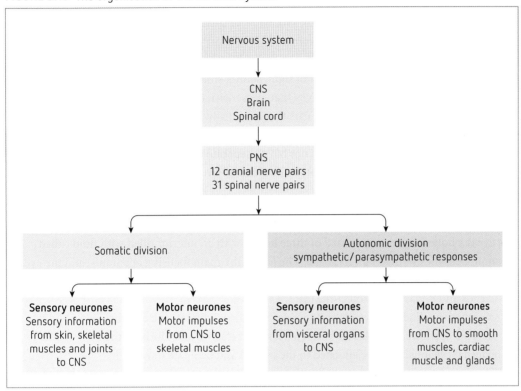

Common tests used to determine neurological disorders include:

- CT scans to view the brain and spine
- electroencephalography (EEG) to monitor the brain activity through the skull
- cerebral angiogram to detect narrowing or obstruction of a blood vessel in the brain or neck.

Maintaining healthy functioning of the nervous system includes:

- remaining at a healthy weight through regular exercise and a balanced diet
- preventing falls in the elderly
- ensuring a balanced diet is consumed that includes B6, B12 and folate
- moderating alcohol intake
- controlling high blood pressure and/or diabetes
- reporting prolonged headaches, neck stiffness or vision problems.

Parkinson's disease

Research the causes and symptoms of Parkinson's disease and answer the following questions:

1   How can Parkinson's disease affect other functions of the body?

2   What nursing care is provided for a person who has Parkinson's disease?

3   What are the treatment options for a person with Parkinson's disease?

4   What are the complications of Parkinson's disease?

3.6 ACTIVITY

Special senses – vision, hearing, smell and taste

The eyes, ears, nose and tongue have sensory receptors or special nerve cells as a part of the peripheral nervous system that extends from the brain and spinal cord. These sensory receptors respond to a stimulus that is then converted into a nerve impulse. The impulse is then sent to that specific part of the brain, which creates the sensation of sight, sound, smell or taste. The sensory receptors are:

- eyesight – photoreceptors in the eyes that are sensitive to light
- hearing – mechanoreceptors in the ears that are sensitive to sound waves or vibrations
- smell and taste – chemoreceptors that are sensitive to various chemicals.

Another sense is touch, which does not have a separate organ where sensory receptors are found; however, there are sensory receptors for touch all over the body, especially in the skin, bowel and sex organs.

Vision

The eye is a hollow sphere composed of three layers, with an interior filled with fluid called *humor* to help the eye maintain its shape. The lens is the main focusing apparatus, and the eye is supported by the following accessory structures and ligaments:

- eyelids and eyelashes – protect the eye
- conjunctiva – lines the eyelids and secretes mucus to lubricate the eyeball
- lacrimal apparatus and glands – secrete tears that cleanse and lubricate the eye
- external eye muscles – are attached to the eyeball and facilitate movement.

The outermost layer of the eyeball is the *sclera*. This thick, white connective tissue is clear at the front to allow light to enter. This transparent section is called the *cornea*. The middle layer of the eyeball is the vascular region and contains the *choroid*, *ciliary body* and *lens*, which is attached by *suspensory ligaments*. The front section of the choroid is the *iris* (coloured part of the eye) and has an opening called the *pupil* through which light passes.

The innermost layer is the *retina*, which contains *photoreceptors* (rods and cones) and the *optic nerve* (see Figure 3.19).

Light enters the eye through the pupil, which contracts or dilates to control the amount of light entering. The light then moves through the lens, which changes shape to adjust for near or far vision (focusing). This process is known as *accommodation*. The light then moves through the humor of the eye to the retina. Here, the photoreceptors detect light and generate a nerve impulse that is transmitted through the optic nerve to the brain.

Hearing

The ear is responsible for hearing and maintaining equilibrium (balance), and it is divided into three major areas (as shown in Figure 3.20):

- outer ear – contains the *pinna* that directs sound waves into the ear via the *external auditory canal*. This canal is lined with ceruminous glands that secrete *cerumen* (earwax). The soundwaves reach the *tympanic membrane* (eardrum) and cause it to vibrate
- middle ear – contains three *ossicles* (small bones) – the *malleus*, *incus* and *stapes* – that transmit the vibratory motion from the tympanic membrane to the *oval window* of the inner ear. The *Eustachian tube* connects the middle ear to the throat and plays a role in equalising pressure within the ear
- inner ear –a maze of bony chambers or labyrinth filled with fluid called perilymph. Inside this chamber sits the *cochlea*, which contains the mechanisms of hearing, along with the *vestibule* and *semicircular canals*, which are involved in balance.

FIGURE 3.19 Anatomy of the eye

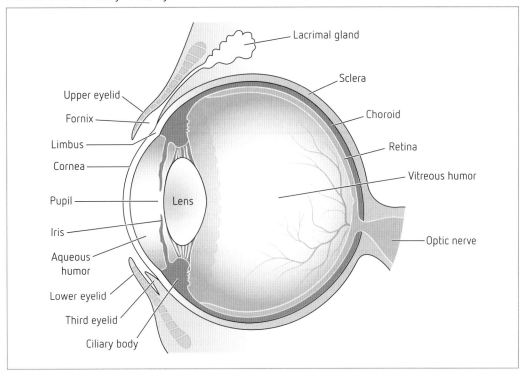

FIGURE 3.20 Anatomy of the ear

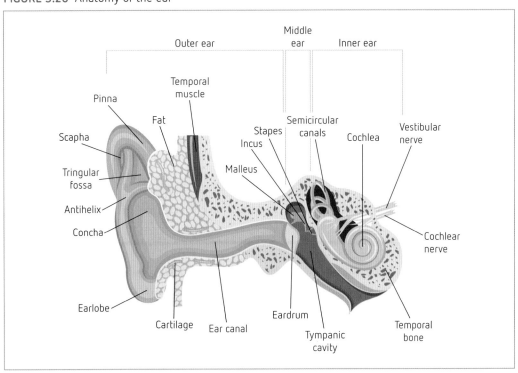

In maintaining hearing, the ear must respond to sound waves. When these sound waves hit the tympanic membrane, it vibrates and causes the ossicles to move. This movement is picked up by the mechanoreceptors in the inner ear, which exist on the hairlike cells on the semicircular canals and vestibule. When these hairlike cells (*cilia*) move, an impulse is sent through the cochlea to the brain, which interprets the information as sound.

In maintaining *equilibrium* (physical balance), the ear must respond to movement. The fluid within the semicircular canals moves as the rest of the body moves. The cilia in the canals detect this movement and transmit impulses to the brain about the vertical, horizontal and rotational planes. This information helps to keep the body in balance.

Smell

Olfactory cells
Passes along smell sensations to the brain.

Receptors for smell line the top of the nasal cavity. These olfactory cells have a direct attachment to the cerebral cortex of the brain. The olfactory cells detect chemicals in the air that we inhale and generate a nerve impulse that is carried up the olfactory nerve to the brain. The brain then interprets this smell. The sense of smell and taste work closely together – if you cannot smell something, you cannot taste it either.

Taste

Taste buds on your tongue contain chemoreceptors that work in a similar way to the receptors in your nose. Each type of taste bud detects different types of taste: sweet, sour, bitter, salty and umami (savoury). Chemicals in food bind to the receptors, which generate a nerve impulse that is carried to the brain.

Body system changes and factors contributing to healthy functioning

As a consequence of the ageing process, the special senses can deteriorate, resulting in the need for eyeglasses or hearing aids. Disease can also affect the senses, with diabetic retinopathy, glaucoma and macular degeneration causing visual disturbances, and otitis media and Meniere's syndrome causing hearing problems including loss of hearing, ringing in the ears or balance disturbances.

Maintaining healthy functioning of the special senses includes:

* avoiding constant exposure to noise
* ensuring a balanced diet is consumed
* avoiding smoking, which can cause taste buds to atrophy
* being aware of medications that can affect the senses
* reporting vision, hearing, taste or smell changes
* ensuring that glasses and hearing aids fit and function correctly.

ACTIVITY 3.7

Macular degeneration

Macular degeneration is the leading cause of visual impairment in our ageing population.

Research the causes and symptoms of macular degeneration and answer the following questions:

1   What are the causes of macular degeneration?

2   What are the treatment options for a person with macular degeneration?

3   What nursing care would you provide for a client who has macular degeneration?

4   What are the complications of macular degeneration?

Gastrointestinal system

The gastrointestinal system enables food to be converted into simpler molecules so that it can be absorbed into the blood for cell energy and function. The system comprises the alimentary tract, which is directly involved in the process of ingestion, digestion and absorption, and 'accessory organs' that aid the process by producing chemical substances to assist with digestion (see Figure 3.21).

Alimentary tract

The alimentary tract is comprised of a 9- to 10-metre muscular tube that extends from mouth to anus. In the *mouth*, saliva helps to moisten the food in preparation for ingestion. Mechanical digestion occurs through the actions of the teeth breaking down food (mastication) to a small size (*bolus*), and chemical digestion occurs with *salivary amylase* breaking down carbohydrates to simple sugars. The tongue then pushes the food to the back of the throat where the swallowing action passes the food down through the *oesophagus* and to the stomach through muscular contractions called peristalsis (see Figure 3.22).

Gastrointestinal system
Responsible for the digestion and absorption of food and liquids into the blood for cell energy and function.

Peristalsis
Involuntary constriction and relaxation of the muscles of the intestine or other canal.

FIGURE 3.21 The gastrointestinal system

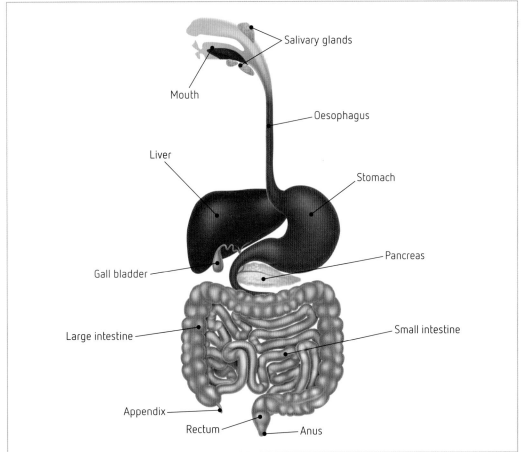

Source: Shutterstock.com/Christos Georghiou

FIGURE 3.22 The peristalsis process

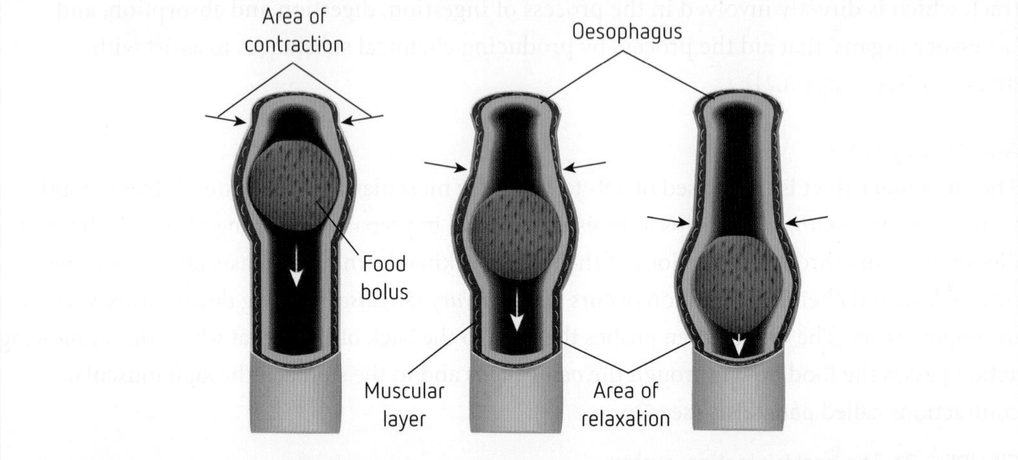

In the *stomach*, peristalsis continues and gastric juices chemically digest the food until it is a thick liquid (*chyme*). This can take up to three hours. The gastric juices also break down proteins in the food into *amino acids*. Chyme passes through to the *small intestine* via the *pyloric sphincter*, which allows a regulated amount of liquid to pass each time. The small intestine consists of the *duodenum*, *jejunum* and *ileum*, and here the digestion of food is complete so that the nutrients can pass through the intestinal walls to the bloodstream.

The material that cannot be digested then passes through to the *large intestine*. Here, water is reabsorbed back into the body so that the liquid chyme is concentrated to form *faeces*. The large intestine consists of the *ascending*, *transverse* and *descending colon* and the *sigmoid colon*. Faeces pass through the rectum and are excreted out of the body through the *anus*.

Accessory organs

Accessory organs help with digestion but are not part of the alimentary tract. They secrete or store substances that pass through ducts into the alimentary canal, and include the:

* tongue – tastes food and helps in swallowing
* salivary glands – secrete salivary amylase that breaks down carbohydrates and lubricates food for ease of passage from the mouth to the stomach
* pancreas – secretes pancreatic juice that breaks down proteins, fats and carbohydrates in the small intestine
* liver – secretes bile that breaks down fats in the duodenum of the small intestine
* gall bladder – stores and concentrates excess bile secreted by the liver.

Physiology

The gastrointestinal system is responsible for converting the food that we eat into energy and nutrients to allow the body to grow and repair. Figure 3.23 outlines the processes involved in digestion.

FIGURE 3.23 The digestive process

PROCESS	DESCRIPTION
Ingestion	Taking in food
Propulsion	Swallowing and peristalsis moving food through the digestive tract
Mechanical breakdown	Chewing, mixing of food by the tongue, stomach churning and segmentation (constrictions in the small intestine). This increases the surface area for absorption and assists in the mixing of food with digestive juices in the small intestine
Digestion	The chemical breakdown of food with assistance from enzymes. By the time the food has left the duodenum, it has been reduced to fatty acids, amino acids, monosaccharides and nucleotides – the chemical building blocks of the body
Absorption	The uptake of nutrients into the bloodstream through the walls of the intestinal tract
Defecation	Elimination of wastes as faeces through the anus

Body system changes and factors contributing to healthy functioning

Developmental changes affect bowel elimination throughout our life. As we age, the rate of peristalsis decreases and the slowing of nerve impulses can delay the urge to defecate, resulting in constipation. Changes to the nutritional status of the person can also impact on elimination. Gastroenteritis, ulcers, irritable bowel syndrome and diverticular disease can all cause gastrointestinal dysfunction. Common symptoms of gastrointestinal disorders include:

* change in bowel habits
* nausea and vomiting
* decreased appetite and weight loss
* abdominal pain or indigestion
* fatigue
* blood in faeces.

    Common tests used to determine gastrointestinal disorders include:

* colonoscopy or endoscopy using a flexible scope to examine the gastrointestinal tract and bowel
* stool specimen testing to check for abnormal bacteria or blood in the faeces
* barium swallow and X-ray to show how well the stomach is working and helps to find emptying problems.

    Maintaining healthy functioning of the gastrointestinal system includes:

* ensuring a balanced diet is consumed that includes fibre, fruit and vegetables and adequate hydration
* regular toileting and reporting episodes of visible blood in faeces, constipation and diarrhoea
* being aware of medications that can affect elimination
* remaining at a healthy weight through regular exercise and a balanced diet
* performing regular oral hygiene.

ACTIVITY 3.8

Nutrition

Awareness of a healthy diet is important because the building of fuel for our body's cells is dependent upon good nutrition. Research healthy diets and/or visit Nutrition Australia at **http://www.nutritionaustralia.org** and answer the following questions:

1. In the following table, list the five food groups that contribute to a balanced diet, examples of each and the nutrients they provide.

FOOD GROUP	EXAMPLE FOODS	NUTRIENTS PROVIDED

2. What is the daily recommendation concerning these five groups that a person should consume each day?

3. What food should be limited or avoided to support a healthy body?

Urinary system

Urinary system

Produces, stores and eliminates fluid waste (urine) from the body.

The **urinary system** is where wastes are filtered from your blood to produce urine for elimination. Because it eliminates fluids from the body, the urinary system also plays a major role in fluid and electrolyte balance (see Figure 3.24).

FIGURE 3.24 The urinary system

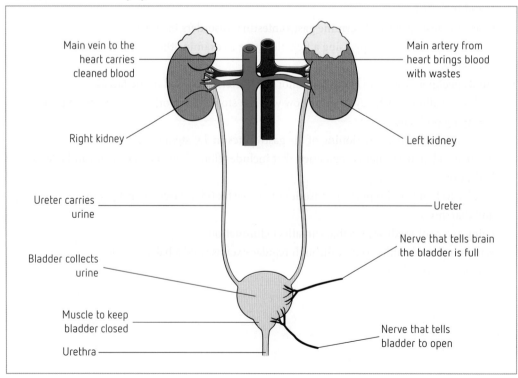

Main vein to the heart carries cleaned blood

Main artery from heart brings blood with wastes

Right kidney

Left kidney

Ureter carries urine

Ureter

Nerve that tells brain the bladder is full

Bladder collects urine

Muscle to keep bladder closed

Nerve that tells bladder to open

Urethra

Kidneys are the major organs of this system, and they form urine, a usually yellow-amber coloured fluid that varies from darker to lighter colour according to diet and hydration status. The concentration of urine is made up of approximately 95 per cent water with the other solutes such as organic molecules and ions.

The functional cells of the kidney are called *nephrons*, which are microscopic tubules. Urine flows from the kidneys through muscular tubes (*ureters*) that convey urine to the bladder through peristalsis and gravity. The urinary bladder is a hollow muscular and elastic organ that collects urine before it is excreted from the body. The average volume that the bladder can hold is 300–450 millilitres of urine, and as it stretches the urge to urinate is initiated. The urethra connects the urinary bladder to the external genitalia for elimination from the body. This process is called *voiding* or *micturition*, and sphincter muscles control the elimination of urine from the body.

Physiology

Blood enters the kidneys through the *renal artery* and then passes through a capillary network within the kidney structure. Pressure forces components of the blood into the renal tubular system where it is then filtered to remove wastes. The kidneys then return important substances back to the circulatory system. These processes can be summarised as:

- filtration – blood is filtered through the capillary walls. Water and solutes are forced through to the renal tubules in the kidneys while blood cells and proteins, which are large molecules, remain in the bloodstream
- reabsorption – water and other essential substances are returned to the blood
- secretion – wastes are secreted to become urine for elimination.

> **Sphincter**
> A circular muscle that constricts a passage or closes a natural orifice. When relaxed, a sphincter allows materials to pass through the opening.

Body system changes and factors contributing to healthy functioning

Destruction of renal tissue can occur due to chronic or acute diseases. This can include acute obstruction due to cancer, calculi, prostate enlargement, infection or chronic kidney disease. Common symptoms of urinary disorders include:

- inability or difficulty in passing urine or incontinence
- painful sensation when voiding
- cloudy, blood-stained or foul-smelling urine
- anorexia
- nausea and vomiting
- hypertension and oedema (which can be associated with renal failure).
  Common tests used to determine urinary disorders include:
- urinalysis to detect blood or abnormal elements in urine
- cystoscopy to visualise bladder for abnormalities
- biopsy to remove kidney tissue for pathologic examination
- intravenous pyelogram where dye is injected to visualise the kidneys, ureters and bladder.
  Maintaining healthy functioning of the urinary system includes:
- ensuring adequate hydration
- regular toileting and reporting episodes of urinary burning or foul-smelling urine
- performing perineal hygiene
- being aware of medications that can affect elimination
- remaining at a healthy weight through regular exercise and a balanced diet.

ACTIVITY 3.9

Fluid and electrolyte (including pH) balance

The kidneys play an important role in water and electrolyte balance, excretion of wastes and maintenance of **blood pH**. For cells to function, blood pH must remain within a narrow range. Research information on acid-base balance of blood and answer the following questions:

1   What is the blood pH range that must be maintained for survival?

2   Define the terms 'alkalosis' and 'acidosis'.

3   What can cause disturbances in acid-base balance?

4   What body systems assist with maintaining acid-base balance?

Blood pH
The acidity or alkalinity of blood.

Reproductive system

The *reproductive* role of the male is to manufacture *sperm* and deliver it to the female reproductive tract. The female produces *ova*, which are fertilised by the sperm to form the first cells of a new individual. Sex hormones play an important role in this process including initiating sexual drives and the growth and development of the reproductive organs.

Structure and function of the male reproductive system

The primary reproductive organs in a male, as shown in Figure 3.25, are the testes, which produce *sperm* and the endocrine hormone testosterone. A ductal system transports sperm from the testes, through the epididymis and vas deferens to the urethra. The *epididymis* is the first part of the ductal system and as the sperm travel along this duct they mature. The *vas deferens* then transfers the mature sperm to the *urethra*. *Seminal vesicles* located at the base of the bladder produce and secrete *semen* to nourish the sperm, and the *prostate gland* secretes a fluid that helps to activate the sperm during *ejaculation*.

FIGURE 3.25 The male reproductive system

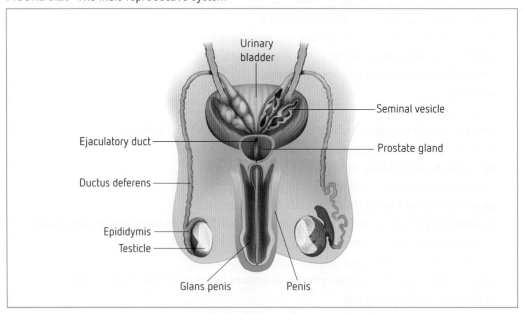

Source: Shutterstock.com/BlueRingMedia

The external genitalia of the male include the *scrotum*, which is a pouch that protects the testes. The *penis* delivers the sperm into the female reproductive tract or expels urine through the urethra. A *foreskin* covers the end of the penis and is sometimes removed through a procedure called *circumcision*.

Structure and function of the female reproductive system

The function of the female reproductive system (see Figure 3.26) is to produce eggs (ova) and support the developing foetus. The primary reproductive organs are the ovaries, which produce *ova* and the endocrine hormone oestrogen. During *ovulation* an egg is transported from the ovary into the *fallopian tube* and through to the *uterus*. If fertilisation occurs, the fertilised egg embeds in the uterus and develops into a foetus. The uterus is a muscular structure lined with *endometrium* that protects and nourishes the foetus as it develops. If fertilisation does not occur, the endometrium sheds its lining and is passed out through the vagina as *menstruation* (period). The narrow end of the uterus is called the *cervix*, which opens to a muscular canal (*vagina*) that opens to the outside of the body, behind the urethra.

The external genitalia of the female include the *labia minora* and *labia majora*. These sets of tissue fold over and protect the vaginal opening. The *clitoris* lies in front of the urethra and has many nerve endings and erectile tissue that swells during sexual arousal.

The *mammary glands* (breasts) contain lobes that produce milk and ducts that transport the milk to the *nipple*. Adult women have 15–20 lobes in each breast.

Body system changes and factors contributing to healthy functioning

As women age, their hormone levels fall to a point where menstruation ceases and menopause is reached. During this time, women may experience hot flushes, irritability, discomfort with sexual intercourse and headaches. Men's testicular function also declines with age, although they can continue to produce sperm.

FIGURE 3.26 The female reproductive system

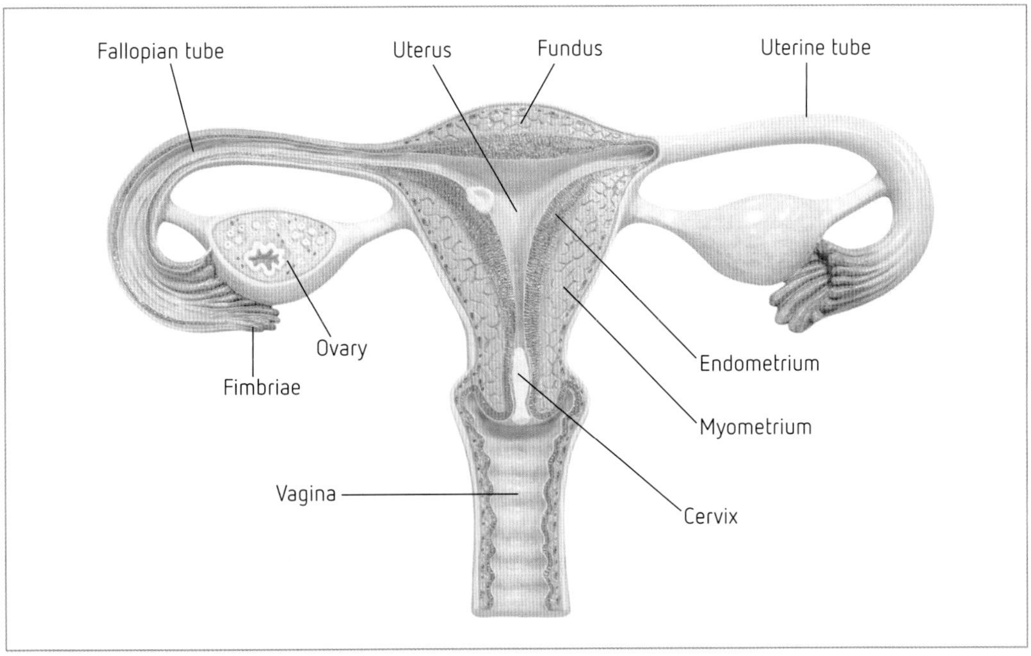

Source: Shutterstock.com/Suwin

Sexually transmitted infections also risk the normal functioning of the reproductive system. They can include chlamydia, gonorrhoea and syphilis, with symptoms including:

- fertility problems
- unusual discharge from vagina or penis
- bleeding between periods
- inability or difficulty passing urine
- painful sensation when passing urine
- pelvic pain
- painless ulcers or body rash.

Common tests used to determine reproductive disorders include:

- mammogram to detect breast abnormalities including tumours
- Pap smear to detect cervical tissue abnormalities
- prostate examination to examine the size of the prostate
- blood tests to detect abnormal hormone levels.

Maintaining healthy functioning of the reproductive system includes:

- undergoing regular Pap smears and breast examinations for women
- observing changes in size, shape or discharge from breasts
- ensuring a balanced diet is consumed with adequate hydration
- undertaking regular testicular and prostate examinations for men
- observing changes in urine output or difficulty in passing urine
- practising safe sex to avoid the potential for sexually transmitted diseases.

ACTIVITY 3.10

Prostate cancer

Prostate cancer is the most common cancer diagnosed in Australia and the third most common cause of cancer death. It is more common in older men, with 85 per cent of cases diagnosed in men over 65 years of age. Research prostate cancer and/or visit the Cancer Council website (http://www.cancer.org.au) to gain more information and answer the following questions:

1 What is benign prostatic hypertrophy?

2 How is prostate cancer detected?

3 What are the causes and symptoms of prostate cancer?

4 What treatment options are available for a person with prostate cancer?

Integumentary system

Integumentary system
The bodily system consisting of the skin and its associated structures, such as the hair, nails, sweat glands and sebaceous glands, all of which protect the body from damage, injury and infection.

The integumentary system includes the skin and its components – the hair, nails and sweat glands that protect the body from damage, injury and infection (see Figure 3.27). The *epidermis* or outer layer of the skin is made up of closely packed epithelial cells and does not contain any blood vessels. The *dermis* is a deep layer of skin under the epidermis that gives skin its strength and elasticity, and it contains nervous tissue, blood and blood vessels. *Subcutaneous* tissue lies under the dermis and contains adipose (fatty) tissue that helps to insulate the body by trapping heat produced by the underlying muscles.

Hair is an accessory organ of the skin and is made up of tightly packed keratin cells. Hair helps to insulate and protect the body from ultraviolet (UV) radiation. *Sudoriferous* (sweat) and *sebaceous* (oil) glands function to lower the body's temperature through evaporative cooling of sweat and to lubricate and protect hairs, while nails protect the distal end of fingers and toes.

FIGURE 3.27 The integumentary system

Stratum corneum
Stratum lucidum
Stratum granulosum
Stratum spinosum
Stratum basale
Basement membrane
Dermis papillary
Meissner's corpuscle of touch
Sebaceous (oil) gland
Hair follicle
Reticular layer
Sensory nerves
Opening of sweat duct
Sudoriferous sweat gland

Hair shaft
Epidermis
dermis
Subcutaneous fat (hypodermis)
Subcutaneous tissue
Vein
Pacinian corpuscle
Artery

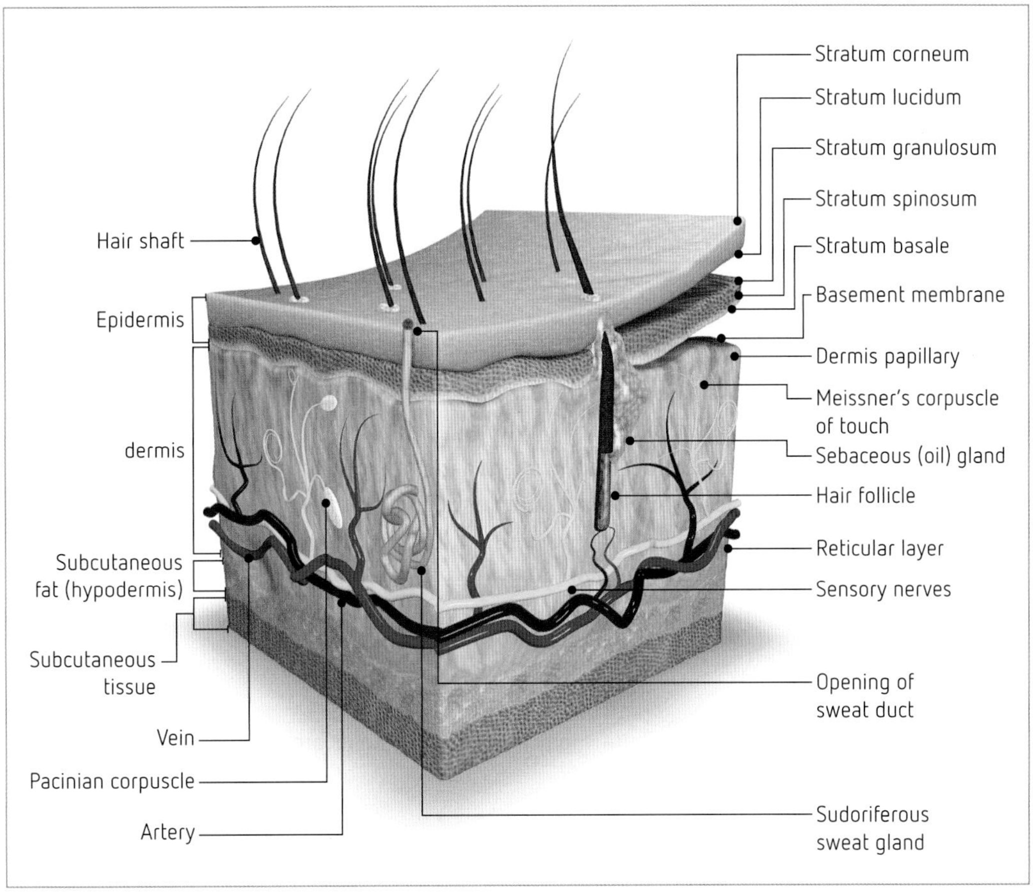

Source: Shutterstock.com/Naeblys

Physiology

The integumentary system functions to protect underlying tissue from pathogens and UV light, regulate body temperature, synthesise vitamin D, provide sensation and excrete substances.

Regulation of body temperature is maintained by the ability of blood vessels to dilate and constrict (*vasodilation* and *vasoconstriction*). The skin is able to lower the body's temperature via evaporative sweat, and vasodilation allows blood to reach the skin, pulling heat away from the body's core. The skin is able to raise the body's temperature through the movement that occurs with shivering and vasoconstriction, which reduces the blood flow to the skin to maintain core body heat.

Vitamin D synthesis is essential for the body to absorb calcium from food. When UV light strikes the skin, it begins the process of converting substances in the epidermis to vitamin D. The nerve endings in the skin also allow the body to *sense* the external environment by responding to touch, pressure, temperature and pain. The density of these receptors varies throughout the body, with some areas being more sensitive than others. *Excretory* functions of the skin include sweat, which contains water and electrolytes.

Vasodilation
Dilation or widening of a blood vessel.

Body system changes and factors contributing to healthy functioning

The structure and function of skin changes with age. The epidermis becomes thinner, wound healing decreases and sweat gland activity decreases, resulting in skin becoming drier, and the dermis losing its elasticity. These changes can contribute to skin conditions in the elderly, including decubitus ulcers, psoriasis, dermatitis and sun damage, causing growths and pigmentation. Signs and symptoms of skin disorders include:

- appearance of growths or bruising
- appearance of rash or blisters after contact with allergens
- itchy skin
- red and scaly skin
- ulceration on legs or feet.

  Common tests used to determine integumentary disorders include:
- biopsy, where a small piece of tissue is removed for microscopic examination
- patch test to determine specific substances that cause allergies.

  Maintaining healthy functioning of the integumentary system includes:
- ensuring a balanced diet is consumed with adequate hydration
- keeping clean and performing skin care
- avoiding excessive exposure to UV light and applying broad spectrum sunscreen and protective clothing and accessories (hats, sunglasses)
- undertaking regular skin checks and reporting abnormal skin growths or changes
- avoiding prolonged periods of sitting or lying without moving position (for elderly people)
- drying skin carefully after bathing.

ACTIVITY 3.11

Burns

When the skin is damaged due to a burn, many other body systems are compromised. Research burns to answer the following questions:

1   How are burns classified?

2   What body systems are compromised when a person experiences a severe burn?

3   What complications can result from a severe burn?

4   How are burns treated?

Lymphatic and immune system

Lymphatic system
Specialised vessels and organs that collect and circulate excess fluid in the body; plays a part in the body's immune response.

The lymphatic system comprises a major part of the body's immune system and consists of organs, lymph nodes, ducts, capillaries and vessels (see Figure 3.28). These structures assist in fighting infection by removing debris and draining excess fluid from the body's tissues. *Lymph nodes* are found in various parts of the body including the neck, armpits, abdomen and groin. Lymphatic vessels move a clear-to-white fluid known as *lymph* from tissues to the bloodstream, and this lymph contains white blood cells (*lymphocytes*) that attack bacteria in the blood. The *immune system* works with the lymphatic system to defend the body from pathogens including bacteria and viruses.

Physiology

The immune system plays a role in allowing the body to defend itself against foreign substances. These defence mechanisms can be classified as non-specific and specific and are described in Figure 3.29.

The specific defence mechanisms also provide *immunity* against foreign substances. This is a result of remembering the foreign substance (*antigen*) that has invaded the body and destroying it when it recurs. Immunity can be *natural* (inherited) or *acquired* through vaccinations, immune serum or breast milk.

FIGURE 3.28 The lymphatic system

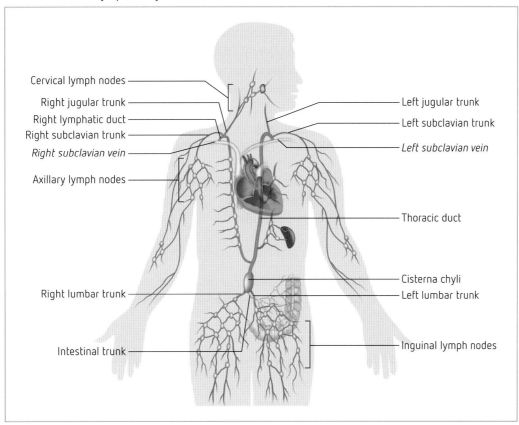

Cervical lymph nodes
Right jugular trunk
Right lymphatic duct
Right subclavian trunk
Right subclavian vein
Axillary lymph nodes
Right lumbar trunk
Intestinal trunk

Left jugular trunk
Left subclavian trunk
Left subclavian vein
Thoracic duct
Cisterna chyli
Left lumbar trunk
Inguinal lymph nodes

Source: Shutterstock.com / Alila Medical Media

FIGURE 3.29 Non-specific and specific defence mechanisms

NON-SPECIFIC DEFENCE MECHANISMS		SPECIFIC DEFENCE MECHANISMS
FIRST LINE DEFENCE BODY'S NATURAL BARRIERS	SECOND LINE DEFENCE BODY'S RESPONSES	THIRD LINE DEFENCE ACT DIRECTLY ON INVADING MICROORGANISMS
Intact skin and mucous membranes protect the body against microorganisms	Inflammatory response prevents spread of harmful agents to other areas and promotes tissue repair	B lymphocytes secrete antibodies that block foreign substances
Secretions destroy microorganisms (saliva, sweat, tears, stomach acid)	Phagocytes engulf and destroy harmful pathogens	Macrophages eat foreign substances
Reflexes prevent microorganisms entering the body (coughing, sneezing, blinking)	Antimicrobial proteins complement the effectiveness of the inflammatory response	
	Fever is increased to fight against microorganisms and speed up the repair process	

Body system changes and factors contributing to healthy functioning

The immune system changes with age. The person becomes more susceptible to infection as fewer antibodies are produced and the skin becomes thinner and less protective. These changes can contribute to immune deficiencies in the elderly. Occasionally the immune recognition system breaks down and it attacks its own tissues. This results in autoimmune disease with the most common being multiple sclerosis, rheumatoid arthritis, systemic lupus erythematosus (SLE) and type 1 diabetes.

Maintaining healthy functioning of the lymphatic and immune system includes:

* ensuring a balanced diet is consumed with adequate hydration
* treating infections promptly
* being aware of allergens and wearing an allergy band for hypersensitivities
* immunising individuals and providing flu injections
* recognising and reporting swollen lymph glands.

ACTIVITY 3.12

Immunisation

Immunisation protects individuals and the community by reducing the spread of disease. Research immunisation and/or visit **https://www.health.gov.au/health-topics/immunisation**, then answer the following questions:

1   What vaccinations are given during childhood and schooling?
2   Who are the 'at risk' groups and what types of vaccinations are recommended for them?
3   What booster shots are recommended for adults?
4   Why is it important for HSAs to have a record of their immunisation status before working in health care?

Relationships between different body systems

The success and survival of the human body is dependent on the ability of each body system to work together. If one function breaks down, it will impact the other systems and functions. The body needs energy for functioning and needs to excrete waste to keep it healthy and this is achieved through the interrelationship between all systems.

The main link between all body systems is the brain, which regulates all of the body systems using a variety of hormones and messages. Energy is provided through food (digestive system) and oxygen (respiratory system) and the nutrients are transported throughout the body via the circulatory system. The waste products are excreted via the urinary system, digestive system and integumentary system. Figure 3.30 outlines additional examples of the interrelationships between various body systems and structures.

2   RECOGNISE AND PROMOTE WAYS TO SUPPORT HEALTHY FUNCTIONING OF THE BODY

The previous section explored the anatomy and physiology of each body system and identified factors that contributed to healthy functioning. This section will expand on that information by looking at how the body's internal environment can maintain stability and how the external

FIGURE 3.30 Interrelationships between body systems

SYSTEM	SYSTEMS IT WORKS CLOSELY WITH
Cardiovascular system	• Respiratory system by supplying oxygen to our body and removing carbon dioxide • Endocrine system to transport hormones through the blood to our body • Nervous system, which regulates heart rate and blood pressure • Urinary system to remove waste products in the blood
Endocrine system	• Reproductive system to regulate reproductive hormones • Gastrointestinal system to release glucose, and the cardiovascular system to supply the body with energy
Nervous system	• Gastrointestinal system to regulate muscles for peristalsis and mechanical digestion • Urinary system to detect a full bladder for elimination • Respiratory system to regulate breathing rate • Musculoskeletal system to control skeletal muscle contraction, with bones providing essential calcium for nervous system function

environment can support healthy functioning through good nutrition, regular exercise and reducing risk factors. You can enhance your work activities by understanding these concepts and sharing the information with your clients to support their healthy functioning.

Review factors that contribute to maintenance of a healthy body

Optimal lifestyle choices and reduction of risk factors help the body to remain healthy, along with the collective coordination between the body systems to maintain a stable internal environment known as *homeostasis*. This process ensures the body's internal environment stays within a 'normal range'. Homeostasis means that the body will regulate variables so that internal conditions remain stable and relatively constant, examples of which include:

- temperature regulation – the body will attempt to correct its temperature if it is above or below the normal range of 36 to 37.2 degrees Celsius. If the temperature is too high, sweating and vasodilation will reduce the temperature, and if it is too low, shivering and vasoconstriction will increase the temperature
- fluid balance – if the body does not have enough fluid (dehydration), the thirst mechanism is activated and the kidneys retain fluid and decrease urine output with dark concentrated urine. Conversely, if the body has too much fluid, it excretes more urine
- glucose maintenance – the body uses glucose as a source of energy and this is regulated by hormones. The release of *insulin* reduces glucose concentration, while glucagon raises its concentration.

Healthy functioning is also based on the principles of good nutrition, regular exercise and reducing risk factors, all of which are outlined in the following.

Nutrition

Maintaining adequate nutrition is essential for sustaining life. The following section outlines important considerations for nutrition.

Eat a healthy, balanced diet

A balanced diet includes as many of the following food groups in each meal or snack as possible:

- vegetables and legumes (e.g., beans) – provide fibre, vitamins and minerals
- fruit – provides fibre, vitamins and minerals
- grain (cereal) – mostly wholegrain and/or high cereal fibre varieties
- lean meats and poultry, fish, eggs, tofu, nuts and seeds, and legumes/beans
- dairy foods – provide calcium and includes milk, yoghurt, cheese and alternatives.
  Fats, oils and sweets provide negligible nutrition and should be kept to a minimum.

Consume fewer processed foods and more food in its natural state

Food provides fuel for the body systems to function effectively. However, processed food contains high amounts of oils, fats and sugars and are quickly excreted from the body without providing many nutrients. It is ideal to eat less processed food and try to consume foods in as close to their natural state as possible so as to provide the required fuel and energy your body needs.

Drink fluids

Water is essential to the body's functioning. It is recommended each person maintain an intake of 1.5 to 2 litres of water a day, and avoid excessive drinking of coffee, tea and sugary drinks.

Exercise

Exercise is any activity that a person participates in that requires physical exertion. The extent to which the exercises provide health benefits will depend on individual health status. A thorough fitness and health status assessment should be conducted before undertaking exercise programs. Regular exercise is important for everyone, and even frail older people can be assisted with passive exercises if they are unable to perform the exercises themselves.

Examples where regular exercise benefits body systems include:

- cardiovascular system – improves cardiovascular health, lowers blood pressure, helps control body weight and protects against a variety of cardiovascular diseases
- lymphatic and immune system – improves circulation, which enables cells and substances of the immune system to move more efficiently throughout the body
- respiratory system – increases the exchange between oxygen and carbon dioxide in the lungs
- gastrointestinal system – promotes gastric motility and reduces constipation.

Reduce risk factors

Many factors influence our health in either a positive or negative way. Determinants that affect our health in a negative way are commonly referred to as *risk factors* and can increase the likelihood of developing disease. Undertaking methods to reduce these risk factors can assist in the management or prevention of health conditions. These include:

- reducing stress
- quitting smoking
- remaining at a healthy weight through regular exercise and a balanced diet
- controlling blood pressure
- regularly reviewing medications

- avoiding alcohol, or only drinking alcohol in moderation
- minimising infections by practising good oral care and hygiene
- conducting regular medical check-ups and screening tests, such as colonoscopies and mammograms, in response to identified risk factors.

Health screening

Reducing risk factors can help maintain the healthy functioning of an individual. Complete the following table by giving examples of the screening tools or tests used for the conditions listed.

3.13 ACTIVITY

CONDITION	SCREENING TOOL OR TEST
Breast cancer	
Cervical cancer	
Colorectal cancer	
High cholesterol	
Prostate cancer	
Osteoporosis	
Diabetes	

Use and share information about healthy functioning of the body

As a member of a team working in acute care, you should be willing to work cooperatively in the pursuit of common goals and objectives. This includes extending your learning and sharing information about the healthy functioning of the human body. Sources you might access to expand your knowledge on recognising healthy functioning include:

- reading books and industry journals about the human body and healthy functioning
- learning from co-workers and other members of your healthcare team based on their experiences
- observing and taking note during handovers of comments, which include information relating to the human body and healthy functioning
- participating in formal and informal industry training; for example, in-service sessions or accredited training that provides a pathway to expanding your understanding of body systems and healthy functioning
- using the internet to obtain more information on the terms covered in this chapter on body systems.

Your basic knowledge will expand as you gain more experience, and this will further assist you in understanding the problems of the people in your care. It will also provide you with a greater understanding of medical interventions and treatments and the importance of the nursing care plan. Your enhanced knowledge of body systems and strategies for healthy functioning will increase the quality of your work activities and complement the work of other members in your healthcare team.

SUMMARY

This chapter has provided relevant knowledge and skills to work with basic information about the human body and to recognise and promote ways to maintain its healthy functioning. The body is a complex organism and by understanding how it works, how its systems are interrelated and how it can be maintained, you can support clients who are under your care.

This chapter used health terminology to identify anatomical features and common symptoms so that you can become familiar with the terms when reporting and recording changes to normal body functioning. It also emphasised the factors that contribute to the maintenance of the body so that healthy functioning can be promoted.

The last part of the chapter highlighted the interrelationships between body systems and outlined the ways in which healthy functioning can be maintained, including nutrition, exercise and reduction of risk factors. By understanding the human body and its functions, you will be able to recognise changes as a result of disease or illness and report effectively to your healthcare team.

APPLY YOUR KNOWLEDGE

Fluid balance disorders

Ewan is an 85-year-old male who lives alone but in recent years has been struggling to maintain his independence. He now relies on his stepdaughter Mina to help him with his medication management and doctors' appointments.

Mina has taken a vacation and Ewan assured her that he would be able to cope whilst she was away. Upon her return, Ewan seemed lethargic, dizzy, slightly confused and complained of muscle cramps and a loss of appetite. Mina took her stepfather to his doctor who found his blood pressure to be very low, his mouth dry and his heart rate high, and organised admission to hospital for investigation. He was diagnosed with severe dehydration and acute renal failure.

1   Describe the structure and function of the urinary system.

2   In what body cavity do the kidneys belong?

Ewan presented to the ward and an HSA was assigned to his care under the supervision of an RN. Ewan had IV therapy and an indwelling catheter in situ. The HSA noted that his urine volume was minimal and the colour was very dark. The HSA was assigned to monitor his fluid balance on a chart, encourage him to drink and take his BP, temp and pulse and urinalysis 4/24. The HSA also emptied Ewan's catheter bag when it was full.

3   What current signs indicate that Ewan has an altered fluid balance causing dehydration?

4   Using the knowledge learnt in Chapter 2, 'Comply with infection prevention and control policies and procedures', what standard precautions would the HSA take when emptying Ewan's catheter bag?

After two days, Ewan's urine was pale coloured and he was passing 1500 millilitres daily. His blood pressure normalised and his appetite had improved. Mina noted that he seemed to be back to his usual cheerful self.

The doctor discharged Ewan with his plan, including education on staying hydrated and instructions to report any unusual urinary symptoms, and that if he felt unwell and unable to drink enough to contact his GP. The discharge nurse made an appointment for the social worker to see Mina. This was to organise a home care package that would enable Ewan to stay at home, with additional support, so that he would not be relying on Mina for all his needs.

5   What urinary system changes would need to be reported and how does the discharge plan ensure healthy functioning of Ewan's urinary system?

6   How could the HSA extend their learning of the urinary system and its healthy functioning?

7   Understanding the scope of your role is essential to performing it effectively within the healthcare team. What was the scope of the HSA's involvement in the care for Ewan whilst he was hospitalised?

◄ REFLECTING ON THE INDUSTRY INSIGHT

1   Mr Ford's injury resulted in a bleed between the skull and the brain. What is this called?
    a   Subdural haematoma.
    b   Sub arachnoid haematoma.
    c   Epidural haematoma.
    d   Pia dural haematoma.

2   Which of the following neurological observations would be performed on Mr Ford?
    a   Pupil size, motor function and level of consciousness.
    b   Coma status, circulation and sensory function.
    c   Verbal response, capillary return and vital signs.
    d   Body temperature, blood pressure and reflexes.

3   Which of the following describes the term 'physiology'?
    a   The chemical make-up of organisms.
    b   The normal functions of organisms and their parts.
    c   The study of disease processes in humans.
    d   How each body part is structured.

SELF-CHECK QUESTIONS

1   Why is it important for an HSA to be able to describe directional terms using medical terminology?
2   Why is the plasma membrane of a cell semipermeable?
3   List and describe the functions of the four basic tissue types.
4   Why do many veins in the body have valves?
5   How does the integumentary system play a role in regulation of body temperature?
6   List the primary glands of the endocrine system and the associated organs that have a secondary function in hormone release.
7   Describe what protects the central nervous system.
8   Describe how food is chemically broken down in the gastrointestinal system.
9   Why is vitamin D essential for the body?
10 What are your definitions of the following key words and terms that have been used in this chapter?

KEY WORD OR TERM	YOUR DEFINITION
Organelles	
Vasodilation	
Homeostasis	
Peristalsis	
Sphincter	
Erythrocytes	
Blood pH	
Menopause	

QUESTIONS FOR DISCUSSION

1   Discuss the chronic diseases of the musculoskeletal system and their implications in terms of medical care and support.

2   How does homeostasis work to maintain the equilibrium of fluid balance?

3   Discuss the differences between the parasympathetic and sympathetic nervous systems and give examples of their effects.

4   Discuss the importance of carbohydrates, fats and proteins in the human diet and where they can be found.

5   Discuss the recommendations that you would make to maintain healthy functioning of the body with regards to reducing risk factors and regular exercise.

EXTENSION ACTIVITY

Aboriginal and Torres Strait Islander peoples' health

Research and data gathered from across Australia on Aboriginal and Torres Strait Islander peoples' health shows significant differences between Aboriginal and Torres Strait Islander and non-Indigenous Australian health. The *Aboriginal and Torres Strait Islander Health Performance Framework – summary report* (AIHW, 2020) contains a summary of the data from the most up-to-date sources, which includes the following facts:

•   In 2015–17, life expectancy at birth was 71.6 years for Indigenous males and 75.6 years for Indigenous females. The gap between Indigenous and non-Indigenous Australians was 8.6 years for males and 7.8 years for females.

- The rate of disease burden among Aboriginal and Torres Strait Islander people is more than double (2.3 times) that of non-Indigenous Australians.
- Between 2006 and 2018, the age-standardised death rate from cancer among Indigenous Australians increased from 205 to 235 per 100 000. A decrease in the cancer death rate among non-Indigenous Australians occurred over the same period, leading to a widening of the gap.
- In 2014–18, the age-standardised death rate for Indigenous Australians with diabetes was more than five times as high as for non-Indigenous Australians.
- Indigenous Australians have lower rates of participation in screening programs than non-Indigenous Australians for breast cancer.

1   What factors might explain why there is such a difference between Aboriginal and Torres Strait Islander peoples and non-Indigenous Australians in terms of healthy body systems?

2   Discuss the relevance of this data in terms of improvements that could be made to narrow the gap between Aboriginal and Torres Strait Islander peoples and non-Indigenous Australians in terms of healthy body systems and diseases.

3   In groups, identify what five things you think would make a positive difference in the future for Aboriginal and Torres Strait Islander peoples.

4   Discuss the importance of this data in terms of your present or future role as an HSA.

REFERENCES

Australian Bureau of Statistics (ABS) (2018). National Health Survey: First results, 2017–18. Retrieved 6 April 2019 from http://www.abs.gov.au/ausstats/abs@.nsf/Lookup/by%20Subject/4364.0.55.001~2017-18~Main%20Features~Asthma~35

Australian Institute of Health and Welfare (AIHW) (2020). *Aboriginal and Torres Strait Islander Health Performance Framework – summary report 2020*. Retrieved 7 October 2022 from https://www.indigenoushpf.gov.au/

COMMUNICATE AND WORK IN HEALTH AND COMMUNITY SERVICES

Learning objectives

By the end of this chapter, you should be able to:

1 communicate effectively with people
2 collaborate with colleagues
3 address constraints to communication
4 report problems to a supervisor
5 complete workplace correspondence and documentation
6 contribute to continuous improvement.

Introduction

This chapter describes the skills and knowledge required to communicate effectively with patients and other members of your healthcare team. Your effective communication skills in a team-based work environment are crucial for the support services that you provide to patients.

As a health services assistant (HSA), by collaborating with colleagues through effective listening and following communication protocols you can carry out workplace instructions that promote positive results in patient care. You can also identify difficult situations when they arise and report effectively. This reporting may be in the form of oral or written documentation, which must be completed according to organisational standards.

This chapter will provide you with an understanding of the importance of effective communication and the ability to identify constraints that can hinder the communication process. By seeking feedback and advice for continuous improvement, you can develop your skills and knowledge to build strong relationships with patients and the entire healthcare team.

INDUSTRY INSIGHTS 💬

Whiteboard communication

My first experience with whiteboard communication was when I was working in the medical assessment unit at a local hospital. The whiteboards were on the wall next to each patient's bed and were marked into sections to provide general and specific information for nursing, medical and allied health staff. Their aim was to provide a quick view of updates to a patient's status and needs without having to look at the patient's notes. Information included discharge date, diet, goals and a space for families to write any information. The people treating the patient might not always be available when the family or carer is there, but they still want to be able to answer their questions.

Confidential information was not displayed on the whiteboard and patients were always asked for their consent to display their information.

An example of the whiteboard in use was when the allied health team wrote the goal of attending daily rehabilitation sessions for mobility for the patient, and their family had written that their mother needed assistance in filling out the food menu form because of her arthritis. The family also wrote a request to arrange transport for their mother upon discharge because there was no-one available to pick her up. With this information, I was able to prepare the patient for her daily rehabilitation sessions and help her by filling out the menu form, and the nursing unit manager was informed to organise transport for the patient on the discharge day.

Whiteboards have been shown to provide an increase in patient and family understanding of treatment and improved communication between staff and patients. The doctors, nurses and allied health professionals interact with the whiteboard individually and occasionally together, and this prevents duplication of tasks and miscommunication between the team (Health Research Funding Organisation, 2019).

When I erase the information once a patient is discharged, I feel a sense of accomplishment that we have completed all the tasks and procedures required for our patient.

1 COMMUNICATE EFFECTIVELY WITH PEOPLE

Effective communication is clearly delivered, received and understood. Each person's communication style is unique, so it is important to use a range of methods to ensure that information is conveyed appropriately. Using a combination of verbal and non-verbal communication, being clear, clarifying meaning and listening effectively will assist with this shared understanding. By exchanging information clearly, and responding appropriately and within confidentiality guidelines, you will be able to effectively communicate in your role as an HSA with a diverse range of people in the healthcare setting.

Use verbal and non-verbal communication to enhance understanding

Communication

Sending, receiving or exchanging information.

The word communication can be defined as the sending or receiving of messages containing meaning. This two-way process involves conveying a message and understanding what others have to say. The message usually contains thoughts, ideas, opinions, feelings and information. Communication can be verbal (spoken), non-verbal (body language) or written. By using effective interpersonal verbal and non-verbal communication in your role as an HSA, you can enhance understanding and demonstrate respect for patients and your healthcare team.

Communication process

The components of the *communication process* include the sender, encoding, the channel, receiver and decoding, and is represented in Figure 4.1.

1 The *sender* is the person who sends the *message*.
2 *Encoding* the message means that it is transformed into a form that can be sent, such as words.
3 The *channel* of communication is the manner in which the message is sent; for example, speaking, writing or body language.
4 The *receiver* must be able to *decode* the message, which means processing it so that it is understood.
5 *Feedback* is the process of ensuring that the receiver has correctly understood the message.

FIGURE 4.1 The communication process

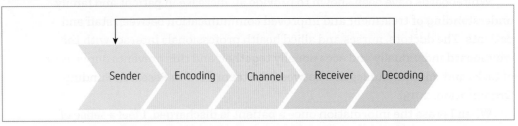

Therefore, communicating not only involves getting the message across but also being able to listen to and understand what others are saying. And it also requires observation of verbal and non-verbal clues in order to monitor the effectiveness of a message.

Interpersonal communication

Interpersonal communication

Face-to-face exchange of information, feelings and meaning through verbal and non-verbal messages.

Interpersonal communication involves exchanging information face to face through a combination of verbal and non-verbal messages. In an acute care setting with ill and vulnerable people, interpersonal communication allows patients to directly express their concerns. By utilising interpersonal communication, an HSA can listen and show concern for the patient's needs, give attention so that the patient feels safe, and improve patient satisfaction and healthcare outcomes.

Verbal communication

Verbal communication involves the use of words and the way they are delivered. This includes tone of voice, the use of pauses, and the rate of speech, all of which provide information about the message and the information obtained. Communicating verbally is important when we are trying to gain information; for example, to obtain the details of a patient's dietary preferences. The words, however, must be understood, so it is important to seek help from an interpreter if language is a barrier.

Tone of voice

Tone of voice involves the volume and emphasis used, and this adds meaning to the words. A loud voice can display anger or aggression, or an expressionless voice can display lack of interest. Placing emphasis on a word can strengthen its meaning. As an HSA, it is important to listen to the patient's tone of voice because it can display important information about a patient's emotions and energy levels. You should also use a positive tone during verbal communication to put patients at ease.

Use of pauses

Pauses can add impact to communication. Adding a pause after a statement gives it emphasis and before a statement gains attention. Also, pausing after speaking gives the listener time to consider their reply.

Rate of speech

If your rate of speech is too fast, the listener will not have time to consider what you have said. It is important to match the rate of speech to that of your patient, and also adjust the rate when speaking with patients who have hearing or cognitive difficulties.

Non-verbal communication

Non-verbal communication refers to all the types of messages that are not expressed in words, including:

- facial expressions
- eye contact
- posture
- gestures
- touch
- proxemics (use of space)
- appearance

Facial expressions

The face is one of the most expressive channels of communication. Being aware of your facial expressions is important because so much of what we are thinking is given away by the expressions on our face. Patients are often sensitive to the facial expressions of the person caring for them, so it is important to make every effort to maintain a neutral facial expression rather than showing negative emotions.

Non-verbal communication
All the messages in a conversation that are not expressed in words.

Proxemics
The space that people feel is necessary to maintain between themselves and others.

For example, a patient asked the HSA looking after him, 'Are you upset with me? You look angry.' The HSA said she was not upset with the patient; but because she was rushed, she had not paid attention to her facial expression while in the room. She had conveyed her negative emotions to the patient, who misunderstood the meaning.

It is important for the HSA to be aware that face masks can muffle sounds and cover facial expressions. The need for face masks and social distancing during the COVID-19 pandemic has had an adverse effect on interpersonal communication. Speaking in a louder tone, making eye contact and emphasising the eyebrows and upper cheeks has been a means to provide effective interpersonal communication, as has explaining the need for the mask-wearing to the patient.

Eye contact

Maintain good eye contact but do not stare. This helps to build rapport and conveys interest in what the patient has to say. A failure to make eye contact can indicate lack of interest or attention. Consider, however, that in some cultures it is rude to make eye contact.

Posture

When possible, sit next to the patient at an angle rather than standing. Bring your face to the same level as that of the patient and lean forward to show interest in the person. A relaxed and open posture, with arms and legs uncrossed and hands relaxed, also lets them know that you are there to listen to their needs (see Figure 4.2).

FIGURE 4.2 Displaying an open posture shows interest in the person

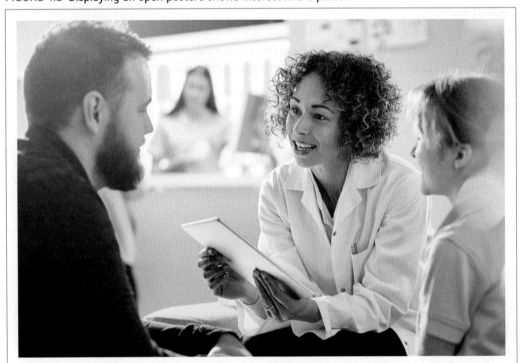

Source: iStock.com/sturti

Gestures

Gestures can clarify and supplement speech. The way a person moves communicates information about mood, attitude and state of health. Wringing hands may indicate fear or pain; a tapping foot may indicate impatience. Avoid making assumptions about these body language gestures and ask the patient what he or she is feeling if there is concern about visual gestures. For example, 'You seem to be pacing the room. Is there something on your mind?'

Touch

Touch is a very powerful means of communication. Lightly touching a person's hand can convey concern and affection for them. However, remember that touch must be appropriate and cultural considerations must be understood. Consent must also be gained when touching patients.

For example, Francesca, the HSA, needs to perform observations on her patient. She begins by obtaining consent and then explains that she will be touching the patient during the procedure: 'I'm going to take your blood pressure, Doris. If you could stretch out your arm I will be able to wrap the cuff around your upper arm. You will feel tightness as the cuff inflates and then the machine will take a reading and the cuff will deflate. Do you have any questions?'

Proxemics

The space that people feel is necessary to set between themselves and others is known as proxemics. This was first described by E.T. Hall in 1966. The required space that needs to be maintained during communication varies from person to person and between cultures.

In traditional Western cultures, the areas of personal space or communication zones are approximately:

* intimate (15–45 cm) – behaviour with loved ones, physical assessment in health care
* personal (45 cm–1.2 m) – interviews, teaching one-on-one, private conversations
* social (1.2–3.6 m) – demonstrations, group interactions
* public (>3.6 m) – lectures, behaviour with strangers.

As an HSA, you will often be required to occupy a client's personal or intimate space to provide care. It is important to be sensitive to the discomfort this may cause and communicate with the person. For example, 'I need to stand close to you when I am assisting you to stand up. You may feel awkward, but it is important that I consider your safety.'

Appearance

Personal hygiene, general appearance, clothing and body ornamentation (including piercings and tattoos) relay information about a person. These non-verbal messages may convey clients' true feelings about themselves, their cultural heritage, or they may give an indication of the state of their physical and emotional health. Lack of personal care may be a reflection of psychological factors, such as depression or mental illness. As an HSA you should also convey professionalism in your appearance at all times by being hygienic and well groomed. It is important to be aware of your healthcare policies regarding piercings, acrylic nails and tattoos, which may vary across sites.

Interpersonal skills survey

Consider the following questionnaire on how well you communicate with others. Think about whether you always, sometimes or never use the described interpersonal skills.

I notice others' body language
I respect people's personal space
I listen carefully and speak clearly
I speak slowly and look at the listener for understanding
I ask for things in a way that is easy to understand
I give brief, clear directions
I position myself at eye level when communicating with a patient
I make sure I obtain consent before touching a patient
I use gestures to help when people do not understand
I make sure my appearance and attire are professional when I am working

Consider the areas where improvements are needed and practise these skills in the workplace.

Communicate service information in a clear manner and confirm understanding

Communication occurs in every aspect of healthcare work: while performing tasks, dealing with problems that need to be solved and during interactions with co-workers. All the information you communicate should be clear and easily understood and reflect organisational policies, protocols and procedures. Using clear oral communication strategies can also help patients to better understand the health information you give them.

Strategies for clear communication with patients include:

- making appropriate eye contact throughout the interaction
- keeping the language simple, using appropriate vocabulary for the patient's age and educational level
- speaking clearly and at a moderate rate
- keeping the messages clear and concise
- repeating and reinforcing key ideas with tone and pauses
- demonstrating how something is done – be it an exercise or position, a demonstration of how to do something may be clearer than a verbal explanation
- using diagrams, pamphlets or videos to reinforce the message
- encouraging patients to ask questions and be involved in the conversation during visits, and also to be proactive in their health care
- seeking feedback to ensure that information has been received correctly.

Protocols
The set of rules that explain the correct conduct and procedures to be followed in formal situations.

Confirm understanding

A key role of any healthcare worker is to ensure that they tailor their message to the knowledge and abilities of the listener so that the message can be understood. Your ability to convey your understanding back to your patients will affect the degree to which your patients feel understood and cared for. This can be achieved by using active and reflective listening, asking questions, paraphrasing, seeking clarification and summarising to check that the message was not only received but also correctly interpreted. Reflection can then be used to mirror the feelings that have been expressed.

Listen

Effective listening relies on clarifying meaning and replying appropriately, and for this to occur there has to be active and reflective listening, which means that the listener is focused on what the speaker is saying. Being *focused* means being free of distraction and maintaining eye contact where culturally appropriate to do so.

Showing a genuine interest in what is being said by a patient can be displayed by the use of phrases such as 'Uh-um', 'I see' and 'I understand what you mean', and the use of body language such as nodding your head. Active and reflective listening skills are especially important with patients who may have communication difficulties due to physical or mental conditions.

Active and reflective listening skills include:
- concentrating completely on what is being said and minimising distractions from other people or any noise
- using an open posture to show interest in what the other person is saying
- listening carefully and not interrupting patients when they are talking
- having an open mind and not disagreeing before the person has finished speaking
- asking appropriate questions about what has been said
- being prepared to summarise or paraphrase what has been heard, especially if there is uncertainty about what has been said
- remaining calm and in control and showing empathy for the person speaking (i.e., concern for their feelings).

Active and reflective listening
Focusing on what someone is saying to you by asking questions, paraphrasing, seeking clarification and summarising.

Clarification
A communication technique used to clear up confusion or uncertainty.

Reflection
Mirroring the feeling or tone of someone's message so that the person can better understand their own thoughts and feelings.

Obtaining information using effective listening

Think about a time when you had to talk to someone who was a bad listener and answer the following questions:

1 What characteristics did the person display that made them a bad listener?

2 How did you feel when you were talking to them?

3 What techniques could you have used to encourage the person to listen to you?

4.2 ACTIVITY

Question

Using questioning helps to gain information about the patient. It can also be an important tool to ensure that patients understand their care and treatment.

Questions can either be open or closed. *Open questions* encourage the exploration of thoughts and feelings because they ask the person to describe something in their own words.

They are useful when you want the patient to expand on an issue that they are talking about. These types of questions often start with 'why', 'what' or 'how'; for example, 'What seems to be the problem?' In contrast, *closed questions* usually lead to a specific 'yes' or 'no' answer or factual comment, and do not encourage the person to talk further. However, they are useful if an answer with limited options is required. They usually begin with 'have/has', 'is/are', 'do/did', 'would/will', 'could/can' and sometimes 'when', 'who', 'which' and 'where'; for example, 'Have you arranged for someone to take you home once you are discharged?' or 'When did you last eat?'

Paraphrase

Paraphrasing is a technique where the listener repeats in their own words what the speaker has said. This can be a useful way to check whether your interpretation of what a patient has said is accurate. By restating the message in your own words you show the patient that you have understood.

Using phrases such as 'What I'm hearing is …' or 'It sounds like you are saying …' gives the patient the opportunity to correct any misunderstandings.

Seek clarification

You may ask for clarification when you cannot make sense of the patient's response. This makes it possible to understand confused and complex issues and reinforces that you have an interest in what the patient has to say. For example, 'I'm not quite sure I understand what you are saying.'

Summarise

When a patient is providing information, such as during an admission history, it is necessary to try to summarise critical pieces of information. Summarising allows you to be sure that you have understood what the patient said and allows the patient to add new information that may have been forgotten. By using frequent summary statements, you can identify misunderstandings that may exist, especially when there are barriers in communication, such as language. The aim of a summary is to review understanding, not to judge or provide solutions. For example, 'So, to sum up, you have mentioned several concerns …'

Reflect

Reflection involves restating both the feelings and words of the patient to allow them to 'hear' their own thoughts. It is important to be non-judgemental and not to add to the speaker's meaning. Effective use of reflective skills can build trust and communicate acceptance and understanding to the patient. For example:

Patient: 'I'm very frightened about the procedure tomorrow.'

Nurse: 'So, you're frightened about the procedure. Can you say more about what's so frightening for you?'

By using effective listening skills, you can develop a **therapeutic relationship** with the patient. This relationship encourages the patient to express their feelings, facilitates trust and reduces the anxiety that they may be experiencing. Applying these skills requires practice but ultimately results in effective communication techniques that allow you to take better care of patients as well as yourself.

Therapeutic relationship
In nursing, a relationship between the healthcare person and the patient that improves physical, social and emotional wellbeing.

Communication strategies for Mrs Romero

Read the following scenario and answer the questions that follow.

SCENARIO
Mrs Romero: 'Where's the doctor? He said he'd be here this morning. And it took you 15 minutes to answer my call button. I expect that when I press the button, I will get some attention.'
Nurse: Sits next to the patient with an open posture and looks at her. 'I can hear that you're feeling very aware of how slowly things seem to move here. It must be difficult. I can imagine how frustrated you must be.'
Mrs Romero: 'It is frustrating! I feel as if I'm not important.'
Nurse: 'So it feels like the delays mean that we are not caring about you.'
Mrs Romero: 'Not really. I know that you are busy [pauses for a moment] but I do feel frustrated, and tired and confused. And having to lie here in bed makes me feel worse.'
Nurse: 'What seems to be making you confused?'
Mrs Romero: 'Well, the doctor says one thing and the nurses say another.'
Nurse: 'I'm not quite sure I understand what you are saying. Can you give me an example?'
Mrs Romero: 'I don't know if I'm going home today or tomorrow.'
Nurse: 'So, to sum up, you're not sure when you are going home.'
Mrs Romero: 'Yes, that's right.'
Nurse: 'How about I find the doctor and clarify your discharge plan. Would that help?'
Mrs Romero: 'Yes, that would make me feel so much better. Then I could ring my daughter and organise for her to pick me up.'
Nurse: 'OK, I'll find out the details now and stop in again to let you know. I know it can be very frustrating to be left waiting.'

4.3 ACTIVITY

1 Identify the communication strategies used by the nurse in this scenario.

2 How has the nurse used effective communication to clarify her understanding, as well as that of Mrs Romero?

Exchange information clearly and within confidentiality procedures

All verbal and written information should be provided clearly and in a timely manner while adhering to confidentiality requirements. Confidentiality relates to patients who expect that any personal information that is conveyed in writing or verbally stays private and secure. This right to privacy is based on international, Commonwealth (*Privacy Act 1988*) and state laws.

Government legislation and regulatory requirements on privacy should be reflected by organisational policies and procedures, as well as codes of practice. As an HSA, you may learn personal information about a patient, including details of their lifestyle, finances, family relationships and medical history. This information is confidential and must not be disclosed to anyone except in an emergency situation when the patient's medical history needs to be known in order to provide the most appropriate treatment.

The *Privacy Act* (Australian Government, 1988) ensures that:

* personal information about patients is collected and used responsibly with their consent, or by their guardian if required (see Figure 4.3)
* patients or their guardians are able to know what information has been collected and how it is being used

FIGURE 4.3 Personal information about clients is collected and used responsibly with their consent

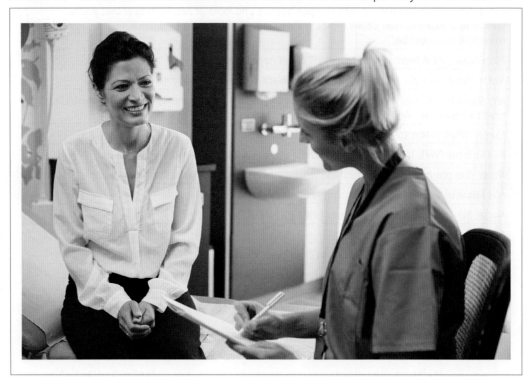

Source: Shutterstock.com/Monkey Business Images

* patients or their guardians are able to request that personal information held by an organisation is corrected if it is incorrect
* information is not to be shared with others unless not doing so involves a risk of harm to the patient.
  Privacy and confidentiality also cover health records, which include a patient's:
* physical, mental and psychological health, including disability
* interventions received, including medications and their effectiveness
* genetic predispositions relating to aspects of health.

2 COLLABORATE WITH COLLEAGUES

Working in an acute care facility requires effective communication and collaboration with colleagues. It is important to be well organised, to listen and to readily respond to all workplace requirements. This involves active listening and, if necessary, clarifying and agreeing on timeframes for carrying out instructions. An awareness of the correct terminology, lines of communication and protocols will ensure that all work undertaken is consistent with the guidelines of the organisation.

Listen, clarify and agree on timelines

Developing good working relationships with your colleagues allows your healthcare team to work together in the interests of the patients to achieve all expected outcomes within agreed timelines. This work should be patient-centred because patients are the prime focus of the tasks that need to be undertaken. Failure to achieve timelines may be caused by a number of factors, which include excessive workloads, unexpected events, or an inability to complete tasks that are outside the scope of practice. By listening and clarifying, you will have a clear understanding of what needs to be achieved.

When agreeing on timelines with colleagues, it is important to consider if they are:

* realistic
* agreed on by your healthcare team
* attainable within the timeframe.

A timeline for an outcome should be achieved with the available resources in the healthcare setting and the available nursing staff. Keep in mind the patient's emotional and physical condition and include them as an active participant when setting timelines because it can assist with reaching the desired outcome.

Your work efficiency

Improving your work efficiency by addressing time wasting is necessary to meet the needs of patients who require your support. These needs should be provided in accordance with workplace instructions.

1 Discuss how you work within timelines and indicate areas where improvements could be made.

2 What tools or techniques can be used to improve your work efficiency?

3 Ask your workplace colleagues, who may be able to suggest additional strategies for improvement.

4.4 ACTIVITY

Identify lines of communication

It is important that you have a clear understanding of the lines of communication within your healthcare facility and with other health-service providers. Lines of communication cover who reports to whom and should be reinforced by the HSA position description and scope of practice.

Communicate within an acute care facility or to other services

In a healthcare team, HSAs work under the supervision of a registered nurse (RN) who is responsible for delegating duties and providing support. As an HSA, it is your responsibility to report concerns and any changes in a patient's condition to the RN. Each facility will also have policies and procedures for communicating to other services outside of the organisation.

By actively cooperating with the entire team and using the correct lines of communication, you will contribute effectively to achieving the best outcomes for the patient and the organisation. It will also enable you to show initiative and use your skills and knowledge to benefit the team. Open communication with all levels of the team is important for total patient care.

Lines of communication in nursing

The provision of safe patient care is the shared responsibility of all those involved in the multidisciplinary team. At all times, HSAs work under the supervision of an RN who allocates patient care activities with predictable patient outcomes. Describe the roles and reporting lines for the following nursing roles:

1   enrolled nurse

2   registered nurse

3   clinical nurse specialist

4   clinical nurse consultant

5   nurse educator

6   nursing unit manager

Use industry terminology correctly in verbal, written and digital communication

Every industry has its own terminology that contains the specialist vocabulary and acronyms or abbreviations that should be used when communicating with colleagues. Medical terminology is used in communications with healthcare teams because this is the language that achieves a shared understanding across the health sector. It is important that you become familiar with the terminology used in your workplace because it may differ according to the type of healthcare facility. Terminology is used in:

- verbal patient handovers
- inter-professional discussions and instructions
- recording in progress notes and care plans
- documentation in forms and charts
- enquiries and telephone calls.

Chapter 5, 'Interpret and apply medical terminology appropriately', describes the appropriate use of medical terminology in verbal and written communication, including the ISBAR handover strategy, in more detail.

Follow communication protocols in interactions with people and authority

It is important to follow standard policies, procedures and protocols on the agreed communication processes that apply in your organisation and the required lines of authority. Protocols are the set of rules that can be documented as formal procedures. Communication protocols cover how, when and to whom HSAs should communicate in relation to their role. All organisations will expect that communication protocols and procedures are understood and applied correctly.

The Australian health system consists of a mix of public- and private-sector health services, including:

- aged and community care services
- family and children's services

- disability services
- public, private hospitals and clinics
- health services for Aboriginal and Torres Strait Islander people
- emergency services for people in crisis.

You need to be aware of the links and interrelationships between these organisations and services as well as their specific communication protocols. You must also be aware of the roles of support services so you can be sure information is communicated to the appropriate people. Refer to your workplace supervisor who will have more specific information regarding communicating with other services.

An HSA communicates with a number of people as a part of their role. This includes patients, team members and the RN. It may also include family members, visitors and people from other sectors in the health system. If you are representing the team in a meeting (for example, a WHS meeting), what you say must have a purpose, and you need to stay on topic. Bring others into the discussion, pay attention to your body language and avoid unnecessary distractions.

Regardless of the protocols and procedures that apply, and the organisation or service involved, the expectation is that all forms of communication should be clear and accurate. In doing so, strategies for meeting the required standards of care for patients can be achieved. Underlying this communication are the interpersonal skills that are used to establish therapeutic relationships with patients for effective care.

Appropriate communication channels

Following communication protocols enables information to be dealt with at the most appropriate level. As an HSA, you need to be aware of the appropriate channels for communication so that outcomes can be achieved.

Match each of the following scenarios to the most appropriate person to contact: registered nurse, nursing unit manager, nurse educator, team member or interpreter. Note that you may use any of these persons as an answer for more than one scenario.

4.6 ACTIVITY

SCENARIO
You are unsure of how to use the stand-up lifter
You hurt your back when assisting a patient to move up the bed
One of your patients is from a Malaysian background and has limited English
You would like to change your roster
You and your colleagues would like to have a professional development refresher on infection control
You have noticed a reddened area on a patient's sacrum
You need assistance to turn a patient in bed

3 ADDRESS CONSTRAINTS TO COMMUNICATION

Communication helps to establish trusting relationships, ensures information is passed on and understood, and provides therapeutic care. However, there are barriers that can impede effective communication and lead to misunderstandings, resentments, frustrations and demoralisation not only for patients but also for the healthcare team. The ability to use communication skills effectively to identify and report issues can help you to diffuse and/or resolve these difficulties.

Identify and report on potentially complicated or difficult situations

Early signs of potentially complicated or difficult situations should not be ignored but should be reported to your supervisor in accordance with organisational protocols and procedures. In order to develop strategies to diffuse potentially complicated situations, it is helpful to identify and recognise:

* patients or staff with culturally and linguistically diverse (CALD) backgrounds
* patients with physical or cognitive difficulties
* bias, stereotyping or discrimination.

Bringing situations out in the open through reporting has the advantage of issues being dealt with rather than allowing them to cause further harm to working relationships or patient care. Reporting early also has the advantage of enabling your supervisor to gather information and to devise strategies to resolve any difficulties. Once the supervisor has been notified of a potentially complicated or difficult situation, there is an expectation within the healthcare team that the issue will be addressed.

SCENARIO

Difficult situations and cultural awareness

Your co-worker, Katia, is a Muslim who wears a traditional head covering. Most of the healthcare team do not have an issue with Katia's attire; however, one co-worker constantly mocks her for her Muslim attire and calls her names. Katia is uncomfortable with the situation and sometimes becomes ill with worry and stays at home. You report this to your nursing unit manager who discusses the situation with both parties. Cultural awareness training is offered to all staff and the relationship with Katia and her co-worker improves considerably.

1   Why was it important to report this situation to the supervisor?
2   How did the cultural awareness training benefit the staff in this situation?

Identify and resolve constraints to effective communication

A communication constraint is anything that prevents you or the patient from receiving and understanding messages. Constraints may lead to the message becoming distorted, causing confusion and misunderstanding. However, this can be resolved by using appropriate communication strategies and techniques, including active and reflective listening and clarification. Effective communication involves overcoming these barriers and conveying a clear and concise message.

Premature assumptions and jumping to conclusions

Assumption

Something taken for granted or accepted as true without proof; a supposition.

In some cases, instead of listening, a person is preparing a response to a message that he or she has not heard. They may also interrupt and finish a person's sentence for them to hasten the conversation. By making assumptions, finishing sentences or jumping to conclusions about the speaker, the listener keeps themselves from paying attention to the real message. Being open and non-judgemental will allow you to truly hear what is being said.

Judgements based on cultural differences

Pre-supposing things about another person based on cultural differences or stereotyping can result in not hearing a message or misinterpreting the message. If you are aware of how your attitudes and values contribute to your identity, you will be more sensitive to the values of others. By revealing and discussing biases and assumptions, it is possible to minimise their negative impact and thereby communicate more effectively. By learning to treat everyone as an individual, you will open up the channels for communication and overcome barriers based on discrimination.

Distraction or lack of attention

When the receiver is preoccupied with other work or thoughts, they do not listen to the message attentively. Distraction can take many forms and can constrain effective communication. Examples of distraction include daydreaming, texting, talking to others, and listening only to the content, not recognising the feelings or non-verbal cues. Try to actively listen to what people are saying and be mindful of the conversation.

Differences in perceptions or attitudes

A common cause of communication breakdown is people with different perceptions or attitudes; for example, the differing perceptions people have of power and status. In healthcare organisations there is a hierarchy of authority, with reporting arrangements at different levels. This difference in status results in some people at less senior levels being reluctant to communicate with authority. This difficulty can be eliminated by managers who relate to and understand their staff. Patients may also feel uncomfortable raising an issue with a doctor due to their status. You should encourage patients to ask questions or write down their questions to be answered by the doctor at a convenient time.

Another way you can avoid barriers to communication is by not criticising or being judgemental. A skilled communicator must be aware of these barriers and try to reduce their impact by continually checking understanding and by avoiding their own negative attitudes or perceptions.

Physiological disabilities

People who have hearing, vision or speech impairment may experience difficulties communicating and interacting with those around them. Cognitive difficulties can also affect a person's ability to understand and make sense of their environment.

Hearing impairment

Individuals who have a hearing impairment may have hearing aids or a cochlear implant. During communication, ensure that the hearing aid is in place and in good working order. Establish with the client where you should sit to best aid effective communication. This is because their hearing may be better on one particular side, or they may lip read and need to be able to see your mouth clearly. If there is background noise you may need to move to a quieter environment. The quality of your voice and the use of clear diction is also important for effective communication. Use of an Auslan interpreter may also be required.

Vision impairment

Individuals who have a vision impairment have limited ability to see another's body language, so clear verbal communication is important. Written communication may need to be adapted for their needs, such as large print, Braille or audio formats to make information more accessible.

Speech impairment

When communicating with individuals who have a speech impairment, a speech therapist can assist to promote effective communication (see Figure 4.4). This can be in the form of sign language, a communication board or the use of an artificial voice box for a person who has had a laryngectomy. You can show understanding by being patient and listening attentively and allowing more time than usual for a response.

FIGURE 4.4 Speech therapists work with patients to promote effective communication

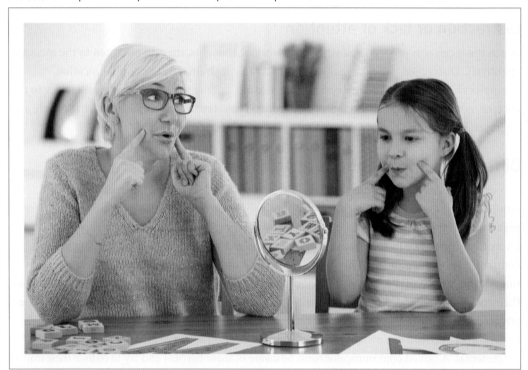

Source: iStock.com/KatarzynaBialasiewicz

Cognitive impairment

Individuals who have a cognitive impairment may suffer from confusion or dementia, among other conditions. The client may feel frustration because they are not able to comprehend the situation or conversation or are struggling to find the words to express their feelings.

Strategies for effective communication include:

- establishing rapport and involving patients in their care planning
- using face-to-face communication
- keeping language simple by using short sentences and avoiding jargon
- breaking the task into a step-by-step process
- raising only one topic at a time
- minimising distractions in the environment.

External barriers

Messages can be blocked by environmental factors, such as the physical setting where communication takes place. You should check that there are no distractions or noises (e.g., a television) and make sure that the environment is comfortable and secure. People need to feel safe before they will listen or offer suggestions.

Language

Language barriers occur when people do not speak the same language or do not have the same level of ability in language. It also occurs when language is too formal, or jargon or slang is used that is not understood by the receiver. Using visuals, such as photographs, drawings and diagrams, and appropriate non-verbal gestures or interpreters can help overcome language barriers.

Sender or receiver barriers

Read each statement and consider whether you think the barrier is caused by the sender or the receiver:

COMMUNICATION BARRIERS	SENDER BARRIER	RECEIVER BARRIER
Interrupting		
Not being aware of non-verbal cues		
Lack of respect for the speaker		
Becoming distracted or daydreaming		
Looking away from you, even as you are talking		
Jumping to conclusions		
Noise from a loud radio		
Making assumptions about people based on their culture		
Confusion due to dementia		
Using slang or jargon		

4.7 ACTIVITY

Use communication skills to avoid, defuse and resolve conflict

Healthcare settings are stressful environments. Workplace stress can cause interpersonal conflicts; and limited time and resources, cultural diversity and differing expectations can cause conflict that can impact on a person's emotions and physical health.

Conflict can be defined as a situation of differing ideas or opinions that results in two people clashing. It can be constructive or destructive, involve patients or staff, and exists in all work environments. Constructive conflict can lead to change because it helps to raise and address problems. However, if not dealt with properly, conflict can become destructive to a point where resolution cannot easily be achieved.

Conflict begins with a difference of opinion and can escalate to tension and high emotional levels. Effective communication skills can result in recognition of the conflict and can help diffuse situations and issues as they arise and assist with their resolution. If communication skills are not effective, deterioration in the relationship can result in dysfunctional healthcare teams, low productivity and ineffective patient care (see Figure 4.5).

FIGURE 4.5 Destructive and constructive conflict

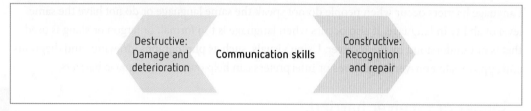

Conflict styles

When using communication skills to deal with conflict, there are a number of styles that can be used to address the issue: competing, collaborating, avoiding, accommodating and compromising (see Figure 4.6). Each of these places emphasis on either goals, relationships or both, as discussed in the following.

FIGURE 4.6 Styles of conflict resolution

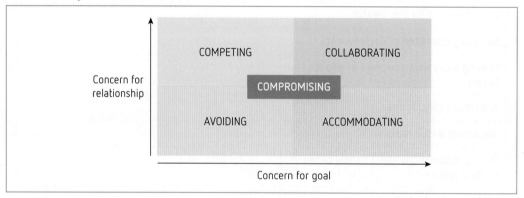

Competing style

The competing style is characterised by a 'win' at all costs attitude with high assertiveness and minimal cooperation. It can be used when goals are important and decisive action is vital. For example, a team leader may take charge and direct an experienced team member to care for a difficult patient.

Collaborating style

The collaborating style is about true problem-solving. The aim is to find a mutual solution to the conflict, with both parties cooperating in an attempt to resolve an issue. This allows for teamwork to help achieve the goals and maintain a healthy relationship. For example, when the nursing unit has insufficient staff for the shift, the healthcare team can work collaboratively to prioritise essential patient care, so that together they can achieve the goals required.

Avoiding style

The avoiding style allows both parties to cool down or can be used to withdraw from a threatening situation where the potential damage outweighs the benefits. This style is generally not advised with major conflicts because these tend to escalate when not addressed. For example, two nurses are having an argument. Either of the nurses may choose to walk away and avoid the situation until they have allowed their emotions to cool down. After this time, each nurse can then revisit the situation in a more positive and respectful way.

Accommodating style

The accommodating style deals with conflict by smoothing things over. The goal is to preserve the relationship at all costs. This is useful when you are in the wrong, when the issue is more important to the other person than to you, or when you want to demonstrate that you are a reasonable person. For example, when a healthcare worker is looking after a dying patient, they may go above and beyond to accommodate the patient's comfort and the family's wishes.

Compromising style

The compromising style relies on concessions by both parties which can result in a win-win situation. It can resolve a conflict quickly and is best used when conflicts are only mild. For example, a senior nurse wants the Christmas/New Year's Eve holidays off and another staff member wants the same holidays. A compromise can be reached where one has the Christmas break and the other has the New Year's Eve break.

Resolve conflict

When dealing with conflict, using open and collaborative communication can help to resolve issues and avoid misunderstandings. It is important to be in control of yourself and your actions towards others who are demonstrating negative behaviours. Strategies include:
- bringing the conflicting individuals together to discuss the problem
- agreeing to ground rules for discussion that are acceptable to all parties
- allowing each person to tell their story from their perspective
- highlighting some common ground that all involved in the conflict can agree on
- helping the individuals to collaborate and develop interventions
- keeping the lines of communication open and respecting differences in attitudes, values and behaviours
- if resolution cannot be achieved, a third party may need to mediate. This may be in the form of confrontation, which is used in some workplace resolution processes.

Communication techniques

How you approach and communicate about conflicts can determine their outcome. Ensuring that your body language and tone of voice convey a positive message is important, and can be achieved by:
- establishing eye contact
- using active and reflective listening
- remaining calm and maintaining an open and relaxed posture
- speaking in a moderate tone and nodding your head
- not interrupting or judging
- identifying the problem
- rephrasing what you hear and acknowledging the other's point of view
- using open-ended questions and asking what you can do to help
- discussing the issue, not the individual.

Assertion

Being emphatic in a calm and positive way, without being either aggressive or passive.

Assertion

Assertion is another skill that can be used in communication to avoid mistakes, focus issues and resolve differences. Being assertive means being able to stand up for your own or another person's rights in a calm and positive way, without being aggressive or passive.

Using 'I' statements to describe your feelings and needs supports assertive communication. These statements focus on the feelings or beliefs of the speaker rather than the thoughts and characteristics of the listener. For example, two nurses are speaking very loudly at the nurses' station and the HSA is annoyed. An assertive comment would be: 'When you are having a loud conversation, I find it hard to concentrate on writing my notes.'

Conflict among colleagues

When it comes to the way you treat and deal with your colleagues, the following suggestions can help to keep the workplace conflict-free:

- Treat fellow workers with the same amount of respect that you expect from them.
- Always have open lines of communication.
- Help out colleagues when necessary, particularly if they are busy and you have time.
- Never talk behind colleagues' backs.
- Air grievances (try assertive communication) before the matter gets out of hand.
- Listen to grievances and try to get to the bottom of the problem by asking questions (see Figure 4.7).
- Try to keep your personal problems away from the workplace.
- Use feedback to improve your relationships with colleagues.

FIGURE 4.7 Resolve conflict before it escalates and impacts on working relationships

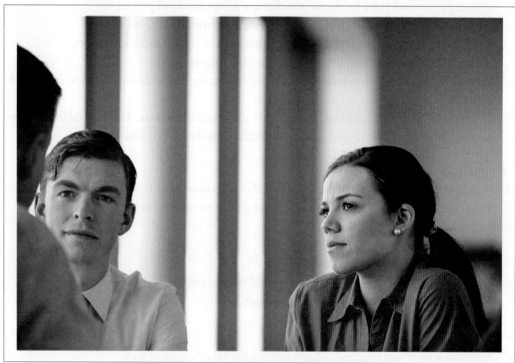

Source: Alamy Stock Photo / Cultura Creative

4 REPORT PROBLEMS TO A SUPERVISOR

As an HSA, you should be able to contribute to the identification and implementation of practical solutions to help maintain a safe working environment. This includes reporting any adverse events, breaches of practice, unresolved conflicts and issues impacting on the achievement of employee, employer and/or patient rights and responsibilities. In doing so, it is important that you comply with legal and ethical responsibilities and discuss any difficulties with your supervisor or appropriate personnel.

Comply with ethical and legal responsibilities

Ethical and legal conduct has particular relevance to the delivery of patient care based on principles that include:

* adhering to the requirements of the National Safety and Quality Health Service (NSQHS) Standards, which aim to improve the quality of health service provision in Australia. The NSQHS Standards provide a nationally consistent statement of the level of care consumers can expect from health service organisations (Australian Commission on Safety and Quality in Health Care, 2017)
* complying with the *Work Health and Safety Act 2011* to take 'reasonable care' to ensure that your acts do not adversely affect the health and safety of yourself and others
* complying with privacy, confidentiality and disclosure requirements
* performing your work role with a duty of care by taking responsibility to avoid injury to a person who is in your care
* ensuring that you demonstrate a non-discriminatory approach to your work in relation to both patients and other workers
* working within your role's boundaries, responsibilities and limitations
* ensuring that all procedures are undertaken with the patient's informed consent.

Follow ethical guidelines

A code of ethics is a set of moral principles and standards that a profession uses to guide practice. Codes of ethics are usually voluntary controls that serve as a means of regulation within a profession.

Ethical principles suggest that all members of the healthcare team have certain obligations and responsibilities to their patients and to each other. This means being able to work together harmoniously and being willing to help each other when needed. For the team, ethics means that all members have certain obligations and responsibilities to their patients (see Figure 4.8).

FIGURE 4.8 Ethics values fairness and doing the right thing professionally

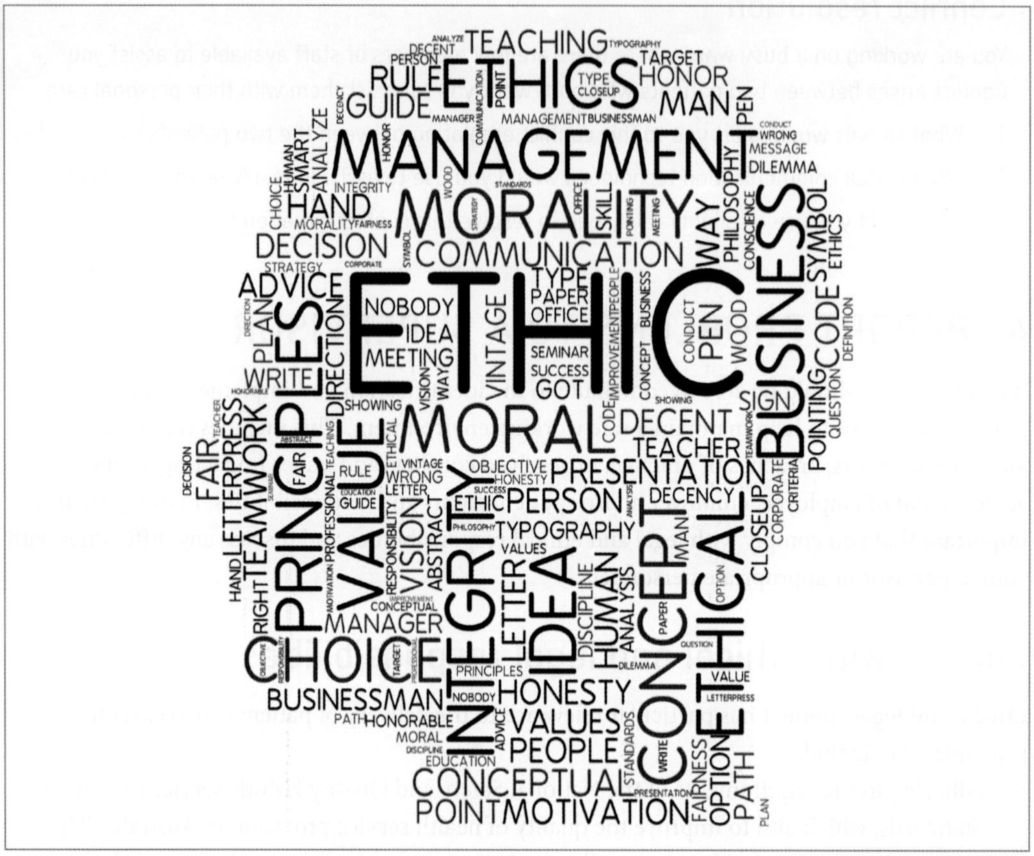

Source: Shutterstock.com/PlusONE

Under this code of conduct an HSA, as an employee, has the following responsibilities:

- Do not accept gifts from individuals.
- Treat everyone and every organisation equally and without preference.
- Provide a supportive professional working relationship for patients that is respectful and caring.
- Perform all nursing and support services in a conscientious manner in accord with the long-term interests of the patient.
- Report any possible conflicts of interest to a supervisor.

ACTIVITY 4.9

Ethical principles – person-centred care

The principle of person-centred care is an ethical consideration maintaining that a person's individual needs and preferences are a central consideration in the provision of nursing care.

Research and answer the following questions related to person-centred care:

1   What attributes enable the HSA to deliver person-centred care?

2   What nursing practices contribute to person-centred care?

3   How can the environment support this care?

4.   What ethical and legal responsibilities do you have as an HSA in providing person-centred care?

Conflict of interest

A conflict of interest is a situation in which someone in a position of trust has competing professional or personal interests. These competing interests can make it difficult to carry out work in an impartial way. For example, the nursing unit manager gives his friends the first choice when rostering work and allocating duties, or always gives preference to a particular nurse when training opportunities arise.

Conflict of interest
A situation in which the concerns or aims of two different parties are incompatible.

Mandatory reporting

The *Family Law Act 1975*, sections 67ZA(1) and (2) require that when persons have reasonable grounds for suspecting that a child has been abused, or is at risk of being abused, they must, as soon as practicable, notify a prescribed child welfare authority of their suspicion and its basis (Australian Institute of Family Studies, 2020). Mandatory reporting is a term used to describe this legislation. The groups of people regarded as mandatory reporters include but are not limited to teachers, doctors, healthcare workers and police. As an HSA, you have a shared responsibility to report to your supervisor any suspected cases of abuse or neglect against children or others at risk.

The laws are not the same across all states and territories (see Figure 4.9); however, 'legislation provides that as long as the report is made in good faith, the reporter cannot be liable in any civil, criminal or administrative proceeding' (Mathews & Scott, 2017).

Mandatory reporting
The legal requirement to report suspected cases of child abuse and neglect.

FIGURE 4.9 Mandatory reporting laws

LEGISLATION
Children and Young People Act 2008 (ACT)
Children and Young Persons (Care and Protection) Act 1998 (NSW)
Care and Protection of Children Act 2007 (NT)
Child Protection Act 1999 (Qld)
Children's Protection Act 1993 (SA)
Children, Young Persons and Their Families Act 1997 (Tas.)
Children, Youth and Families Act 2005 (Vic.)
Children and Community Services Act 2004 (WA)

Source: Adapted from: Mathews, B. & Scott, D. (2017). Mandatory reporting of child abuse and neglect. Melbourne, Vic.: Australian Institute of Family Studies. Retrieved 18 March 2017 from https://aifs.gov.au/cfca/publications/mandatory-reporting-child-abuse-and-neglect

Refer breaches of procedures and issues impacting on employer, employee or client rights to appropriate people

Professional conduct refers to the manner in which a person behaves in a professional capacity. When performing duties as an HSA, you are required to practise ethically and in accordance with legislation and organisational policy, procedure and guidelines. When a fellow worker breaches procedure or behaves unethically, it is your responsibility to report to the supervisor. In some instances, speaking with the person directly can resolve the issue; however, it is also important to report to the supervisor because additional training may need to be undertaken by the person. How you report should be consistent with your organisational policies and procedures.

Reporting should occur if you have any concerns about any breach of professional standards in terms of patient care or legal responsibilities involving workers in an organisation, including harassment, bullying and discrimination. You have a responsibility to ensure that you do not tolerate such behaviour, by raising your concerns.

When reporting breaches of procedure or unethical conduct, you need to be clear about:

*   who was involved
*   when the incident occurred
*   how you believe the conduct to be a breach of standards or unethical behaviour
*   what actions you have taken (i.e., speaking directly to the worker or supervisor)
*   policies and procedures for reporting.

Being able to respond appropriately and knowing when to refer issues to your supervisor is an important decision. This particularly applies to any concerns about your scope of practice that impact on the boundaries of your role. You need to be always mindful of the standard of care provided to patients and any concerns should always be referred to your supervisor.

By using constructive methods of conflict resolution, accepting people's right to hold different points of view and being willing to work collaboratively, a trusting and respectful workplace can be built. Building positive relationships ensures that many issues in the workplace can be minimised.

ACTIVITY 4.10

Report on breaches of standards

Outline how and who you would report to in the following three examples. What are the potential risks of these breaches of standards?

Example 1

An HSA notices that the RN breaks sterile technique when performing a complex dressing on a patient.

Example 2

During the day shift, the HSA notices the cleaner taking chocolates from a patient's bedside. When she confronts the cleaner, they state, 'Everyone takes chocolates from the patients. They just get thrown away when the patient is discharged anyway.'

Example 3

During your lunch break in the cafeteria, you are concerned that one of the newer members of the healthcare team, who is your personal friend, is openly discussing the mental health records of a patient.

Refer unresolved conflict situations

Any unresolved conflict situations should be referred to your supervisor because they can have a destabilising impact on the healthcare team. Unresolved conflict is likely to occur when:

* workloads become excessive
* there are difficulties in deciding priorities
* there are disagreements on how a situation was or should be resolved
* communication or interpersonal skills are ineffective
* work roles and allocated tasks lack clarity.

An unresolved conflict can escalate to a dispute if there is a major disagreement with another person. The dispute can then become a grievance if no action is taken, and result in formal notification requiring resolution by a third party. It is for this reason that a supervisor needs to be informed of underlying harmful conflict that could undermine working relationships.

Early indicators of unresolved conflict can include:

* an increase in the number of people off sick
* people being irritable and getting easily upset with each other and with events that occur
* poor communication in the healthcare team
* poor work performance.

Most organisations will have procedures that need to be used in resolving conflict, especially when there is notification of an actual dispute or when it escalates and becomes a grievance. However, if a supervisor is alerted to the problems or is aware of the early indicators, they can intervene before it undermines the effectiveness of the healthcare team.

Unresolved conflicts

Outline the impacts of the following three unresolved conflicts for the individual and/or patient and the healthcare team:

4.11 ACTIVITY

Example 1

The ward has been busy all day. Your healthcare team is experiencing a consistently high workload and you notice that your co-worker appears to be overwhelmed by the task requirements of two demanding patients. None of the other team members have come to offer him assistance, so you assume that they are equally busy with their own patients. He appears visibly upset.

Example 2

You observe a confrontation at the desk area, where the doctor has just reprimanded an HSA in front of others for not having toileted a patient prior to her scheduled appointment at the radiology department. The HSA is upset and embarrassed because she had been busy with another patient. She later states that this doctor has shouted at her before, but she did not want to discuss it with him because he never listens anyway.

Example 3

You are working in the short stay ward and a patient is admitted for observation following a fall. You have not received a proper handover from the nurse and are not sure of your designated responsibilities with regard to this patient's care. The patient wants to go home and becomes agitated and uncooperative towards you.

5 COMPLETE WORKPLACE CORRESPONDENCE AND DOCUMENTATION

Written and electronic documentation should be completed according to legal requirements and organisational guidelines. All workplace documents should be read in relation to your role, and when documenting events you should use clear, accurate and objective language. When unsure, it is important to clarify understanding with your supervisor, especially in relation to digital media, which should be used according to your facility's policies and procedures.

Complete documents using clear, accurate and objective language in accordance with legal and organisational requirements

As an HSA, workplace documents that you should read that relate to your role might include:
- work health and safety (WHS) responsibilities and procedures
- information provided by your employer regarding the conditions of your employment
- your position description and any organisational directives concerning your scope of practice
- policies and procedures impacting on the tasks of your work unit
- patient care plans and charts
- patient notes, assessment tools and incident reports.
    If you are unclear on the boundaries of your role, your scope of practice, or the legal and organisational requirements, you should seek advice from the RN.

Follow written instructions

Reading notices and instructions is an important responsibility in every workplace. The information given can be important for carrying out your job. An example is the policy and procedure manuals that contain information about practices and standards in the workplace and how they are implemented. Remember to ask for clarification if you do not understand what you are reading.

Take notes or messages

Some people find that it assists them to remember details of what a speaker has said if they write down a few notes as they listen. Others prefer to simply listen first and then summarise what they hear. It is important that you try each method and decide what best suits you. When taking messages, you must maintain privacy and confidentiality and check the person's name, position and contact details. Write a short summary of the message and include what the receiver is required to do (e.g., call back). Be clear and concise and communicate only the relevant information in a logical order. Remember that an HSA must not take medication orders over the telephone and must refer these calls to the RN.

Complete documentation

If you are involved with writing or electronically documenting progress notes, you should maintain the following:

* be clear and accurate so that other members of your healthcare team can assume care of the patient or to provide ongoing service at any time (for example, 'Client was observed to be agitated in session as evidenced by clenched fist, shouting and pacing.')
* distinguish between what was observed or performed, and what was reported by others as happening (for example, 'Relatives stated that Mr Jamison fell in the bathroom and bruised his leg.')
* use correct terminology and write in plain English with correct grammar, spelling and punctuation
* avoid using subjective and emotional language (for example, words such as 'feel', 'believe', and 'think' are subjective)
* remember that under freedom of information legislation, patients can request to obtain and read their records
* use a pen and not a pencil to record written comments – dark ink should be used that is readily reproducible, legible, and difficult to erase and write over
* make sure that all notes are countersigned by an RN.

All written reports should comply with the policies and procedures of your organisation and should be sequential and objective. Refer to Chapter 10, 'Provide non-client contact support in an acute care environment', for more information on completing written reports and documentation.

Follow organisation communication policies and procedures for using digital media

Digital media covers workplace correspondence and documentation that can be created, viewed, distributed, modified and preserved on a computer, tablet or mobile phone. This covers internet and organisational intranet, videos, podcasts, emails and newsletters (see Figure 4.10). The growing use of digital media is providing opportunities for organisations and individuals to communicate and share information with staff, external stakeholders and the community. Your organisation is likely to have a policy regarding digital media and in particular social media, and it is your responsibility to adhere to all organisational policies and regulations.

The purpose of communication and the content of the message to be delivered should be considered when deciding on the appropriate channel of delivery. For example, if it is a sensitive or complex issue, face-to-face dialogue may be more appropriate. The use of social media must not interfere with an employee's effective and efficient performance of their work responsibilities. It is your responsibility to not engage in or allow others to engage in inappropriate, irresponsible, offensive or harmful communication activities.

Social media
Websites and other online means of communication that are used by large groups of people to share information and to develop social and professional contacts.

FIGURE 4.10 Types of digital media

DIGITAL MEDIA	USAGE
Intranet	Helps improve communication to management and healthcare staff through blog posts, broadcasts, departmental subsites, centralised policies and employee applications
Email	Used for contact between healthcare professionals and health services. Healthcare providers should receive informed consent before sharing protected health information with patients through this medium
Internet	Used for information about patient care, medical and health education, and research. It can also be used to source national and state legislation, policies and guidelines.
Social media	The Australian Department of Health (2021) uses social media (Facebook, Twitter and YouTube) to share links and information about health policies and programs. The Department of Health has policies that govern the way they use social media as well as policies for departmental staff to guide and support them in their use of social media, both at work and outside work. The Australian Health Practitioner Regulation Agency (AHPRA, 2019) also has a policy to help practitioners understand their obligations when using social media

ACTIVITY 4.12

Digital media in health care

Look up the Department of Health guidelines on social media at **https://www.health.gov.au/ using-our-websites/social-media** and respond to the following:

1   List the requirements when commenting on social media pages.

2   How does the Department of Health moderate social media pages?

3   How is privacy maintained on the platforms or sites?

6   CONTRIBUTE TO CONTINUOUS IMPROVEMENT

Continuous improvement is an ongoing cycle of review and evaluation of the processes and procedures in an organisation. It helps to refine the way things are done to make them as effective and efficient as possible. As an HSA, you should contribute to identifying and voicing improvement suggestions and promote and model changes in work practices. Feedback and advice should be sought from others, including your supervisor, to further develop your skills and knowledge.

Contribute to identifying, improving, promoting and modelling work practices

Organisations involved in the delivery of health services emphasise continuous improvement and opportunities for healthcare workers to contribute to the review and development of policies and procedures. In some organisations, this opportunity can be provided through the forming of quality work teams (see Figure 4.11) that actively seek improvements in the workplace. These teams are an acknowledgement that managers are not always the people with the best ideas. Also, by combining everyone's ideas, there is a greater likelihood that the organisation will gain genuine improvements in the workplace.

FIGURE 4.11 A quality team contributing to continuous improvements in work practices

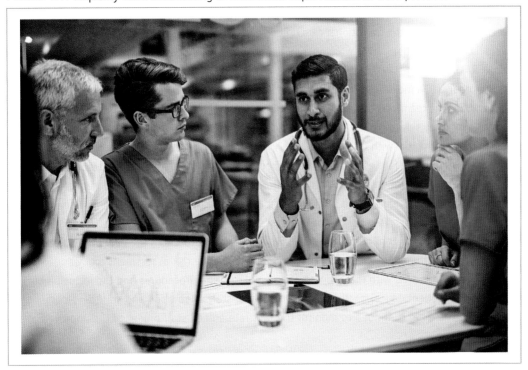

Source: iStock.com/Cecilie_Arcurs

Quality work teams can identify areas for improved work practices and procedures through:

- reading reports
- seeking and addressing feedback
- ongoing monitoring of tasks
- distributing surveys and questionnaires
- assessing, observing and measuring environmental factors
- checking equipment in a range of work environments.

Once changes are brought about by continuous improvement, it is the responsibility of all staff to participate in their implementation. By promoting and modelling changes to improved work practices and procedures, the effectiveness of work teams is enhanced.

The benefits of promoting and modelling best practice in a work team include:

- information is shared about the needs of patients, particularly in relation to problems that arise and strategies for dealing with them
- strong working relationships are created and sustained in the workplace
- innovation and creativity in the carrying out of tasks is encouraged
- conflict between team members and frustration with existing work practices and procedures can be resolved
- services to patients who need your support are improved.

Identifying and improving work processes

The new manager of the transitional care unit was concerned that the statistics for patient falls were increasing. He decided to work on a model of improvement using a falls risk assessment tool (FRAT).

He organised a meeting with staff including the manager, an RN, an enrolled nurse (EN) and an HSA. The team was tasked with finding the most appropriate tool for the facility. After consultation they selected a risk assessment tool that had been used in a similar facility and they began trialling the tool with the patients.

After a month, the falls episodes had been reduced and the team then started working on how the risk assessment tool could be integrated into the policies and procedures for the organisation. They decided to add protocols for patient mobility awareness, strength training and medication review as an addition to the risk assessment tool.

The falls episodes continued to reduce, and the team incorporated the new policies and procedures into the orientation program for all new staff. The risk assessment tool was continuously improved with the addition of new policies and procedures and the inclusion of protocols on patient education. It also became part of staff orientation and staff development programs. The team continued to monitor the falls rate and all staff modelled the improved work practices.

1   Why was it important for the manager to include the RN, EN and HSA in the consultation process?
2   What is the benefit of continuous improvement in this scenario?

Seek feedback and advice and consult a manager to develop skills and knowledge

Seeking feedback and advice on areas for skill and knowledge development from your supervisor, team members and other co-workers will help to develop and maintain your competence level. Health services assistants work in a team-based unit; and working alongside other people provides an opportunity to include their feedback as a part of your self-assessment on areas that require development (see Figure 4.12).

Seeking feedback and advice should relate to your overall performance and include:

* what you are doing well, and what you are doing not so well
* why you are doing well in some areas and not in others
* areas where your performance could be improved.

Seeking feedback and advice should also provide options in terms of where, when and how skill and knowledge development can best occur. Refer to Chapter 7, 'Organise personal work priorities and development', where personal skill development and formal and informal learning is outlined in greater detail.

FIGURE 4.12 Participating in a staff development opportunity to improve knowledge and skills

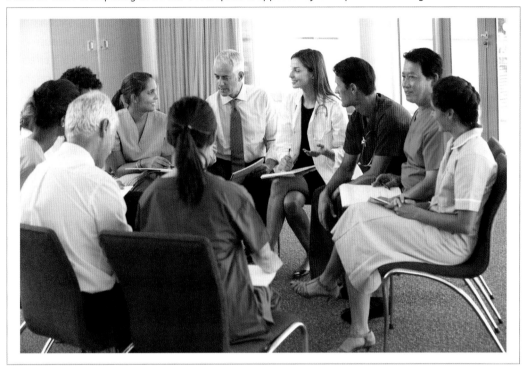

Source: iStock.com/bowdenimages

Skill and knowledge development

1   Identify any new skill development areas appropriate for your present or future role as an HSA working in acute care.

2   Explain why this skill and knowledge development is required.

3   Investigate the mandatory training requirements in your workplace and identify those that can assist with your professional development.

4   Outline other training options for gaining these skills or knowledge.

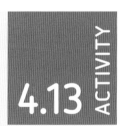

4.13 ACTIVITY

SUMMARY

This chapter outlined how to effectively communicate with people including patients, co-workers and the multidisciplinary team. Therapeutic communication is an important skill to learn because it assists in identifying the patient's needs and determining positive health outcomes. By using effective communication to collaborate with patients and colleagues, misunderstandings and conflicts can be avoided, and constructive workplace relationships can be achieved.

Communication needs to be tailored to the diverse needs of the patients and it is essential that as an HSA you are mindful of constraints that can hinder its process. By considering alternative approaches to these constraints, the quality of support will be enhanced. This chapter also examined when it is necessary to report communication problems to your supervisor, and the importance of completing workplace correspondence and documentation with clarity and accuracy according to organisational policies and procedures.

The last part of the chapter considered the significance of continuous improvement and how you can contribute to this by seeking to improve your own knowledge and skills through feedback and advice. This benefits not only your healthcare team but also the organisation in achieving quality outcomes for all.

APPLY YOUR KNOWLEDGE

Communication constraints

Adriana was a middle-aged woman on our ward who had been admitted for a hysterectomy. She also had a hearing impairment. As the HSA looking after Adriana, I was required to assist with her admission. I felt that I could communicate effectively with her as my grandmother also had difficulty hearing and I had learnt that communicating involves not only what is heard but also what is seen. For people with hearing loss, the visual clues of speech become very important.

1   What are some examples of non-verbal communication that the HSA could use to enhance Adriana's understanding?

Adriana let me know that she found it difficult to hear in the busy ward, so I took her to the patient lounge when asking her the admission questions.

2   What constraints affected Adriana's ability to understand the questions and how could the HSA make it easier for Adriana to comprehend?

I spoke clearly and not too fast and paraphrased the sentences to make sure Adriana understood. She told me that she was anxious and expressed her fear about the operation to me. I sat closer to her and touched her hand.

3   What is paraphrasing and how did it confirm Adriana's understanding?

4   How did the non-verbal techniques of touch and proximity help Adriana's anxiety?

As part of my role, I recorded Adriana's anxiety in her notes and reported the interaction during handover to the next shift. My colleagues acknowledged my effective communication skills and gave me feedback that they had contributed to Adriana's ongoing care. I reflected on this and it gave me a great sense of satisfaction and a willingness to continue to improve my skills.

5   Why is it important to complete documents using clear, accurate and objective language?

6   How did the feedback from colleagues help to develop competence and contribute to continuous improvement for the HSA?

7   Using the knowledge learnt in Chapter 1, 'Participate in workplace health and safety', how would you use Gibbs' reflective cycle to analyse your response to Adriana's anxiety?

8   Understanding the scope of your role as an HSA is essential to performing your role effectively within the healthcare team. How did the HSA demonstrate the scope of their role in supporting Adriana?

◄ REFLECTING ON THE INDUSTRY INSIGHT 💬

1 Why is it important to gain the patient's consent prior to writing information on a whiteboard?
   a   To prevent the patient from suing the nurse for breach of privacy.
   b   So that confidential information is not written for all staff and family to view.
   c   Consent is not required for writing patient information on a bedside whiteboard.
   d   It is compulsory to write information and this is not the patient's decision.

2 Which of the following is an example of a goal that was written on a whiteboard for the patient in the industry insight?
   a   To attend daily rehabilitation sessions for mobility.
   b   To perform ECG monitoring every four hours.
   c   To minimise the average length of stay in hospital.
   d   To communicate with the surgeon regarding anaesthetic dosage.

3 Why is it important for the multidisciplinary team to interact regarding the patient's condition and progress?
   a   So that they do not have to individually communicate with the patient.
   b   So that one team member can write all the patient notes for every member of the multidisciplinary team.
   c   To prevent miscommunication between the team and duplication of tasks.
   d   To share confidential information between the entire health team.

SELF-CHECK QUESTIONS

1   Outline the attributes of effective verbal communication.

2   Explain the benefits of therapeutic communication for patients.

3   What is reflection and how can you demonstrate this technique in communication?

4   What are open-ended questions and why are they an effective form of communication?

5   Outline the barriers to communication that may occur in healthcare settings.

6   What are the important considerations when agreeing on timelines with colleagues?

7   What communication techniques can be used to resolve workplace or patient conflicts?

8   What considerations do you need to make when taking messages in the workplace?

9   Describe the importance of skill development opportunities in your role as an HSA.

10 What are your definitions of the following key words and terms that have been used in this chapter?

KEY WORD OR TERM	YOUR DEFINITION
Interpersonal communication	
Proxemics	

KEY WORD OR TERM	YOUR DEFINITION
Clarification	
Reflection	
Assumption	
Assertion	
Social media	
Conflict of interest	

QUESTIONS FOR DISCUSSION

1 Discuss how a person's culture can influence your choice of communication strategies.
2 Discuss the importance of displaying empathy when communicating with patients.
3 Identify the workplace documentation used in your facility for communication and discuss why it is important to your role as an HSA.
4 Discuss the importance of receiving feedback as it relates to your work as an HSA.
5 Discuss how continuous improvement can be applied to communication with the healthcare team.

EXTENSION ACTIVITY

Communicating appropriately with new clients and colleagues

You have applied for a new position in acute care as an HSA. The following questions have been given to you 15 minutes before the interview for your consideration. With reference to the information covered in this chapter and from your own experience, outline the answers you would give to these questions. Note: this extension exercise may be completed in groups as a verbal response. Practise being an interviewer and interviewee and ask your colleagues to comment on your non-verbal and verbal communication techniques.

1 What techniques would you use to communicate appropriately with patients and other workers?
2 This position requires the ability to collaborate with colleagues. Describe how you would apply this in the workplace.
3 Under what circumstances would you report problems to your supervisor?
4 How can you best contribute to continuous improvement?

REFERENCES

Australian Commission on Safety and Quality in Health Care (ACSQHC) (2017). National Safety and Quality Health Service Standard. Retrieved 4 May 2019 from https://www.nationalstandards.safetyandquality. gov.au/3.-preventing-and-controlling-healthcare-associated-infection

Australian Department of Health (2021). Social media policy. Retrieved 3 July 2022 from https://www. health.gov.au/using-our-websites/social-media

Australian Digital Health Agency (2020). National Nursing and Midwifery Digital Health Capability Framework. Retrieved 17 February 2022 from https://www.digitalhealth.gov.au/sites/default/ files/2020-11/National_Nursing_and_Midwifery_Digital_Health_Capability_Framework_ publication.pdf

Australian Government (1988). *Privacy Act 1988*. Retrieved from https://www.legislation.gov.au/Details/ C2014C00076/Download

Australian Government (2011). *Work Health and Safety Act 2011*. Retrieved 13 March 2017 from https:// www.comlaw.gov.au/Details/C2011A00137

Australian Health Practitioner Regulatory Agency (AHPRA) (2019). New social media guide. Retrieved 17 February 2022 from https://www.nursingmidwiferyboard.gov.au/News/2019-11-11-Social-media-guide.aspx

Australian Institute of Family Studies (AIFS) (2020). Mandatory reporting of child abuse and neglect. Retrieved 3 July 2022 from https://aifs.gov.au/sites/default/files/publication-documents/2006_ mandatory_reporting_of_child_abuse_and_neglect_0.pdf

Edward T. Hall and proxemics. (n.d.), The Free Library (2014). Retrieved 3 July 2022 from https://www. thefreelibrary.com/Edward+T.+Hall+and+proxemics.-a0247338951

Health Research Funding Organisation (2019). Why whiteboards improve patient communication. Retrieved 3 March 2019 from https://healthresearchfunding.org/whiteboards-improve-patient-communication/

Mathews, B. & Scott, D. (2017). Mandatory reporting of child abuse and neglect. Melbourne, Vic.: Australian Institute of Family Studies. Retrieved 18 March 2017 from https://aifs.gov.au/cfca/publications/ mandatory-reporting-child-abuse-and-neglect

Mheidly, N., Fares, M.Y., Zalzale, H. & Fares, J. (2020). Effect of face masks on interpersonal communication during the Covid-19 pandemic. *Frontiers in Public Health*, 9 December. Doi: 10.3389/ fpubh.2020.582191.

INTERPRET AND APPLY MEDICAL TERMINOLOGY APPROPRIATELY

Learning objectives

By the end of this chapter, you should be able to:

1 respond appropriately to instructions that contain medical terminology
2 use medical terminology correctly to carry out routine tasks and seek appropriate assistance as required
3 use appropriate medical terminology in oral and written communication.

Introduction

This chapter describes the relevant knowledge and skills you will require to understand and respond to instructions, to carry out routine tasks and communicate with a range of internal and external patients in a medical environment, and to use appropriate medical terminology.

Effective use of medical terminology is essential in health care because it is the professional language used in records, reports and correspondence. As a health services assistant (HSA), you will need to understand this language to provide continuity of care and collaborate effectively in your healthcare team.

This chapter will provide you with a thorough understanding of medical terminology so you are able to confidently undertake tasks and communicate through written or oral means in the workplace. Commonly used medical terminology and abbreviations are also listed in the appendix at the end of the chapter.

INDUSTRY INSIGHTS 💬

Bedside handover and medical terminology

I found my first experience of bedside handover very informative because both the nurses and the patient, Mr Bianco, participated in the sharing of knowledge.

The computer-generated handover sheet had real-time information about all the patients in the ward, including Mr Bianco. This sheet detailed each individual's condition, treatment, current nursing care and planning.

Our team leader began the handover by introducing Mr Bianco to the oncoming team: 'Good afternoon Mr Bianco. This is the team that will be looking after you this evening. Mary the registered nurse and John the assistant nurse.'

She then gave detailed information about Mr Bianco to us: 'Mr Bianco was admitted with a fractured left neck of femur. He had a total hip replacement yesterday. Mr Bianco's BP is 125/70, he is afebrile with a temp of 36.8 and a pulse of 86.'

She asked Mr Bianco about his pain, showed the registered nurse (RN) the medication chart and discussed his pain medication. She also discussed his discharge planning.

While some medical terminology was used, it was explained to Mr Bianco along the way. Our team leader used the ISBAR (identify, situation, background, assessment and recommendation) acronym to provide structure to the handover and finished by asking Mr Bianco if he wanted to add anything, if he needed any clarification or had any questions to ask. We were also asked if we needed any more information and I asked about his mobility requirements. Afterwards, I spent some time reviewing the medical terminology used on the handover sheet and wrote notes next to words I was unfamiliar with to research later.

Using bedside handover made Mr Bianco feel valued because it allowed for his participation, and it made us approach the nursing care with a patient-centred focus.

1 RESPOND APPROPRIATELY TO INSTRUCTIONS THAT CONTAIN MEDICAL TERMINOLOGY

In the healthcare industry, you will be required to read and write reports and understand and give verbal instructions, most of which contain medical terminology. This terminology has Greek or Latin origins and many terms are a combination of components of these languages. In an acute or community healthcare setting, the ability to respond appropriately using this language has a significant impact on the ongoing care of the patient.

Receive, interpret and document written and oral instructions using medical terminology

Written and oral instructions are used extensively by healthcare teams. It is important for you to listen and clarify the message to ensure that you have a full understanding of what is required. Written and oral instructions may include:

- patient notes
- medication orders

- nursing care plans
- referrals
- reports
- telephone calls
- test results
- operation lists
- verbal instructions.
  Medical terminology used in these instructions may include:
- abbreviations for medical and pharmacological terms
- systems, locations and organs of the body
- common medical conditions including illnesses, injuries and diseases
- departments and sections of a hospital
- health insurance terminology
- medical specialities and occupations
- medical equipment and instruments
- medical investigations and procedures.

You must be able to understand medical terminology by learning the three basic word parts (prefix, root and suffix) and the rules for combining them to create words. By understanding the three basic parts of words and how you combine them, you will determine the meaning of the word. Generally, terms dealing with **diagnosis** and surgery have Greek origins and anatomical terms have Latin origins. This understanding will assist you to communicate effectively with your healthcare team, patients and their families. There is a glossary in the appendix at the end of this chapter for you to refer to that contains common prefixes, root words and suffixes used in health care. The following sections will cover these concepts in more detail.

Diagnosis

Identifying a disease, illness or problem.

Prefixes

Prefix

A one- or two-syllable word part placed before a word to modify or alter its meaning.

Prefixes always come at the beginning of a word, as shown in Figure 5.1. They usually indicate location, time, number or status and refer to a one- or two-syllable word part placed before a word to modify or alter its meaning. Prefixes keep the same meaning whenever they are attached to words.

FIGURE 5.1 Prefixes

PREFIX	MEANING	EXAMPLE
Anti	Against	Antibiotic
Dys	Painful, difficult	Dysmenorrhoea
Hemi	Half	Hemicolectomy
Hypo	Below, deficient	Hypotension
Tachy	Rapid	Tachycardia

Commonly used prefixes

Referring to the list of commonly used prefixes in the appendix at the end of this chapter or in a medical dictionary, complete the following table by filling in the correct prefixes and their meaning:

5.1 ACTIVITY

PREFIX	MEANING	EXAMPLE
		Hypertension
		Leukocyte
		Antenatal
		Suprapubic
		Microbiology

Root words

Root words contain the basic meaning of the term, as shown in Figure 5.2. They usually indicate the involved body part and refer to the main body of the word. All medical words have at least one root word, and by adding prefixes and suffixes it changes the meaning of the word.

Root word
Usually indicates the involved body part and refers to the main body of the word.

FIGURE 5.2 Root words

ROOT	MEANING	EXAMPLE
Arthr	Joint	Arthritis
Cardi	Heart	Cardiogram
Derm	Skin	Dermatology
Gastro	Stomach	Gastroenteritis
Osteo	Bone	Osteoporosis

Suffixes

Suffixes always come at the end of a word, as shown in Figure 5.3. They usually indicate the procedure, condition, disorder or disease, and are a one- or two-syllable word part attached to the end of a word to modify or alter its meaning.

Suffix
A one- or two-syllable word part attached to the end of a word to modify or alter its meaning.

FIGURE 5.3 Suffixes

SUFFIX	MEANING	EXAMPLE
-ectomy	Removal	Appendectomy
-itis	Inflammation	Bronchitis
-ology	Study of	Haematology
-plasty	Repair of	Rhinoplasty
-scopy	Visualisation	Laparoscopy

ACTIVITY 5.2

Commonly used suffixes

Referring to the list of commonly used suffixes in the appendix at the end of this chapter or in a medical dictionary, complete the following table by filling in the correct suffixes and their meaning:

SUFFIX	MEANING	EXAMPLE
		Paraplegia
		Polydipsia
		Colostomy
		Anorexia
		Intravenous

Combining vowels

A combining vowel is used in-between two or more elements in a medical term and assists with its pronunciation. Figure 5.4 provides some examples of how combining vowels are used.

FIGURE 5.4 Combining vowels

EXAMPLE						MEDICAL TERM
Electr /	o	/ cardi /		o	/ graph	Electrocardiograph
root /	vowel	/ root /		vowel	/ suffix	
Arthr /	o	/ scopy				Arthroscopy
root /	vowel	/ suffix				
Abdomin /	o	/ centesis				Abdominocentesis
root /	vowel	/ suffix				

Eponyms

An eponym is a term that represents such things as a structure, disease or a drug, and which is based on the name of a person, place or thing. Examples of eponyms are shown in Figure 5.5.

FIGURE 5.5 Eponyms

TERM	ORIGIN
Achilles tendon	Named after Achilles, a Greek mythological character
Adam's apple	Named after Adam, a biblical character
Alzheimer's disease	Named after Alois Alzheimer, 19th-century German psychiatrist who first described the disease
Branxton-Hicks contractions	Named after Dr John Branxton who first described it in 1872
Eustachian tube	Named after Bartolomeo Eustachi, the 16th-century Italian anatomist

TERM	ORIGIN
Mantoux test	Named after Dr Charles Mantoux who created the test in 1907
Parkinson's disease	Named after James Parkinson, 18th-century English surgeon whose research was the basis for later discovery
Ross River fever	Named after Ross River, Townsville, Queensland, where it was first identified

Body systems and conditions

It is important that you understand the body and its systems, as well as the conditions that can occur. The following sections provide an overview of common medical terminology related to body systems and conditions, including short practical examples. The examples apply the terminology to healthcare practice to help contextualise the terms. For details on the anatomy and physiology of each system, see Chapter 3, 'Recognise healthy body systems'.

Cardiovascular system

The cardiovascular system consists of the heart, arteries, veins, capillaries and blood. Figure 5.6 lists the common medical terms for the cardiovascular system along with their definitions.

FIGURE 5.6 Cardiovascular system terms

TERM	DEFINITION
Anaemia	A condition of deficient oxygen
Angina	Sensation of chest pain due to insufficient oxygen and blood to the heart
Arrhythmia	Abnormal heart rhythm
Arteriosclerosis	Hardening of the arteries
Cardiologist	A doctor whose speciality is management of heart disorders
Defibrillation	Delivering an electric shock to stop the ventricles from fibrillating
Hypertension	High blood pressure
Ischaemia	Decreased blood supply to a body part
Septum	The wall that separates the right and left side of the heart
Thrombocyte	Platelets or blood clot cells

Example: Cardiovascular system terminology in practice

Phillip presented to his general practitioner (GP) with headache and angina. On examination he was found to have hypertension with a BP of 195/110. His ECG indicated an arrhythmia and blood tests indicated elevated enzymes. He was referred to a cardiologist who made a provisional diagnosis of arteriosclerosis. He was commenced on antihypertensive medication and follow-up with a nutritionist.

Respiratory system

The respiratory system consists of the nose, throat, larynx, trachea, lungs, bronchus and alveoli. Figure 5.7 lists the common medical terms for this system along with their definitions.

FIGURE 5.7 Respiratory system terms

TERM	DEFINITION
Asthma	A respiratory disease causing narrowing and swelling of the airways
Bronchodilator	A drug that dilates the bronchi
Cyanosis	Bluish discolouration of the skin due to poor circulation
Dyspnoea	Difficulty breathing
Emphysema	A long-term, progressive disease of the lungs
Febrile	Having a fever
Larynx	Voice box
Pleura	The membrane surrounding the lungs
Tracheostomy	The formation of an opening through the neck to the trachea to enable breathing
Wheeze	A whistling sound made while breathing

Example: Respiratory system terminology in practice

John, a smoker for 40 years, presented to the medical centre with dyspnoea, fever and cough. He had a history of emphysema and had been taking bronchodilators. The doctor noticed that he used his accessory muscles to breathe, had an audible expiratory wheeze, and cyanosis around his lips. His respiratory rate was 32 resps/min and he was febrile with a temperature of 37.8. He was commenced on antibiotics and educated on the need to cease smoking.

Musculoskeletal system

The musculoskeletal system consists of bones, joints, muscles, tendons, cartilage and ligaments. Figure 5.8 lists the common medical terms for this system along with their definition.

FIGURE 5.8 Musculoskeletal system terms

TERM	DEFINITION
Arthroscopy	Using an endoscope to visualise and examine a joint
Arthritis	An inflammatory joint disorder
Contracture	Abnormal shortening of muscle tissue leading to deformity
Dislocation	When a bone slips out of a joint
Fracture	A broken bone
Ligament	Fibrous tissue that holds bone to bone
Osteoporosis	A condition causing weak and fragile bones

TERM	DEFINITION
Physiotherapist	A healthcare professional who treats disease or injury through physical means
Prosthesis	Replacement of a missing body part using an artificial part; e.g., leg prosthesis
X-ray	Using electromagnetic radiation to take a picture inside the body

Example: Musculoskeletal system terminology in practice

Lola is 78 years old and recently noticed that her knee and hip joints ached when she walked. Her doctor diagnosed osteoporosis and osteoarthritis and advised an exercise and diet program. Earlier today Lola was admitted with an injured left leg after slipping in the shower. X-ray revealed a fractured hip, which has since been repaired by an orthopaedic surgeon. She has been referred to a physiotherapist to assist with her mobilisation once she has been discharged.

Endocrine system

The endocrine system consists of glands and hormones. Figure 5.9 lists the common medical terms for this system along with their definitions.

FIGURE 5.9 Endocrine system terms

TERM	DEFINITION
Adrenaline	A hormone released in response to stress
Diabetes	A group of different conditions in which there is too much glucose in the blood
Endocrinologist	A doctor whose speciality is management of disease of the endocrine system
Homeostasis	Having a consistent internal environment in the body
Hormones	Chemical messengers that are secreted into the bloodstream to control many body functions
Hyperglycaemia	Too much glucose circulating in the blood
Hypothyroidism	Disease resulting from insufficient thyroid hormone
Islets of Langerhans	The hormone-secreting portion of the pancreas
Metabolism	The physical and chemical processes that occur in the body which keep us functioning normally
Pancreas	A large gland behind the stomach that secretes digestive enzymes into the duodenum
Steroids	Drugs that help the growth and repair of muscle tissue

Example: Endocrine system terminology in practice

Maria is a 47-year-old woman who has put on weight over the last year. On a recent visit to her GP she complained of feeling tired. She was found to be hyperglycaemic with a BGL of 13.5 mmol/L; and after further blood tests she was diagnosed as having type 2 diabetes mellitus. She asked her GP what diabetes is and was told that it is a disease where the hormones in the pancreas do not metabolise sugar effectively. She was advised to have follow-up tests with an endocrinologist.

Nervous system

The nervous system consists of the brain, spinal cord and nerves. Figure 5.10 lists the common medical terms for this system along with their definitions.

FIGURE 5.10 Nervous system terms

TERM	DEFINITION
Aneurysm	Weakening or bulge in the wall of a blood vessel
Cerebrospinal fluid	Clear fluid that surrounds the brain and spinal cord
Consciousness	The state of awareness
Encephalitis	Inflammation of the brain
Intracranial	Within the skull
Neurone	Nerve cells that transmit nerve impulses
Neuropathy	Disease or damage to nerves
Neurosurgeon	A doctor who performs surgery on the brain and spine
Sedative	A drug used for its calming effect
Subdural haematoma	A blood clot between the layer of the skull and the brain

Example: Nervous system terminology in practice

Con has had a persistent headache since he knocked his head on the garage door two days ago. His doctor prescribed a mild sedative and gave him instructions to return if the headache did not improve. He has since presented to the hospital with an altered level of consciousness and nausea. Tests indicated raised intracranial pressure and CT scan confirmed a subdural haematoma, which was then successfully drained in the operating theatre by a neurosurgeon. He was discharged four days later.

Gastrointestinal system

The gastrointestinal system consists of the mouth, oesophagus, stomach, and small and large intestine. Figure 5.11 lists the common medical terms for this system along with their definitions.

FIGURE 5.11 Gastrointestinal system terms

TERM	DEFINITION
Cholecystectomy	Surgical removal of the gallbladder
Cirrhosis	A degenerative disease of the liver
Colonoscopy	Visual examination of the colon via a scope
Constipation	Difficulty in emptying bowels
Diverticulitis	Inflammation of diverticula in the bowel wall
Enema	Fluid injected via the rectum to evacuate the bowel
Gastroenterologist	A doctor whose speciality is management of disease of the gastrointestinal tract
Nausea	Sensation of discomfort in the stomach
Suppository	A drug delivered via the rectum, vagina or urethra

Example: Gastrointestinal system terminology in practice

Raymond has recently been experiencing abdominal pain and bloating, nausea and constipation. He presented to the medical centre and the GP prescribed a suppository, which had no effect. He was admitted for further tests including a colonoscopy that indicated diverticulitis. He was commenced on a healthy lifestyle plan to manage his condition that included a high-fibre diet, exercise and decreasing his consumption of processed foods.

Urinary system

The urinary system consists of the kidneys, ureters, bladder and urethra. Figure 5.12 lists the common medical terms for this system along with their definitions.

FIGURE 5.12 Urinary system terms

TERM	DEFINITION
Cystitis	Infection of the bladder
Dialysis	A procedure in which a machine is used to separate waste material from the blood
Dysuria	Painful urination
Haematuria	Blood in the urine
Incontinence	Accidental or involuntary loss of urine from the bladder (urinary incontinence) or faeces from the bowel (faecal incontinence)
Indwelling catheter (IDC)	A tube inserted into the bladder
Micturition	The act of passing urine (urination or voiding)
Nephrologist	A doctor whose specialty is management of disease of the kidneys
Prostatic hypertrophy	Enlargement of the prostate gland
Renal calculi	Solid particles in the kidney (stones)

Example: Urinary system terminology in practice

Robert recently began suffering from urinary retention. His family has taken him to the local hospital in the hope that this problem could be relieved. Tests were ordered and an indwelling catheter was inserted to facilitate micturition. He was diagnosed with cystitis, haematuria and renal calculi. The nephrologist used a type of shock therapy to crush the stones and ordered antibiotics for his urinary tract infection.

Reproductive system

The reproductive system consists of the male and female reproductive tracts. Figure 5.13 lists the common medical terms for this system along with their definitions.

FIGURE 5.13 Reproductive system terms

TERM	DEFINITION
Endometriosis	Lining cells of the uterus (endometrium) growing outside of the uterus
Fallopian tubes	Two tubes leading from the ovaries to the uterus
Gynaecologist	A doctor who specialises in the health of the female reproductive system (vagina, uterus and ovaries) and the breasts
Mastitis	Inflammation of the breast
Menopause	The stage when the ovaries stop producing reproductive hormones
Ovaries	The female reproductive organ in which ova (eggs) are produced
Pap smear	A test used to check for changes in the cells of the cervix that may lead to cervical cancer
Prostatectomy	Removal of the prostate gland
Sperm	Male reproductive cells
Testosterone	Male sex hormone

Example: Reproductive system terminology in practice

Wendy was diagnosed with endometriosis in her late 30s; however, since menopause began in her 50s, she has been experiencing increased pelvic pain. Her gynaecologist ordered a Pap smear, which showed Wendy had cancer. She underwent a hysterectomy, whereby her ovaries, uterus and fallopian tubes were removed. She is now having yearly checks and has had no ill effects from her surgery.

Integumentary system

The integumentary system consists of the skin, hair, nails, sweat and oil glands. Figure 5.14 lists the common medical terms for this system along with their definitions.

FIGURE 5.14 Integumentary system terms

TERM	DEFINITION
Allergy	Hypersensitivity of the immune system to something in the environment
Anti-inflammatory	Medication that suppresses inflammation
Debridement	Medical removal of dead, damaged or infected tissue
Decubitus ulcer	Damage to the skin and underlying tissue – also known as a pressure ulcer, pressure sore or bed sore
Dehydration	Abnormal water loss from the body
Dermatologist	A doctor whose speciality is management of disease of the integumentary system
Eczema	Chronic inflammatory skin condition
Jaundice	Yellowish pigmentation of the skin and sclera
Necrotic tissue	Dead tissue that usually results from an inadequate local blood supply
Sacrum	A large, triangular bone at the base of the spine

Example: Integumentary system terminology in practice

Claudia is 85 years old and was admitted to hospital from a local nursing home with dehydration. She presented with decubitus ulcers on her sacrum and heels and a rash on her elbows. The medical staff debrided the necrotic tissue from her ulcer sites and covered them with a medicated wound dressing. The doctor prescribed anti-inflammatory cream for her rash, which was diagnosed as eczema. She was referred to a dermatologist for follow-up treatment.

Specialised areas and occupations

It is essential for HSAs to be able to interpret oral and written orders from specialised areas in health organisations. This includes medical specialities and the occupations associated with them.

Complete the following table by filling in the blank fields – use a medical dictionary to assist you if needed:

5.3 ACTIVITY

SPECIALISED AREA	PERTAINING TO:	OCCUPATION
Endocrinology		
Paediatrics		
Anaesthetics		
Geriatrics		
Orthopaedics		
Oncology		
Pathology		
Pharmacology		
Immunology		

Medical investigations and procedures

Medical investigations and procedures are used to gather information to confirm a diagnosis and treat a condition. Important areas that are concerned with diagnostic and treatment procedures include:

- nuclear medicine
- pathology
- radiology
- screening clinics – for example, breast screening clinics
- general operating room (GOR)
- emergency department (ED) or accident and emergency department (AED)
- intensive care unit (ICU)
- medical centre.

Figure 5.15 lists common suffixes and words related to these procedures and treatments.

FIGURE 5.15 Investigations and procedures

SUFFIX/WORD	DEFINITION	EXAMPLE
-opsy	medical examination or inspection	Biopsy
-scopy	viewing, examining using an instrument	Bronchoscopy
-metry	measuring	Spirometry
-graphy	recording in form of drawing, writing, tracing	Electroencephalography
-ectomy	surgical removal of	Mastectomy
-ostomy	artificial opening	Colostomy
-otomy	cut into a part of the body	Tracheotomy
-plasty	repair of, plastic surgery, refashioning	Rhinoplasty
-rrhaphy	surgical suturing	Herniorrhaphy
anastomosis	surgical connection between two structures	Arterial anastomosis
fusion	fusing together two or more separate parts	Spinal fusion

ACTIVITY 5.4

Current medical terminology

Sandra has just commenced work as an HSA in a rural hospital. She is eager to learn about the medical procedures and processes so that she can become a valuable member of the healthcare team. The hospital is quite busy and Sandra has been asked to fill in at the radiology department. The radiologist takes a professional interest in Sandra and lets her assist with patients when her duties allow. Sandra enjoys learning new information each day and writes down the new medical terminology in her diary so that she can look it up after hours.

1   Why is it important for Sandra to keep up to date with medical terminology?

2   What type of medical procedures would a radiologist perform?

Medical equipment

It is important that you have knowledge of medical equipment and related terminology because you may be required to prepare for a procedure or order stock. Figure 5.16 lists common terms for medical equipment and their definitions.

FIGURE 5.16 Medical equipment

SUFFIX/WORD	DEFINITION
Autoclave	An apparatus used to sterilise materials by steam under pressure
Cannula	A metal or plastic tube for insertion into the body to draw off fluid or to introduce medication. While a needle is used to insert the cannula, it is not always left in place; e.g., for medications or IV fluids
Catheter	A flexible tube inserted through a narrow opening into a body cavity
Scalpel	A knife with a small, sharp, sometimes detachable blade (see Figure 5.17)

SUFFIX/WORD	DEFINITION
Sphygmomanometer	A device used to check blood pressure and which comes in two types: manual or digital
Stethoscope	A medical instrument for listening to the action of a person's heart or breathing
Syringe	A device used to inject fluids into or withdraw them from the body or its cavities

FIGURE 5.17 A scalpel

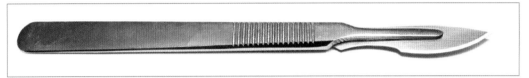

Source: iStock.com/bjolo

Use checklists where appropriate

Healthcare facilities use checklists to maintain consistency of information or tasks. Many tasks are recorded through checklists and these ensure that an accurate record is kept of a process and can be referred to by the team to provide continuous holistic care of the patient. In many facilities, checklists are found in the procedure manuals. Figure 5.18 shows an example of a work health and safety induction checklist used in many healthcare facilities.

FIGURE 5.18 Work health and safety induction checklist

INDUCTION TOPIC	STUDENT INITIAL	STAFF INITIAL
Tour of ward or department area		
Fire evacuation plan, fire stairs and doors, extinguishers		
Emergency alarm		
Emergency evacuation area		
Emergency procedures guide		
Location of resuscitation trolley		
Security procedures and key issue		
Duress alarms		
WHS intranet site		
WHS-related policies to read		
Hazard management register and reporting procedure		
How to refer – incident/injury		
Safety data sheet (SDS) folder		
Out of order tag procedure		
Needlestick injury or blood exposure procedure		
Location of manual handling equipment		

Checklists in your workplace

1   Find a checklist in your organisation.
2   List the medical terminology used in the checklist and the meanings.
3   In what situation is this checklist used and who is it used for?
4   Critique the checklist and suggest any improvements.

Interpret abbreviations for specialised medical terminology

Medical terms can be long when translated or described in plain English. Therefore, commonly used terms are abbreviated when used in patient notes, care plans and charts. This helps the healthcare team write quickly and efficiently in records so that they can continue with patient care. It also allows you to read and understand the records quickly.

Abbreviations and symbols

Acronym

A word formed by the initial letters of each word in the complete phrase.

Acceptable abbreviations

Abbreviations that are approved for use by each health organisation.

Acronyms are words formed by the initial letters of the complete phrase, while symbols and abbreviations are a shortened form of a word or phrase. Most abbreviations and acronyms are written in uppercase if they mean a word or term in English, whereas lower case is used for terms in Latin. Please be aware that some facilities have medical or acceptable abbreviations that are specialised for their areas, and you should be familiar with the acceptable abbreviations used in your workplace. Figure 5.19 lists common symbols used in health care.

FIGURE 5.19 Common symbols used in health care

SYMBOL	MEANING
<	less than
>	greater than
♂	male
♀	female
1°	primary, first degree
2°	secondary, second degree
3°	tertiary, third degree
Rx	treatment

Use abbreviations with care because even frequently used abbreviations can have additional meanings that you may be unaware of. When you do use abbreviations, use them in context to help determine the meaning that is intended; for example:

*   FBC (full blood count) – The doctor requested an FBC to determine Mrs Jones's haemoglobin.
*   FBC (fluid balance chart) – Mrs Jones was commenced on an FBC to monitor her oral intake and urine output.

Figures 5.20–5.23 list some of the abbreviations commonly used in healthcare settings for units of measurement, time, types of medication and medication routes.

Metric system

The metric system is a decimal system based on weights and measures. The three basic units of measurement are *volume*, *length* and *weight*, with volume and weight being used frequently for medication dosages.

FIGURE 5.20 Abbreviations for units of measurement

WEIGHT	VOLUME
grams = g	litre = L
kilograms (kilo) = kg	millilitre = mL
microgram = microg	millimole = mmol
milligram = mg	

Time abbreviations

FIGURE 5.21 Abbreviations for time

TIME	ABBREVIATION
4 hrly	every four hours
6 hrly	every six hours
ac	before meals/food
bd	twice a day
mane	in the morning
nocte	at night
pc	after meal/food
prn	as required
qid	four times a day
stat	immediately
tds	three times a day

Medication type abbreviations

FIGURE 5.22 Abbreviations for types of medications

TYPE OF MEDICATION	ABBREVIATION
capsules	cap
metered dose inhaler	MDI
ointment	oint

TYPE OF MEDICATION	ABBREVIATION
patient controlled analgesia	PCA
pessary	pess
suppositories	supp
tablets	tab

Medication route abbreviations

FIGURE 5.23 Abbreviations for medication routes

METHOD OF DRUG ADMINISTRATION	ABBREVIATION
intramuscular	IM
intravenous	IV
nasogastric	NG
nebulised	NEB
oral	PO
per rectum	PR
percutaneous enteral gastrostomy	PEG
subcutaneous	subcut

ACTIVITY 5.6

Abbreviations in your workplace

Source the list of approved abbreviations used in your organisation and answer the following questions:

1   How can you develop your understanding of the abbreviations and acronyms used in your workplace?

2   Interpret the abbreviations and acronyms that are in bold in the following:

Jocelyn is to be admitted to hospital to have her gall bladder removed. Jocelyn is to be **NBM** for six hours **pre-op**. The Dr has ordered an **MSU** and **FBC** and **Hb** to be taken.

Post-op, Jocelyn will be on an early discharge program. She will need mouth care **p.c.** She must also have pressure area care **(PAC) 2nd hrly** and be encouraged to do **DBC** exercises **qid** or **prn**.

Interpret and adhere to the policies and procedures of the workplace

You must adhere to all policies and procedures within the workplace to ensure compliance with current legislation, regulations and ethical requirements (see Figure 5.24). Policies are guidelines that outline what to do in particular situations. For example, the *Australian guidelines for the prevention and control of infection in healthcare* (NHMRC, 2019) outline practices required to minimise the risk of patients, visitors, volunteers and health workers acquiring a healthcare-associated infection, multi-resistant organism colonisation or communicable disease.

FIGURE 5.24 A policy and procedure manual

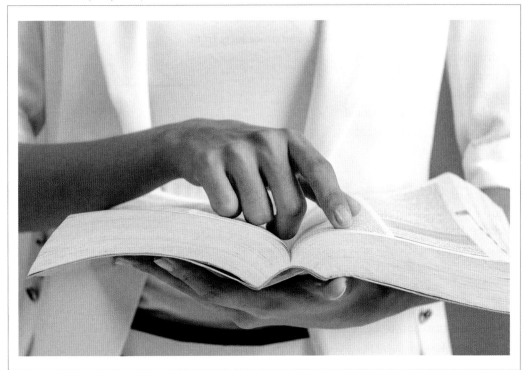

Source: iStock.com/psphotograph

Policies are often associated with procedures that support them by describing how the policies will be put into action. Procedures can be in the form of guidelines, checklists, instructions or flowcharts. Both policy and procedure clarify what the organisation wants to do and how to do it.

Policies and procedures may be for:

- privacy and confidentiality
- advanced care directives
- complaints management
- transport for health
- infection control
- hand hygiene
- incident management
- record management
- manual handling
- evacuation.

All staff need to be aware of the policies and procedures in their workplace, where they are located and when there are changes to them. Speak with your supervisor and attend staff meetings because these sources can provide you with the most relevant information.

Seek clarification when necessary

The ability to interpret and clarify these policies and procedures is essential for the healthcare team so that everyone recognises and adheres to the requirements, and practice variation is reduced across all health areas.

You can seek clarification on policies and procedures from:

* drug information databases
* medical staff
* medical dictionary
* policy and procedure manual
* supervisors
* hospital intranet.

ACTIVITY 5.7

Seeking clarification from a supervisor

You are the HSA looking after Mr Jones, who is being discharged today. His discharge summary indicates that he must keep his dressing intact for six days and then return to the doctor's surgery for suture removal. He asks you what 'intact' means and if he can have a shower and wet the dressing. You are not familiar with his surgical history.

Answer the following questions regarding Mr Jones's discharge summary:

1 Who would you seek clarification from for Mr Jones's question?

2 List the questions you would ask.

3 What is the meaning of the word 'intact' in this scenario?

4 Where would you find procedures for wound management in your organisation?

2 CARRY OUT ROUTINE TASKS

As an HSA, you can be responsible for a wide variety of tasks, from recording information to providing quality care for the patient. Embedded in all these tasks is medical terminology that must be used correctly so that consistency of information is maintained.

The tasks that you will be involved in while working in routine hospital, community care and medical practice environments include:

* reporting and recording in nursing care plans, progress notes and individual plans
* admission, transfer and discharge notes
* patient enquiries and complaints
* patient care tasks
* appointments and accounts.

A sound understanding of terminology is important so that you can answer patient enquiries about procedures and care. You should ask your supervisor or an appropriately qualified professional if unsure, so that misunderstandings are less likely to occur. It is also important to remember to communicate at a level that the patient can understand. This may mean simplifying some words or phrases to clarify information.

Medical practice tasks

A medical practice office worker is responsible for a wide variety of daily tasks, which range from making appointments, filing records and answering enquiries to ordering and recording information. These tasks help to maintain an organised and safe working environment and all require the use of medical terminology so that the health team understands what is required and to avoid misunderstandings.

Appointments and bookings

When you are making appointments and bookings, you may be communicating with outside professionals who are an extension of your healthcare team. It is therefore important to use correct medical terminology at all times. Bookings may be made with local GPs, rehabilitation centres, physiotherapists or other allied and community professionals. The type of medicine a practice is involved with will determine the range of medical terminology that staff need to understand.

Patient records

Correct medical terminology in compiling patient records is essential so that follow-on treatment can be initiated. Transcribed patient records become part of a patient's permanent medical record. These documents can be admission and discharge summaries, patient histories, operative reports, diagnostic studies, consultations or referral letters.

> **Patient history**
> Information gained by asking specific questions, either of the patient or significant others.

Accounts

Medical billing and coding are complex and require extensive knowledge of the healthcare system, medical terminology and medical code sets. There are many software applications that generate accounts for clients, and you must have the knowledge required in order that the correct information is recorded. Private health insurance funds, Medicare, WorkCover and the Department of Veterans' Affairs are agencies that require correct information so that accurate accounts can be processed.

Equipment and supplies

Knowledge of medical equipment and supplies is essential if you are to be responsible for ordering stock or checking orders against an invoice. You must be aware of the names of standard medical supplies and equipment used by your organisation so that items are not ordered that are technically unsuitable or incompatible with existing equipment.

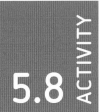

Types of routine tasks

Answer the following questions regarding routine tasks in your workplace or when undertaking work experience:

1   List the routine tasks that you undertake in your organisation as an HSA.
2   Categorise the tasks under:
   a   routine tasks
   b   patient care
   c   reporting and recording.
3   List the medical terminology used when performing these tasks.

5.8 ACTIVITY

3 USE APPROPRIATE MEDICAL TERMINOLOGY IN ORAL AND WRITTEN COMMUNICATION

As an HSA, communicating with a range of community or hospital professionals on patient-related matters is part of everyday practice. A thorough knowledge of appropriate medical terminology is essential in these communications to ensure accurate and timely transfer of information, responsibility and accountability.

Use appropriate medical terminology in oral communications with patients, fellow workers and health professionals

When passing on oral instructions or communicating with other team members, correct pronunciation ensures that accurate information is received. In addition, oral communication must be adjusted according to a patient's ability to understand. This may mean substituting or simplifying medical terms into words that your patients can understand. It is important for you to seek clarification if unsure of the information. Oral communication may include:

- clinical handovers
- answering telephone enquiries
- paging staff
- reporting at staff meetings
- giving verbal instructions to patients and co-workers.

Clinical handover

Clinical handover

Transfer of information, accountability and responsibility for patients from one healthcare worker to another.

Clinical handover is the transfer of information, accountability and responsibility for a patient or group of patients from one healthcare worker to another (see Figure 5.25). It ensures that the person taking over the care of the patient has information concerning the most current needs of the person. It can occur:

- during a change of shift
- when a patient's care is transferred to another healthcare provider
- when the patient's condition changes.

Health facilities across Australia use the ISBAR communication strategy to enhance structural communication and referral between healthcare professionals and healthcare teams. The ISBAR mnemonic contains essential elements to guide healthcare workers and avoid misunderstandings in the process of face-to-face handover, as follows:

- **I**dentify – yourself, your role and your patient
- **S**ituation – state the patient's diagnosis or reason for admission and current problem
- **B**ackground – give patient history, clinical background or context
- **A**ssessment – current problems, observations and treatments
- **R**ecommendation – actions required after handover.

FIGURE 5.25 Clinical handover

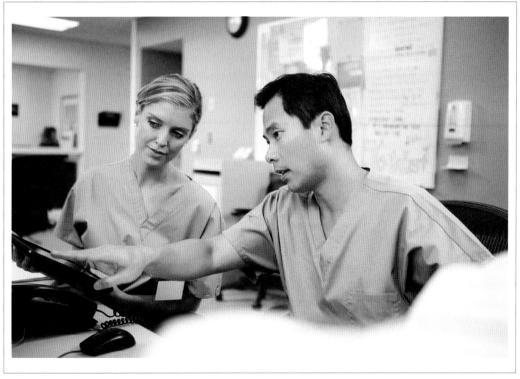

Source: iStock.com/monkeybusinessimages

Telephone communications

You will be required to verbally communicate information over the telephone in a variety of contexts, from paging staff to conveying information regarding the status of a patient. The ISBAR tool is used when identifying someone, and in discussing patient situations, history and actions. Correct use of medical terminology is essential for clear and accurate reporting. Check with your organisation regarding policies for telephone reporting.

ISBAR scenarios

For each of the following four scenarios:

1   categorise the communication strategy using the ISBAR mnemonic

2   describe the meaning of the medical terminology and abbreviations used.

Scenario 1: Telephone enquiry

Hello, my name is Patricia Hennessey. I'm an HSA working at the Bonella Medical Centre. I'm calling about your client, Mr Erik Costello, a 48-year-old man who was due for his six-week appointment next Thursday as a follow-up after his knee replacement. He has come into the centre today and looks pale and feels nauseous and his knee is swollen. He is hypotensive with a blood pressure reading of 105/72 and he is febrile with a temperature of 37.6. Could you please advise if you could see him sooner or recommend another physician?

5.9 ACTIVITY

Scenario 2: Clinical handover to RN

Hello, I'm Sarah Roscoe, the HSA who has been looking after Mr Parker today. He's the 84-year-old diabetic in bed 7 who was admitted with confusion and gangrene in his right toe. While I was giving him a shower this morning he complained of shortness of breath. I took him back to bed and he was tachycardic with a pulse of 102, and he looked pale. Could you come and have a look at him please?

Scenario 3: Discharge handover

Hello, I'm Mauricio Gavaro, the HSA who has been looking after your mother, Mrs Elham, in the short-stay ward. She is now ready for discharge after her operation this morning. She is awake and alert and is eating some sandwiches and having a cup of tea while she waits for you to come and pick her up. The discharge nurse has made a follow-up appointment with her physician for next week.

Scenario 4: Reporting at staff meeting

I'm Brian Nickels, the HSA who has been looking after Mrs Smith this week. She has Alzheimer's dementia and mild right-sided weakness due to a CVA. Today she has been continuously swearing and speaking loudly in the activities room. She walked over to Mr Porteous and punched him in his left arm. I spoke gently to her and guided her back to her room, sat her in a chair and gave her a cup of tea. She stopped swearing and was quiet. Can you please keep an eye on her this afternoon?

Use appropriate medical terminology in written communication with patients, fellow workers and health professionals

An understanding of medical terminology in health records and documentation is critical to the HSA role. Through written communication you will convey the status of patients, the care given and outcomes of interventions (see Figure 5.26). This ensures quality outcomes for patients.

Recording information in written format is also used for:

* appointments and telephone messages
* patient care plans
* clinical forms and charts
* patient histories (admission, discharge, transfer)
* patient progress notes.

When filling out forms and documents, it is important to not only use correct medical terminology but also to comply with organisational policy and procedures regarding reporting and recording, and to use accepted terminology and abbreviations only. Remember that written reports are legal documents. As an HSA in an acute setting, the patient notes you make will always be checked and countersigned by a supervisor.

FIGURE 5.26 Patient form: discharge checklist

TRANSFER OF CARE (DISCHARGE) CHECKLIST

Facility:

FAMILY NAME

GIVEN NAME

D.O.B. _____ / _____ / _____   M.O.

☐ MALE ☐ FEMALE

MRN

ADDRESS

LOCATION / WARD

COMPLETE ALL DETAILS OR AFFIX PATIENT LABEL HERE

BARCODE HERE

SMR000000

Holes punched as per AS2828-1999
BINDING MARGIN - NO WRITING

Destination: Home ☐   RACF ☐   Other (specify facility/ward) ☐ _____

Transport mode: Self/Relative/Carer ☐   Ambulance ☐   Patient Transport ☐
Arranged/booked ☐   Confirmed ☐

Notification: To (named person) _____   Time _____   Date _____

Personal items returned	Yes	No	NA	Date
Valuables	☐	☐	☐	_____
Medical Imaging (e.g Films/CDs)	☐	☐	☐	_____
Equipment (e.g. walking aid)	☐	☐	☐	_____
Dentures	☐	☐	☐	_____
Hearing Aids	☐	☐	☐	_____
Spectacles	☐	☐	☐	_____
Medications	☐	☐		_____

Transfer of care plan	Yes	No	N/A	Comments/notes
Medications list/scripts provided	☐	☐	☐	_____
IV cannula removed	☐	☐	☐	_____
Medical devices removed	☐	☐	☐	_____
Medical Discharge Summary Completed	☐	☐	☐	_____
Resuscitation plan	☐	☐	☐	_____
Follow Up Appointments				
GP	☐	☐	☐	_____
Specialist	☐	☐	☐	_____
Outpatient clinic/community referrals	☐	☐	☐	_____

Patient Instructions and Information (note what education provided and what format)

_____
_____
_____
_____

**Transfer of Care Plan agreed
(sign after discussion)**
Patient/Carer _____   Date/time _____
Clinician _____   Date/time _____

Transfer Checklist Completed by (Name & sign) _____

Designation _____   Date/time _____

Discharged by (name & sign) _____   Date/time _____

XXX0000 - 00/0000

This form is being tested in XX between XX and XX

Page 1 of 1

TRANSFER OF CARE CHECKLIST

FORM #

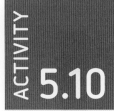

Understanding appropriate medical terminology in written communication

For each of the following scenarios, describe the meaning of the medical terminology and abbreviations used.

Scenario 1: Patient admission

Mr Jones, 52 years of age, presented to the emergency department with palpitations and an uncomfortable feeling in his chest. On admission, he was hypertensive with a BP of 180/110 and tachycardic with a pulse of 130 bpm. He had a previous history of an MI with atypical chest pain. An ECG was taken that showed atrial fibrillation. As a result, he was booked in for cardioversion to restore normal heart rhythm.

Scenario 2: Patient history

Ten-year-old Jack Smythe was admitted via the casualty department. He presented with right lower quadrant pain, nausea, vomiting, anorexia and dysuria, and was slightly febrile. On palpation rebound tenderness was present. Diagnostic evaluation included a U/A, full blood count that demonstrated an elevated leucocyte count, and an ultrasound. Jack was booked in for an emergency appendectomy to prevent the potential complication of perforation, which could lead to peritonitis.

Scenario 3: Pre-operative instructions

Mrs Cordina was to be admitted to hospital from the Forestville Nursing Home for a laparoscopic cholecystectomy. She was advised to be NBM for eight hours pre-op. The doctor ordered an ECG, chest X-ray, complete blood work-up and U/A. Mrs Cordina also wore TED stockings on her legs. Post-operatively, she had to have IV therapy, which could be discontinued once she began drinking fluids. She was on 4th hrly TPR and was required to do DB&C and leg exercises. Pain relief had been ordered – paracetamol 500 mg qid.

Scenario 4: Provisional diagnosis

Urinalysis was performed on Mr Rod Parker, 64 years of age, who had a history of dysuria with urinary retention. It revealed the presence of haematuria. An IVP and cystoscopy confirmed the diagnosis of prostatic hypertrophy. A prostatectomy was performed. Three days post-operatively, Mr Parker was febrile with a temp of 38.2 and was commenced on Amoxicillin PO, tds. He was discharged for follow-up with his GP.

Present written communication to a designated person for verification

A medical record provides a complete history of the patient for all the healthcare team, and when accurately written it helps to provide the best possible care for a patient. The findings in the patient notes or records can offer clues to diagnosis or verify test results to augment clinical findings. With this data, treatment modes can be chosen. Healthcare workers can ensure continuity of care for their patients by reading the records to determine the prior care that has been given and the care that is to follow, even from one facility to another.

It is important to verify written records with your supervisor, practice manager or doctor to enable:

- continuity of care
- legal compliance
- statistics for research
- financial medical claims.

Medical records are also legal documents and verifying the correct terminology can support any legal situation that may occur. Correctly written and verified medical terminologies also facilitate data collection at the point of care and this data can be used for multiple purposes; for example, statistics for disease investigation, clinical decision-making and patient safety reporting.

Continuity of care
Where health care is provided for a person in a coordinated manner by a health team.

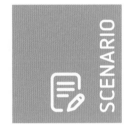

SCENARIO

Diagnosis for Mr Bolton

An initial diagnosis can change as more information is obtained through examination of a patient's history and updating the health complaints. Therefore, it is important to make sure all your written communication about a patient is verified for accuracy.

Laura works in the urology ward as an HSA. She has been looking after Mr Bolton and writes in his notes that he is occasionally confused regarding time and place. She adds to the notes that he is febrile with a temperature of 38.7 and feeling nauseous. On verifying his notes with the RN, blood tests and MSU were taken. Mr Bolton was diagnosed with a UTI and commenced on antibiotics. His confusion, fever and nausea were reduced.

1   What other sources can the healthcare team use to verify information regarding Mr Bolton?
2   Why is it important to write objective information in Mr Bolton's notes?
3   What is the meaning of the abbreviations in this scenario?

Spell and pronounce medical terminology correctly

Correct spelling and pronunciation of medical terms is crucial for accurate communication among healthcare professionals. It is important to check the accuracy of your work to avoid incorrect details, wrongly spelt names or misunderstandings. This can result in a document being filed incorrectly or misinterpretations and can seriously undermine a patient's confidentiality.

Spelling

Accuracy in spelling medical terms is vitally important. Many words look or sound alike but have slightly different spelling, which results in different meanings. For example, arterio means artery and arthro means joint. All documentation should be checked using a medical dictionary for correct spelling and grammar if there is uncertainty. Creating a personal dictionary of commonly used medical terminology is also a useful way to remember spelling and terms.

American English spelling differs from the British English spelling, which is predominantly used in Australia. Many medical terms spelt with 'ae' or 'oe' in British English are spelt with 'e' in American English. American spelling of medical words does not acknowledge any silent vowels, which means an 'o' or an 'a' that is not pronounced is not included in the written word. American spelling may also be phonetic, whereby the word is spelt the way it sounds. Examples include fiber not fibre, and center not centre. Be aware of these spelling differences when using an American textbook.

Figure 5.27 outlines some examples of the differences between the two types of English.

FIGURE 5.27 British English and American English spelling

BRITISH	AMERICAN	MEANING
haem	hem	blood
gynae	gyne	female reproductive system
faeces	feces	excrement
oedema	edema	collection of fluid
diarrhoea	diarrhea	loose bowel movements

Pronunciation

When you are learning new medical terms, say them out loud to your team to ensure your pronunciation is correct. By practising, memorising and using medical terminology as much as possible, your vocabulary will improve and grow. Figure 5.28 outlines some guidelines for pronunciation.

FIGURE 5.28 Pronunciation

SPELLING	GUIDELINE	PRONUNCIATION	EXAMPLE
ch	h is silent	'K'	chronic
ps	p is silent	'S'	psychotic
pn	p is silent	'N'	pneumothorax
pt	p is silent	'T'	ptosis
oe	o is silent	'ee'	coeliac
i	at the end of a word	'eye'	glomeruli

ACTIVITY 5.11

Using correct spelling for medical terminology

Select the correctly spelt word to make the following statements true:

1   Low blood pressure is also called hypotension/hypertension.

2   The ileum/ilium is located at the lower portion of the small intestine.

3   The serous lining of the abdominal cavity is called the peritoneum/perineum.

4   The main artery in the neck is called the carotid/parotid.

5   The surgical removal of the colon is defined as a colectomy/colostomy.

6   Aural/oral pertains to the ear or sense of hearing.

7   Positioning the patient in the prostrate/prostate position means lying them prone.

8   Difficulty swallowing is called dysphagia/dysphasia.

SUMMARY

This chapter outlined the importance of interpreting and applying medical terminology in all healthcare tasks. As the universal language of the healthcare and medical industry, this specialist language helps workers to completely understand what is happening or what has to be done to help a patient.

By standardising the communication between health professionals through medical terminology, you are able to understand and respond to instructions and carry out tasks that assist you to care for your patients and to be an effective member of the healthcare team.

The last part of the chapter emphasised the importance of using this terminology in oral and written communications, including spelling and pronouncing correctly to report and record a patient's condition. This enables all members of the health team to provide continuity of care for the individual.

APPLY YOUR KNOWLEDGE

Medical terminology in disease treatment

Terri (♀) presented with a non-tender breast lump in the (R) upper outer quadrant of her breast which was also seen on mammogram. She had thought it was mastitis as she was breastfeeding her new baby. A targeted ultrasound scan of the right breast was performed that demonstrated an area of change, which could be due to infection; however, the diagnosis was Ca breast.

A core biopsy was then performed under local anaesthesia which identified an invasive lobular carcinoma. Terri was then referred for CT scan staging of her chest, abdomen and pelvis, and a bone scan. This was performed by the radiologist.

℞ for her cancer followed and Terri underwent a local excision of her right breast and axillary clearance which was followed by radiotherapy. Side effects experienced by Terri from the radiotherapy were nausea and localised erythema.

1   Identify the root words, suffixes and meanings used throughout this case history.

2   Describe the medical terms used throughout this case history.

As the HSA looking after Terri, my role included recording and reporting changes to Terri's condition. I recorded the side effects of the radiotherapy in her progress notes and verified these with the RN.

3   Using the knowledge learnt in Chapter 4, 'Communicate and work in health and community services', describe why it is important for the HSA to report concerns or changes to a patient's condition.

During clinical handover to the next shift, I used the ISBAR mnemonic with medical terminology throughout.

4   Identify the mnemonic and outline why it is important for the HSA to use this structured approach during clinical handover.

Terri was prescribed Tamoxifen PO 20mg/day by the doctor to reduce the risk of the cancer recurring. The doctor also advised her not to breastfeed as the medication could pass through the bloodstream into the breast milk. Terri was later discharged and recovered well and was required to attend further outpatient radiotherapy sessions for the next 3/12.

5   Abbreviations and symbols were used extensively throughout this case history. Define the abbreviations and symbols used.

6   Understanding the scope of the role as an HSA is essential to communicating effectively within the healthcare team. What was the scope of the HSA role in this case study and why is it important for the HSA to have a sound understanding of medical terminology to perform their role effectively?

◀ REFLECTING ON THE INDUSTRY INSIGHT 💬

1   Which of the following information was described in Mr Bianco's handover sheet?
    a   The client's diagnostic-related group.
    b   Current problems, observations and treatments.
    c   Audit of client care procedures.
    d   Future discharge guidelines.

2   In the industry insight, what does the acronym ISBAR stand for?
    a   Identify, situation, background, assessment and recommendation.
    b   Information, status, backup, analysis and reasoning.
    c   Issue, state, backdrop, acuity and response.
    d   Introduction, site, baseline, argument and reply.

3   Which of the following is a reason why using computer-generated documentation for bedside handover is advantageous?
    a   It improves spreadsheet skills.
    b   It can be edited by the ward clerk as required.
    c   It can be given to the patient to read easily.
    d   It contains real-time data regarding the patient's condition.

SELF-CHECK QUESTIONS

1   What are the forms of oral and written instructions used in your organisation?

2   What is the purpose of checklists for patient care procedures?

3   Why is it important to check the approved abbreviations used in your organisation?

4   What should you do if you do not know a word or how to spell, pronounce or use it?

5   What are some of the routine tasks you might undertake in your workplace that would require an understanding of medical terminology?

6   What resources are available within a healthcare organisation to help staff use and check medical terminology?

7   What is the difference between a policy and a procedure?

8   Where would you find the policies and procedures in your workplace?

9   Why is it important to be aware of the names of standard medical supplies and equipment used by your organisation?

10 What are your definitions of the following key words and terms that have been used in the chapter?

KEY WORD OR TERM	YOUR DEFINITION
Prefix	
Root word	

KEY WORD OR TERM	YOUR DEFINITION
Suffix	
Acronym	
Policy	
Clinical handover	
Diagnosis	
Patient history	
Continuity of care	

QUESTIONS FOR DISCUSSION

1   Discuss the importance of non-clinical staff having a rudimentary knowledge of appropriate medical terminology.

2   Discuss the importance and use of verified written records for health care.

3   Abbreviations should not be documented on the patient's consent form and procedures must be written in full words. Why is this important?

4   Discuss the strategies that could be used by healthcare workers who come from CALD backgrounds and have strong accents, when reporting the patient's condition?

5   Discuss the different types of medical terminology and abbreviations typically used in rehabilitation, aged care and community settings.

EXTENSION ACTIVITY

Medical terminology in orthopaedics

Adam Cordner, 24 years old, felt a snap inside his knee when changing direction while playing soccer with his local team. He was taken off the field with a visibly swollen left knee and complaining of acute pain. He was evaluated by the athletic trainer who performed hamstring and quadriceps strength tests and neurovascular assessment of the affected limb. He was taken to the local hospital where diagnostic testing included an X-ray and MRI. The X-ray taken did not show a break, but the MRI showed a torn ACL, medial meniscal tear and a bone contusion. Mr Cordner underwent arthroscopic surgery on his knee, with the orthopaedic surgeon performing an autograft reconstruction as well as repair to the torn meniscus. Post-op he was commenced on Panadeine QID. He was discharged the next day on crutches, with a firm bandage applied to the injury in order to protect the site, apply compression and control swelling. Adam followed his rehabilitation protocol, which consisted of ROM and strengthening exercises. After 12 weeks he began slow forward and backward jogging on a level surface and isotonic exercises with low resistance and high repetition. He recommended competitive soccer after 12 months of rehabilitation.

1   Fill in the definitions for each of the related terms and abbreviations in this scenario in the following table.

MEDICAL TERM/ABBREVIATION	DEFINITION
ACL	
Acute	
Arthroscopic	
Autograft	
Compression	
Contusion	
Crutches	
Diagnostic	
Hamstring	
Isotonic	
Medial	
Meniscus	
MRI	
Neurovascular	
Orthopaedic	
Post-op	
Qid	
Quadriceps	
Rehabilitation	
Resistance	
ROM	
X-ray	

2   In pairs, practise rephrasing this case study by describing the abbreviations and medical terms in language that a non-medical person could understand.

3   Discuss with your colleagues the ISBAR communication strategies that were used in this case study.

4   Why is it important for members of the healthcare team to explain medical terminology in easy-to-understand language for the patient and their families or significant others?

REFERENCES

National Health and Medical Research Council (NHMRC) (2019). *Australian guidelines for the prevention and control of infection in healthcare*. Retrieved 17 October 2022 from https://www.nhmrc.gov.au/sites/default/files/documents/infection-control-guidelines-feb2020.pdf

New South Wales Health (2017). Infection prevention and control policy. Retrieved 1 January 2019 from https://www1.health.nsw.gov.au/pds/Pages/doc.aspx?dn=PD2017_013

NSW Agency for Clinical Innovation (2014). *Critical Led Discharge (CLD)*. Retrieved 17 October 2022 from https://aci.health.nsw.gov.au/__data/assets/pdf_file/0004/235264/ACI-ACT-CLD-Resource.pdf

Walker, S., Wood, M. & Nicol, J. (2020). *Mastering Medical Terminology*, 3rd edition. Elsevier, Australia.

COMMONLY USED MEDICAL TERMINOLOGY AND ABBREVIATIONS

COMMON PREFIXES

PREFIX	DEFINITION
a/an	Without, lack of, not
ab	Away from, negative
ad	Towards, near to, addition to
ante	Before, prior to, in front of in time or place
brady	Slow
circum	Around, surrounding
co	With, together
contra	Against, opposite
di	Two, twice, double, reversal, separation, apart from
dia	Through, across, between
ecto	Out, outer, out of place
endo	Inside, within, into, in
epi	Upon, on the outside, over
ex/exo	Outside, out, to protrude
hom/homeo	Like, same
hyper	Above, beyond, excessive
intra/intro	In the middle of, within, inward, into
leuco/leuko	White, colourless
mal	Bad, abnormal
megalo	Huge
melan	Black

PREFIX	DEFINITION
micro	Small
multi	Many
neo	New, immature
olig	Scant, deficient, few, little
peri	Around, about, beyond
poly	Many, much, generalised
pre	In front of, before
quad	Four
retro	Backward, located behind
semi	Half, partial
steno	Narrow or constricted
sub/sup	Under, less than, partial
supra	Over, above, upon, exceeding
trans	Across, through, beyond

COMMON ROOT WORDS

ROOT WORD	DEFINITION
angi	Vessel
arter	Artery
arthr/articul	Joint
axilla	Armpit
carcino	Cancer
cardi	Heart
cerebr	Brain
chol	Gall, bile
cilia	Hair, hairlike
crani	Skull
cyst	Bladder, sac of fluid
cyt	Cell
derm	Skin
enter	Intestine

ROOT WORD	DEFINITION
febri	Fever
gastro	Stomach
glossa	Tongue
gyn	Female, female reproductive organs
haem	Blood
hepat	Liver
hyster	Uterus
mammo/mast	Breast
my	Muscle
nephr	Kidney, renal
neur	Nerve
ophthalmo	Eye
orch/orchid	Testes
osteo	Bone
oto	Ear
path	Disease
pulm	Lung
rhin	Nose, noselike
stoma	Mouth, opening
thorac	Chest
thrombo	Clot
trache	Trachea
tympan	Eardrum
urethro	Urethra
uter	Uterus (womb)
vertebr	Spinal column or vertebrae

COMMON SUFFIXES

SUFFIX	DEFINITION
-aemia/aemic	Condition or presence of blood
-agra/algia	Pain

SUFFIX	DEFINITION
-carcinoma	Malignant tumour
-cele	Hernia, tumour, swelling
-centesis	Puncture to remove fluid
-dermia	Condition of the skin
-desis	Binding, fixation
-dipsia	Condition of thirst
-edema	Swelling
-genesis	Origin, reproducing
-glycaemia	Condition of sugar in the blood
-graph	Product of writing or drawing
-kinesia	Condition involving movement
-logy	Study or science of
-megaly	Enlargement
-mentia	Condition of the mind
-neural/neuria	Pertaining to the nerves
-oma	Growth (tumour)
-orexia	Condition of appetite
-otic	Pertaining to the ear
-oxia	State of oxygen in the blood
-paedic/pedic	Treatment of children
-paenia/penia	Deficiency
-pathy	Disease of, therapy
-pepsia	State of digestion
-phagia	Eating or desire to eat
-phasia	Speech
-plegia	Paralysis
-rrhoea/rrhea	Flow, discharge
-sclerosis	Hardening
-scope	Instrument used to examine
-sect	To cut
-sepsis/septic	Condition of decay

SUFFIX	DEFINITION
-stasis	To stand, stoppage of flow, control
-stenosis	Condition of narrowing
-stoma	Mouth or opening
-stomy	Artificial opening
-venous	Pertaining to the veins

COMMON ABBREVIATIONS

ABBREVIATION	DEFINITION
ADL	Activities of daily living
BGL	Blood glucose level
BNO	Bowels not open
BO	Bowels open
BP	Blood pressure
CAL	Chronic airways limitation
CCF	Congestive cardiac failure
CNC	Clinical nurse consultant
CVA	Cerebrovascular accident
DBC	Deep breathing and coughing
DVT	Deep vein thrombosis
ECG	Electrocardiogram
FBC	Fluid balance chart
GP	General practitioner
HNPU	Has not passed urine
HSA	Health services assistant
IDC	Indwelling catheter
IDDM	Insulin-dependent diabetes mellitus
MD	Medical doctor
MI	Myocardial infarction
MSU	Midstream specimen of urine
NBM	Nil by mouth
NGT	Nasogastric tube

ABBREVIATION	DEFINITION
NIDDM	Non-insulin-dependent diabetes mellitus
NUM	Nursing unit manager
PAC	Pressure area care
PRN	[Pro re nata] as required
PU	Passed urine
RN	Registered nurse
TPR	Temperature, pulse and respiration
UA	Urinalysis

WORK WITH DIVERSE PEOPLE

Learning objectives

By the end of this chapter, you should be able to:

1 reflect on your perspectives of cultural diversity
2 appreciate the benefits of diversity and inclusiveness
3 communicate with people from diverse backgrounds and situations
4 promote understanding across diverse groups.

Introduction

This chapter describes the skills and knowledge required to work respectfully with people from diverse social and cultural groups and situations, including Aboriginal and Torres Strait Islander people.

Identifying your own social and cultural perspectives allows you to work as a health services assistant (HSA) with an awareness of your limitations as well as understanding how to be inclusive towards others. By valuing and respecting diversity, you can develop relationships with co-workers and patients that contribute to cohesion and culturally competent care.

Using effective communication by showing respect for diversity develops trusting relationships. Being aware of issues that may cause communication misunderstandings can lead to strategies for resolution. As an HSA, you need to be aware of culture as a factor in all human behaviour and to use work practices that show respect for people from culturally and linguistically diverse (CALD) backgrounds. This chapter will allow you to reflect on your own perspectives and appreciate diversity in order to communicate effectively with people from diverse cultures.

INDUSTRY INSIGHTS ➕

Cultural safety

SafeWork NSW (2020) defines cultural safety as

> creating a workplace where everyone can examine our own cultural identities and attitudes, and be open-minded and flexible in our attitudes towards people from cultures other than our own … [It] demands actions that recognise, respect and nurture the unique cultural identity of a person and safely meets their needs, expectations and rights. It means working from the cultural perspective of the other person, not from your own perspective.
>
> SafeWork NSW, 2020

My first experience with cultural safety as an HSA was when I started working in a rural hospital. In my first week I attended a cultural safety training and development program, which gave me some knowledge and skills to work effectively with my colleagues and patients from culturally diverse backgrounds. We were shown techniques for ensuring we respected the cultural and social differences in the provision of health care. We were also taught self-reflective practices, and our instructors reinforced the need to provide feedback to management relating to cultural tension issues that could arise in the workplace. There was great emphasis on the concept of holistic health care for Aboriginal and Torres Strait Islander patients and the need to recognise and respect local Aboriginal history, customs, cultures and kinship structures.

This training prepared me well so that I could become more confident in delivering effective care to a person or family from another culture. I was able to examine my own cultural identity and attitudes, and become open-minded, respectful and flexible in my attitudes towards people from cultures other than my own. I was also able to recognise stereotypical barriers and plan to avoid these in my interactions with my patients.

Cultural safety
'Creating a workplace where everyone can examine our own cultural identities and attitudes, and be open-minded and flexible in our attitudes towards people from cultures other than our own.' (SafeWork NSW, 2020)

1 REFLECT ON OWN PERSPECTIVES

In an acute healthcare setting you will be exposed to many different cultural groups, including co-workers and the people in your care. It is important to identify and improve your social awareness to provide culturally competent care. Developing an awareness of your own perspectives on diversity will help you understand how these have shaped your attitudes, values and beliefs. This in turn will help you work more effectively with others.

Identify and reflect on own social and cultural perspectives and biases

Each person has their own cultural identity, which is formed by the society that they belong to and their life experiences. Reflecting on your own cultural perspectives, including your cultural identity and biases, can help you develop skills in providing culturally competent care.

Cultural identity

You can define the culture of a group of people in terms of the way they act, their beliefs and the principles that they live by. Being able to associate with and feel like part of such a group forms part of a person's cultural identity. It can include:

Cultural identity

The feeling of belonging to a group.

- nationality
- location
- ethnicity
- social class
- gender
- religious or spiritual beliefs.

Visible culture includes those aspects of your culture that can be readily seen by others, such as appearance, diet, dress, behaviour and customs. These aspects make up a small part of your cultural identity and do not necessarily represent the most important information to help others understand your needs. The less visible aspects include values, attitudes, beliefs (see Figure 6.1) and perceptions. These represent the larger part of your identity and can give greater insight into your needs.

FIGURE 6.1 Attitudes, values and beliefs

Attitudes	Values	Beliefs
A way of thinking or feeling about certain idea or issues Attitudes can be revealed in thoughts, actions, body language, dress etc.	A measure of the worth or importance a person attaches to something Our values are often reflected in the way we live our lives	A feeling that something is true. It can relate to spiritual, cultural or moral principles

Cultural bias

Each person has their own cultural identity, and often these culturally based attitudes, values and beliefs are learnt through socialisation. While these attitudes and values are useful in terms of living in society, they may also act as a barrier to adapting to change and in working with people from other cultures. For example, you may have developed assumptions about other cultures or about a particular cultural group. These assumptions may influence your perception of other cultures and so are known as cultural bias. It is therefore important to identify and reflect on your own cultural self in terms of your social and cultural perspectives and biases in order to understand how to provide culturally appropriate care to the diverse groups in our society.

Cultural bias

Assumptions about other cultures or about a particular cultural group that affects related perceptions.

Cultural diversity

Within every culture, there is diversity. A culturally diverse society is characterised by differences in the visible and less visible aspects of culture. There will also be differences in economic background, age, education, history, geographical background, political affiliation, sexual orientation and religious beliefs (see Figure 6.2). Appreciating the differences between individuals and embracing the diversity within each group can influence your attitudes and values and help reduce your bias. Recognising this diversity creates tolerance in the workplace, where everyone can benefit from the qualities and experiences that these diverse groups can bring.

FIGURE 6.2 Everyone is a part of the diversity of culture

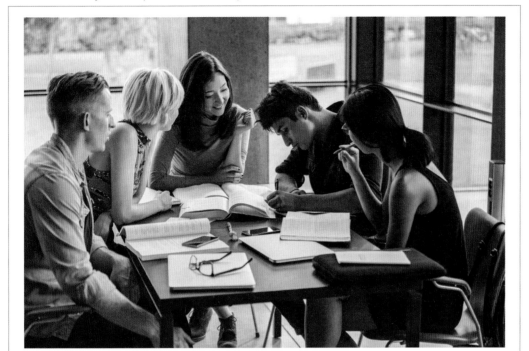

Source: Alamy Stock Photo/Ammentorp Photography

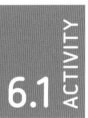

Reflection on cultural perspectives

Cultural values are what shape society, and shape and influence the people who live within that society. Reflect on your personal social and cultural perspectives and answer the following questions:

1   What biases have you identified?

2   How might your perspectives impact on your work as an HSA?

3   How could you improve on any negative bias you may have?

Work with an awareness of your limitations

If you lack cultural awareness it is likely to have a harmful effect on your working relationships and may find expression as:

*   stereotyping – when one person judges another person or group based on the opinions or experiences of themselves or others that are not necessarily accurate and are often oversimplified and offensive

*   discrimination – when a person is treated in an unfair or different manner to others because of defining factors including, but not limited to, gender, race, sexuality, religion, age and marital status (discussed in more detail later in this chapter).

> **Discrimination**
> Treating a person or people unfairly due to their age, gender, race, religion, sexuality, marital status etc.

Stereotyping

Negative or stereotypical comments can cause conflict with other workers and patients and should be avoided. Stereotyping happens when people have a limited understanding of differences and is based on unfair or untrue assumptions about a particular group of people. Though there are both positive and negative **stereotypes**, many are offensive and should be avoided. Applying stereotypes can mean that assumptions are made, often incorrectly, about individuals. It can lead to particular cultural groups being treated as a single entity rather than as being made up of individual people.

Stereotype

A generalised idea or image about a person or thing that is often oversimplified and offensive.

As you work with other team members, you need to be aware of any negative comments and stereotyping. You need to show some understanding of the cultural background of the person making the comments and be conscious of the impact of the comment in terms of the hurt and stress it can create. Stereotypical comments show a lack of respect to team members and those in your care.

ACTIVITY 6.2

Stereotyping

Every race, culture, country, religion and community has a stereotype. It is a way of oversimplifying how groups of people behave. Examples of stereotypes include:

- all Italians are good cooks
- all Americans are obsessed with guns
- all Africans can dance
- girls play with dolls and boys play with trucks
- people who wear glasses are smart.
  Consider stereotyping and respond to the following:

1 List any additional positive or negative stereotypes in society you can think of.

2 Evaluate the positives and negatives of using stereotypes in society, such as understanding an individual based on common characteristics (positive) to racism (negative).

Personal assumptions

You should not allow your own assumptions to determine the level or type of support that you provide to patients. You need to remain non-judgemental about the needs and preferences of the people in your care. The care you give should be based on your patient's culture, not your bias. This is known as **transcultural strategies of care**.

Transcultural strategies of care

Care that acknowledges an individual's culture, values, beliefs and practices.

Transcultural care is based on the following principles:

- Patients are there to receive appropriate care and support.
- Patient differences are based on their diverse backgrounds and they have varying attitudes, values and beliefs that can be expressed in a number of ways.
- Individualised care plans should consider these differences so as to provide the best outcomes for patients.
- It is important to identify the specific culture and other aspects of the patient's cultural diversity when developing their individualised care plan.

Transcultural strategies of care include discovering what is different and what is similar about individuals in terms of their culture, and using this information to provide the most appropriate standard of nursing support. Being aware of your personal assumptions and avoiding stereotyping will help you improve your understanding of diversity and promote appropriate transcultural care.

Use reflection to support inclusivity and understanding of others

To use inclusive work practices means that you actively support and embrace people from a diverse range of backgrounds – see Figure 6.3; statistics from the Australian Bureau of Statistics (ABS) (2022a; 2022b). Valuing the benefits of diverse cultures can improve the workplace and performance of the organisation. By reflecting and recognising individual and cultural differences, you are developing cultural competence and positively contributing to the wellbeing of the patients in your care.

FIGURE 6.3 Just over a quarter (27.6%) of the Australian population were born overseas, and almost half have a parent who was born overseas (48.2%). Over 5.5 million people use a language other than English at home

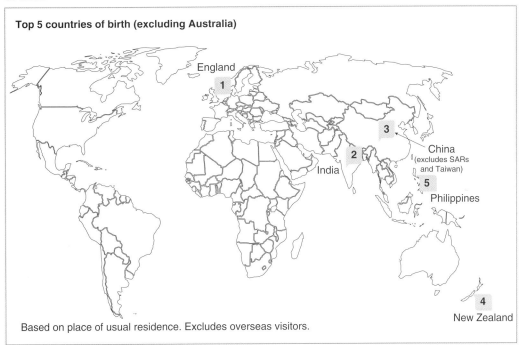

Top 5 countries of birth (excluding Australia)

Based on place of usual residence. Excludes overseas visitors.

Source: Australian Bureau of Statistics (2022). Cultural diversity: Census. Retrieved 17 October 2022 from https://www.abs.gov.au/statistics/people/people-and-communities/cultural-diversity-census/latest-release. Licensed under a Creative Commons Attribution 4.0 International licence, https://creativecommons.org/licenses/by/4.0/

Cultural competence

Cultural competence is the ability to understand, communicate with and effectively interact with people across cultures. It is based on:

- valuing cultural diversity through your interactions with patients and co-workers
- being aware of your own cultural attributes
- being aware of the dynamics when different cultures interact
- having a knowledge of different cultures and their attributes
- being able to adapt care to reflect an understanding of different cultures.

Cultural competence
The ability of systems to provide care to patients with diverse values, beliefs and behaviours.

ACTIVITY 6.3

Self-assessment of your cultural competence

Explore your cultural competence by indicating 'Never', 'Sometimes' or 'Always' against each awareness statement. How you answer will help you identify both areas of strength and those that need further development to help you develop cultural competence. Remember that cultural competence is a process, and that learning is a lifelong process.

AWARENESS
I view human differences as positive
I have a clear sense of my own ethnic, cultural and racial identity
I am aware that to learn more about others I need to understand and share my own culture
I am aware of the assumptions I hold about people of different cultures
I am aware of the stereotypes I believed to be true and have developed personal strategies to reduce the harm they may cause
I am aware of how my culture informs my judgements
I take advantage of learning opportunities about cultural differences

Identify and act on ways to improve your own self and social awareness

Social awareness allows you to understand and respond to the needs of others. It can improve our judgement and help us identify opportunities for professional development and personal growth. Identifying and acting on ways to improve yourself and your social awareness can be helped by the following strategies.

Develop empathy

Empathy is being aware of and sensitive to another's feelings and emotions. You can use a range of strategies to develop empathy, including:

- putting aside your views and trying to see things from the other person's point of view
- having an open mind and attitude
- thinking about the feelings of others
- being prepared to change direction as the other person's thoughts and feelings also change.

Develop emotional intelligence

Emotional intelligence

The ability to both manage your own emotions and understand the emotions of people around you.

Emotional intelligence is about being able to manage both your own emotions and others' emotional responses. To develop emotional intelligence, you must be willing to reflect on your own performance and behaviour, and then manage your responses. Strategies include:

- managing your negative emotions so that they do not affect your judgement
- identifying situations that make you feel uncomfortable, and trying to change your behaviour to make the best of the situation
- managing stress
- demonstrating positive body language

- listening and delaying your responses
- expressing your thoughts and feelings
- identifying your strengths and weaknesses for improvement.

Participate in informal learning

If you have open, trusting relationships with the people who know you, you can ask them for feedback about your social awareness. This will help you develop your strengths and identify your weaknesses. As a lifelong learner, you should also take part in any discussions and workshops on cultural diversity issues. This is particularly important where informal learning examines cultural issues that impact on the support you provide for the patients in your care.

Participate in formal learning

It is essential that formal learning in health care incorporates education about cultural diversity. Many organisations include cultural training as part of their mandatory training requirements, and qualifications now include information on working with people from diverse backgrounds, including co-workers and patients and their families. Studying this subject matter can improve cultural awareness.

Access resource material and networks

You can access a great amount of material on cultural diversity on the internet. There are cultural profiles specifically developed for the health sector that provide useful information on aspects of culture including diverse values and attitudes, pre-migration experiences and communication preferences. The departments of health in each state and territory have a variety of multicultural resources for health professionals. There are also many networks that you can access for cultural advice, including ethnic-specific organisations, community groups and multicultural organisations. The Australian Department of Health Partners in Culturally Appropriate Care (PICAC) provides training, workshops and resources to assist 'aged care service providers to deliver care that meets the needs of culturally and linguistically diverse (CALD) people' (Australian Department of Health and Aged Care, 2022).

Multiculturalism
Incorporating ideas, beliefs or people from many different countries and cultural backgrounds.

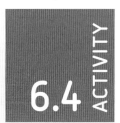

6.4 ACTIVITY

Support networks

There are many national, state and territory organisations that you can source when developing your cultural awareness.

1   Identify three examples of consultation and support networks that can help provide culturally appropriate services in your workplace.

2   What informal learning can you undertake to develop your social awareness?

3   Identify any formal cultural awareness programs or training activities in the facility where you are working or undertaking work experience.

2 APPRECIATE DIVERSITY AND DEMONSTRATE INCLUSIVENESS

Healthcare providers need to demonstrate an appreciation of diversity and inclusiveness by recognising and using the unique insights, perspectives and backgrounds of people from CALD backgrounds. This will promote a more harmonious workplace in which people can be understood and accepted for their different backgrounds and beliefs. Avoiding discrimination and providing equal opportunities will lead to a safer environment for both patients and the healthcare team.

Value and respect diversity and inclusiveness

As an HSA, you need to be aware of the cultural and diverse backgrounds of the people in your care, as well as of your co-workers, and to be sensitive to their values and attitudes. You can demonstrate how you value and respect diversity and promote inclusive practice by:

Inclusive practice
Not discriminating against people or treating them unfairly on the basis of differences when caring for them.

- learning about and showing respect for diversity
- listening to the narratives that patients and team members tell about their lives
- valuing and celebrating different cultures and diversity in work teams
- ensuring cultural consideration is shown in patient care plans
- ensuring cultural consideration is shown in palliative care
- showing an awareness of religious and spiritual beliefs
- showing an awareness of legislation and policies
- identifying risks and promoting protective factors for marginalised groups.

Show respect for diversity

Do not assume that everyone shares the same cultural values as you. Do not automatically assume you know where someone was born, what language they speak or their cultural or health practices. Statements or comments about your assumptions may create confusion or hostility, which may then impede working relationships. Consider that each person's attitudes and values are a product of their experiences and learning. This may be reflected by their attitudes on issues such as the role of women, immigration and sexual orientation, which may be quite different from your attitudes as an individual. However, you should approach such differences as areas for understanding, and respect people's diversity.

Sexual orientation and gender identity

This includes lesbian, gay, bisexual, transgender, queer, intersex and asexual people. Showing respect for these diverse genders and orientations is vital in providing effective support and can include:

- asking how a patient or colleague would like to be addressed
- avoid assuming a patient's gender identity or sexual orientation
- being open-minded about each person's orientation or background
- expanding your own knowledge about sexual orientation and gender identity.

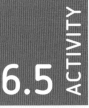

Respecting diversity

Andrew Cummings is aged 89. He served in the infantry during the Vietnam War. He was extremely fit and healthy but is now in acute care after a major stroke that has affected his mobility. The registered nurse (RN) has designated Sophie Chang, the HSA, to look after Andrew and to provide support for his showering, dressing and eating. Sophie was born in Australia and is of Asian descent.

Andrew is quite rude to Sophie when she assists him with his shower. He makes some inappropriate statements that include referring to his wartime service as 'fighting Asians'. Finally, he comments that he doesn't know how he can put up with one of them looking after him.

After this outburst, the RN gives Sophie the option of being reallocated to other patients where she will not be subject to Andrew's prejudice. Sophie declines and decides to talk with Andrew about his views and his attitude towards her. She explains to Andrew that she respects his army service and can understand his anger but that she does not approve of his racist views. She mentions that her father also served overseas and was a flight sergeant in the RAAF during the Vietnam War.

One week later, the RN asks Sophie how she is getting on with Andrew. Sophie states that Andrew no longer treats her badly but is now showing her respect and has even apologised for his previous behaviour.

1   How does this case study show that age and generational factors are important to consider when caring for a person with different attitudes and beliefs?

2   Why was it important for Sophie to ask Andrew about his experiences and views?

3   Why is it important to acknowledge differences in attitudes and values even though they may differ from your own?

4   Discuss the importance of not overreacting because of your own cultural values.

Listen to the narratives

People like to be storytellers. Narratives are stories, and the narratives that people outline about past and present events that affect them are intended to help them make sense of what is happening around them. They are important clues to cultural identity.

Within the narratives, there are values and attitudes that support rituals and celebrations that may be ethnic in origin. Listening to the stories helps you establish a better understanding of the patient's needs and identify future requirements for their care plans, such as diet and providing for spiritual needs. Listening to the narratives told by team members also helps you understand their attitudes, values and traditions, which will improve your working relationships with the team.

Value and celebrate different cultures and diversity within work teams

It is important to value and openly celebrate the multicultural aspect of your work team. Acknowledging religious celebrations, rituals, national holidays and festivals is one important way of bringing the work team together, with a full appreciation of the culture of the event (see Figure 6.4). Valuing and celebrating different cultures and diversity also helps overcome feelings of isolation by individuals who may be in a small minority and feel ignored by others.

FIGURE 6.4 One way in which cultural diversity is celebrated in Australia

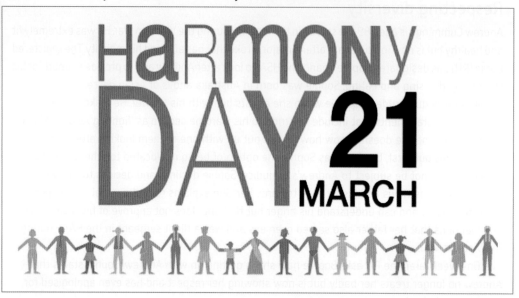

Source: © Commonwealth of Australia, released under a CC BY 3.0 AU licence

Celebrating cultural diversity

1 Identify three religious and/or national celebrations relating to various ethnic backgrounds that would be appropriate to celebrate in the workplace.

2 Explain what you could do to acknowledge religious and/or national celebrations in a healthcare environment.

3 Explain the benefits of valuing and celebrating diverse cultures.

Ensure cultural considerations are shown in patient care plans

The nursing theorist Madeline Leininger believed that cultural assessment was necessary before planning and implementing care. This included conducting cultural assessments on all patients and creating collaborative networks. She stated that patient satisfaction with nursing care and outcomes would be positively related to nursing care that incorporated cultural values and practices (Nursing Theory, 2016).

In assessing cultural beliefs, healthcare providers should consider a range of areas, including the patient's perception of illness and treatment; their social organisation, including family; communication behaviours and expressions of pain; healthcare beliefs; and past experiences with care. Healthcare providers should start systematic cultural assessments and culture-specific care plans at the first patient contact and should regularly re-evaluate and modify these during interactions with patients, families and communities.

Some examples of cultural considerations in care plans include:

- ensuring that food preparation is based on required religious considerations such as halal or kosher certification
- positioning a bed so that the immobile patient is facing the correct way for praying to Mecca

- spending time with an Aboriginal patient and their family and/or Elders to understand the patient's needs and integrate tradition-based views on medical treatment and nursing into their care plan
- using same-gender personal care (showering, bathing) support for female patients, when possible
- placing a Koran in an incubator or cot, or rosary beads on top of an incubator or cot, to accommodate religious requests.

For long-term patients, you can embrace cultural diversity by celebrating rituals, national holidays and festivals. This can create a culturally and psychologically safe environment for them.

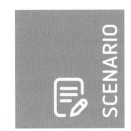

Appropriate cultural considerations

Brian, an HSA, was delegated care of Mrs Abad, who is a Muslim. Mr Abad, her husband, refused to allow Brian to enter his wife's room to take her to the shower. Brian recognised the cultural beliefs of the couple, where modesty and sexual segregation must always be maintained. He realised that it was inappropriate for him to perform care that intruded on Mrs Abad's modesty and asked a female healthcare worker to assist with the shower. In this way, Brian demonstrated culturally respectful care. He raised the issue at handover and it was noted in the patient's care plan.

1   What other adjustments to his practices could Brian consider for the Muslim culture in a healthcare environment?
2   What other healthcare staff should be made aware of Mrs Abad's culture?

Ensure cultural considerations are shown in palliative care

Culturally appropriate palliative care requires you to understand and respect death, dying and bereavement from different cultural perspectives. Suggestions for the healthcare team to understand culturally relevant palliative care include the following:

- be willing to allow individuals and their families to discuss issues around death and dying
- support the cultural, linguistic and spiritual needs of individuals and their families, including rituals and practices around death and dying
- support the cultural and religious attitudes to prescribed treatments and medications
- support the need for family members to participate in decision-making about care and treatment
- ensure palliative care patients and their families have access to culturally appropriate emotional and spiritual support.

You need to ensure that cultural factors are considered and respected at the end of life. If a patient or the family notifies a healthcare worker about religious or cultural needs about death, the worker needs to document these in the care plan and communicate them to the entire health team (Palliative Care Australia, n.d.). Refer to Chapter 15, 'Deliver care services using a palliative approach', for more on beliefs and patient care at death.

Show an awareness of religious and spiritual beliefs

Culturally appropriate spiritual support helps patients express their spirituality in an open and non-judgemental environment. While religious and spiritual beliefs vary widely, it is important to help maintain the practices, beliefs and networks for each specific religion. You can demonstrate this by ensuring religious resources, clergy or chaplains are readily available.

SCENARIO

Showing spiritual awareness

When Heather, the HSA, entered the room of her Iranian patient, she found her huddled on the floor, mumbling. When she tried to help her up, the patient became visibly upset. She spoke minimal English, so Heather listened and spent time understanding her needs. The patient said that she had been praying and was practising her religion in the traditional manner. Heather reported this to the RN and they provided the patient with some privacy and a floor mat during certain times of the day so she could pray.

1 How could the religious beliefs of this patient be considered if they were bed-bound?
2 How could Heather accommodate the prayer practices of the patient's visitors?
3 Why is it important for the HSA to report the incident to the supervisor?

Show an awareness of international, national and state or territory government policies

Under most international agreements and Commonwealth and state or territory legislation, it is illegal to discriminate against people because of their cultural background. The Universal Declaration of Human Rights (United Nations, 1948) preserves the humanistic ideals of equality and freedom of the individual in international law. This is reflected in the Commonwealth Government's (2018) statement, 'Multicultural Australia: United, strong, successful', which 'renews and reaffirms the Government's commitment to a multicultural Australia, in which racism and discrimination have no place' (p. 3). This statement emphasises:

- sharing of values, rights and responsibilities
- building a safe and secure Australia with a shared vision for the future
- encouraging economic and social participation of new arrivals
- continuing to build harmonious and socially cohesive communities.

State governments actively promote the benefits of cultural diversity. In Western Australia, all public sector agencies are expected to provide high-quality services and programs for all people. This is highlighted by their Multicultural Policy Framework (WA Government, 2020), which creates inclusive and welcoming communities for everyone to participate equitably and has the following priority areas:

- harmonious and inclusive communities
- culturally responsive policies, programs and services
- economic, social, cultural, civic and political participation.

As an HSA, you need to be aware of:

- the principles of cultural diversity, which are now embraced by all governments
- any state or territory reporting requirements that apply to your health facility
- policies and strategies on cultural diversity as they apply within your health facility.

Universal Declaration of Human Rights
The internationally agreed declaration stating that all people everywhere have the same human rights that no-one can take away from them.

Identify risks and promote protective factors in marginalised groups

Marginalised groups are a mix of people with economic, social, early-life and health disadvantage. This can include people from CALD backgrounds, people with disability and people with mental health issues. It may also include those who are socially isolated or suffering financial hardship. These groups can be at risk of physical, emotional and mental health problems because of exclusion and negative attitudes. Promoting resilience, social support, self-esteem and positive coping strategies may help mitigate some of these factors.

Marginalised groups
Specific groups of people who have been pushed to the lower or outer edge of society.

Contribute to workplace and professional relationships based on diversity and inclusiveness

Professional relationships should include an appreciation of diverse cultures. A workplace team that has diverse backgrounds and cultural values is helpful for ensuring transcultural care. These cross-cultural teams have wide-ranging skills and knowledge necessary to complete all patient tasks involving care and support. They are often more adaptable and achieve goals more efficiently.

As a member of a work team, you should develop workplace and professional relationships based on an appreciation of diversity and inclusiveness by:
- acknowledging and caring about cultural differences, including the attitudes, values and beliefs of other team members
- sharing your understanding of cultural diversity
- developing trust and support with individuals to make it easier for them to talk to you
- encouraging discussion of diversity to avoid conflict in the work team
- prioritising professional development on working with diversity
- developing professional relationships with experts in various cultures to increase the cultural competence of individuals and the work team.

Developing cultural competence should be emphasised during orientation, during team meetings and during handover when issues of cultural diversity can be raised.

Workplace diversity

1   Identify the cultural and diverse groups in your workplace or classroom environment. These diversities can include culture, gender, expertise, language, ethnicity and spiritual beliefs.

2   Identify the benefits of diversity within these groups.

3   Identify challenges that could be faced within these groups

6.7 ACTIVITY

Use work practices that make environments safe

Work practices must comply with legislation so that the patients and healthcare team are in a safe environment that is free from discrimination. Legislation includes anti-discrimination, equal employment opportunity, and work health and safety regulations. You need to ensure that work practices are based around duty of care, which is aimed at preventing harm or injury to the people in your care. You may cause harm to cultural groups through omission or deliberate action, as outlined in Figure 6.5.

Discrimination

You should be aware that the Commonwealth *Racial Discrimination Act 1975* makes it unlawful to publicly offend, insult, humiliate or intimidate another person or group of people because of their race, colour, or national or ethnic origin. This includes making gestures or producing drawings, images or written publications such as in newspapers, leaflets and websites.

FIGURE 6.5 Harm caused by omission or by deliberate actions

CAUSE OF HARM	EXAMPLE
Omission	Failing to allow certain rituals involving bereavement and the care of the recently deceased
	Ignoring these practices can create psychological stress, which may also lead to physical illness
Deliberate actions	Telling insulting jokes about particular racial groups
	Allowing this can harm a person and cause them to feel unsafe
	Statements about discrimination, bullying and harassment are covered under the Commonwealth *Work Health and Safety Act 2011*, as well as the *Australian Human Rights Commission Act 1986*

All Australian states and territories have racial discrimination legislation similar to the *Racial Discrimination Act 1975*. Penalties for breaches of Commonwealth, state and territory legislation will depend on the severity of the offence. For instance, in New South Wales there is a maximum penalty of a $10 000 fine or six months' imprisonment for an individual and $100 000 for a corporation.

Work-based practices should make environments safe and culturally appropriate, non-discriminatory, and free of bias, stereotyping, racism and prejudice. Strategies to eliminate bias and discrimination may include:

- encouraging involvement in cross-cultural work teams
- ensuring that cross-cultural employees are represented on health and safety committees
- contributing to a workplace free of culturally insensitive literature, posters and signage
- ensuring that decision-making on cultural events and occasions reflects the cultural diversity of patients and team members
- acknowledging and celebrating differences as being positive
- encouraging individuals to seek advice from supervisors and/or referring to other professionals when required.

Equal employment opportunity

Federal, state and territory equal employment opportunity (EEO) laws state that it is unlawful to discriminate against a person in the area of employment. This includes recruitment, during employment and termination of employment. Recruitment, selection and promotion practices must be open, competitive and based on merit. This ensures that every employee regardless of race, religious belief, age or gender is given the same opportunities and advantages.

Human rights

The Australian Human Rights Commission, formed in 1986, has an important role in promoting and safeguarding diversity by:

- resolving complaints of discrimination or breaches of human rights under federal laws
- holding public inquiries into human rights issues of national importance
- developing human rights education programs and resources for schools, workplaces and the community

- providing independent legal advice to assist courts in cases that involve human rights principles
- providing advice and submissions to parliaments and governments to develop laws, policies and programs
- undertaking and coordinating research into human rights and discrimination issues.

Australian Human Rights Commission, n.d.

Direct and indirect discrimination

Direct discrimination means that a person is very obviously being treated unfairly or unequally. Indirect discrimination is not as obvious and occurs when a work condition or rule disadvantages one group of people more than another.

Identify whether each of the following examples is direct or indirect discrimination.

6.8 ACTIVITY

EXAMPLE
All information about workplace health and safety is written in English
The facility refuses to hire an aged person
An organisation refuses to employ a person because he has disclosed his mental health disorder
Culturally insensitive signs are displayed in the workplace
Failure to provide kosher food for a Jewish patient
Refusal to provide same-gender care for a person even though their religious or cultural beliefs require it

3 COMMUNICATE WITH PEOPLE FROM DIVERSE BACKGROUNDS AND SITUATIONS

Respecting people from diverse backgrounds includes using all forms of communication to develop and maintain effective relationships, mutual trust and confidence. This includes both verbal and non-verbal forms of communication, and engaging interpreters to assist where there are language barriers. Knowing, respecting and understanding another culture can help with the communication process and also develop your skills.

Show respect for diversity in your communication

Culturally appropriate communication helps to develop and maintain effective relationships and mutual trust and confidence with your co-workers, patients and significant others. An awareness of different cultural traditions in the form of beliefs, behaviours and celebrations will enable you to communicate more effectively. The following list contains some examples of different cultural traditions that should be considered when communicating in the health environment:

- In hospital, Muslim women may wish to remain as fully clothed as possible, and many will choose to be seen only by female health professionals. Men may prefer to keep covered from waist to knee and be cared for only by male staff.

- Mediterranean people tend to express their emotions and use gestures and vocalisation to express joy, sadness and grief more openly and freely than other cultures. For many Mediterranean people, a high level of physical contact is natural and normal.
- Vietnamese people consider that the body operates in a delicate balance between the hot and cold qualities of food and medicine. Before seeking or complying with treatment, Vietnamese people may consider the effect that the treatment will have on the balance of these elements.
- Among some Asian cultures, maintaining harmony is an important value. Therefore, there is a strong emphasis on avoiding conflict and direct confrontation. Because of respect for authority, disagreement with the recommendations of healthcare professionals is often avoided.
- Among Chinese patients, because the behaviour of the individual reflects on the family, mental illness or any behaviour that indicates lack of self-control may produce shame and guilt. As a result, Chinese patients may be reluctant to discuss symptoms of mental illness.
- The extended family of Pacific Islanders has significant influence, and the oldest male in the family is often the decision-maker and spokesperson. Older family members are respected and their authority often goes unquestioned.
- Australia's healthcare system is quite different from that in Latin America, and patients from Latin American countries may expect different care. They may not be used to having to obtain referrals to see specialists or prescriptions for medications.

Communicating with Aboriginal and Torres Strait Islander people

Healthcare workers need to understand the history and story of Aboriginal and Torres Strait Islander peoples and how it impacts on their lives. This can help when developing culturally appropriate programs and ways of servicing Aboriginal and Torres Strait Islander communities. By understanding Aboriginal and Torres Strait Islander patients' needs and considering all aspects of their lives, including cultural traditions and commitments, positive outcomes can be achieved.

Some Aboriginal and Torres Strait Islander people do not speak, read or write English fluently, so consider using alternative methods of communication, such as pictures, sign language or interpreters if available. Where possible, it is recommended that services are provided by a healthcare worker of the same gender as the patient because gender-related barriers can lead to difficulty in obtaining information.

Extended periods of silence during conversations can be considered normal in Aboriginal and Torres Strait Islander cultures. These periods are used to listen and show respect. It is important to observe the silence and body language to determine when to start speaking (Queensland Health, 2015). The aspects of Aboriginal and Torres Strait Islander cultures in Figure 6.6 need to be considered when communicating with Aboriginal and Torres Strait Islander patients and their families.

FIGURE 6.6 Aboriginal and Torres Strait Islander cultural considerations

Kinship	Care for someone is traditionally covered by the framework of the kinship system through family connections and the Elders as the leaders of the communities
	Health facilities should expect women to have many visitors because this is a custom of kinship. This should be supported as best as possible
Health care	Do not expect clients to discuss scars and wounds on their bodies. These could represent initiation, conflict or grief
Sociocultural barriers	Different cultural understandings based on language, or the emotional consequences in accepting the need for support, may create barriers
Knowledge about rights and services	Poor knowledge of entitlements, rights and powers of appeal, and a poorly developed system of advocacy, are consistently identified as barriers to obtaining services
Limited access to services	Even when services are available, their use can be limited by factors that may include a reluctance to use mainstream medical services

Source: Adapted from Deakin Rural Health (2019). Practical considerations for health professionals working with Aboriginal clients. Retrieved 17 October 2022 from http://www.deakinruralhealth.com.au/practical-considerations-for-health-professionals-working-with-aboriginal-clients/

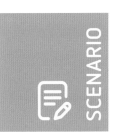

SCENARIO

Aboriginal cultural traditions and effect on patient care strategies – Joseph, DjaDjaWurrung Elder

Joseph is an active and highly respected DjaDjaWurrung Elder living north of Bendigo in Wedderburn, Victoria. He is 45 years of age and has suffered a brain haemorrhage. This has led to his individualised support plan involving rehabilitation and reliance on others for some activities of daily living. His plan includes help from local Aboriginal health workers in Bendigo and strategies that still allow Joseph to pass on stories and fulfil his role as an Elder. The plan also includes visiting cultural sites on traditional DjaDjaWurrung land in parts of north-western Victoria, such as Mount Korong near Wedderburn (see Figure 6.7). This provides positive benefits for Joseph's social and emotional wellbeing.

FIGURE 6.7 Mount Korong

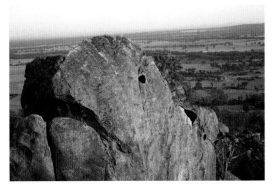

Source: Darryl Arnott

1   Why is it important to take a holistic approach to Joseph's care?
2   How does visiting cultural sites benefit Joseph's social and emotional wellbeing?

Use verbal and non-verbal communication for effective relationships

Verbal and non-verbal communication is used to establish, develop and maintain effective relationships. Verbal communication includes choice of words and how they are spoken in terms of clarity, tone, pitch and the pause between words. When working with CALD clients and co-workers you may need to use a range of specific strategies to support communication. It is also important not to make assumptions about a person's language proficiency, which can vary.

Important strategies include:

* actively listen to what has been said and respond appropriately
* use questions to start conversations, to solve problems and to demonstrate an interest in what others have to say
* seek clarification when you are unsure of responses
* use interpersonal skills to relate to and bond with other people and be considerate and respectful
* do not over-emphasise the language barrier; treat it in the same way as all other communication barriers
* use non-verbal communication to reinforce spoken words, such as facial expressions, eye contact, gestures and the position of yourself physically in relation to others.

While these features of effective communication are common to most cultures, there are some differences that apply across cultures, especially to non-verbal communication. These are highlighted in Figure 6.8 and include posture, gesturing (head nodding, handshakes, pointing), eye contact and touch.

FIGURE 6.8 Perception of non-verbal communication

ACTION	AUSTRALIA	OTHER CULTURES
Posture	Indicates how you feel	Hands in pockets shows disrespect in different cultures Sitting with crossed legs is considered offensive in some cultures
Head nodding	Yes or no	Could be different; for example, in the Middle East, down is agreement and up is disagreement Head up and down in Japan indicates someone is listening
Handshake	Used as a greeting	May be frowned upon in some cultures and an embrace may be preferred
Pointing	Use of a finger or hand to indicate a location, thing or person	Pointing with one finger is considered to be rude in some cultures; Asians typically use their entire hand to point to something
Eye contact	Shows you are listening	In many Asian cultures, avoiding eye contact is seen as a sign of respect
Touch	Used as affectionate gesture	In the Middle East, the left hand is reserved for bodily hygiene and should not be used to touch another or transfer objects

Source: Adapted from Adetunji, R. & Sze, K. (2012). Understanding non-verbal communication across cultures: A symbolic interactionism approach. i-Come International Conference on Communication and Media 2012, Penang, Malaysia, 1–3 November 2012.

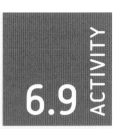

Listening skills

Active listening is a valuable tool to enhance communication. Answer the following questions regarding listening.

1   What is the impact on communication when the person just listens and does not exchange information?

2   What could be the cause of a listener not contributing to the communication?

3   How can non-verbal signals encourage the speaker?

6.9 ACTIVITY

Use effective strategies to communicate where there are language barriers

Each culture has its own verbal and written language for communication. Language barriers can exist where there are differences in accent due to speed and pronunciation of language, grammar and sentence structure. This can make it difficult to understand what the speaker is saying. Other barriers include jargon, which is the language peculiar to a particular trade, profession or group; or slang, which includes words that are not a part of standard vocabulary and are used informally. Other language barriers and strategies for communication are discussed in the following. You can also refer to Chapter 4, 'Communicate and work in health and community services', for more on effective communication.

People with inadequate language skills

Where barriers exist due to inadequate language skills, use effective strategies to communicate in the most efficient way possible by:

- speaking slowly and enunciating words carefully
- using short, rather than complex, sentences
- pausing to check for understanding and to obtain a response
- rephrasing your words
- using appropriate gestures and facial and physical expressions to support meaning
- asking simple questions.

People with limited or no vocal ability

Other communication barriers will occur if patients have to rely on augmentative or alternative communication techniques. Augmentative communication refers to the use of aids or techniques to enhance speech if words are not clearly articulated and understood. Alternative communication refers to communication techniques that are used if vocal ability is lacking. However, the terms are often used together, and an augmentative and alternative communication (AAC) system consists of a combination of methods used for communication based on the particular needs of each patient.

Effective strategies should aim to meet each individual's needs by selecting whatever is required to enable communication. For example, one individual might use cards with written words, while another might require a device with speech software activated by pointing at symbols (see Figure 6.9). A head pointer enables a patient with limited mobility to activate the computer by using a pointer attached to their head instead of using the mouse or the arrow keys.

FIGURE 6.9 A tablet with symbol-based speech software can aid communication

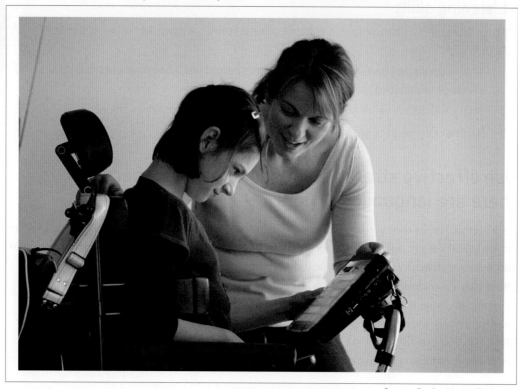

Source: Fairfax Media/Eddie Jim

Communicating with signs and images

1   Many signs are designed to communicate with people regardless of the language they speak. Identify and describe the meaning of signs in your workplace that use symbols instead of words.

2   The national interpreter symbol is endorsed by the Commonwealth, state and territory governments. What is the purpose of this symbol?

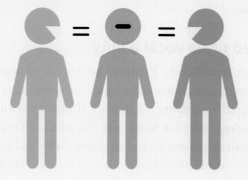

People with disabilities

You should always be conscious of any barriers to communication due to diseases and/or developmental and acquired disabilities. This includes patients with physical, intellectual, vision and hearing disabilities. In general, you should:

- respond positively to all attempts at communication
- provide plenty of time for patients to communicate to you
- support the patient to lead the conversation, rather than yourself
- do not take control and finish off the conversation; not only does this show a lack of respect, it also creates a situation where the message is likely to be misinterpreted
- avoid distractions that might interfere with a patient's communication and your ability to listen to what is being said
- focus only on the patient with whom you are communicating
- check for understanding by asking open-ended questions that require an extended response
- be prepared to rephrase information by using different words
- make sure that you are facing a person if they are hearing impaired so that they can read your lips if required
- be mindful of the sound level of your voice with those who are visually impaired.

Seek assistance from interpreters or others

If you are unable to communicate effectively because of a language difficulty, you may need to seek assistance from a professional interpreter (see Figure 6.10). However, you should recognise that the use of an interpreter does not always reflect the non-verbal aspects of the translation. It also needs to be acknowledged that, even when a professional interpreter is being used, it is unlikely that there will be an exact match between the words in different languages.

FIGURE 6.10 Professional interpreters can assist communication

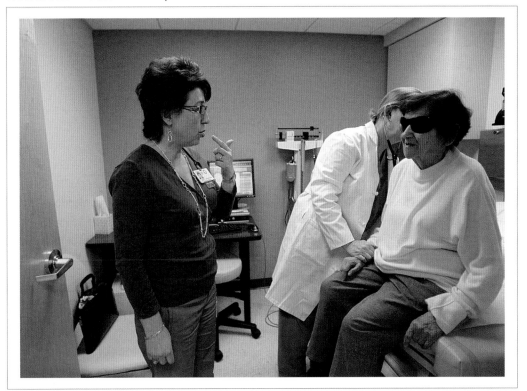

Source: Getty Images / Suzanne Kreiter / *The Boston Globe*

Interpreters are not responsible for the analysis of information; their role requires that they do not comment or provide advice but only relay information. Professional interpreters are part of the healthcare team and are bound by professional ethics such as confidentiality and impartiality. When using an interpreter, the following suggestions are recommended:

- Find out what language, dialect or ethnicity your patient prefers. Patients might reject a particular ethnic group within their country.
- A professional interpreter should be used to increase the likelihood that the translation will be accurate. They are likely to be highly fluent in both languages and understand the importance of interpreting the verbal *and* non-verbal communication (body language).
- Make sure that the interpreter is briefed on the purpose of the communication and understands the context of the meeting and the outcomes being sought.
- Avoid using family members or children as interpreters.
- Try to use an interpreter of the same sex as the patient. For instance, there is likely to be less embarrassment if the interpreter is a female when a female patient is talking about personal problems.
- Remember that the communication is not with the interpreter. Look at the patient you are communicating with, not the interpreter. The role of the interpreter is to assist the communication process and not to take over the role of communicating from the patient.
- Where an on-site interpreter is not available, you may be able to use a telephone interpreter.

ACTIVITY 6.11

Role of professional interpreters

Respond to the following regarding professional interpreters:

1. Look up the health interpreting service in your area and list the services that they provide.
2. Find out the circumstances where professional interpreters are used as well as the procedures that are followed.

4 PROMOTE UNDERSTANDING ACROSS DIVERSE GROUPS

Miscommunication can occur because of a lack of cultural sensitivity and can result in conflict within the workplace. When healthcare providers are aware of the causes of these miscommunications, they can develop effective strategies to prevent the problem escalating. Resolving differences requires consideration of cultural diversity, tolerance from all involved and professional support when situations escalate beyond your control. Through acknowledgement of culture and collaboration, an understanding can be achieved for the person and the healthcare team.

Identify causes of miscommunication while considering social and cultural diversity

Miscommunication can occur whenever there are cultural differences. They can be due to differences in cultural practice or perception, conflict between different ethnic groups, ethnocentrism, and lack of awareness of illness or treatment. When misunderstandings occur in the workplace, the causes must be identified before a resolution can be achieved.

Communication can also break down because of different perceptions of body language, using jargon, literacy issues or poor listening skills. The stress and/or fear of a hospital environment can also intensify the communication breakdown.

Ethnocentrism

The belief that your own group or culture is better or more important than others is termed ethnocentrism. This leads to making incorrect assumptions about others' behaviour based on your own values and beliefs. It is important to recognise that not everyone shares the same beliefs as you and to treat everyone as individuals.

Figure 6.11 lists some instances of cross-cultural misunderstanding and conflict and provides examples of the identified cause of the conflict. These examples highlight where cultural ignorance and insensitivity can cause misunderstandings.

Ethnocentrism
The belief that your own cultural or ethnic group is superior to others.

FIGURE 6.11 Examples of cross-cultural misunderstanding

MISUNDERSTANDING	EXAMPLE OF IDENTIFIED CAUSE
A family is resentful towards staff	The family had been told not to speak too loudly or to disturb other patients, and not to bring their own food when visiting their son in the hospital
A female patient is embarrassed to be around a male nurse	The HSA was a young male who felt it necessary to look people in the eye when he spoke, and often sat alongside people when he explained how to complete tasks The female patient was recently from Iran where eye contact is not encouraged. She was also expecting a female nurse in accord with her cultural background
A middle-aged patient is dissatisfied with the meals provided to him	The patient was Jewish and would only eat kosher food
A work team has feelings of resentment towards an HSA	The conscientious HSA explained to her team leader that she would need to work her shifts around the Jewish holidays. This needed to be explained to other members of her work team so that it did not become an issue
A 35-year-old patient is fearful and panicking	The patient was told that she needed to go for a dental check at the dental health clinic. Her last experience with a dentist was in Laos, where it was not unusual for teeth extractions to occur without an anaesthetic
A patient who does not speak English is angry	The father had difficulty speaking English, so the RN used his daughter as an interpreter, which caused translation difficulties and was felt not to show respect for the status of the father in the family
The patient is dissatisfied about his care planning	The patient resented the involvement of a male HSA because he felt nursing and other support roles should be carried out by females
A patient is being non-cooperative with showering	Showering was seldom used as a form of cleansing in this patient's country of origin
An Aboriginal family refuses to seek medical help	The family was living a traditional lifestyle and felt that the service did not acknowledge their traditional views on bush medicines
A family whose son died after suffering a stroke is extremely angry	The priest was not called in until it was too late to take confession

Checking communication

Cross-cultural misunderstandings can cause problems with communication. Answer the following questions regarding these misunderstandings:

1   Search the internet to identify cultural differences that can hinder the development of trusting, supportive and helpful relationships.

2   What are the different cultural attitudes towards:
   *   conflict
   *   time management
   *   decision-making
   *   disclosure
   *   pain?

Resolve differences and address difficulties with appropriate people

There are a number of ways to resolve cultural misunderstandings and conflict. Some misunderstandings can be easily resolved when the people involved have an opportunity to explain and clarify. Your approach to resolving misunderstanding and conflict should consider cultural considerations. When promoting understanding across diverse groups, you should take the following four steps:

1   Define the problem by identifying issues that may be causing the conflict, ideally from the viewpoint of both parties.

2   Examine the cultural interpretation by considering the impact of cultural differences and explain to all parties how it is seen from the various viewpoints.

3   Resolve the conflict by gaining commitment and addressing any difficulties. This should bring about a change to the situation that is to the satisfaction of everyone involved. Try to resolve differences sensitively and avoid letting bias or emotions lead the responses.

4   Evaluate and monitor changes to check that conflict no longer applies. If you feel unable to confront the situation directly, or if you are unsure about whether to act on something you have seen, discuss the issue with your supervisor. It is important that action is taken promptly, no matter who is involved in the conflict, or whether the offensive behaviour is directed at you or you witness it happen to someone else.

In some instances, you could use a mediator to avoid direct confrontation. This has the advantage of involving a neutral third party who is more able to remove the emotion and allow each party to focus on a resolution. The mediator will clarify cultural influences by talking privately to each party involved in the misunderstanding in order to avoid direct confrontation. It may be necessary to consult a cultural leader, Aboriginal or Torres Strait Islander Elder, pastoral carer or interpreter, who can assist to resolve misunderstandings in a sensitive way.

Identifying strategies for team members

After reading each of the following cultural issues, identify strategies that may assist the individuals with their needs.

6.13 ACTIVITY

CULTURAL ISSUE
An HSA from Afghanistan is showing signs of considerable stress and anxiety and you suspect it is based on previous traumatic experiences
A young HSA confides to you that he is homosexual, but he is reluctant to tell his other team members
An HSA feels that the acute care facility may have responded to the needs of Muslim patients in terms of transcultural care, but his team has failed to respond to the patient's religious obligations as a Muslim
Joe is from the Torres Strait Islands and claims that he has been subject to racial vilification by another team member

SUMMARY

This chapter examined the importance of diversity as a factor that should be considered when working with patients and the healthcare team. The importance of reflecting on your own cultural perspectives and biases, and using your reflections to promote cultural safety and to work inclusively with patients and team members, was discussed.

By being culturally aware, the healthcare team can form effective workplace and professional relationships and use these diverse skills and knowledge to provide unique patient care. An important aspect included in this chapter was how to communicate effectively by using both verbal and non-verbal communication where language barriers exist.

The last part of the chapter highlighted that cross-cultural misunderstandings and conflict can occur if there is a lack of awareness of the cultural background of individuals. By using the strategies for how to resolve cultural misunderstandings, you will have the necessary tools to provide better support and services to culturally diverse people.

APPLY YOUR KNOWLEDGE

Refugee health services

My experience with refugees started when I accepted a role as an HSA working with a community health team to provide culturally appropriate health care and support in the early periods of settlement.

The African refugees that we looked after had experienced traumatic events such as prolonged periods of deprivation, loss of identify and culture, human rights abuses and the loss of family members. The aims of the community health team were to improve the refugees' health through referral to health networks and offer support and orientation programs.

1   What visible aspects of the refugees' culture would be seen by the HSA and the health team?

2   Working with refugees was a new experience for me and I recognised that I needed to improve my cultural awareness for this group of people. How could this be achieved?

We found that the refugees had needs that were difficult to resolve due to language barriers, anxiety, unfamiliarity with our health system and financial constraints. The community health team worked closely with support networks to help with these challenges.

3   Using the knowledge gained in Chapter 4, 'Communicate and work in health and community services', what strategies could be used where language communication barriers exist?

4   If interpreters are used, what suggestions are recommended to assist with communication?

I found that working in this service gave me an understanding of the complexities that these refugees faced. The entire team worked on reflecting and recognising individual and cultural differences to improve their cultural competence and positively contribute to the care of these groups.

5   What is cultural competence and how can the HSA improve their cultural competence?

6   Understanding the scope of your role as an HSA is essential to performing your role effectively within the healthcare team. How did the HSA demonstrate the scope of their role when working with the refugee services?

◄ REFLECTING ON THE INDUSTRY INSIGHT 💬

1 Which of the following best describes cultural safety in health care?
   a Objectively examining the values, beliefs, traditions and perceptions within other cultures.
   b Our way of life and the values, beliefs and attitudes that we use in health care.
   c Ensuring respect for cultural and social differences in the provision of health care.
   d Knowledge, awareness and acceptance of other cultures.

2 Why is self-reflection important when caring for a person from another culture?
   a Because we may hold attitudes and beliefs that can cause cultural tension and detrimentally influence our care.
   b It allows us to deliver care that is the same for every patient.
   c It will assist in a speedy recovery for the patient.
   d We can discuss our reflections with the team during handover.

3 How can an HSA provide holistic health care for Aboriginal and Torres Strait Islander patients?
   a Allow the family to assist in the provision of health care.
   b Recognise history, customs, cultures and kinship structures when providing health care.
   c Look after the chronic as well as the acute symptoms.
   d Refer the patient to a social worker for further care.

SELF-CHECK QUESTIONS

1 How can stereotyping cause conflict with other workers and patients?

2 Outline how you can improve your cultural competence.

3 How can an HSA improve their social awareness when working with people from different cultures?

4 How can the healthcare team promote inclusivity in the workplace?

5 What are strategies to eliminate bias and discrimination in the workplace?

6 Explain how to overcome communication misunderstandings for clients with intellectual disabilities?

7 Describe the importance of recognising a person's cultural preferences when completing the individual care plan.

8 What are the causes of miscommunication between people from different cultures?

9 How should misunderstandings be resolved where there are cultural differences in work teams?

10 What are your definitions of the following key words and terms that have been used in this chapter?

KEY WORD OR TERM	YOUR DEFINITION
Cultural competence	
Cultural identity	
Discrimination	
Ethnocentrism	
Inclusive practice	
Marginalised groups	
Multiculturalism	
Stereotype	
Transcultural care	
Universal Declaration of Human Rights	

QUESTIONS FOR DISCUSSION

1   Discuss the reasons why Australia has one of the most culturally and linguistically diverse (CALD) populations in the world.
2   Discuss the cultural considerations that should be shown in palliative care.
3   Discuss the experiences that place marginalised CALD groups at risk and how they compensate to minimise these experiences.
4   Discuss how the Australian Human Rights Commission promotes and safeguards diversity.
5   Discuss the issues affecting lesbian, gay, bisexual, transgender, queer, intersex and gender diverse (LGBTQI+) people and how inclusive practice might be achieved.

EXTENSION ACTIVITY

Case study – Dr Elsie Wawelberg

Dr Elsie Wawelberg is 89 years of age. She came to Australia as a 17-year-old refugee and studied medicine at Melbourne University as a mature age student. After graduation, she became a general practitioner in north-eastern Victoria until she retired at the age of 70. She was an extremely popular country GP, was active in her community in the local drama group and was president of the local historical society. After living in the country, Elsie moved to Croydon in the outer eastern suburbs of Melbourne. She has recently had a severe fall and broke her hip and is now in an acute care facility.

Elsie becomes very aggressive when she has to be showered and almost hysterical whenever she sees the ambulance staff in the hospital. The HSA decides to investigate further. She checks with Elsie's nephew and learns that Elsie is Jewish and spent some time as a very young child in a concentration camp in Poland, where she lost both her parents. This resulted in her fear of having showers and a hatred of uniforms. As a result of these findings, the HSA reports to her supervisor and Elsie's care plan is changed. Sponging and bathing is used as opposed to showering, and staff provide plenty of reassurance whenever they attend to her needs. Her care plan reflects her cultural needs and the staff display a respectful attitude when providing personal support and in implementing her care.

1 How does this case study highlight the importance of transcultural patient care?

2 Discuss how Elsie's care plan should be formed with a consideration of her cultural background.

3 Discuss the importance of diversity and inclusiveness in healthcare settings.

4 In groups, choose a culture and research the inclusive care that you would provide in an acute care facility for a patient of this culture.

REFERENCES

Adetunji, R. & Sze, K. (2012). Understanding non-verbal communication across cultures: A symbolic interactionism approach. i-Come International Conference on Communication and Media 2012, Penang, Malaysia, 1–3 November 2012.

Australian Bureau of Statistics (2022a). 2021 Census: Nearly half of Australians have a parent born overseas. Retrieved 17 October 2022 from https://www.abs.gov.au/media-centre/media-releases/2021-census-nearly-half-australians-have-parent-born-overseas

Australian Bureau of Statistics (2022b). Cultural diversity: Census. Retrieved 17 October 2022 from https://www.abs.gov.au/statistics/people/people-and-communities/cultural-diversity-census/latest-release

Australian Department of Health and Aged Care (2022). Partners in Culturally Appropriate Care (PICAC). Retrieved 17 October 2022 from https://www.health.gov.au/initiatives-and-programs/partners-in-culturally-appropriate-care-picac

Australian Government (2018). Multicultural Australia: United, strong, successful. Retrieved 30 March 2022 from https://www.homeaffairs.gov.au/about-us/our-portfolios/multicultural-affairs/about-multicultural-affairs/our-statement

Australian Human Rights Commission (n.d.). About the Commission. Retrieved 13 October 2019 from https://www.humanrights.gov.au/our-work/commission-general/about-commission

Deakin Rural Health (2019). Practical considerations for health professionals working with Aboriginal clients. Retrieved 17 October 2022 from http://www.deakinruralhealth.com.au/practical-considerations-for-health-professionals-working-with-aboriginal-clients/

Milosevic, D., Smith, M. & Cheng, I.-H. (2012). The NSW Refugee Health Service: Improving refugee access to primary care. *Australian Family Physician*, 41(3). Retrieved 17 October 2022 from https://www.racgp.org.au/afp/2012/march/the-nsw-refugee-health-service

Nursing Theory (2016). Cultural care theory. Retrieved 17 October 2022 from http://nursing-theory.org/theories-and-models/leininger-culture-care-theory.php

Palliative Care Australia (n.d.). Palliative care and culturally and linguistically diverse communities – Position Statement. Retrieved 17 October 2022 from https://palliativecare.org.au/wp-content/uploads/2015/08/PCA-Culturally-and-Linguistically-Diverse-Communities-and-Palliative-Care-Position-Statement.pdf

Queensland Health (2015). Communicating effectively with Aboriginal and Torres Strait Islander people. Retrieved 17 October 2022 from https://www.health.qld.gov.au/__data/assets/pdf_file/0021/151923/communicating.pdf

SafeWork NSW (2020). What is cultural safety? Retrieved 11 June 2022 from https://www.safework.nsw.gov.au/safety-starts-here/our-aboriginal-program/culturally-safe-workplaces/what-is-cultural-safety

United Nations (1948). *The Universal Declaration of Human Rights*. Retrieved 5 April 2017 from http://www.un.org/en/universal-declaration-human-rights/

Western Australia Government (2020). WA Multicultural Policy Framework. Retrieved 11 June 2022 from https://www.omi.wa.gov.au/resources-and-statistics/publications/publication/wa-multicultural-policy-framework

ORGANISE PERSONAL WORK PRIORITIES AND DEVELOPMENT

Learning objectives

By the end of this chapter, you should be able to:

1   organise and complete your own work schedule
2   monitor and adjust your own work performance
3   coordinate your personal skill development and learning.

Introduction

This chapter describes the skills and knowledge required to organise work schedules, to monitor and obtain feedback on work performance and to maintain the required levels of competence.

Your work schedule as a health services assistant (HSA) should be based around team and organisational goals and objectives. When prioritising tasks, it is important to do so in terms of the tasks that are considered urgent and important, look at contingencies and use the available business technology equipment efficiently. By implementing these strategies, including self-assessment and responding to feedback received from supervisors and co-workers, you can achieve optimal work performance. It is important to be aware of any stress-related work factors that could impede your performance and use stress management strategies or access the appropriate supports.

The last part of the chapter outlines how personal learning and professional development can improve performance, and the importance of lifelong learning in gaining additional knowledge and skills to improve your workplace practices.

Contingencies
An outline of what you are going to do when something does not go to plan.

Self-assessment
Reflecting on the quality of the work you have done, including strengths and weaknesses.

1 ORGANISE AND COMPLETE OWN WORK SCHEDULE

Your tasks as an HSA should be within your scope of practice as outlined in the position description. Many of these tasks will be based on routines while others will be in response to events that develop while you are working on your shift. All tasks should be prioritised based on achieving important and urgent work goals to ensure that they are completed on time. Completing a schedule for your work with timeframes and priorities can enable you to work effectively in the healthcare team and achieve the organisation's strategic goals.

Ensure work goals, objectives or key performance indicators are understood

Key performance indicator (KPI)

A measurable value that demonstrates how effectively objectives and goals are being met.

When planning work goals, it is important to consider the requirements of the organisation that you work for. Organisational or strategic goals and operational or work goals are the plans of what needs to be achieved; objectives are the actions taken to achieve the goals; and **key performance indicators (KPIs)** measure their effectiveness (see Figure 7.1). In your role as an HSA, you will be working as a member of a multidisciplinary team with registered nurses (RNs) who are responsible for delegating the tasks that allow you to achieve specific goals.

FIGURE 7.1 Goals, objectives and key performance indicators

Goals	Objectives	Key performance indicators
General guidelines that explain what you want to achieve	The strategies or implementation steps to achieve the specific goals	A measurable value that demonstrates how effectively the objectives are being achieved

Organisational or strategic goals

Strategic goals are long-term statements that are often found in the organisation's mission statement or business plan and communicate the general purpose of the organisation and its direction. An example is the Australian Government Department of Health (2019) long-term national health plan to build the world's best health system.

Operational or work goals

Work goals are short-term statements that are designed to achieve the goals of the organisation. They are detailed so that the staff understand what is expected of them, and should be categorised as SMART (specific, measurable, actionable, realistic and time-based) goals (see Figure 7.2). Consideration needs to be given to the resources required and the most effective strategies (objectives) for achievement when planning work goals.

FIGURE 7.2 SMART goals

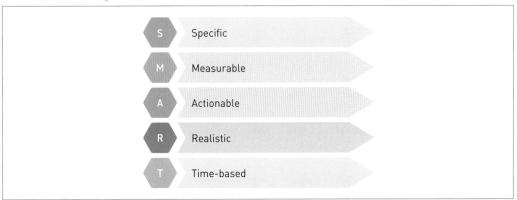

S — Specific

M — Measurable

A — Actionable

R — Realistic

T — Time-based

For example, a hospital has the organisational goal of providing safe and holistic health care to all patients. The work goal may be to reduce pressure areas on patients by improving the pressure area risk assessments. The team objectives would be to complete risk assessments on all patients and implement strategies for pressure sore prevention. These tasks could include regular turning and the use of pressure-relieving devices.

Key performance indicators

A KPI is a measurable value that demonstrates how effectively objectives and goals are being met. In the example we discussed previously, the KPI might be a reduction in pressure areas.

This could be measured through observation of the patient's skin and completion of risk analysis documentation.

Other examples of KPIs in a healthcare setting include:

- increased staff compliance with hand hygiene
- reduction in falls incidents
- reduction in the number of outbreaks of infection
- increased compliance with staff mandatory training
- reduced emergency department waiting time
- increased patient satisfaction.

Data resulting from this measurement contributes to the operational and strategic decision-making for an organisation. It is therefore important that you understand the significance of KPIs in identifying where performance is at the required level or where improvements are needed. As an HSA, your role is to be guided by the RN in implementing steps to achieve the goals and required performance for both the team and the organisation's benefit.

ACTIVITY 7.1

Work goals and objectives

Identify objectives or strategies to achieve the required goals:

GOAL	OBJECTIVES OR STRATEGIES TO ACHIEVE THE GOAL
Ensuring confidentiality of information	
Providing culturally competent care	
Building team skills	
Working within scope of practice	
Maintaining patient privacy	
Preventing spread of infection	
Ensuring safety and security	
Promoting self-care	

Assess and prioritise workloads to ensure tasks are completed

As an HSA, you will be expected to complete many tasks and it is important that you are able to assess and prioritise your workload to ensure that tasks are completed within the time allocated. Some of these tasks may be directly patient related, such as assisting with feeding or showering, or non-patient related, such as completing forms. However, all tasks need to be completed on time. There are a number of advantages in assessing and prioritising workloads, including:

- clarifying what is important and has high priority for the patient's wellbeing; for example, a high priority would be patient preparation before an early morning operation
- establishing necessary timeframes and resources; for example, a bed bath takes longer than a shower and may need additional support from co-workers
- helping to communicate issues that may need attention; for example, the need for support when tasks are outside the scope of practice

- allowing the healthcare worker to identify all the tasks that are required for the patients over a shift or period of time; for example, the number of showers, observations, assists with feeds or transfers during a shift
- providing motivation when workloads have been achieved.

Work tasks are recorded by you during handover and clarified with the RN at the commencement of the shift. In some healthcare facilities, patient data sheets are printed with relevant details regarding the patients' condition and treatment. It is then up to the healthcare worker to add additional information that will help in the completion of tasks for the shift. Another alternative is to use a shift planner, an example of which is shown in Figure 7.3. This can be used to write down important information regarding your patients. It organises all the information and routine tasks that you need to undertake on each patient for the duration of the shift.

FIGURE 7.3 Shift planner

TIME MANAGEMENT SHEET FOR NURSES — DAY SHIFT				DATE:
Patient History	Patient 1	Patient 2	Patient 3	Patient 4
7:00 am – 8:00 am				
8:00 am – 9:00 am				
9:00 am – 10:00 am				
10:00 am – 11:00 am				
Handover Notes				
11:00 am – 12:00 pm				
12:00 pm – 1:00 pm				
1:00 pm – 2:00 pm				
2:00 pm – 3:00 pm				
Handover Notes				
Key: M = Medications OBS = Observations W = Wound care FBC = Fluid Balance Chart ★ = Progress Notes				

Source: https://www.ausmed.com/articles/time-management-for-nurses/

Tasks can include:
- handover at the start and end of the shift
- completing clinical assessments on patients; for example, observations, BGL measurements
- administrative tasks; for example, documentation in notes
- attending meetings or training sessions
- transporting or transferring patients from one area to another
- assisting patients in their activities of daily living (ADLs)
- breaks for lunch or dinner.

Initially, the RN or enrolled nurse (EN) may provide assistance with assessment and the prioritising of tasks, but as you become more familiar with planning, you will develop confidence in determining where and how to allocate your time. Consider that time spent on urgent goals may be based on a deadline that may be non-negotiable, and if this is not achieved it will have an impact on other members of the health team. Learning to prioritise what is urgent or non-urgent and how it impacts on other tasks takes practice and can be clarified by discussion with supervisors.

> **Deadline**
>
> An urgent goal that is non-negotiable and has to be met by a certain time.

Important considerations when assessing and prioritising tasks include:

- making sure that the tasks are clear and have definite timeframes
- ensuring that timeframes are realistic enough to complete the task
- ensuring that tasks are ranked in order of importance
- involving others in determining priorities if unsure
- identifying any difficulties in achieving tasks and resolving them with your supervisor or co-workers.

There may be a number of unforeseen events that affect the completion of work tasks. Planning cannot account for all aspects of work, so there is a need to be flexible in coping with unexpected events. Interruptions are part of everyday work and you may need to re-establish your priorities if these occur.

ACTIVITY 7.2

Your work plan

With the support of your facilitator, develop a work plan for a morning shift in an acute care facility as described in the following.

You are working with a team including an EN and an RN and are delegated nursing care for six patients:

- Bed 1: Mr Jones requires a sponge bath. His temperature, pulse and respirations need to be taken 4/24 and he will be sitting out of bed for lunch. He requires assistance with mobility.

- Bed 2: Mr Nielson is a shower with assist. He has a skin tear on his shin that requires dressing after his shower. He is able to manage his hygiene and nutritional needs but often gets confused and wanders.

- Bed 3: Mr Nguyen is self-caring and will be going to theatre for a prostatectomy. He will be taken to the operating theatre at 0900 hrs. He is NBM and needs an early shower and pre-operative observations to be recorded.

- Bed 4: Mr Angelatos is a diabetic who requires BGLs to be taken before meals. He requires assistance with his shower and feeding and finds walking difficult. He is on a fluid balance chart and requires 4/24 temperature, pulse and respirations.

- Bed 5: A new admission will arrive after morning tea at 1000 hrs. The bed area has not been prepared and he will require orientation to the ward and admission observations of temperature, pulse, respirations and weight.

- Bed 6: Mr Cohen has been admitted with nausea and vomiting for investigation. He is very worried about his condition and has no family support.

  You are expected to attend in-service training on manual handling at 1500 hrs.

  Include in your work plan any priorities, suggested timeframes and support from co-workers required. Also include incidental events; for example, meal breaks, handover, documentation updates and review.

Identify factors affecting achievement of work objectives and incorporate contingencies

The priorities which have been set as part of a work plan can change at any time. Urgent tasks, emergencies, complications and unexpected delays can all impact on the achievement of work objectives. It is important to identify the factors that can affect the achievement of objectives and incorporate contingencies into all work plans. Contingencies describe what to do when something does not go to plan. It may include arranging with the supervisor for someone else to complete a task or rescheduling a task to be completed at a later date if it cannot be completed on time and is not considered urgent.

Factors affecting the achievement of work objectives

There are a number of factors that may make it difficult to plan and complete work objectives; however, through contingency planning, these difficulties can be minimised. Examples of factors and contingency planning for those factors are discussed in the following.

Unclear instructions

At times, you may not have enough information to enable you to perform a task. This may be due to poor communication, misinterpretation or language difficulties.

Contingency planning – be prepared to summarise or paraphrase what you have heard, especially if you are unsure what has been said. Ask appropriate questions about what has been said and concentrate completely by minimising distractions from other people or environments.

Competing demands

As an HSA, you work under the guidance of the RN or EN. There may be times when you are conflicted with the demands of the patients and your supervisors or other co-workers who may require your assistance.

Contingency planning – prioritise tasks and consider what is most urgent. Knowing your scope of practice will help to determine what tasks you are able to perform. When in doubt, ask the supervisor to clarify what they would like to be prioritised.

Lack of staff

Absent staff members or staff being moved to another section can place pressure on the remaining staff to complete tasks.

Contingency planning – prioritise tasks based on achieving important and urgent work goals first and then non-urgent tasks if you are able. It is important to clarify the urgent tasks with the RN and report regarding all tasks that have not been completed.

Lack of physical resources

In healthcare settings, resources are often in high demand; for example, manual handling devices may be required by multiple clients during a morning shift. Observation equipment may be wanted by several staff members at the same time.

Contingency planning – preplanning is important before tasks are undertaken. This means discussing with your co-workers what their priorities are and negotiating the best times for the use of resources. It can also mean sharing loads and assisting others with their tasks so that they can help you with yours. It is important to identify any difficulties in achieving tasks and resolve them with your team leader or co-workers.

Equipment failure

Equipment failure can occur unexpectedly, perhaps due to uncharged batteries or breakages. This can impact on monitoring and patient care.

Contingency planning – checks should be completed on all equipment so that incidents of equipment failure can be reported and orders for new equipment or their repair can be arranged. You need to be aware of the location of replacement batteries and know how to use manual equipment if required. For example, use a manual blood pressure sphygmomanometer and stethoscope if the automated equipment does not work. In urgent situations, equipment can be borrowed from other areas.

Incidents and emergencies

Examples of incidents include errors in treatment, a breach of duty of care, a fall or a sharps incident. Emergencies include acute patient episodes (e.g., cardiac arrest), aggression, fire and threats.

Contingency planning – a response to an incident or emergency should comply with the policies and procedures of the organisation and be within your scope of practice. You should obey all directions from designated personnel and consult with the team leader to re-establish your workload after the incident or emergency has been resolved (see Figure 7.4). This may include providing immediate care to a patient or completing required documentation.

FIGURE 7.4 Follow all instructions from designated personnel

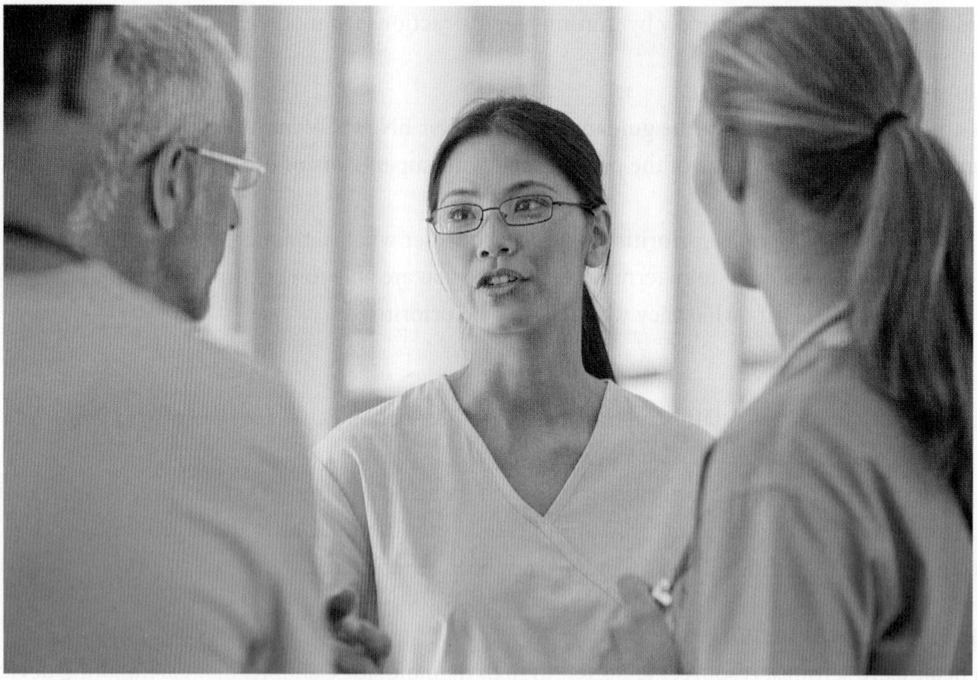

Source: Alamy Stock Photo / Juice Images326

Time management

Using time effectively requires careful planning. Time management skills can be improved by identifying any unnecessary time-wasting activities that affect the achievement of individual goals. Time wasting occurs at three levels:

1 *Organisational time wasting* – inefficiencies in the way work is organised. Examples include too many individuals allocated to set tasks and poor supervision by others. If you consider that work could be improved and can be done in less time, suggest improvements that can benefit the work team.

2 *Work group time wasting* – distractions and time wasting caused by the actions of others within a work team. Examples include excessive time spent discussing life outside work, people being late for meetings or not listening to others, and supervisors not clarifying roles and responsibilities.

3 *Individual time wasting* – consider whether you waste time when undertaking work tasks by asking yourself the following questions:
   - Did I forget to do things and then spent more time catching up?
   - Could I have been better organised?
   - Did I spend time on private matters in work time?
   - Did I allow myself to be distracted?
   - Did I spend too much time finding the negatives and not getting on with it?
   - Did I try to meet the deadlines?

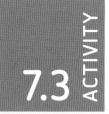

Use of time

1 Document the time spent during daily activities either while studying or in the workplace.

2 Identify any unnecessary time-wasting activities.

3 Identify any work activities that can be completed with a colleague to maximise use of time.

4 Explain how you can apply effective time management skills to better manage your time during work or study activities.

5 Practise these time management skills in the classroom or workplace.

Use business technology efficiently and effectively

A range of business technology has been developed to manage and monitor scheduling and the completion of tasks in the healthcare sector, including equipment and software applications (see Figure 7.5 for examples). These provide improved communication and efficiency and reduce the amount of time that healthcare workers need to spend on tasks.

As an HSA, you should ensure that you are familiar with all business technology (see Figure 7.6), especially where it can be used to help you manage and complete tasks. Operators of all electronic equipment should receive training and instruction in the use of technology according to the manufacturer's instructions and also by:
- face-to-face or online training sessions provided by the organisation
- training by a colleague who is competent in the use of the technology
- referring to an up-to-date manufacturer's manual.

FIGURE 7.5 Equipment and software to improve communication and efficiency

Paging systems	Wireless-based paging systems ensure ongoing contact with team members at different locations during the workday
	These systems allow team members to be readily located at all times while on duty and to be directed to important and urgent tasks
Tablet computers, desktop PCs and mobile carts	Computer-based tools allow you to enter and retrieve information without leaving the bedside
	These systems can operate wirelessly and connect to databases containing care guidelines and other resources
	They reduce the amount of time that you need to access patient notes in set locations, so less time is spent away from urgent and important tasks involving patient care
Clinical information systems	These systems enable access to patient records, laboratory results and data, resources and other information
	Clinical information systems provide you with integrated information that can assist in completing or monitoring tasks efficiently. An example is the Victorian Health Incident Management System (VHIMS), which collects and classifies clinical incidents, occupational health and safety incidents, hazards and consumer feedback (Safer Care Victoria, 2019)

By becoming familiar with the basic troubleshooting requirements for any technology that you regularly use, you will be able to rectify any problems if they arise. Report the problems to the appropriate person if they cannot be rectified by yourself or others.

FIGURE 7.6 An HSA should be familiar with all business technology

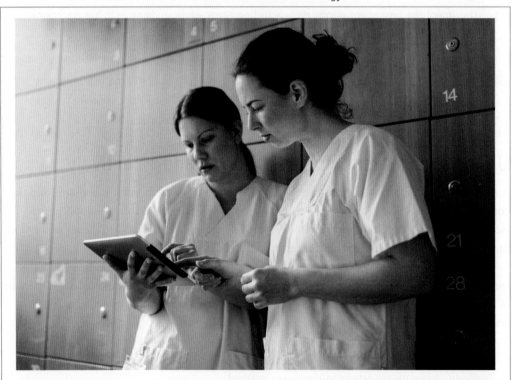

Source: Getty Images/Hinterhaus Productions

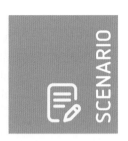

Communication technology in the hospital

Melissa works in a busy private hospital as an HSA. The hospital uses a range of technologies to support efficient communication. An integrated database and scheduling system have been customised for use on all computers in the hospital. The patient's history, diagnostic test results and medical imaging are consolidated into a single set of records that is easily accessible via any computer. Melissa is able to add patient information including observations and reports (which are electronically countersigned by the RN). When doctors are needed, the calendar allows staff to view their schedules so that they can be called when needed. The staff rosters can also be viewed and requests for a change of shift can be logged into the system for review.

This management system enables Melissa to deliver more patient-focused care and provides simplified communication and streamlined workloads for the entire multidisciplinary team.

1   Can you think of any other health, community or allied industries in which the use of integrated data would be a useful tool?
2   Why is it important for the RN to countersign Melissa's notes?
3   Why is it important to log out after each computer interaction?

2   MONITOR OWN WORK PERFORMANCE

Monitoring work performance to ensure that it complies with legislation is an important aspect of any healthcare worker's role. This can be achieved by working to your scope of practice and completing healthcare tasks safely and competently. Monitoring for improved performance includes self-assessment and obtaining feedback from supervisors, co-workers and clients. Stress can also affect performance, so it is important to recognise signs of stress and access the appropriate support systems so that nursing care is not compromised.

Monitor and adjust work performance through self-assessment

Self-assessment is one way to monitor work performance. It involves looking at the quality of the work done based on the goals that have been set. The work undertaken by an HSA occurs in a health setting with a multidisciplinary team that has the following features:

*   defined roles and responsibilities
*   different levels of accountability in accordance with roles and responsibilities
*   mutual respect shown for the contribution of individuals
*   collaborative practices to ensure high-quality and safe patient care
*   policies and procedures to support work tasks.

Your performance is dependent on this team, and when you are supported, encouraged and valued it will be reflected in your work and your interactions. Self-assessment enables you to monitor and evaluate your performance and should be based on:

*   a clear understanding of the outcomes you are expected to achieve
*   the agreed standards at which the tasks are to be completed
*   the time available for the completion of the work.

Self-assessment needs to be ongoing rather than an occasional exercise. It should involve keeping a diary or a reflective journal to monitor your performance and checking for feedback. Your self-assessment and the feedback received from your supervisor, co-workers and patients should enable you to continuously improve in terms of the performance of tasks and in meeting the needs of patients.

Ask yourself the following questions to help you reflect on your work as part of a self-assessment:

- Are there things that I do well and other things that I don't do so well?
- How well do I work with other people?
- Do I manage my time efficiently?
- Am I showing improvement?
- Do I use my initiative?
- Have I shown an awareness of and complied with legislation?
- Have I worked towards the team goals?

SWOT analysis

A strategic planning technique used to help a person or organisation identify strengths, weaknesses, opportunities and threats.

A SWOT analysis is a useful tool that can be used to identify your strengths, weaknesses, opportunities and threats. After completing a SWOT analysis, you can consider how to:

- build on your strengths
- work on your weaknesses
- take advantage of opportunities
- respond to threats.

A self-assessment and SWOT analysis can identify how you positively contribute to the team or show you where you need more development. An example may be:

- Strengths – you have strengths in performing the clinical skills of taking blood pressure, temperature and blood glucose levels.
- Weaknesses – you require more practice in patient handover.
- Opportunities – taking advantage of professional development opportunities in ISBAR (identify, situation, background, assessment and recommendation) training.
- Threats – time required to undertake this professional development training, fitting it into your schedule.

This analysis can give you a clear idea of the type of opportunities or clinical training you require and can give you satisfaction when you recognise areas of weakness and improve on them.

ACTIVITY 7.4

SWOT analysis

Complete your individual SWOT analysis (see Figure 7.7):

- Consider your strengths and weaknesses from your own reflections and those of others.
- When looking at opportunities, look at your strengths and ask yourself whether these open up any opportunities. Alternatively, look at your weaknesses and ask yourself whether you could open up opportunities by eliminating them.
- Threats can be obstacles or changes in technology or policies and procedures that can impact on your work. Recognition of threats can open up professional development opportunities.
  Once completed, you will have a plan for your own professional development needs.

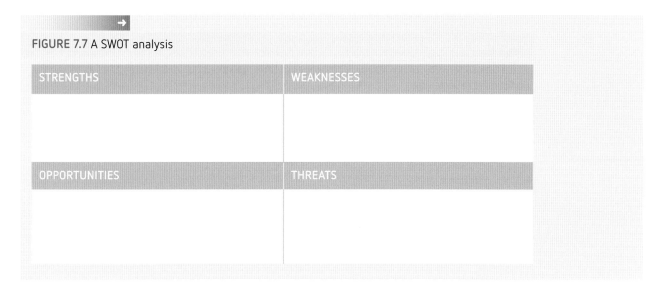

FIGURE 7.7 A SWOT analysis

STRENGTHS	WEAKNESSES
OPPORTUNITIES	THREATS

Self-assessment and compliance with legislation

Self-assessment of your performance should also consider your compliance with the following:

- scope of practice
- privacy and confidentiality
- duty of care
- harassment, bullying and discrimination
- work, health and safety.

Scope of practice

Scope of practice refers to the broad frameworks and context of healthcare workers including (1) the range of roles, and (2) functions and responsibilities. Self-assessment for the HSA includes knowledge of their scope of practice and work/role boundaries. Figure 7.8 outlines an example position description and accountabilities for an HSA.

FIGURE 7.8 Sample position description and accountabilities of a health services assistant

POSITION DESCRIPTION – HEALTH SERVICES ASSISTANT (HSA)
Reports to: Nurse Unit Manager
1 POSITION OBJECTIVE
The health services assistant works as an assistant to the healthcare team, assisting the registered and enrolled nurses to provide delegated aspects of patient care. Elements of direct and indirect patient care will be delegated in accordance with the professional judgement of the supervising registered nurse.

2 POSITION ACCOUNTABILITIES

Under the supervision of the nurse unit manager or their registered nurse delegates, the health services assistant is expected to:

- contribute to positive patient outcomes by ensuring all elements of delegated work are completed accurately and in accordance with policies and procedures
- participate in delegated aspects of care to assist activities of daily living for selected patients, including, but not limited to, assistance with:
  - personal hygiene
  - nutritional needs
  - mobility, transfers and positioning within the ward
  - elimination needs.
- ensure patient privacy and dignity is maintained at all times
- observe and report patients considered at risk of harm to self/others
- maintain a safe patient environment and report incidents promptly to the supervising RN and other relevant member/s of the nursing team
- assist with making beds and keeping the unit environment tidy
- communicate effectively with patients, families and the interdisciplinary team
- participate in documentation as relevant
- ensure relevant infection-control policies are adhered to at all times
- assist to maintain stock levels of ward supplies.

3 GENERIC

- abide by organisational policies and procedures
- participate in performance appraisal programs
- undertake not to reveal any confidential information relating to patients and employees, policies and processes
- undertake organisational annual mandatory competencies
- participate in emergency incident response activities at the direction of management
- ability to work collaboratively as part of an interdisciplinary team
- willingness to contribute to quality patient care
- utilise well-developed interpersonal skills, including an ability to communicate effectively with other staff, patients and families
- commit to ongoing professional development
- commit to a professional work ethic
- apply basic computer skills.

Privacy and confidentiality

Patients have the right to expect that their personal information will stay private and secure. Privacy and confidentiality include:

- a patient's physical, mental and psychological health, including disability
- treatments a patient has received and their effectiveness
- any necessary medications and treatment based on an illness, injury or disability.

Self-assessment for the HSA includes maintaining this privacy and confidentiality at all times both within and outside the workplace. Refer to Chapter 4, 'Communicate and work in health and community services', for more on privacy and confidentiality.

Duty of care

Healthcare workers have a legal obligation to take reasonable care to avoid causing harm to a patient. This means ensuring the safety of patients by complying with work health and safety requirements, and reporting any present or potential hazards. Self-assessment means that you understand these requirements and practise duty of care accordingly.

Harassment, bullying and discrimination

Under the *Equal Opportunity Act 2010*, it is illegal to discriminate against a person on the basis of their gender, race, age, physical or mental disability, pregnancy, having children, marital status or religious beliefs. Showing an awareness of, and compliance with, this legislation is an important part of self-assessment.

Work health and safety

Chapter 1, 'Participate in workplace health and safety', discussed work health and safety requirements for employees and employers in organisations. If, through self-assessment, you find that your performance needs improvement, it is your responsibility to ask your supervisor for additional training.

Ensure feedback on performance is actively sought and evaluated

It is important to seek feedback on your performance from your supervisors and colleagues in the context of your individual and teamwork requirements. As an HSA, you will work alongside others as part of a multidisciplinary team. This provides an invaluable opportunity to include their feedback as part of your own self-assessment. If the self-assessment is done in isolation, without consideration of what others feel about your performance, it may lead to incorrect conclusions as to how best to improve your skills and abilities.

Self-assessment needs to be combined with monitoring of your interactions with other people who are significant members of your team. These include your supervisor, other team members and patients. As part of your interaction with team members you should assess what worked well and what did not work well. To learn from your experiences and develop your skills in the workplace, you need to analyse your positive and negative interactions. With positive interactions, you need to examine the reasons why they were positive and whether your approach can be applied to similar situations that may come up in the future. With the negative interactions, you need to spend time analysing why they were negative and whether other approaches may have been better.

When asking for feedback, ask for specific examples rather than generalisations and ask for suggestions that can improve areas of weakness. Feedback from your supervisor and co-workers can help determine your answers to the self-reflection questions outlined previously.

You should also seek feedback from patients with questions regarding whether the care that you have provided them has addressed their needs.

Mentoring

Mentoring

Assisting an individual in terms of achieving their work goals with the use of a more experienced person.

Stretch target

A target that cannot be achieved by small improvements and requires extending oneself.

Performance appraisal

A review of your job performance with feedback on further growth and development.

Your future workplace may provide you with a mentor – a more experienced worker who can assist you to learn on the job and help in your long-term career development. Mentoring is aimed at improving performance and may occur formally or informally. It is based on assisting an individual in terms of achieving their work goals. These work goals should be in the form of stretch targets, which provide a real challenge to achieve.

Performance appraisal

Performance appraisal may occur in your organisation when a supervisor meets with you to discuss your performance in your role. This aims to provide feedback on the positive aspects of your performance and areas where you need to improve (see Figure 7.9). An outcome of performance appraisal might include learning new skills or improving techniques.

FIGURE 7.9 Supervisors give valuable feedback during performance appraisal

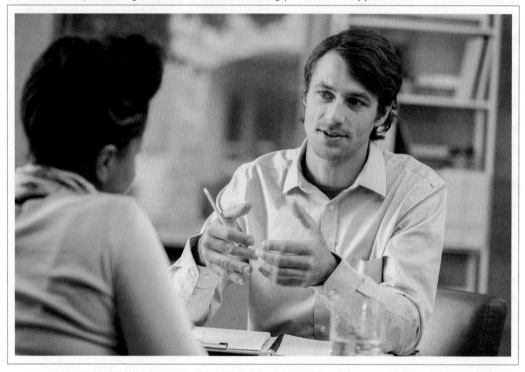

Source: iStock.com / Steve Debenport

A performance appraisal considers the following questions:

- What are the positive features of my performance?
- Are there any issues or problems that impact on performance?
- What can be done to improve my performance on the job?
- What are my future goals and how could they be achieved?

Feedback you receive from your supervisor on your performance will allow you to be more aware of your strengths and weaknesses. These observations cannot be ignored – you need to consider them when undertaking your self-assessment.

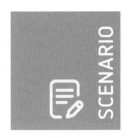

Kelly's performance appraisal

Kelly, the HSA, was having trouble with her relationship skills and asked the RN for feedback on her interaction with Mrs Baker while she was admitting the patient to the unit. The RN replied, 'I observed that when you spoke to Mrs Baker, your arms were crossed and you avoided eye contact with her. You need to work on developing open body language, maintaining eye contact and concentrating on what the patient says.'

This gave Kelly a clear understanding that she was not achieving the required standard and what she needed to do in order to achieve this. The feedback was specific and clearly identified the aspects of the communication skills with which Kelly was having difficulty.

Kelly continued to practise her communication skills and used the RN as a mentor. She continued to seek feedback and her communication skills with patients improved.

1   Why was it important for Kelly to seek feedback on her communication style with Mrs Baker?
2   How does feedback play a role in education and learning?
3   How does open communication benefit the nurse–patient relationship?

Routinely identify and report on variations in the quality of products and services

Health facilities routinely evaluate and review new technologies and procedures and develop guidelines for use based on evidence-based practice. This can improve patient outcomes and allow resources to be used more effectively. Identifying and reporting on variations in the quality of products and services can help continuous improvements to be made.

Variations in products may be due to:

* changes in the quality of supplies or supplier
* changes in equipment due to improved technology
* changes in regulations or standards
* the age and condition of equipment.

Variations in services may be due to:

* new staff members
* reduction in staff
* availability of equipment
* changes to policy and procedures
* varying instructions.

Whether assistance is available or not, the most common initiative to reduce unwanted variation in clinical practice is the implementation of clinical practice guidelines, evidence-based pathways and clinical protocols. Implementation of guidelines needs to be supported by education, equipment, promotion and awareness. Initiatives to implement best practice and reduce variations require local and national approaches. All healthcare workers should identify and report any variations so that quality management and continuous improvement processes can be used to determine how changes should be made.

ACTIVITY

7.5

Definitions

Define the following terms related to variation of processes and provide an example of each:

- Controlled variation
- Uncontrolled variation
- Quality management
- Continuous improvement
- Process variation.

Identify signs and sources of stress and effects on personal wellbeing, and access appropriate supports

Working in acute care settings involves a high level of intensity and emotion. The dynamics of the work environment involve pressure situations, which cause your body to react by releasing hormones that increase heart rate, breathing and metabolism. At times this adrenaline rush may keep you motivated and alert to the challenges that occur during your work. However, the same pressures that caused the rush of energy can negatively impact health and wellbeing.

Signs of stress in the workplace may be shown by:

- frequent absence from work
- alcohol or other substance abuse
- conflict with others
- poor work performance
- accidents or incidents.

Refer to Chapter 1, 'Participate in workplace health and safety', for strategies to deal with stress.

Conflict in the workplace

Stress can be caused by traumatic or post-traumatic incidents, a reaction to workplace demands or conflict in the workplace. Conflict often goes through a number of phases that can challenge the work team and create a range of unhelpful stressful emotions for the individuals involved.

Phase 1 of workplace conflict

This phase refers to the underlying causes of conflict such as dissatisfaction over roles, communication problems or competition for scarce resources.

Phase 2 of workplace conflict

The next phase occurs when the conflict is observed by other members of the team. The perception of conflict is shown by feelings of threat, hostility, fear or mistrust.

Phases 1 and 2 can damage the dynamics of the work team. It may lead to a failure to achieve goals, which may have a harmful effect on patient care. Initiatives may be ignored and an enormous amount of energy can be used in trying to resolve the issues rather than concentrating on achieving outcomes. Morale may be affected as individuals become dragged into the conflict, which may impact on their own stress levels.

At this stage, the conflict may be acceptable and even positive if different views inspire necessary change. However, if the conflict is observed as negative and a cause of stress, it needs to be resolved.

Phase 3 of workplace conflict

This is where attempts are made by another person, who is likely to be a supervisor, to resolve the conflict for everybody concerned.

Phase 4 of workplace conflict

This final phase involves the implementation of strategies to resolve the conflict.

Formal grievance resolution procedures

In some cases, a more formal grievance resolution procedure will be used with a different mediator, who may not be the immediate supervisor. The aim of the procedure is to hear from everyone involved with the dispute, to attempt mediation and to make a resolution if the individuals cannot agree.

Support services

Support services can assist the person to manage their stress when they cannot manage it themselves. This is important because it ensures that you and the people in your care are safe. Various support services are available, including:

*   supervisors or managers within the workplace
*   counselling services; for example, through employee assistance programs (see Figure 7.10)
*   training courses on handling stress.

FIGURE 7.10 Counselling services can assist a person to manage their stress

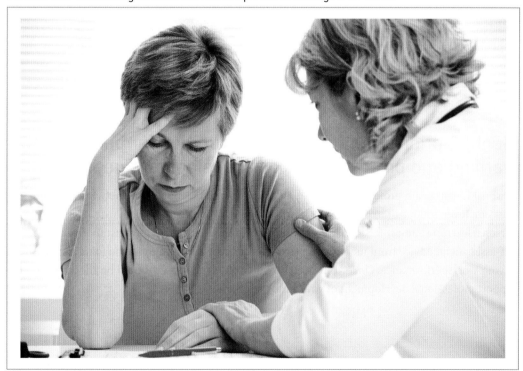

Source: iStock.com/AlexRaths

Build resilience

Building resilience may reduce levels of stress and can be achieved through:

- developing your relationships with family and friends so that you can discuss problems and jointly resolve issues of concern that may be causing you stress
- developing a positive attitude
- keeping issues in perspective
- considering that stressful situations are an opportunity for you to learn
- proactively facing the difficult issues head-on
- maintaining a healthy diet with regular exercise
- learning from your mistakes and reflecting on how you managed stressful situations.

ACTIVITY 7.6

Dealing with conflict

Refer to a conflict situation that has occurred in your workplace either with a patient, carer or with staff. If this has not occurred, think of a conflict situation as an example.

1   Outline the impact it had on working relationships and/or patient care.

2   Discuss how this was resolved and who contributed to the resolution.

3   Reflect on the experience with a focus on lessons to be learnt.

---

3 COORDINATE PERSONAL SKILL DEVELOPMENT AND LEARNING

Patient care and technology are often changing in healthcare settings, so it is important to update your skills through personal skills development. This means becoming a lifelong learner by planning and prioritising opportunities for personal and professional skill development. By liaising with your supervisor, co-workers and other relevant personnel, including the human resources department of your organisation, you can source opportunities to maintain your competence and develop new skills.

Identify, prioritise and plan opportunities for personal learning and professional skills development needs

Personal learning and professional development are a shared responsibility between you and your employer and result in continuous improvement and improved patient care. Your personal learning and professional development requirements should be a result of your own self-assessment; advice from mentors, supervisors and co-workers; and the ongoing monitoring of your work performance. Once your needs are identified, resources should be allocated to support professional development of your knowledge and skills.

Two types of skill sets exist for healthcare workers and other professions:

- Hard skills – hands-on procedural skills that you use to perform your job effectively; for example, performing simple dressing changes, mobilising and transferring clients, and checking vital signs.
- Soft skills – interpersonal skills that you need to facilitate communication and work successfully; for example, work ethic, dependability, reliability, communication style, problem-solving and conflict management.

As a lifelong learner, you should be willing to improve on your hard and soft skills and regularly review and monitor your performance against work plans, organisational objectives and feedback from others. Based on this analysis, you should seek opportunities for formal and informal development of your knowledge and skills in order to optimise your performance.

Formal professional development activities

Formal professional development activities may include the following:

- career planning or development, which identifies a progression into other roles and responsibilities in the health sector and may include a pathway into enrolled and registered nursing
- coaching, mentoring and/or supervision, which provide one-on-one support and guidance to improve performance
- workplace skills assessment or recognition of prior learning (RPL), which is used to acknowledge existing skills or to assess skills learnt in an existing study program
- on-the-job training with the specific purpose of developing and enhancing skills
- work-shadowing experienced HSAs and/or other staff
- formal programs provided within your organisation or from training providers. Formal programs are based around structured learning that may be accredited in terms of a unit of competence or completion of a qualification. The methods of delivery may vary and include facilitated workshops, online learning and workplace delivery and assessment.

Informal learning opportunities

Opportunities for incidental or informal learning can be identified through experiential learning, which is based on learning through experience and reflecting on what has been learnt. This reflection can be unconscious or facilitated by others through a discussion or a debriefing session and may involve individuals or a group. The debriefing session should reinforce what has been learnt and provide feedback and reflection. It can also include discussion of how the newly acquired knowledge and skills can be applied to new situations.

Informal learning:

- is unplanned and has no predetermined learning objectives
- provides an opportunity for interaction with others
- applies learning in everyday situations.

Informal learning
Incorporates applied learning in everyday situations.

Experiential learning
Learning process based on 'learn by doing' and by reflecting on the experience.

Taking advantage of learning opportunities

As an HSA, Toby had classroom training in understanding the theory of blood pressure and the technique in measuring it. He practised on his classmates and in the workplace. Over the months and using the technique with many different types of patients in a variety of medical situations, he became confident and familiar with its use. Now taking blood pressure is almost second nature. From the formal learning in the classroom to the informal learning in everyday nursing situations, this skill has been developed to become part of Toby's normal repertoire as a health professional.

1   What are some examples of informal learning in everyday nursing situations that Toby could learn to become proficient in his work as an HSA?

2   Why is debriefing important for Toby after he has performed skills appropriately?

Formal learning

Structured learning programs that may be accredited in terms of a unit of competence or completion of a qualification.

Access, complete and record professional development opportunities

Continuing professional development (CPD) is one way that healthcare workers improve and broaden their knowledge, expertise and competence, and develop the personal and professional qualities needed to be an effective member of a multidisciplinary team. It involves not only accessing and completing development opportunities but also recording them as workplace evidence of competency. Recording evidence of activities can be in the form of an iFolio or written document, as shown in Figure 7.11.

FIGURE 7.11 Continuing professional development (CPD) document

DATE	PROVIDER DETAILS	TYPE OF LEARNING ACTIVITY	TOPICS COVERED	EVIDENCE
x/x/xx	College of Nursing	Infection control workshop	Standard and additional precautions	Certificate of completion
x/x/xx	Bargo Hospital in-service	Introduction to ISBAR	Reporting and recording	Reflective journal

Learning activities can be formal or informal and may include:

- enrolling in an accredited course of study
- completing self-directed eLearning packages
- attending an in-service in the workplace
- one-to-one skills instruction by a supervisor with observation followed by an opportunity to demonstrate skills
- direct supervision sessions in the wards on job tasks, with feedback provided by a supervisor.

You should access all sources of learning not only to improve your skills but also to ensure that you become aware of any updates in legislation, codes of practice, and policies and procedures.

Recording continuing professional development (CPD)

7.7 ACTIVITY

1   Reflect on the professional development activities you have undertaken in your role as an HSA, both within the classroom and the workplace. This includes online training, workshops and readings from journals, websites and textbooks.

2   Develop a template and begin documenting any continuing professional development you have undertaken through these formal and informal sessions.

3   Access your CPD record throughout your studies and workplace experience and add events as they arise.

4   Consider using this record of professional development when applying for future employment and during interviews.

Incorporate formal and informal feedback into review of further learning needs

Once you have completed professional development, you should provide feedback on the effectiveness of the training program as to whether your learning needs have been met. A useful model to determine the effectiveness of learning for the workplace is Kirkpatrick's Four-Level Training Evaluation Model (outlined in Figure 7.12), which examines training effectiveness in terms of reaction, learning, behaviour and results.

FIGURE 7.12 Kirkpatrick's Four-Level Training Evaluation Model

LEVEL	TRAINING EFFECTIVENESS
Level 1 – Reaction	Was the training presented well and was it valuable in terms of instruction methods, knowledge and skills covered?
Level 2 – Learning	Did the training increase your knowledge and skills?
Level 3 – Behaviour	Have you changed your work performance due to the training?
Level 4 – Results	Are you applying the newly learnt skills in the workplace with positive results?

Source: Mind Tools (n.d.). Kirkpatrick's Four-Level Training Evaluation Model Analysing Training Effectiveness. Retrieved 17 October 2022 from https://www.mindtools.com/pages/article/kirkpatrick.htm

Feedback for levels 1 and 2 can be provided as soon as the training is completed. This may involve completion of a survey or formal questionnaire that is distributed at the end of the training program.

It is more difficult to determine whether there is an impact with levels 3 and 4 of the evaluation; however, a few months after the end of the training, the effectiveness these levels will be evident in feedback from your supervisor and your co-workers. It is important that you also provide feedback on impacts or changed behaviour and results. This may involve a meeting with your supervisor where you discuss the changes in work performance and how they have resulted in positive benefits to the workplace (see Figure 7.13).

FIGURE 7.13 Meeting with supervisor to discuss effectiveness of training

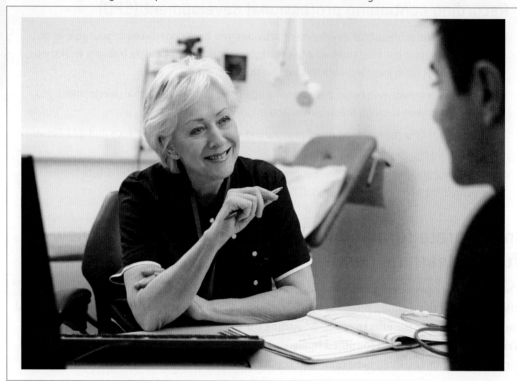

Source: Shutterstock.com/Monkey Business Images

When discussing the evaluation of behaviour (Level 3) and results (Level 4), it is important to look at reasons why there may have been no change. This may be because:

- the training was irrelevant
- barriers prevented the training from being implemented at the workplace; for example, due to lack of support, communication issues or lack of resources
- the HSA lacked the desire to apply their newly acquired knowledge and skills.

ACTIVITY 7.8

Applying Kirkpatrick's Four-Level Training Evaluation Model

Apply the Kirkpatrick model to your training as an HSA by evaluating:

1. how the training and instructional methods were presented in the classroom
2. what knowledge and skills you have developed as a result of the training
3. how you have changed your work performance due to the training
4. what newly learnt skills you are applying in the workplace.

SUMMARY

This chapter outlined the importance of organising your personal work priorities and undertaking professional development opportunities to enhance your skills and knowledge in the workplace. It highlighted the importance of developing a work schedule in terms of work goals and objectives, and to prioritise the tasks for yourself and your patients and to assist the healthcare team. The chapter emphasised the need to identify factors impacting on the achievement of work goals and the contingency plans that can be considered. The importance of effectively using time management and technology was outlined to help manage and monitor scheduling for the completion of tasks.

Self-assessment of performance and seeking feedback was covered, as was the importance of identifying and addressing signs of stress, which may impact on your personal wellbeing and work performance.

The last part of the chapter identified the importance of personal skill development and learning to assist in career development and to improve individual and team performance. By recording continuing professional development, you can monitor your lifelong learning and seek to improve your personal attributes and work performance.

APPLY YOUR KNOWLEDGE

Conflict with self

Ashleigh, an HSA, was working an evening shift and was looking after eight patients with the help of the RN, who was busy giving out medications. Two patients needed her at the same time; however, she had to choose which patient she was to see and take care of first. She had to make the right decision and prioritise correctly. Mr Arnold required assistance to go to the toilet and Mr Tauson required his BSL to be taken before dinner.

1   What contingency planning could Ashleigh adopt in this situation?

This situation made Ashleigh reflect on her own time management skills and if she could have been better organised. She spoke with her manager to find out if there were any professional development opportunities to further develop her skills.

2   How could Ashleigh have managed her time more effectively to ensure all tasks were completed without delays?

3   What type of formal or informal professional development opportunities could Ashleigh undertake?

4   Why is it important to provide feedback once professional development has been completed?

After Ashleigh had helped her patients, the RN told her that the ward would be understaffed for the next two hours as one of the staff had been called to fill in on another busy ward. This caused conflict for Ashleigh as she did not have the capabilities to manage the additional patients whose care was outside of her scope of practice.

5   Using the knowledge gained in Chapter 4, 'Communicate and work in health and community services', how could Ashleigh address her concerns in an assertive manner to her supervisor?

6   Understanding the HSA scope of practice is essential when caring for patients. How did the HSA demonstrate an understanding of the scope of her role in this case study?

◄ **REFLECTING** ON THE INDUSTRY INSIGHT ➕

1   In the 'Industry insight' at the start of this chapter, a new HSA is paired up with an enrolled nurse and learns to put her training into effect. This transference of learning to the workplace needs to occur for training programs to be successful. Which of the following can help with this process?

   a   Support from colleagues.

   b   Outsourcing the procedure.

   c   An authoritarian management style.

   d   A lack of sufficient mentors.

2   How did the new HSA enhance her personal skill development?

   a   By talking to friends.

   b   By being unprepared.

   c   Through constant practice.

   d   By ignoring change.

3   The HSA's colleague commented on a 'job well done'. How does this influence a positive reaction to feedback on performance?

   a   By giving the feedback well after the event has occurred.

   b   By giving feedback outside your scope of practice.

   c   By providing a positive orientation to the feedback.

   d   By ignoring relevant information about the performance.

SELF-CHECK QUESTIONS

1   Describe the importance of achieving work goals and objectives as an HSA.

2   Describe how an HSA can assess and prioritise their workload.

3   Outline the factors that may impact on the achievement of work objectives and the importance of contingency planning.

4   Explain how technology can be used to save time and to manage and monitor the scheduling of work.

5   Outline how a SWOT analysis can be used to monitor performance.

6   Describe how mentoring can improve performance.

7   Sometimes, stress in the workplace does not arise from the patients but from the relatives and carers at the bedside. Identify any potential stressors in these situations.

8   Explain the importance of professional development for the individual, the healthcare team and for health and safety regulations in Australia.

9   What is the difference between hard and soft skills?

10 What are your definitions of the following key words and terms that have been used in this chapter?

KEY WORD OR TERM	YOUR DEFINITION
Key performance indicators (KPIs)	
Operational goals	
Contingencies	
Deadline	
Experiential learning	
Formal learning	
Informal learning	
Performance appraisal	
Self-assessment	
Resilience	

QUESTIONS FOR DISCUSSION

1   Look up the South Australian State Public Health Plan at **https://www.sahealth.sa.gov.au/ wps/wcm/connect/public+content/sa+health+internet/resources/state+ public+health+plan+2019-2024** and discuss how the vision incorporates the organisational goals for health in South Australia.

2   Discuss why taking ownership of your job, using your initiative and efficient time management are three critical factors when working in an acute care environment.

3   Discuss how you would identify any gaps in knowledge or skills and what actions you would take to improve performance.

4   Discuss the causes of work-related stress and how an organisation can take steps to ensure work-related stress is reduced.

5   Identify and discuss the mandatory training requirements of your organisation or health district. Discuss how you can incorporate the training in your work plans, organisational objectives and patient care.

EXTENSION ACTIVITY

Case study – United Health Care Services

United Health Care Services (UHCS Inc.) is a provider of small-to-medium hospitals in New York State, Illinois, Florida, California, Arizona and Idaho. United Health Care Services intends to establish a number of hospitals in various locations in New South Wales. But before any expansion of the organisation occurs in Australia, the company aims to complete a brief feasibility study on the nature of its expansion. The feasibility study would consider the importance of multidisciplinary teams in acute care, based on the importance of nursing care support provided by HSAs.

For the first part of the initial feasibility study, you have been asked to put together a brief summary of points that will contribute to the paper. Your summary needs to detail how HSAs should organise their personal work priorities and development in the acute care setting, while showing initiative and ownership of their work role.

1   With reference to the information outlined in this chapter and to an organisation where you presently work or may work in the future, describe how the HSA should organise their work priorities in an acute care setting.

2   Develop a template that could be used to organise and time-manage typical work priorities (e.g., activities of daily living, clinical observations, reporting) in an acute care setting.

3   Form groups and role-play a handover that considers the work priorities of an HSA. Your team will use the template that you have just developed to record the activities. Once completed, discuss how the template assisted you with your handover.

4   How could the template be improved?

REFERENCES

Australian Government Department of Health (2019). Australia's Long Term National Health Plan. Retrieved 31 March 2022 from https://www.health.gov.au/sites/default/files/australia-s-long-term-national-health-plan_0.pdf

Health, Education and Training Institute (HETI) (2022). My health learning. Retrieved 22 May 2022 from https://www.heti.nsw.gov.au/Placements-Scholarships-Grants/clinical-placements/my-health-learning-and-mandatory-training

Mind Tools (n.d.). Kirkpatrick's Four-Level Training Evaluation Model Analysing Training Effectiveness. Retrieved 17 October 2022 from https://www.mindtools.com/pages/article/kirkpatrick.htm

Safer Care Victoria (2019). Victorian Health Incident Management System (VHIMS). Retrieved 19 October 2019 from https://www.bettersafercare.vic.gov.au/our-work/incident-response/VHIMS

Victorian Government (2010). *The Equal Opportunity Act 2010*. Retrieved 19 October 2019 from http://www.legislation.vic.gov.au/Domino/Web_Notes/LDMS/PubStatbook.nsf/f932b66241ecf1b7ca256e92000e23be/7CAFB78A7EE91429CA25771200123812/$FILE/10-016a.pdf

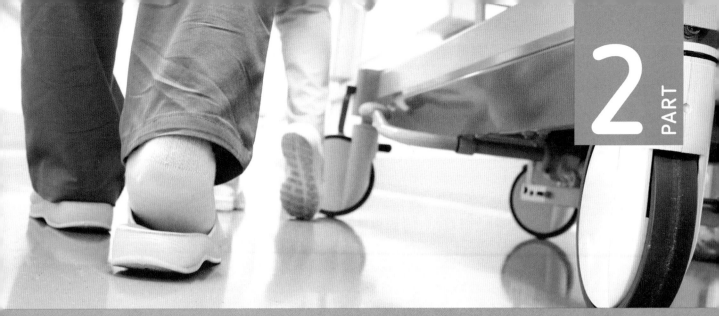

ELECTIVES – ACUTE CARE SPECIALISATION

Acute care nursing is usually performed in hospital when the patient has an acute illness or injury, or they are recovering from surgery. As part of the healthcare team, health services assistants support acute care nursing and are supervised by the registered nurse according to the guidelines, policies and procedures of the acute care environment.

Chapters 8 and 9 apply this knowledge so that you understand instructions and respond appropriately when conducting routine tasks. These include supporting clients who require assistance with basic physical movement, and the safe, timely and efficient transport of clients from one location to another. By providing this support, and being able to communicate effectively, strong relationships with clients and the entire healthcare team can be developed.

Chapters 10 and 11 provide an overview of nursing care and the equipment used in an acute care environment. Clinical assessment, measurement and nursing interventions are described. These chapters will give you knowledge of the techniques, appropriate equipment and processes to support a client who has acute healthcare needs.

Chapter 12 identifies the strategies required to respond to behaviours of concern that can arise in acute care settings. Minimising the impact of these behaviours can make the workplace safer for both the patient and the healthcare team

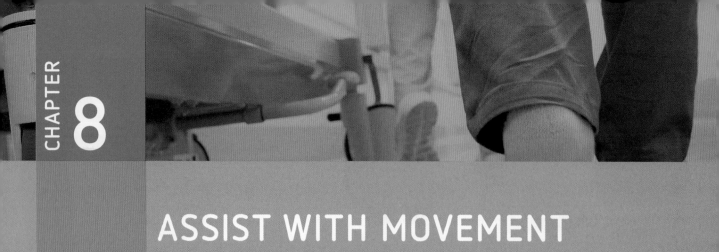

ASSIST WITH MOVEMENT

Learning objectives

By the end of this chapter, you should be able to:

1 prepare to assist a person with movement, confirming requirements and risk factors, and prepare the environment and select appropriate equipment according to organisational policies and procedures and safe work practices

2 assist a person with movement using safe handling techniques, appropriate equipment and communication to ensure comfort and safety

3 complete assistance with movement, return and clean equipment, and report faults in accordance with organisational policy and procedure.

Introduction

People who are frail or debilitated from illness or have been immobilised due to their condition require assistance with movement. This is the most effective measure to prevent complications, such as pressure ulcers and contractures, and also to boost their confidence and reduce their time spent in the healthcare facility.

This chapter describes the relevant skills and knowledge required to assist people with basic physical movement, which may be due to incapacity. As a health services assistant (HSA), you will need to understand the importance of risk assessment in preparing the person and the environment, before carrying out the movement safely and with the appropriate equipment.

This chapter also highlights the procedures used to assist a person with mobilisation in a number of situations while maintaining their comfort and safety. It also discusses the organisational policies for both reporting on assisting clients with movement and the cleaning and returning of equipment used.

INDUSTRY INSIGHTS ➕

Early mobilisation post-operatively

Yesterday was my first shift in the orthopaedic ward. I was looking after 69-year-old Keith Bradshaw, who had been admitted with severe osteoarthritis of the right knee and had a total knee replacement the following morning. Prior to Mr Bradshaw's first post-operative walk with the physiotherapist, the registered nurse (RN) gave him pain relief so that he could undertake the mobilisation without undue distress. When the physiotherapist arrived, I assisted with Mr Bradshaw's mobilisation.

Even though Mr Bradshaw was hesitant to attempt to walk, the physiotherapist used clear communication and was very patient. The physiotherapist explained that the reason for early ambulation is to lower the chance of complications related to being bed-bound, such as clots, pneumonia, bladder infections and pressure sores, and it also possibly reduces the time spent in hospital.

To begin with, I made sure that the environment was clear, lowered the bed and, after Mr Bradshaw sat up slowly, ensured that he had non-slip socks on and helped put a transfer belt on him. He waited a moment and took some deep breaths to clear his light-headedness and then the physiotherapist positioned the forearm support frame in front of him. We both grabbed the handles on the transfer belt to support Mr Bradshaw, and on the physiotherapist's count of 'one, two, three' we assisted him to stand. He only took a few steps, but I could see from the look on his face that he was as astonished as I was about being able to walk so soon after surgery.

Early walking after surgery is one of the most crucial things a patient can do to prevent complications. I am sure Mr Bradshaw's early mobilisation will hasten his recovery, minimise his complications, and as his confidence grows, he will be able to mobilise independently and be discharged earlier from hospital.

1 PREPARE TO ASSIST A PERSON WITH MOVEMENT

Before commencing any new task, it is important to make an initial assessment, source the available equipment and the available personnel, and ensure that the plan of action to be implemented is safe and effective. When undertaking movement, one of the main responsibilities is to ensure that the workplace does not risk a person's health or safety. This can be confirmed through communicating with your healthcare team, consulting the person and their care plan, and complying with organisational policies and procedures. Selection of the appropriate equipment can then be made to move the person while maintaining their comfort and minimising risk.

Confirm movement requirements and risk factors with relevant personnel, plans or organisational policies and procedures

By confirming the movement requirements with your healthcare team, the person's care plan and relevant protocols, you ensure that you have the correct equipment for and instructions about the move. This includes considering ethical and legal responsibilities such as duty of care, reporting any incidents and adhering to infection control procedures. Organisational policies such as 'no lift' policies need to be maintained and additional training undertaken if necessary.

Legal and ethical considerations

The law in all Australian states and territories sets out the legal requirements for health and safety at work. The *Work Health and Safety Act 2011* describes employer and employee responsibilities when assessing the risks posed by hazards in the workplace and determining how best to modify or eliminate work processes to control or eliminate the risk.

Duty of care

Employers have a primary duty of care that requires them to ensure health and safety by eliminating risks to health and safety. This includes providing appropriate equipment to assist with the movement of individuals. If it is not reasonably possible to eliminate the risk, it must be minimised so far as is practicable.

Employees also have a duty of care and must take reasonable care to protect their own and others' health and safety. They must use the equipment provided by the employer to protect their health and safety while following correct techniques, and report hazards and faults or injuries. For any healthcare worker, it is important to inform their supervisor if they have an existing back problem that may interfere with their ability to assist a person with movement.

All employees are obliged to report any hazard by using the accepted protocol for that workplace. Online or paper-based forms can be completed, retained and acted upon as a record of risk management processes within the organisation. If an employee feels that hazards are not dealt with appropriately and adequately through available channels in the workplace, the matter can be reported for further investigation.

Incident reporting

As an HSA, you are responsible for ensuring that you are capable of undertaking manual handling tasks and reporting any injuries or instances of back pain that occur when assisting a client to mobilise. This is done by completion of an incident report as soon as possible after the event. Avoiding repetitive strain and using correct manual handling techniques and equipment will reduce the likelihood of this occurring. Incident reporting should also be carried out for a 'near miss', when an incident or accident is narrowly avoided. Reporting helps to prevent a similar incident in the future. Refer to Chapter 1, 'Participate in workplace health and safety', for details on completing incident report forms.

Infection control

You may need to take specific precautions when moving a person who has a wound or infectious disease. The wounds should be appropriately covered and you will need to wear gloves during the manual handling procedure. Additional personal protective equipment (PPE) (masks, gowns) may be necessary depending on the condition of the person. Check with the RN or organisational policies and procedures if unsure. Equipment will also need to be appropriately cleaned after the procedure according to your organisation's policies. Refer to Chapter 2, 'Comply with infection prevention and control policies and procedures', for more information on PPE and cleaning equipment.

Incident
An event or particular occurrence; for example, a falls incident.

Duty of care
The requirement to ensure health and safety by eliminating risks.

No lifting policies

Many healthcare facilities have introduced 'minimal lifting' or 'no lifting' policies as a part of their manual handling risk management. The Australian Nursing and Midwifery Federation (2018) endorses a safe patient handling policy, which states that the manual lifting of people must be eliminated in all but exceptional circumstances, such as life-threatening situations. This policy promotes the use of mechanical lifting aids and other equipment to assist staff in moving, transferring and lifting individuals to reduce injuries. You should make yourself aware of organisational policies related to manual handling and lifting in your workplace.

Training

All organisations must provide ongoing training to ensure that any healthcare worker who is involved in manual handling activities is aware of the risks, and to ensure that he or she is carrying out their work activities safely. This includes:

- educating and training staff in the correct use of aids and equipment, in manual handling techniques and in individual assessment
- providing an adequate number of appropriately skilled staff
- enforcing the use of equipment through supervision and post-training support
- ensuring that the manual handling and equipment needs of the patient are assessed and amended at each stage of the patient journey if required.

Organisational policies and procedures

Source the incident management policy that is used in your workplace and answer the following questions regarding the policy:

1   What is an example of a near miss when assisting with movement?

2   Why is it important to report a near miss on an incident report?

3   Why is it important to source feedback from staff and patients after a manual handling incident?

8.1 ACTIVITY

Select, prepare and adjust equipment according to person's requirements and individualised plan

Assessment of the client will be undertaken by a qualified person, such as an RN or physiotherapist, before equipment is selected. This will then be documented on an individual's care plan or notes. The appropriate equipment or assistive devices must be used even in situations where the patient and/or family preference is for it not to be used. In some instances, equipment will need to be adjusted to accommodate the needs of the person (e.g., the height of a walking stick) and for your safety (e.g., applying brakes on a bed before repositioning a person). The following outlines the various types of equipment that can be selected when assisting a person to move.

Assistive device

Any device that is designed, made or adapted to assist a person to perform a particular task.

Rope ladder, pull straps and bed trapeze

Ladders and straps are used to assist a person to pull up from a lying to a sitting position in a bed (see Figure 8.1). The strap attaches to the foot end of the bed and the loops or rungs can be

FIGURE 8.1 Ladders are used to assist a person to pull up from a lying to a sitting position in a bed

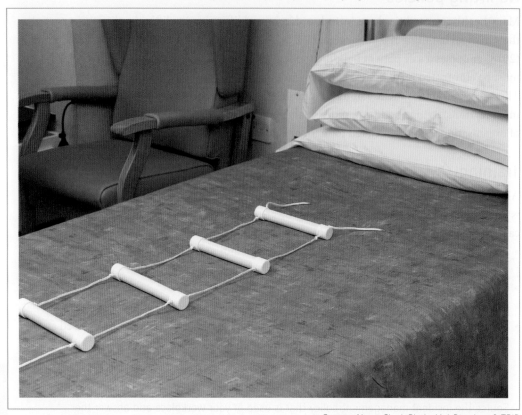

Source: Alamy Stock Photo / Art Directors & TRIP

grasped or the elbow or forearm can be placed through the openings so that the individual can 'climb' to a sitting position. You should ensure that the ladder is firmly secured to the foot of the bed and that it is adjusted to the correct length for the person.

A bed trapeze/triangle is designed to assist the person to sit up in bed and reposition themselves. It is usually fixed to the head of the bed as an overhead attachment. It can be adjusted in length and should be moved to the side when not in use. Please refer to your organisational policy regarding the trapeze as these are being phased out in some healthcare facilities.

Slide sheet

Slide sheets are very smooth sheets made from strong, thin, synthetic material, and are used to:
- reposition a person in bed
- sit the person up in bed
- turn a person to their side or back
- swing the person's legs in or out of a bed
- assist in other transfers such as to a chair, wheelchair or vehicle.

The top sheet slides against the bottom sheet to create a smooth and easy movement. This reduces friction so that less force is required to move the person. Slide sheets come in various sizes to suit each individual – they can be a single sheet or a tubular configuration (see Figure 8.2).

FIGURE 8.2 Slide sheet

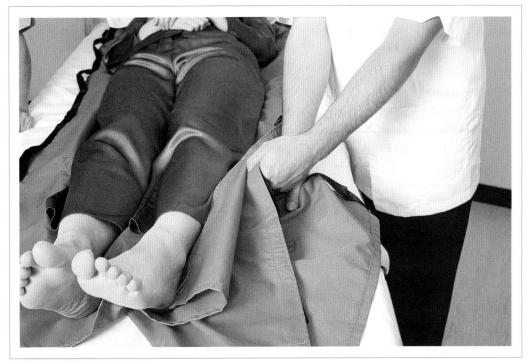

Source: Alamy Stock Photo/Mediscan

Swivel and transfer boards

Swivel boards are portable rotating discs that assist a person to transfer out of a vehicle or chair or pivot 360 degrees with the assistance of a healthcare worker (see Figure 8.3).

FIGURE 8.3 Swivel board used in cars

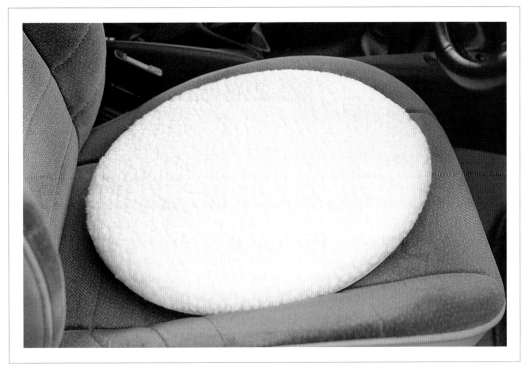

Source: Reproduced with permission of Performance Health

Transfer boards are large boards with shiny surfaces that allow a supine person to be transferred from bed to trolley. Smaller boards have tapered edges and can be used to slide a seated person from one surface to another. Boards can vary in size and you should refer to the information on the board to determine its load capacity.

Transfer belts

Transfer belts are worn around the waist by patients who require minimal assistance to walk (see Figure 8.4). The belt can be used to assist a person to move from sitting to standing, sitting to sitting, and for support while standing and walking. They have grab handles for healthcare workers to grasp and are fastened by Velcro or buckles. They come in various sizes to suit the person.

FIGURE 8.4 Transfer belts are worn around the waist by individuals who require minimal assistance to walk

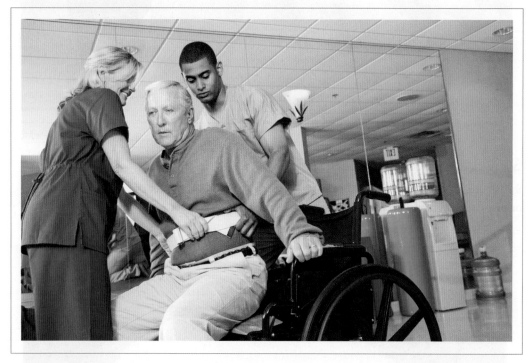

Source: iStock.com / AlexRaths

Mechanical lifters

There are many types of mechanical lifters used to help with the mobility of a person who is unable to weight-bear. These battery-powered or manually controlled devices have various-sized slings that lift and support the person and maintain their safety and comfort during the procedure. To provide stability, the base can be adjusted to get closer to the load or to avoid obstructions; for example, splaying the legs to fit closer to the person in a chair. It is important to be aware of the safe working load before undertaking manual handling tasks with mechanical lifters.

Hoists help move a person with reduced mobility from one location to another or in lifting a person from the floor. They can be ceiling-mounted or portable devices. They should not be used to transport a person over long distances (see Figure 8.5). Stand-up lifters are used to stand up and transfer individuals who may only be able to weight-bear on one leg but have balance and control of their upper body. Transfers can be from one seating surface to another; for example, bed to chair or chair to commode. Manual stand-up lifters require some effort on the part of the patient, which makes them ideal for rehabilitation.

FIGURE 8.5 Hoist

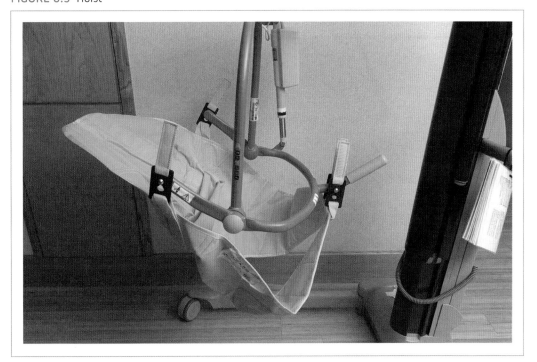

Source: Alamy Stock Photo / Art Directors & TRIP

Sit to stand transfer platforms can be used to ensure safe, active standing support during short transfers, such as between beds and wheelchairs/shower chairs.

Walking frames, crutches and walking sticks

Walking frames provide stable support and are used when the person has an unsteady gait or is partially weight-bearing. Crutches enable the person to ambulate by taking the weight off their body through one or both legs. Walking sticks can be used for a person with one-sided weakness and to provide balance and support. A single-stem walking stick is most common, but tripod or quad canes are available, which have three to four feet to offer extra balance and stability. Some necessary adjustments to these types of equipment include ensuring that the aid is the correct height for the person and that rubber tips are in good repair and all screws are tight. Figure 8.6 identifies different types of walking sticks.

FIGURE 8.6 Examples of different types of walking sticks

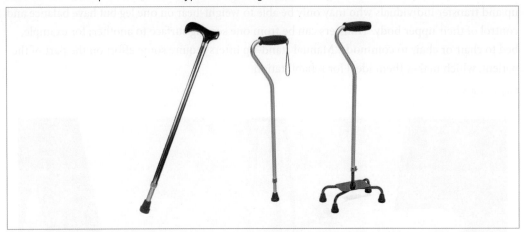

Source: Shutterstock.com/vvoe; Shutterstock.com/AlexLMX

Wheelchairs and commode chairs

Wheelchairs are used by individuals for whom walking is difficult or impossible due to illness, injury or disability. Commode chairs are placed near a bed for ease of toileting at night. The bedpan is concealed within the frame of the chair and is accessed by lifting up the seat. They can be static or portable for use in a shower. Adjustment to these types of equipment includes ensuring that the wheelchair or commode chair fits the individual and that all components are in working order; for example, tyres, wheels and brakes, and armrests and footrests.

Raised toilet seat

These plastic raised toilet seats fit to toilet bowls using adjustable screws or brackets. They are available in different heights and decrease the distance that a person needs to lower themselves down to, or raise themselves up from, a toilet.

ACTIVITY 8.2

Selecting appropriate equipment

Match the appropriate equipment to their clinical scenarios:

Equipment

- transfer belt
- hoist
- stand-up lifter
- slide sheet
- walking frame
- rope ladder
- transfer board
- raised toilet seat.

Clinical scenario

- The person needs to be repositioned on their side in bed and has limited mobility.
- The person has limited ability to bend over the toilet seat.
- The person needs minimal assistance to stand up from a chair.
- The person needs to be transferred from the bed to a trolley.
- The person has upper body control but can weight-bear on only one leg and requires assistance to stand.
- The person cannot weight-bear and needs to be moved from bed to chair.
- The person wishes to walk down the corridor and has an unsteady gait.
- The person has good upper body strength and needs to sit up in bed.

Appropriately prepare the environment

The first step in initiating safe movement of a person is ensuring that the environment is clear and ready. Make sure that the bedside area is clear to lift or pivot a person and that the bed is the correct height for the procedure. Adjustable beds are manually or hydraulically operated with position adjustments to the back rest, leg rest area and bed height. Environmental safety considerations include ensuring that the bed brakes are on, the floors have no tripping hazards and that the route is free from obstructions. The destination must also be prepared so that the manual handling equipment and person can be manoeuvred effectively.

Grab rails are applicable to both wet and dry areas and can be used both indoors and outdoors. They assist a person to maintain their balance and provide support while a person is manoeuvring; for example, a grab rail can be used in a bathroom to assist a person to stand up from the toilet seat. A bathroom or corridor with grab rails can provide independence for a person with instability.

Considerations when the environment is not custom fitted with aids

When there are no mobility aids in the facility to assist with the movement, you must determine the patient's ability to assist you with the move. Additional support can be gained from another co-worker. Alternatively, the patient may have existing mobility aids in their home that can be brought in for the duration of their stay in hospital.

Preparing the environment

Mrs Baker has just been admitted into the ward from a nursing home. She is booked for theatre tomorrow and will undergo a cholecystectomy. She weighs 110 kg, is mildly disorientated and is unsteady on her feet.

1   What are the risk factors for Mrs Baker and how can they be reduced?
2   How would you prepare the bed to ensure that Mrs Baker is safe and comfortable?
3   What mobility equipment would you use when Mrs Baker needs to use the bathroom?
4   What assistive devices could help Mrs Baker in the bathroom?
5   How can Mrs Baker's relatives assist you in making the environment risk-free for her?

8.3 ACTIVITY

Explain the procedure and gain consent and cooperation according to appropriate communication protocols

Prior to moving a person, it is important to communicate to explain the procedure, assess the person's ability to assist, and gain their consent. A person may be resistant to being moved in a particular way if they have not been consulted or if it is culturally inappropriate. Check that they understand what you are going to do and ask if they have any concerns. If assistance is required, you must discuss the procedure with your co-worker so that your movements are coordinated.

Communication considerations when preparing to assist a person with movement include:

- checking if the person has cognitive, vision or hearing disturbances that could interfere with communication
- identifying yourself and addressing the person by name
- communicating in simple language and using gestures or an interpreter if there are language barriers
- explaining the move to the person and allowing them to ask questions, then provide clear, concise answers
- making sure that the person is in a comfortable state; for example, pain relief may need to be administered by the RN/EN prior to the procedure
- planning the move by determining the lead person and instructing your partner to mirror your movements, which will ensure that the load is equally shared.

Confidentiality, privacy and disclosure

You must respect the confidentiality and privacy of the person while assisting them with mobility. Make sure you close the bedside curtains and cover the person appropriately during the procedure. Always maintain confidentiality by not disclosing any confidential information other than in the course of your professional duties.

Disclosure
Revealing or uncovering information that was intended to be private.

Cultural and religious considerations

Moving a person requires you to touch them, even when mechanical aids are used, and some techniques also require close body contact. In some cultures and religions, it is considered inappropriate to touch a person or to have physical contact between men and women; therefore, communication is essential to overcoming these barriers to moving and handling. Explain to the person how you are going to move them, emphasising that it is for their safety. It may also be useful to provide an explanation of the move to family members who may be present.

SCENARIO

Lifting Mrs Flora with a hoist

Claudia, the HSA, needs to use a hoist to lift Mrs Flora from the bed to a chair. She begins by identifying herself to Mrs Flora and then assessing the environment to make sure it is clear of obstructions. She makes sure that Mrs Flora is pain-free and gains consent for the lift. An assistant is required, so Claudia explains the procedure step by step to both Mrs Flora and her co-worker in clear, simple language. She asks if Mrs Flora can understand her instructions and if she has any questions or concerns.

1   Why is it important for one of the healthcare workers to act as a 'lead' when undertaking this lift?
2   How can Mrs Flora assist with this procedure?

Carry out preparation and procedures according to safe working practices

When preparing for a manual handling procedure, you should identify any factor that could cause danger, injury or adverse consequences so that safe work practices can be undertaken. This is part of the risk management process and includes identification of the hazard, assessing the risk and attempting to eliminate or minimise the risk.

Hazard identification

It is important that you are aware of manual handling hazards prior to undertaking any movement. A *hazard* is a source or situation with the potential for harm. Safework SA (2020) defines a hazardous manual task as one that

> requires a person to lift, lower, push, pull, carry or otherwise move, hold or restrain any person … or thing that involves one or more of the following:
> * repetitive or sustained force
> * high or sudden force
> * repetitive movement
> * sustained or awkward posture
> * exposure to vibration.

Hazardous manual tasks in an acute care setting include pushing and pulling loads and handling people. Once a hazard has been identified, the staff member must assess the risk, determine how significant the risk is, and how often it might occur.

Risk assessment

This involves analysing the risk factors that have been identified and the potential for an injury to occur. With manual handling, the health and safety of the person being handled needs to be considered as well as your own health and safety. Risk factors can include:

* physical and cognitive state; for example, weight, disease state, ability to assist and ability to cooperate
* history of falls
* medications
* environment; for example, workplace layout, equipment attached to the person, and distance to be moved
* your skill level and experience
* posture required or repetitive actions.

Once the risk assessment is complete, management of the process can be commenced to determine the measures that are needed to eliminate or reduce the risk.

Risk elimination or control

The risk elimination or control process should be done in consultation with staff. The first goal of risk management is the elimination of the risk, and if this is not possible, minimisation of risk to the lowest level possible. Since the manual handling of individuals cannot be eliminated, the provision and use of appropriate equipment along with training can help with risk control.

Safe Work Australia (2020) has developed a code of practice for hazardous manual tasks. For an HSA undertaking manual handling tasks, this means:

Risk control

A hazard management process aimed at identifying risks and eliminating or reducing the likelihood of injury.

- pushing rather than pulling because it involves less work by the muscles of the lower back
- using slide sheets to reduce friction when moving individuals
- positioning trolleys with wheels in the direction of travel
- using the large, powerful muscles of the legs to initiate the push or pull of a load
- not fully lifting a person (other than a small infant) unaided
- using mechanical aids, assistive devices or another worker wherever possible and ensuring staff are adequately trained in equipment use
- maximising the person's ability to assist in the move as much as possible
- ensuring the location and storage of mechanical and assistive devices allows easy access
- providing grab rails, bath seats and toilet seat raisers to help the person to help themselves.

ACTIVITY 8.4

Hazards and risk controls in the acute care environment

Figure 8.7 identifies potential sources of hazards that may be found when assisting a person to mobilise. Beside each hazard, provide an assessment of it and consider the risk control measures to eliminate or reduce the risk. The first row has been provided as an example.

FIGURE 8.7 Hazards and risk controls in the acute care environment

HAZARD	ASSESSMENT OF HAZARD	RISK CONTROL MEASURES
Furniture	Check for obstruction or congestion	Move furniture to organise for clear access
Flooring		
Power cords		
Lighting		
Cognitive state of person		
Physical state of person		
Person's clothing		
Infectious diseases		
Healthcare workers' skills and knowledge		

SCENARIO

Assisting Mr Amponsem with a walk belt

Phillipe, an HSA, needs to help Mr Amponsem to the shower using a walk belt. Potential hazards include the environment, the person or equipment, so he checks that the path is clear from bed to bathroom, that the bathroom is unoccupied and has no clutter, and that the shower chair is in place and the floor is clean and dry. He makes sure that Mr Amponsem understands the procedure and gains his permission, and that the walk belt is the appropriate size and in good order. In preparation for the shower, Phillipe makes sure that Mr Amponsem has appropriate footwear, and that his toiletries, clothing and towels are ready in the bathroom.

1 What communication techniques could Phillipe use if Mr Amponsem has poor understanding of English?
2 What precautions were used in the scenario to maintain safety and security for Mr Amponsem?

2 ASSIST WITH MOVEMENT

When assisting a person to move, it is important for you to encourage the person to be as independent as possible while assisting you so that they feel safe and secure. This means using correct body mechanics for each type of move, using the correct equipment and communicating throughout the procedure.

Carry out movement using safe handling methods and equipment using a range of techniques

It is important to examine the principles of safe handling to give you the information you need to look after your own health and safety before moving a person. A manual handling injury can impact the workplace through the loss of an experienced and skilled staff member. An understanding of basic body mechanics is the first step in ensuring that the movement is carried out in the safest manner for both you and the person being moved.

Basic body biomechanics

You should have the knowledge and skills to assess your own actions and movements in relation to manual handling tasks so that you may reduce the risks and likelihood of injury. This includes knowledge of the body and basic body mechanics, as well as the range of motion of body parts, and an understanding of why it is important to have correct posture and balance.

The spinal column supports the nerves and spine, and is made up of:

- vertebrae – provide structural support for the back and protection for the spinal cord
- discs – located between each vertebra; they provide cushioning for the spinal column and compress when bending forward and backwards
- ligaments – tough, fibrous tissue that connects the vertebrae to each other
- muscles – give the entire structure strength and stability.

By applying good body mechanics and planning movement, you can avoid muscle strain and reduce the risk of injury. This can be achieved by:

- gentle exercises to help prepare the muscles prior to lifting
- planning the lift or movement (person, environment, co-worker)
- ensuring footwear is protective and non-slip
- having a wide base of support by keeping feet shoulder-width apart
- pointing toes in the direction you are going to move, with knees slightly bent
- keeping objects close to the body and close to waist/hip area (centre of gravity)
- using smooth movements and avoiding twisting, stretching and bending if possible
- keeping the back straight while lifting and carrying (avoid stooped positions)
- pushing or sliding an object rather than lifting
- transferring your weight from one leg to another during movement, using the large leg muscles
- bracing abdominal muscles when moving a person
- using mechanical devices or assistance if the load is too big, heavy or awkward
- using the words of coordination – the command 'ready, steady, slide' or 'one, two, three'.

Body mechanics
The way a person moves and holds their body when they sit, stand, lift, carry and bend.

Range of motion
The measurement of movement around a specific joint or body part.

Centre of gravity
The point at which the entire mass of the body is assumed to be concentrated – waist/hip height.

Body mechanics

For each of the following principles of good body mechanics, describe the rationale (the reason for its use):

- Maintaining a wide base of support by keeping feet shoulder-width apart
- Pointing your toes in the direction of movement
- Keeping a load close to the centre of gravity
- Keeping your back straight
- Pushing rather than lifting
- Bracing your abdominal muscles when moving a person
- Using smooth movements
- Transferring weight from one leg to another
- Using leg muscles when moving.

Techniques to assist with mobility

Figure 8.8 outlines the standard procedures used to assist any person with mobility. These standard procedures should be used when repositioning, mobilising or transferring a person. This is followed by the specific steps for each procedure.

FIGURE 8.8 Standard procedures to assist a person with mobility

Before the procedure
- Identify yourself to the person and determine their identity is correct
- Undertake risk assessment
- Review care plan and consult with the healthcare team
- Explain the procedure to the person and gain consent and/or ability to assist
- Ensure the person's confidentiality and privacy

During the procedure
- Consider infection control precautions (wash hands, apply appropriate PPE)
- Prepare the environment and remove obstructions
- Organise equipment and/or personnel
- Check equipment safety – brakes, batteries, cleanliness and functional working order of equipment
- Communicate clear instructions at each stage to both the person and your partner if required
- Adhere to relevant legislation, policies and manual handling principles

After the procedure
- Confirm the person's satisfaction and comfort before leaving
- Clean and return equipment as required by organisation
- Wash hands
- Evaluate your own body biomechanics and safety
- Document the procedure in the client's notes
- Report completion of the procedure to the RN or supervisor

Repositioning

Prolonged immobility can cause a number of disorders, including pressure ulcers, constipation and muscle weakness. By assisting a person to reposition you promote self-care practices and reduce these complications. Maintaining good body alignment when repositioning helps to prevent pressure points, contractures or unnecessary discomfort for the person. Pillows can support the person on their side, and they can be made secure by raising the bed rails.

When sitting a person up, encourage them to assist where possible; for example, to bend their knees to push themselves up in bed or to use equipment to help themselves sit up in bed. They can do this with the aid of a:

- rope ladder – the person pulls themselves up by gripping along the ladder until they are sitting up
- overhead bed trapeze/triangle – the person hangs onto the trapeze/triangle with both hands and pulls themselves forward until sitting up.

Reposition a person using a slide sheet

Ensure the bed is at hip height of the tallest worker present if possible before commencing the move. The preparation of the patient includes placing their arms over their chest and bending their knees. This makes the move easier for both the patient and the healthcare workers. The following steps can then be undertaken:

1. The first worker places one of their hands on the patient's hip and the other on the back of the patient's shoulder.
2. The second worker places one of their hands on the patient's elbow and the other on the patient's knee.
3. Roll the patient onto their side or ask if they can assist.
4. Position the open side of the slide sheet on the same side that the pulling action is to occur and place the partially folded sheet under the person OR position the open side towards the shoulders of the person for pulling up the bed.
5. Roll the person back and ensure the slide sheet covers the heaviest part of the person at least from their shoulders to past their hips.
6. If you are moving a person up the bed, encourage them to assist by bending their legs up and pushing down with their feet.
7. Hold the top fold of sheet and slide the person into position while transferring your weight from your front foot to back foot with feet placed in a lunge position. Keep your knees slightly bent and back straight.
8. To retrieve the slide sheet, gently remove the bottom half of the slide sheet from under the person, pulling the corner diagonally away from the person and towards the head of the bed.

Mobilising

The level of assistance required to assist with mobility will depend on the condition of the person. Risk assessment includes appropriate footwear for the person. Non-slip socks are used in many healthcare facilities and are a safe option for people walking on potentially slippery surfaces; alternatively, make sure that the person is wearing supportive non-slip shoes.

Assist a person to walk with a belt

Walking or transfer belts can help a person to stand and allow them to be assisted to walk. It is important the user has good balance when standing and can move their feet independently when walking.

When walking with the person, stand to the side with your hands holding onto the handles of the belt; keep your back straight and feet pointed in the direction of where you are walking. If the person needs further assistance, two carers can be used, with each holding onto the handles of the belt. Good communication between the healthcare workers and the client will ensure a safe procedure.

Assist a person to use crutches

Ensure that the person has the heel of their hand resting on the hand piece of the crutch, while keeping the wrist and elbow bent slightly. Their body weight should be supported by the palms of the hands, and when standing with arms loosely by the side, each crutch should be two finger widths below the armpit.

Safety considerations include the following:
- Ensure screws are fully tightened and rubber stoppers are intact.
- Make sure any weight goes through the hands, not the armpits.
- Crutches should be kept close to the feet, not far out to the side.

The four-point gait sequence, as shown in Figure 8.9, can be performed when the person can move and bear weight on each leg:
1 move the right crutch
2 move the left foot
3 move the left crutch
4 move the right foot.

FIGURE 8.9 The four-point gait sequence

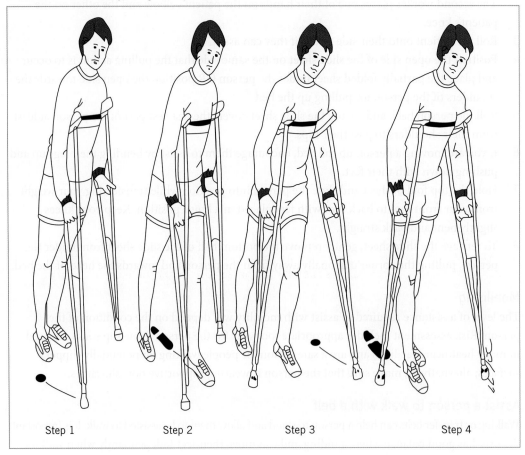

| Step 1 | Step 2 | Step 3 | Step 4 |

Source: https://nursing-skills.blogspot.com/2014/02/four-point-gait-walking.html

The three-point gait sequence, as shown in Figure 8.10, is fairly rapid and requires strong extremities and good balance:

1 balance weight on the crutches
2 move both crutches and affected leg forward
3 move unaffected leg forward.

FIGURE 8.10 The three-point gait sequence

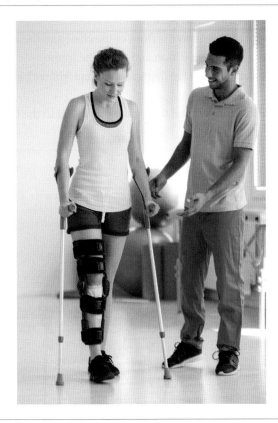

When going down a flight of stairs:

1 put crutches on the first step
2 put weight on the crutch handles and transfer the unaffected extremity onto the step where crutches are placed.

When going up stairs:

1 put weight on the crutch handles and lift the unaffected extremity onto the first step of the stairs
2 put weight on the unaffected extremity and lift the other extremity and the crutches onto the step.

Assist a person to use a walking stick

When assisting a person to use a walking stick, make sure that the stick is held in the opposite hand to the weaker leg and ensure that the rubber tip is intact and not worn. The person should:

• align their wrist with their hip joint
• bend their elbow slightly with the handle at hip level
• stand as straight as possible when they walk

- pay attention when walking with the walking stick on slippery or uneven surfaces
- not walk with the walking stick too far ahead.

Assist a person to use a walking frame

Walking frames (see Figure 8.11) provide greater support and security for a person who is unsteady on their feet or when partial weight-bearing is recommended. When assisting a person to use a walking frame:

- place the frame in front of the seated person
- advise the person to move forward to the front of the chair and then use the chair arms to push themselves up to a standing position and grasp the frame
- stand beside the person and encourage them to stand upright with eyes looking forward when walking
- make sure the person moves the frame then moves their feet to the frame.

FIGURE 8.11 Walking frames provide greater support and security

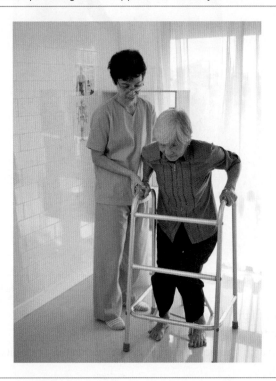

Source: Shutterstock.com / StudioByTheSea

Move a person by wheelchair or trolley

The essential requirements for wheelchair or trolley transport are to make sure that the chair or trolley fits the person correctly and that they can be transported safely. This means ensuring brakes are applied when positioning the person and footrests or trolley side rails are raised when the individual is being transported. Chapter 9, 'Transport individuals', outlines in more detail the process for moving a person by wheelchair or trolley.

Transfer a person

Planning a transfer involves communication with the patient as well as other workers. Transfers can occur between beds, chairs and cars and it is important that you have a sound understanding of the use of equipment in your facility. When a person has been lying down, it is recommended that they move slowly to a sitting position and sit there for several minutes before transfer. This allows their blood pressure to adjust, which can help prevent them feeling faint.

Chair/bed to chair transfer using a transfer belt

When undertaking a transfer using a transfer belt (see Figure 8.12), start by preparing the environment and positioning the chair, wheelchair or commode so the distance of the transfer is at a minimum. Ensure the brakes are on and any footplates are taken off or swung away. The following steps can then be undertaken:

1 Ask the person to slide forwards on the chair or bed and attach a transfer belt.
2 Make sure the person's feet are positioned under the edge of the chair or bed; that is, just behind their knees.

FIGURE 8.12 Bed to chair transfer

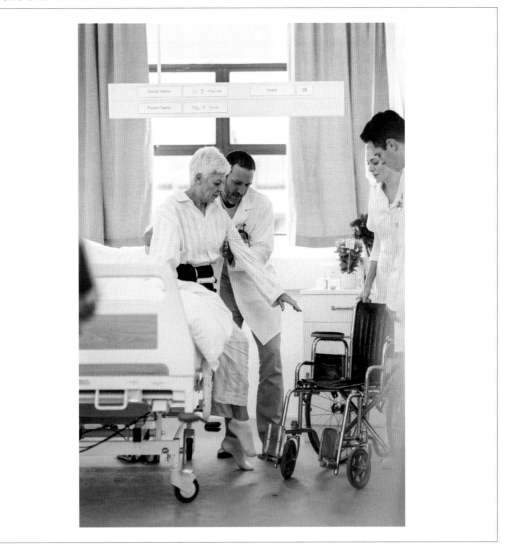

Source: Alamy Stock Photo/Westend61 GmbH

3   Ask the person to move their shoulders forward (nose over toes) and, if possible, position their hands on the armrest or bed so they can assist lift. Never let anyone pull on your arms or your neck!

4   *For a one-person assist*, stand in front of the person and grasp the handles on either side of the transfer belt. *For a two-person assist*, each healthcare worker should stand either side of the person grasping one handle at the front and one handle at the back of the transfer belt. You can block the person's foot with your own if this is comfortable and does not compromise your balance.

5   When the person is ready, keep your back straight, bend at knees, keep the load close and guide the person forwards and upwards. The command 'ready, steady, go' or 'one, two, three' can be used for coordination.

6   Slowly guide the person to the chair, and when the backs of their legs touch the chair, tell them to hold onto the chair arms and gently lower themselves to a seated position.

Chair to chair/bed transfer using a slide board

Before using a slide board (see Figure 8.13), ensure that you are transferring between surfaces of similar height, or transferring to a slightly lower surface. Position the chair as close to the commode or bed as possible, at about a 30-degree angle to the bed.

FIGURE 8.13 Patient using a slide board

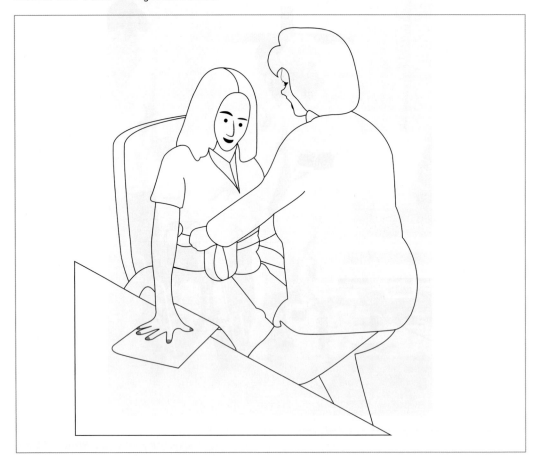

Lock the wheels of the chair or commode, move both footrests out of the way and remove the armrest nearest to you, then undertake the following steps:

1   Slide one end of the transfer board beneath the person's thigh. Point it downward to avoid pinching the skin. Ask them to lean their upper body in the opposite direction from the board to make placing the board easier.
2   Place the other end of the board flat on the seat or bed.
3   To move across the board, the person will push up with their arms and carefully move their body towards the second surface. This may have to be repeated using several short movements instead of one long movement.
4   Once the person is settled fully on the second surface, the transfer board can be removed. When transferring a person into a car using a slide board, the following needs to be considered:
•   Move the car seat as far back as possible before beginning the transfer to allow more room to move.
•   Slightly recline the back of the car seat if more headroom is needed.
•   Roll down the window to provide a surface for the person to grip while moving.
•   After the person's buttocks are positioned on the car seat, fasten the seat belt. This will give more stability when moving their legs into the car.
•   Move the legs into the car one at a time.

Bed to trolley transfer

It is important to ensure that equipment, such as intravenous infusion lines and catheters, are appropriately positioned so that they do not hinder the procedure and are not at risk of being tugged and dislodged when moving the person. During the risk assessment, identify if additional staff are required to maintain the safety of the person's head.

The steps for using a slide sheet and transfer board (see Figure 8.14) from bed to trolley are as follows:

1   Insert the slide sheet under the patient.
2   Insert the transfer board halfway under the patient so that the rest of the board bridges the gap between the two surfaces the patient is being transferred between.
3   Once the transfer board is in place, make sure the cot sides are lowered on the trolley, its height has been adjusted so that it is the same height as the bed, and it is alongside the bed.

FIGURE 8.14 Patient using a transfer board

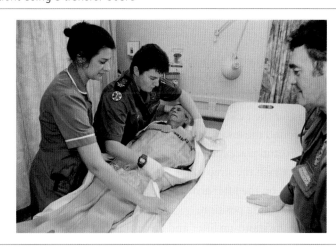

Source: age fotostock / John Birdsall

Then bring the trolley alongside and next to the bed. Make sure that the brakes on both the trolley and the bed are on.

4   Place the patient's arms crossed against their chest.

5   Two workers should position themselves on the far side of the receiving surface (trolley) and two should be by the bed. The handlers positioned nearest the patient's head will take a lead role in the transfer.

6   The worker by the patient's head places one hand on the patient's shoulder and one on the bed. The other worker on this side places one hand on the patient's hip and one on the bed.

7   The workers on the receiving side reach and grasp the slide sheet.

8   On the command, the workers positioned by the receiving surface pull the slide sheet, and the workers nearest the patient help to initiate the transfer by slightly pushing the patient across.

9   It may be necessary to undertake the procedure in two stages; for example, when the patient needs to be transferred across a wider surface, such as from one bed to another, or if there are significant lines and tubing to be kept stable or to be moved in a controlled way.

10 Once the patient is on the trolley, raise the sides.

Transfer a person with a hoist

When you need to move a person from the bed to a chair or commode and they cannot weight-bear, they will need to be transferred using a hoist. Safety is improved and the person feels more secure if the hoist lift is performed by two people. Check regarding the correct procedure for using a hoist within your facility. These general steps can be followed:

1   Refer to the hoist's instructions for operation and ensure the battery is charged.

2   Select the correct sling and place it underneath the person. If the person is in bed, apply the sling by rolling them to each side; if the person is sitting, rock them forwards and then sideways to get the sling underneath them.

3   Secure the brakes on the hoist and the destination; for example, a bed or chair.

4   Position the hoist, lower the boom and attach the sling at all points, ensuring that the sling is not squeezing the person's skin.

5   Ensure the person's arms are contained within the sling and they are holding onto the spreader bar.

6   Raise the person in the hoist and lower them at the destination.

7   Release the slings and remove them.

Transfer a person with a stand-up lifter

The person must be able to partially weight-bear and have good upper body strength for this procedure (as shown in Figure 8.15). Preparation of the person to use the stand-up lifter starts with them in a sitting position on the side of the bed or edge of the chair and requires a minimum of two workers for the task:

1   Place the lifter belt around the lower back of the person.

2   Bring the lifter forward and place the person's feet on the foot plate.

3   Position the lifter and attach the strap loops.

4   Place the person's hands on the lifter arms and prepare to lift.

5   Raise the person to a standing position.

6   Move the person with the stand-up lifter and lower it at the destination.

7   Release the loops and remove the stand-up lifter.

It is essential to always move in same direction as the lifter when walking it; do not twist.

FIGURE 8.15 Patient using a stand-up lifter

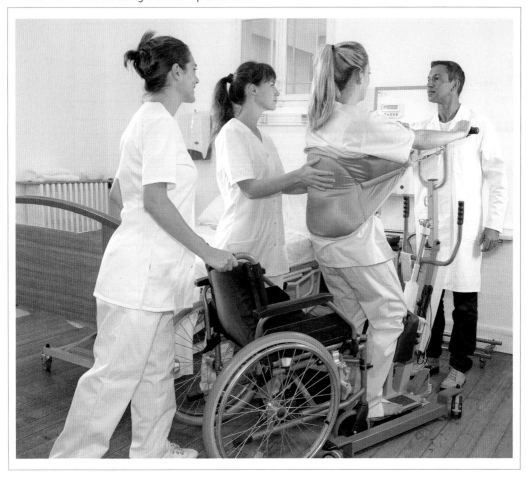

Source: Alamy Stock Photo/Phovoir

Ensure the person's comfort and safety throughout positioning or transfer

It is important to undertake risk assessment and use safe manual handling techniques to ensure the safety and comfort of the person and to avoid possibly injuring them while they are being moved. You should never attempt to manually lift a fallen person because further injury to the person can occur.

Skin integrity

Maintaining skin integrity is an important consideration while moving a person. In particular, elderly people may have thin skin that is easily damaged through rubbing or catching on equipment during the move. It is important to check that your watch, ID band or belt buckle does not accidentally damage the person's skin and that sharp edges on the equipment do not cause cuts or abrasions. Maintaining skin integrity can be ensured by not dragging the person's buttocks on a slide board, making sure they are always clothed before moving them or making sure that a slide sheet is used.

Skin integrity
Skin that is whole, intact and undamaged.

Falls management

Many healthcare organisations have falls risk assessments that help to identify people at risk so that they can develop appropriate strategies. Figure 8.16 gives an example of a falls risk screening tool.

FIGURE 8.16 Ontario falls risk screening tool

	NSW Health	FAMILY NAME	MRN

Facility:

ONTARIO MODIFIED STRATIFY (SYDNEY SCORING) FALLS RISK SCREEN

GIVEN NAME ☐ MALE ☐ FEMALE
D.O.B. ___/___/___ M.O.
ADDRESS
LOCATION / WARD
COMPLETE ALL DETAILS OR AFFIX PATIENT LABEL HERE

	Value	Date / / Score	Date / / Score	Date / / Score
Complete on Admission (A), Post Fall (PF), Change of Condition (CC), or When Appropriate (W)	Value	A	PF ☐ CC ☐ W ☐	PF ☐ CC ☐ W ☐
1. History of Falls Did the patient present to hospital with a fall or have they had a fall since admission?	Yes to any = 6			
If not, has the patient fallen within the last 6 months?				
2. Mental Status Is the patient confused? (i.e. unable to make purposeful decisions, disorganised thinking and/or memory impairment)	Yes to any = 14			
Is the patient disorientated? (i.e. lacking awareness, being mistaken about time, place or person)				
Is the patient agitated? (i.e. fearful affect, frequent movements and/or anxious)				
3. Vision Does the patient require eyeglasses continually?	Yes to any = 1			
Does the patient report blurred vision?				
Does the patient have glaucoma, cataracts or macular degeneration?				
4. Toileting Are there any alterations in urination? (i.e. frequency, urgency, incontinence, nocturia)	Yes = 2			

5. Transfer Score (TS) [means from bed to chair and back]		Add Transfer Score (TS) and Mobility Score (MS)	Total of TS+ MS	Total of TS+ MS	Total of TS+ MS
Independent - use of aids to be independent is allowed	0	If total between 0-2, then score = 0			
Minor help - one person easily or needs supervision for safety	1				
Major help - one strong skilled helper or two normal people; physically can sit	2				
Unable - no sitting balance, mechanical lift	3				
6. Mobility Score (MS)					
Independent (but may use any aid, e.g. walking stick)	0	If total between 3-6, then score = 7			
Walks with help of one person (verbal or physical)	1				
Wheelchair independent including corners, etc	2				
Immobile	3				

≥9 = HIGH RISK OF FALLS	**TOTAL SCORE**			

If a patient scores <9, a clinician using clinical judgment can determine a high level of risk risk for that patient.

☐ Clinical Judgement ☐ High Risk Reason: _____

If any falls risk factors are identified, complete the relevant section on the Falls Risk Assessment and Management Plan (FRAMP) and implement actions.

	Name:	Name:	Name:
	Designation:	Designation:	Designation:
	Signature:	Signature:	Signature:

(Papaioannou A. et al. Prediction of falls using a risk assessment tool in acute care setting BMC Medicine 2004 2:1)

MEDICATIONS: Is the patient on antipsychotics, antidepressants, sedatives/hypnotics, or opioids?
YES ☐ Complete medication section on Falls Risk Assessment and Management Plan.

Provide patient/family/carers with information about Falls Prevention

Holes Punched as per AS2828.1: 2012 BINDING MARGIN - NO WRITING

SMR060911

NH606658 170718

ONTARIO MODIFIED STRATIFY (SYDNEY SCORING) FALLS RISK SCREEN SMR060.911

NO WRITING Page 1 of 2

Source: © State of New South Wales NSW Ministry of Health. For current information go to www.health.nsw.gov.au CC 4.0

The use of active and passive exercises is one strategy that can help a person to regain their strength, improve their mobility and reduce their risk of falls. If the person is unable to move, you can help them by performing passive exercises. Important points to remember while performing these exercises include:

- support all joints during the exercise activity
- use slow, gentle movements when performing exercises
- stop if the person complains of pain or discomfort
- do not overstretch joints.

In an acute care setting, however, falls may result following a stroke, a heart attack, an epileptic fit, a bleeding wound or a fracture. The following steps should be undertaken after a fall:

1 check for responsiveness and make them comfortable
2 call for assistance
3 make sure that the area surrounding the person is safe and that no further harm can occur; for example, spills or hazardous objects
4 assess the person for possible complications, bleeding and consciousness, and stay with the person until help arrives.

If you find the person sitting on the floor after a fall, you should call for help. In assisting the person to stand, ask them to roll on their side, then onto all fours and then into a kneeling position. Using a chair as a prop, help the person up and onto the chair. Should the person be unable to do this with light assistance, then appropriate lifting equipment should be used.

In an emergency situation, where the person shows no signs of life, lay the person flat without pillows, call for help and activate the emergency buzzer if nearby. In an acute care setting, the emergency response team will arrive and bring the necessary equipment to manage the person. Stay with the person until help arrives.

Falls risk screening tools

8.6 ACTIVITY

Falls risk screening is a process of estimating a person's risk of falling and classifying them as being at either low risk or high risk. Falls risk screening should occur as soon as practicable after a person is admitted to hospital.

These tools score clinical factors associated with falling and include management strategies according to the person's overall score. The outcomes of the falls risk assessment, together with the recommended strategies to address identified risk factors, are documented, reported to other healthcare staff, and discussed with the person and their carers.

Source a falls risk assessment tool from the facility where you work or undertake work experience, or source commonly used tools – for example, the Falls Risk Assessment Tool (FRAT) or Falls Risk Assessment and Management Plan (FRAMP) – and complete the following questions:

1 Identify the risk factors that are associated with falling.
2 How is the person scored and/or categorised?
3 List the management strategies and care actions that can be implemented to reduce the risk of falls for these people.
4 How often are the falls risk screens reviewed for the patient?

Adapted from: Australian Commission on Safety and Quality in Health Care (ACSQHC) (2009). Guidebook for preventing falls and harm from falls in older people: Australian hospitals. Retrieved 14 May 2016 from http://www.safetyandquality.gov.au/wp-content/uploads/2009/01/30459-HOSP-Guidebook.pdf

Encourage the person to assist and communicate during movement according to appropriate protocols

Communicating during a movement procedure ensures a smooth and coordinated approach for both the patient and the healthcare workers. Encouraging the person to assist not only reduces the efforts required by the healthcare workers but also increases the person's confidence and independence. Examples of ways in which the patient can assist during movement include:

- putting their hands on the armrests of the chair when standing or sitting
- leaning forward when moving from a sitting to a standing position
- turning their head in the direction of a turn or roll and placing their arm over their chest so that they do not roll onto it
- bending their knees and digging their heels into the bed, ready to push themselves up the bed
- moving in a sling to get comfortable.

Communication throughout the move involves talking through the steps and asking if the person is comfortable. Some individuals may resist being moved because they feel their dignity and safety may be compromised. Communicating the benefits for the person regarding safety and dignity may allay those fears and increase the person's confidence. Alternatively, demonstrating the move with another worker or showing the person how the equipment works can reassure them that the procedure is safe. Speak at a slower pace if the individual has difficulty understanding.

If more than one person is assisting with the move, choose a lead person who will coordinate the move. This lead person will be responsible for giving instructions to both the person being moved and the assistant. This includes who will carry out each step of the move and what the patient can do to assist with the move. Examples of strategies that promote coordination include:

- ensuring that all instructions and commands are consistent throughout the organisation; for example, 'ready, steady, stand' or 'one, two, three'
- making eye contact with your co-worker so that the move is synchronised
- using clear speech so that misunderstandings do not occur.

ACTIVITY 8.7

Communication for safety

1   What communication strategies can you use when the person to be moved has cognitive impairment?

2   What communication strategies can you use when the person has a visual Impairment?

3   What impacts can an uncoordinated approach have on the person to be moved?

4   Your facility has just purchased a new stand-up lifter and you are unsure about how to use it. What actions should you take?

3   COMPLETE ASSISTANCE WITH MOVEMENT

At the completion of a move, it is important to make sure that the person feels safe and secure. An evaluation of the technique used includes communication on any issues that affected the person during the procedure. Ask the person how they felt after the move because feedback is useful to verify that they were comfortable or whether improvements could be made. This can provide continuous improvement when next undertaking manual handling and should be recorded in the person's care plan.

Clean and return equipment in accordance with organisational policy and procedures

All equipment should be wiped clean before it is returned to the storage area in order to prevent contamination for both staff and patients. Make sure you clean the equipment according to the instructions from the manufacturer or the organisation you work for.

Transfer belts and slings are machine-washable, with some facilities using disposable slings as an infection control precaution. Spills and stains on machine-washable belts and slings should be treated as soon as possible. Gently scrape away any soils or mop away liquid from the surface of the fabric with a damp cloth before placing it in the laundry receptacles.

Return all equipment to the designated area in your ward. Some equipment may have specific check-in–check-out protocols and you must be aware of your organisation's procedures. You may also find that patients are allocated their own slide sheets and transfer belts as an infection control measure. If this is the case, the equipment must be returned to the person's bedside area.

Report equipment faults in accordance with organisational procedures, industry standards and guidelines

It is important that you are proactive in maintaining a safe and risk-free environment. This includes maintaining the equipment that you use and notifying any malfunction to an RN or supervisor. Any faults or damage should be reported according to the organisation's procedure, and equipment may be disposed of, tagged or sent to maintenance for repair.

Check transfer belts, straps and slings regularly, and look for wear and damage on seams, fabric, straps, handles and buckles. Slings or straps should be withdrawn from use and replaced where fabric is torn, worn through or shows signs of thinning. Attachment clips should be replaced if they are damaged or have sharp edges that could wear through fabric.

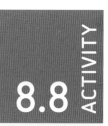

Equipment storage and faults

Locate where hoists, wheelchairs and stand-up lifters are stored in your facility. Answer the following questions:

1 Undertake a risk assessment of this space and suggest ideas for improvement.

2 Why is it important to return equipment to this location on completion of procedures?

3 What is your facility's policy for when you find a fault in the equipment?

8.8 ACTIVITY

SUMMARY

This chapter outlined methods for supporting people who require assistance with basic physical movement. From identifying the movement requirements and risk factors to complying with organisational policies and procedures, this chapter highlighted the importance of preparation of both the environment and equipment to ensure the safety and comfort of the person.

The chapter emphasised the importance of using clear communication and a coordinated approach to encourage the person to reposition and move. The steps involved in repositioning, mobilising and transferring a person using a variety of equipment were outlined. The use of good body mechanics to reduce the risk of injury to the healthcare worker was also emphasised.

The last part of the chapter explained the importance of recording and reporting procedures including faults in equipment. By gaining an understanding of the correct use of equipment and techniques required for movement procedures, you will be equipped with the skills required to perform manual handling tasks effectively.

APPLY YOUR KNOWLEDGE

Falls management

Katerina is 82 and lives in a nursing home. Ten years ago she was diagnosed with osteoporosis and osteoarthritis after complaining of aching leg joints after exercise. She has been mobilising independently using a walker as recommended by her GP. Recently she has been experiencing bouts of dizziness.

She has been admitted to hospital for investigation and her blood pressure on arrival is 85/48. You are the HSA who is looking after this new admission and your first action is to explain to Katerina how to use the buzzer before getting out of bed so that someone can help her with walking. As an additional precaution you raise the bed rails and lower the bed. Despite these precautions, Katerina is found lying on the floor a few hours later. She states that she didn't want to bother anyone as they all looked too busy.

1   What are the initial steps that you should take when you find Katerina on the floor?

2   Using the knowledge learnt in Chapter 1, 'Participate in workplace health and safety', specify what type of documentation is required for this incident and what information is required.

As an HSA, you report the incident to the RN and the doctor assesses Katerina and indicates that there are no significant injuries.

Your colleague helps you to assist Katerina back to bed using a hoist for the transfer.

3   Outline how a hoist can be used to transfer a person back to bed from the floor.

4   How could you communicate to encourage Katerina to assist during the movement?

5   How can Katerina's comfort and safety be ensured throughout the procedure?

Once Katerina is back in bed, you re-explain the importance of contacting staff if she needs to get out of bed. Katerina apologises and reassures the HSA that she will not do this again.

6   After the procedure is complete, what measures do you take to make sure that the hoist is ready for the next transfer?

7   Understanding the scope of practice as an HSA is essential to working effectively within the healthcare team. How did the HSA demonstrate the scope of their role with the actions in this case study?

Katerina was discharged two days later back to the nursing home. She has been prescribed medication for her hypotension and encouraged to maintain adequate hydration. The nursing home has since reported that Katerina is compliant with her treatment and back to walking again with the help of nursing staff, until she feels confident enough to mobilise independently again.

◄ REFLECTING ON THE INDUSTRY INSIGHT 💬

1   Why was it important to allow Mr Bradshaw to sit at the side of the bed and take
    some deep breaths before standing up and walking?
    a   So he could avoid an episode of light-headedness when standing up.
    b   To allow time for him to take pain medication before standing up.
    c   To allow the nurse to kneel behind him and push him up to a standing position.
    d   So that effective communication of information could take place.

2   The physiotherapist called 'one, two, three' before Mr Bradshaw stood up. Why is
    this important?
    a   This is the standard call when undertaking all tasks in nursing.
    b   It ensures a coordinated approach to the manoeuvre by the staff and patient.
    c   It allows the patient to prepare by rocking back and forth prior to standing up.
    d   So that the HSA is aware of who is in charge for the procedure.

3   What were the benefits in giving Mr Bradshaw pain relief prior to his
    early mobilisation?
    a   Pain relief masks the signs of inflammation at the wound site.
    b   The pain relief allowed for comfort and relieved stress prior to the procedure.
    c   The pain relief could be administered by the HSA to relieve the
        patient's anxiety.
    d   The 'top up' provided muscle relaxation to assist with mobilisation.

SELF-CHECK QUESTIONS

1   What is your duty of care before undertaking any manual handling procedure?
2   Why is it important to gain better information about the person's history from families/carers
    prior to assisting a person to move?
3   How can you maintain privacy when transferring a person from bed to chair using the
    stand-up lifter?
4   Define body mechanics and describe why it is important to apply good body mechanics when
    moving a patient?
5   What are some examples of strategies that the HSA could use to promote coordination with their
    colleague when undertaking a move?
6   How can the patient assist the nurses when they are required to slide up the bed with the
    support of a slide sheet?
7   Identify the type of person and situations that would require the use of a stand-up lifter.
8   Identify situations when a person would require the use of a walk belt and outline the risks
    associated when you are helping them to mobilise.
9   What are your responsibilities when a person soils the hoist sling used in a transfer procedure?
10 What are your definitions of the following key words and terms that have been used in
    this chapter?

KEY WORD OR TERM	YOUR DEFINITION
Risk control	
Hoist	
Near miss	
Gait	
Centre of gravity	
Skin integrity	
Assistive device	
Range of motion	

QUESTIONS FOR DISCUSSION

1   Discuss your responsibilities and actions when you need assistance to move a person and there:
    a   are untrained staff
    b   is a negative workplace culture regarding safe practices.
2   Consider the situation of having to assist an elderly person who has minimal English language skills to move up in the bed. Identify the risks and discuss how you would control them.
3   Discuss the procedure when you find tears in the hoist sling used for transfers.
4   Discuss the actions you would take to ensure equipment safety when the client has their own walking frame.
5   Discuss how you would maintain the skin integrity of an elderly person when you are moving them on a hoist from the bed to a commode.

EXTENSION ACTIVITY

Risk assessment for manual handling tasks

When conducting risk assessment for manual handling tasks, the person's medical, personal and cultural needs should be considered. Work in groups to read the scenarios that follow and discuss how you would make the move safe for the person and your co-workers by identifying the:

- risks involved
- communication techniques used
- manual handling aids used and rationale
- control measures to ensure a safe procedure.

Role-play each of the scenarios, with one member being the patient and one or two members being the HSAs undertaking the manual handling tasks. Utilise the appropriate clinical equipment required for each task.

- Scenario 1: A 98-kilogram person has fallen to the floor in a confined bathroom.
- Scenario 2: An unconscious person has soiled the bed and the sheets need to be changed.
- Scenario 3: An elderly non-English-speaking person has just had bilateral knee replacements and needs to go to the bathroom.
- Scenario 4: An elderly person on oxygen therapy needs to sit out of bed for lunch. She has IV therapy and an indwelling catheter in situ.
- Scenario 5: An aggressive and disorientated person who weighs 145 kilograms needs to be turned second hourly to prevent pressure injuries.
- Scenario 6: A person who has just had cataract surgery needs assistance to go to the bathroom. He is slightly deaf.

REFERENCES

Australian Commission on Safety and Quality in Health Care (ACSQHC) (2009). Guidebook for preventing falls and harm from falls in older people: Australian hospitals. Retrieved 14 May 2016 from http://www.safetyandquality.gov.au/wp-content/uploads/2009/01/30459-HOSP-Guidebook.pdf

Australian Nursing and Midwifery Federation (2018). Safe patient handling. Retrieved 7 May 2016 from http://www.anmf.org.au/documents/policies/P_Safe_Patient_Handling.pdf

Government of South Australia (2020). Safe work instructions. Retrieved 15 February 2022 from https://dhs.sa.gov.au/services/disability/safe-work-instructions

Safe Work Australia (2020). Model code of practice: Hazardous manual tasks. Retrieved 17 May 2022 from https://www.safeworkaustralia.gov.au/doc/model-codes-practice/model-code-practice-hazardous-manual-tasks

Safework SA (2020). Hazardous manual tasks: Code of practice. Retrieved 17 May 2022 from https://www.safework.sa.gov.au/__data/assets/pdf_file/0005/136265/Hazardous-Manual-Tasks.pdf

Worksafe Victoria (2021). Hazardous manual handling: Safety basics. Retrieved 15 February 2022 from https://www.worksafe.vic.gov.au/hazardous-manual-handling-safety-basics

TRANSPORT INDIVIDUALS

Learning objectives

By the end of this chapter, you should be able to:

1   prepare a person for transport, take steps to confirm with relevant personnel and the person to determine their support needs, and select and check appropriate equipment for the safe and timely transportation of the person

2   transport the person and equipment in accordance with transportation requirements and organisational policy, ensuring the person's safety and minimising risk to self

3   deliver the person, accurately complete reporting requirements and return equipment appropriately.

Introduction

This chapter describes the knowledge and skills required to enable you to help transport individuals from one site to another in a safe, timely and efficient manner. This includes the preparation of the person and equipment for their safe delivery.

Across each state and within health services, individuals regularly need to be moved in order to access the most appropriate care for their clinical condition. This may involve diagnostic or interventional testing or relocation to an alternative care facility. As a member of the healthcare team, a health services assistant (HSA) needs to provide continuity of care throughout the entire process of transporting a patient.

This chapter will provide you with a thorough understanding of how to prioritise the needs of the individual, undertake risk assessments, prepare appropriate equipment and transport individuals safely. It will also highlight the importance of communication and documentation during this process.

INDUSTRY INSIGHTS ➕

Patient transport services

Non-emergency patient transport is a health service for patients who require transportation to or from a health facility but do not need an emergency ambulance. Patients must be assessed by a medical practitioner or registered nurse as medically unsuitable for community, public or private transport before being eligible for this service.

My patient, Mrs Brennan, required this service because she was leaving the hospital and being transferred back to her nursing home. She was unsuitable for community transport because she required a stretcher, had limited mobility and was incontinent. The registered nurse had used the online patient transport booking system, which automatically populates information from the patient administration records, with the nurse entering in transfer type (outgoing), transport mode (road), facility type (nursing home) and address. Clinical requirements included patient weight and mobility status, which determined the correct equipment to use, with the last information required being the time for the patient to be picked up. My role was to prepare Mrs Brennan for her transfer by helping her change her clothes, toileting her and ensuring that her observations had been taken.

Mrs Brennan was successfully transported back to her nursing home and I learnt how valuable the online booking system was for both the patient and staff. The user-friendly tool improved the coordination of patients requiring non-emergency transport, aligned the resources to ensure that Mrs Brennan received the most appropriate level of care during her transportation, and created a standardised and consistent level of service.

1 PREPARE FOR TRANSPORT

Transporting individuals can involve moving them to or within healthcare facilities to attend diagnostic or treatment services, or as part of an interfacility transport where a patient is moved to an alternative health, rehabilitation or community care location. Prior to preparing the person for transportation, a thorough assessment needs to be made to determine the appropriate mode of transport, and support and equipment requirements. This can be achieved by discussing the individual's needs with the person and relevant personnel.

> **Interfacility transport**
> Transport from one facility to another.

Confirm transport with relevant personnel

It is important to ensure that all people involved in the transportation of the patient have been notified. This includes the client, nursing and/or medical staff, transport personnel and the receiving facility. Kitchen staff might also need to be notified if alternative meal arrangements need to be made. The person's family or advocate should be notified well in advance when the person is being transported to another facility. In some instances, the information regarding transportation can be relayed over the telephone.

If the person is to be discharged or transferred to another facility, it is important to check with the discharge planner who may have already made these communications and completed a patient transfer summary form (see Figure 9.1). This form accompanies the transport personnel and outlines details regarding destination, transport mode, contact details and patient management, including

FIGURE 9.1 Patient transfer summary

FOR MEDICAL RECORD USE ONLY MEDICAL RECORD COPY	SURNAME: _____ MRN: _____ OTHER NAMES: _____ D.O.B. ___/___/___ SEX: _____ AMO: _____ AFFIX ADDRESSOGRAPH LABEL HERE
South Eastern Sydney Illawarra Area Health Service	
INTERHOSPITAL TRANSFER SUMMARY	Original to remian in patient's medical records, copy to transfer with patient.

Transfer Details

Transfer Date: ___/___/___ Transfer from: _____ To: _____

Diagnosis: _____

Patient's current condition: _____

Accepted by Dr: : _____

Mode of Transport: SVH Transport ☐ NSW Ambulance ☐ NSW PTS ☐ Air Ambulance ☐ Wingaway ☐

SHSEH Transport ☐

Bed availability confirmed by receiving facility: Yes ☐ No ☐   Date: ___/___/___ Time: _____ Hrs: _____

Management/intervenion Assessments

Oxygen therapy: Yes ☐ No ☐ Specify: _____	IV therapy: Yes ☐ No ☐ Type: _____ Site: _____
Dietry requirements: Yes ☐ No ☐ NMB: Yes ☐ No ☐ NGT/PEG: Yes ☐ No ☐ Type: _____ TPN: Yes ☐ No ☐	Mobility Issues: Yes ☐ No ☐ Falls Risk score: _____ Walking Aid: Yes ☐ No ☐ Type: _____
Incontinent: Yes ☐ No ☐ Specify: _____ Urinary Catheter: Yes ☐ No ☐ Specify IDC ☐ SPC ☐ Other: _____	Risk of cross infection: Yes ☐ No ☐ Precautions: _____ Contact ☐ Droplet ☐ Airborne ☐ Infection: (Type): _____

Assessment prior to transfer

	Yes	No	Comments
Patient ID bands in place	☐	☐	
Alert Bands in place	☐	☐	
Pain management on route	☐	☐	Score: /10, last dose given at: , Pain medication due: _____
Observations	☐	☐	Obs on discharge: Time:
	☐	☐	T P Resp BP
Glasgow coma scale if required	☐	☐	Score:
Blood sugar level if required	☐	☐	Current BSL: Next due:
Wound care chart	☐	☐	Waterlow score:
Pressure Ulcer Assessment	☐	☐	
Dentures	☐	☐	
Prosthesis	☐	☐	
Communication deficit	☐	☐	
Personal / Valuables / Spectacles	☐	☐	
X-rays / scans (pts own)	☐	☐	
Appropriate Sustenance provided	☐	☐	Sandwiches and drinks required for road travel outside metro Sydney

Handover of Patient's condition

special needs (e.g., non-English-speaking or an intellectual disability). Many of these forms are now online and completed using computerised patient management systems.

The mode of transport used will depend on the needs of the individual, and, as an HSA, your scope limits you to transporting a stable individual only. The registered nurse (RN) or medical practitioner is responsible for assessing the physical and cognitive state of the person prior to transportation. This is to ensure the client is clinically and behaviourally stable and not at risk of experiencing any adverse event, either during transportation or while in another department. Your health facility will have policies regarding the level of escort and mode of transport required. Figure 9.2 outlines the various modes of transport and when they are used.

FIGURE 9.2 Modes of transport and when they are used

TRANSPORT MODE	WHEN USED
Evacuation sheet	Fire or other emergency when speed of evacuation is required
Wheelchair	Individuals who require assistance and cannot weight-bear or can only partially weight-bear
Bed	Individuals who are: • bedridden • cognitively impaired • unconscious or sedated • bariatric • difficult to move due to size or existing conditions; e.g., wounds, recent surgery • attached to equipment for monitoring; e.g., cardiac monitors
Cot	For a baby or infant
Trolley	In rooms where the area is small and will not accommodate a bed In departments with high turnover of patients; e.g., emergency department Deceased people
Motor vehicle/ aeroplane	When the person needs to be taken to another facility Note: These modes of transport can accommodate wheelchairs or trolleys

Relevant personnel for escort

9.1 ACTIVITY

All patients requiring transport within the hospital campus will be escorted by an appropriately qualified person as determined by the medical officer or registered nurse. This decision is based on:

• the need for an escort
• the skill level of the escort
• the number of staff required to perform the escort safely.

Canberra Hospital and Health Services (CHHS) identify that registered nurses must escort patients who are ventilated, have drains or intravenous therapy in situ or have an altered neurological status (ACT Health, 2021). An assistant nurse can escort a patient who is assessed as being physiologically and psychologically stable and the decision is documented in the clinical records.

1 Discuss with your workplace supervisor the clinical circumstances that would require an assistant in nursing (AIN) escort.

2 Find your workplace transfer and transport policy to determine the appropriate personnel for escorting patients.

Check with the person to determine the level of support required, explain the procedure and answer any questions

Clinical constraints

Clinical restrictions that need to be taken into consideration when giving care; for example, IV, IDC, drain.

The person's physical and cognitive state, communication barriers and clinical constraints should be considered when determining their ability to assist during transportation. Your communication with the healthcare team and the person can give an indication of what type of transport mode to use, if assistance is required and if any additional equipment is needed. The care plan will also outline their clinical support needs.

Each individual has the right to know of the plans for transfer. If you notice any signs of anxiety regarding the transfer and transportation, spend time with the individual and/or family and allow them to voice their concerns. Be aware of their level of understanding and clarify any concerns with simple language. Encourage the individual to ask questions and write down the information to reduce uncertainty and misunderstandings.

Communication regarding the person's ability to assist

Prior to transportation, each person will have their individual mobility requirements taken into consideration. The mobility of the person can be classified as:

- ambulant – capable of walking independently, with a walking stick or with minimal assistance
- non-ambulant – require a wheelchair or trolley/bed because they can only partially or non-weight-bear.

As well as considering mobility, you should also identify whether the person is 'able to assist' or is 'dependent'. Worksafe Victoria (2009) identifies a patient 'as 'able to assist' if they are able to understand instructions, are cooperative and would be physically able to assist the process. If they do not meet these criteria, they would be classified as 'dependent' and therefore require extra support.

Communication with the healthcare team, observation of the person and reviewing the care plan can all determine the person's ability to assist with the transportation process. This communication can clarify whether the person has:

- physical conditions which may restrict mobility; for example, pain, contractures, paralysis, amputations, balance problems or stroke
- clinical constraints; for example, wound or urinary drainage devices, intravenous (IV) therapy, monitors or oxygen therapy
- existing conditions that could affect their endurance, for example, asthma, cardiac or lung disease
- cognitive needs that can make it difficult to understand or follow directions; for example, intellectual disability, dementia or challenging behaviours
- language barriers, including aphasia or a non-English-speaking background, that may require an interpreter.

Care plans that determine a person's support needs

Examine the care plans in your organisation and discuss the extent to which they provide the information required to determine the support needs in transporting an individual. Answer the following questions regarding care plans:

1   What information can the care plan provide to assist the healthcare team in identifying the person's Individualised mobility needs?

2   How do cognitive constraints impact on determining the person's support needs for transport?

Prepare for the safe and timely transportation of the person

Transporting a patient within a healthcare facility usually involves passing through corridors, lifts and other noisy and crowded areas that can be unpleasant environments for a person who is unwell. It is, therefore, important to prepare the person to maintain their privacy, dignity and safety for the transportation.

Personal privacy and dignity

You have a responsibility to ensure that the privacy and dignity of the person is respected during their healthcare experience. When transporting an individual this can be achieved by:

*   introducing yourself and acknowledging the person by his or her preferred name
*   explaining the transportation process clearly so that they know what to expect
*   asking if they have any concerns or questions and discuss ways to meet their needs
*   closing the bedside curtains when moving them onto the wheelchair or trolley
*   covering them appropriately during transportation (NSW Health, 2009).

Confidentiality and disclosure

Individuals trust healthcare workers and have a right to expect that their personal information will be kept private. This legal and ethical obligation not to disclose confidential information about a person, except in the course of your professional duties, is an important consideration when providing care. As an HSA, you often need to exchange information about the person in your care with other workers and other services. This allows teams to have up-to-date information about the person and their needs and is an important part of providing quality care.

To maintain confidentiality, avoid talking about the person where you may be overheard by others, and share information only with your healthcare team. Disclosure of confidential information may result in legal action against the healthcare facility. This means that you should be aware of confidentiality when giving a verbal handover report to the arrival facility so that only relevant personnel can hear.

Work role boundaries – responsibilities and limitations

As an HSA, you will be providing direct care activities to individuals under the supervision of an RN. The RN will assess the individual prior to them being transported to ensure that they are stable and not at risk of deteriorating, and that your knowledge and skill level can accommodate the transfer. You must always work within your work role boundaries and not undertake actions that are beyond your scope of practice.

Duty of care

Duty of care means that healthcare workers must anticipate risks for people under their care to prevent them coming to harm. It must be remembered that harm can be both physical and emotional. The employer also has a duty of care to ensure a safe working environment, provide equipment for staff to carry out procedures, and monitor the workplace for hazards and unsafe practices (Victorian Government, 2004).

Prior to the person being transported, ensure the equipment is in safe working order and that the person is safely secured for transport. Transport personnel must be qualified, and any vehicles used must be suitable and roadworthy.

> **Work role boundaries**
> The clear definition of a healthcare worker's duties, rights and limitations.

> **Scope of practice**
> Procedures, actions and processes that a healthcare worker is permitted to undertake.

ACTIVITY 9.3

Scope of practice

Look up the scope of practice for an HSA at the facility where you work or are undertaking work experience.

1 Discuss the responsibilities of an HSA when undertaking transportation.

2 What would be the appropriate action when the transportation task is outside the HSA scope of practice?

Select equipment and check to ensure it is clean and functioning

Once an assessment of the person's physical and cognitive condition has been determined, an assessment of the required equipment should be made. All equipment must be functioning and clean. Your facility will have policies and procedures to ensure that the correct maintenance and safety checks are undertaken with all vehicles, equipment and mobility aids. It is your responsibility to report equipment faults or defects so that the person is transported safely.

Check a wheelchair

Before transporting a person in a wheelchair, it is important to make sure that the chair fits the person and that they can be transported safely. The following checks should also be made.

- Tyres, wheels and brakes:
  - Ensure the pressure in the tyres is adequate for the weight of the person.
  - Inspect for flat spots or wear on the tread.
  - Ensure the wheels spin freely.
  - Check for loose or broken spokes.
  - Test the brakes to make sure they lock the wheels tightly as the person gets in/out of the chair and are free of the wheels when pushing.

- Push handles, armrests and footrests, and upholstery:
    - Check that handles are secure.
    - Check that arm and leg rests can be easily removed, swung away and adjusted.
    - Inspect for damage, wear or excessive stretch of back rest or seat upholstery.
- Attachments:
    - Check the capacity for attachment of additional equipment that is necessary during transportation.

Check a bed or trolley

Before transporting a person in a bed or trolley. the following checks should be made:
- the mattress is in good condition
- the wheels move freely in all directions
- brakes are functioning correctly
- the bed/trolley can be raised or lowered for transferring the person
- the bed or trolley has the capacity to attach equipment; for example, oxygen cylinder, intravenous (IV) pole
- the safety rails can be raised and lowered easily
- there are no sharp edges or protruding parts.

Safety procedures

1 Describe the safety checks that you would undertake with the transport equipment used in your organisation.

2 Where would you find the equipment manuals in your organisation?

3 What is the policy when faults are found in the equipment?

9.4 ACTIVITY

Check additional equipment to ensure it is attached correctly and safely

Part of the assessment of the person includes the identification of devices or therapy equipment that must be transported with the person to support their care. Checking this equipment and ensuring that it is correctly attached is an important safety aspect in any transportation process.

The types of additional equipment that may accompany a person during transportation include:
- portable IV stands for IV therapy
- electronic IV infusion pump
- cardiac monitors
- oxygen cylinder and holder
- indwelling catheter (IDC; see Figure 9.3) or wound drainage and holder
- personal belongings
- X-rays, scans or medical records.

FIGURE 9.3 Indwelling catheter holder

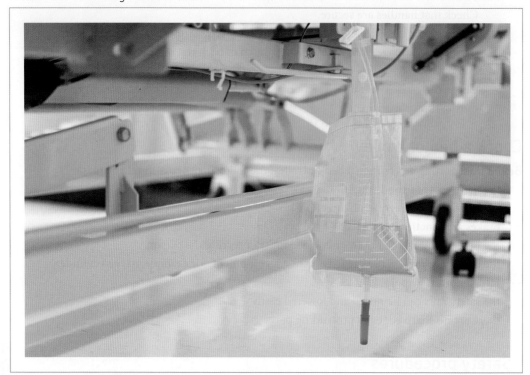

Source: iStock.com / surasak petchang

Before the person is transported, you should ensure that the additional equipment is fixed securely on the trolley, bed or wheelchair. When transportation has commenced, it is important for you to avoid sudden movements that could dislodge the equipment onto the person, potentially causing injuries. It is also important for you to be aware of the person interfering with the equipment, which could lead to disconnection of lines and tubes, or injuries.

Equipment for bariatric people

Bariatric person
A person who is obese or severely obese.

Transporting bariatric people presents a number of logistical difficulties. These include trolley dimensions and strength, as well as stability. Specially designed, heavy-duty trolleys and vehicles are being introduced. You will need to check with your facility regarding any customised equipment for bariatric people.

ACTIVITY 9.5

Equipment to reduce risks for the bariatric person

Read the Safe Work Australia (2020) publication 'Manual handling risks associated with the care, treatment and transportation of bariatric (severely obese) patients in Australia' (**https://www.safeworkaustralia.gov.au/resources-and-publications/reports/manual-handling-risks-associated-care-treatment-and-transportation-bariatric-severely-obese-patients-australia**).
Now answer the following questions regarding bariatric care:

1   What measures (e.g., plans, policies, processes and equipment) have been introduced in Australia to reduce or eliminate the risks in transporting bariatric clients?

2   Identify any bariatric transport equipment at the facility at which you are working or undertaking work experience.

2 TRANSPORT THE PERSON AND EQUIPMENT

During transportation, you must make sure that the person remains safe and secure and that risks to yourself are minimised. This includes the application of standard or additional precautions and the security of any additional equipment that is attached to the wheelchair, bed or trolley. You must also stay alert for unexpected complications, such as disconnections of lines or changes in the clinical condition of the person.

Transport the person to a location in accordance with organisational policy

Organisations have policies and procedures for transporting individuals regarding level of escort required, documentation and responsibilities of personnel. As an HSA, you need to attend to the following considerations during transportation:

* ensure that your scope of practice encompasses the care for the person's condition and equipment
* make sure that you have received a full report on the condition of the person beforehand
* ensure that you have the correct equipment and attachments necessary to assist with the person's care
* use correct body mechanics throughout the process
* continue to check the stability of the person
* make sure that you are aware of the instructions for the receiving facility and have the person's records and supporting documents with you.

Manoeuvre and transport equipment to ensure the person's comfort and safety and minimise risk

The physical and emotional comfort and safety of the person is paramount during the transportation process. This can be achieved by effective communication and manoeuvring the transport equipment in a safe manner while adhering to correct body mechanics. The identification of potential hazards through careful risk assessment and implementation of precautions to minimise risk must also be considered, not only for the person being transported but also for yourself.

Risk assessment

You should complete a risk assessment before and during transportation of the person. This should take into consideration your needs, as well as those of the client, and all other safety aspects involved, including:

* clinical condition of the individual to be transported
* level of assistance required
* additional equipment that needs to be attached for transporting the person safely
* knowledge of equipment and checking that it is in safe working order
* appropriate footwear for the individual if transported in a wheelchair
* clearing the area to allow for the transport equipment to be manoeuvred
* consideration of additional precautions required due to the person's clinical condition.

WHS, including body mechanics

Body mechanics should always be considered when transporting individuals so that you do not sustain any injuries. Many facilities have a 'no lift' policy, which means that no manual lifting should be done. Instead, workers are required to use mechanical aids to move a person so that they can be safely transported. This may include mechanical or electronic lifting devices.

You must learn how to use mechanical or electronic lifting devices before you can safely handle this equipment. Facilities use a wide variety of devices and will teach you how to use the devices and match them to each individual and their needs.

The equipment that you use will allow you to perform the task easily and safely so that the person is transported in comfort. Review body biomechanics in Chapter 8, 'Assist with movement', because this is the key to injury prevention.

Infection control

Your workplace will have infection control policies and procedures that you must adhere to when transporting clients. Communication regarding a person's infection status must be done prior to the transfer to another ward or department. Standard or additional precautions must be followed for all people during transportation. The precautions for patient transport are outlined in Figure 9.4, and the 'Scenario' box highlights important additional precautions to consider when transporting infectious people.

FIGURE 9.4 Precautions for patient transport

STANDARD PRECAUTIONS	ADDITIONAL PRECAUTIONS

These are the basic levels of infection control required for the general care of all people:
• Hand hygiene and cough etiquette
• Incorporating safe practices for handling blood, body fluids and secretions as well as excretions. This includes additional personal protective equipment (PPE) precautions
• Make sure that impervious dressings cover lesions or drainage from affected area
	These need to be followed when the person is infectious or immuno-compromised:
	• Use PPE barriers, such as mask, gown and gloves
	• Notify in advance staff at the receiving area or vehicle personnel of the individual's condition and the precautions taken to prevent transmission or maintain isolation
	• Do not enter a lift with the person if there are already other people in the lift. If the lift stops at another floor, ask the people waiting to refrain from entering it
	• If transferring a COVID-19 patient:
	  – the patient should wear a surgical mask
	  – the receiving department should be notified in advance
	  – cleaning and disinfection of the lift must be completed after the transfer
	  – all staff should wear clean PPE during the transit

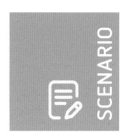

Infection control for Florence Burton

An imaging study has been requested for a patient, Florence Burton. Radiology staff have called the ward to confirm the request and arrange transport, and the RN has asked you to assist with the patient's wheelchair transport. Florence's notes indicate that she has a methicillin-resistant *Staphylococcus aureus* (MRSA) infection in her leg wound. You check with your RN to determine the correct precautions that need to be taken for Florence and begin by ensuring that the infected area is contained and covered with an impervious dressing. You ask Florence to perform hand hygiene prior to her transportation and notify the receiving facility of her condition. You check that the documents accompanying Florence clearly state details relating to her MRSA status.

The RN informs you that gowns and gloves need not be worn because direct patient care is not anticipated and the MRSA is isolated to her leg wound only; however, she reminds you that you need to perform hand hygiene before and after completing the transportation task. The most direct route is selected for the transportation to avoid unnecessary contact with employees or visitors during the transportation, and when you arrive, you restate Florence's condition at the receiving facility and hand over her documents.

1 Why was it important to check the correct infection control precautions in this scenario?
2 Why was it important to notify the receiving facility of Florence's condition and infectious status?

Safe transportation procedures

Safe wheelchair transport

Safety and comfort during transportation in a wheelchair is a priority for both the individual and transport personnel. You may need to use pillows or adaptive devices to ensure that the person remains in a safe position. For example, a person with a fractured arm or poor limb control due to a stroke may need a pillow under their arm during the transportation process. It is important to always keep the person informed about what you are intending to do.

The following points will ensure that the risks are minimised:

- ensure that if a safety strap is fitted, it is secured to the person
- replace the arm of the wheelchair if it was removed during the transfer
- ensure brakes are applied and footrests raised when the individual is getting in or out of the wheelchair
- position the person with feet supported on the footrest
- check the person's body alignment during the transportation and reposition when necessary – lock the brakes before repositioning
- ensure blankets, clothing and person's hands are free from the wheels
- guide the wheelchair from behind using both handgrips
- approach corners slowly and be aware of passing traffic
- prop doors open before entering rooms if possible or back through doorways
- back over thresholds and when entering and leaving elevators if possible.

Source: From Hegner/Acello/Caldwell, 3P-EBK:NURSING ASSISTANT A NURSING PROCESS APPROACH, 11E. © 2016 Cengage.

Negotiate kerbs

Whenever possible, it is best to avoid kerbs. Instead, always try to use ramps. If a kerb is unavoidable then the following precautions should be taken:

- Pushing an occupied wheelchair down a kerb:
    - Back the wheelchair over the edge of the kerb, making sure that both wheels touch down at the same time to balance the wheelchair and its occupant on the rear wheels.
    - Check that the road is clear. Carefully pull the wheelchair further back into the road and, when the occupant's feet are clear of the kerb, gently lower the front to the road.
- Pushing an occupied wheelchair up a kerb:
    - When the occupant's feet are nearly touching the kerb, pull back on the handles to balance the wheelchair and its occupant on the rear wheels, then push the wheelchair forwards until the wheels rest on the pavement.
    - Push the wheelchair forwards until the back wheels touch the kerb and then lift up on the handles as you continue pushing forwards to place the wheels on the pavement.

Wheelchair in car transport

Whenever possible and practical, it is strongly recommended that wheelchair occupants transfer out of their wheelchair onto a vehicle seat and use the vehicle seatbelt system. This is generally the safest mode of transport.

Wheelchair tie-down systems secure the wheelchair firmly to the floor of the vehicle at specified tie-down points, as shown in Figure 9.5. Alternatively, a docking system may be used.

FIGURE 9.5 Wheelchair tie-down system

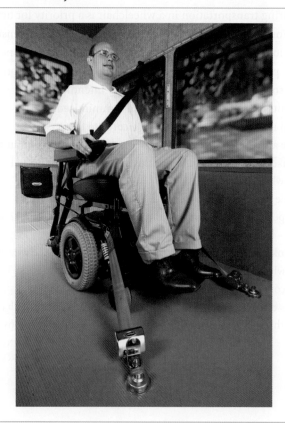

Source: Q'Straint

The occupied wheelchair should face forwards during transportation and the wheelchair user must be restrained independently of the wheelchair (Independent Living Centre WA, 2015). Check the regulations that apply to wheelchair transport in your locations or source Independent Living Centres in each state, which provide information and advisory services to help wheelchair users choose the right safety products.

Safe trolley or bed transport

Many facilities have transport officers to assist with the transportation of people in beds or trolleys (see Figure 9.6) and, as an HSA, you may be required to accompany them during transportation. Family members may also accompany the person during transportation – for example, to operating theatres or imaging rooms – so it is important that you communicate all aspects of the transportation clearly. This can reduce anxiety for both the individual and their relatives or support person.

FIGURE 9.6 Hospital trolley

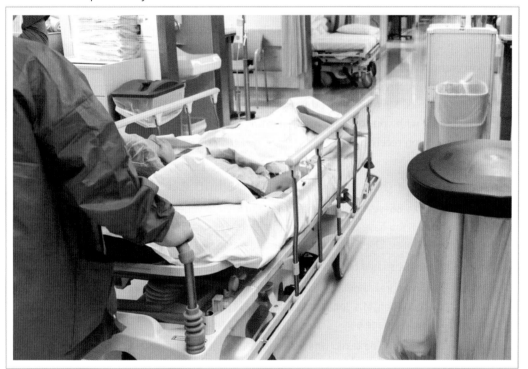

Essential safety considerations include the following:
- raise the side rails on beds, trolleys or cots
- raise the head of the trolley or bed for the person's comfort, if possible
- push the head of the trolley so you can see potential hazards
- approach corners slowly and be aware of passing traffic
- prop doors open before the trolley or bed enters the rooms, or back through doorways
- push the stop button to lock doors open when entering or leaving elevators
- back trolleys or beds through elevators

- stand by the person's head while the elevator is moving
- walk backwards when transporting a trolley or bed down a ramp, while guiding from the head end
- apply brakes when parking a trolley or bed.

Source: From Hegner/Acello/Caldwell, 3P-EBK:NURSING ASSISTANT A NURSING PROCESS APPROACH, 11E. © 2016 Cengage.

Safety with catheters, tubing and drainage devices

When transporting a person with catheters, tubing or drainage devices, you need to ensure that the flow is not impeded and that the line and insertion site are not compromised. General guidelines during the transportation process include:

- keep tubing off the floor
- avoid putting any tension on a catheter, nasogastric tube or drainage device
- prevent drainage from back-flowing into the person by keeping the drainage bag lower than the insertion site
- keep the drainage receptacle upright
- do not drape the tubing over the upright rails of a trolley or bed
- do not allow tubing to dangle near wheels
- report complications to the RN.

If the person is receiving oxygen therapy, ensure an uninterrupted flow through the tubing by checking for kinks. Make sure that the oxygen cylinder is secured safely to the transportation equipment. Check with your organisation regarding the scope of practice for an HSA when transporting a person receiving oxygen.

ACTIVITY 9.6

Transporting a person with an indwelling catheter

Mrs Johansson is an 86-year-old who has been admitted to your department with a fractured tibia and confusion. You have been asked by the RN to assist with her transportation to the X-ray department on a trolley. She has an indwelling catheter in situ:

1 What precautions should be undertaken prior to transportation?

2 What safety measures should be considered during the trolley transportation?
   During transportation, Mrs Johansson accidentally pulls on the tubing and it becomes dislodged from the drainage bag.

3 What actions need to be taken when the indwelling catheter becomes dislodged from the drainage bag?

4 What are the potential complications from this incident for the patient and HSA?

Transport a critically ill person

Check with your organisation for the policy regarding the intra- or inter-hospital transportation of a critically ill person to an intensive care unit, operating theatre or high care cardiac ward. Many hospitals will have dedicated persons who have the specific skills and training for these transports, including dedicated wards persons or porters. As an HSA you may be required to assist with the transport by organising the required equipment (e.g., IV pole, transfer board, medical records) and assisting with other ward duties whilst the transfer is taking place. Ensure that you understand the communications and maintain a calm approach.

The critically ill person will have experienced staff who are able to resuscitate and provide appropriate emergency care and they may also use a priority elevator in the facility. Consider debriefing with supervisors after any stressful incident or accessing appropriate resources to ensure your health and wellbeing.

In regards to COVID-19 transfers, all staff involved in the transport, or in close contact with patients being transferred, must be fully vaccinated. They must also implement full airborne droplet and contact personal protective equipment (PPE) (gloves, fluid-resistant gown, P2/N95 mask and eye protection) that have been fit-tested and fit-checked (NSW Agency for Clinical Innovation, 2021).

Transport a deceased person

Check with your organisation for the policy regarding the transportation of a deceased person. In a hospital facility, the person may be transported to a holding facility or mortuary. In a community setting, arrangements may be made with a funeral director for transport. The deceased person must be placed in a body bag prior to transportation, with identification clearly written on the outer surface of the bag. The RN or doctor will arrange for the deceased person to be removed from the facility with the appropriate transport personnel. Refer to Chapter 15, 'Deliver care services using a palliative approach', for more details regarding care of the deceased.

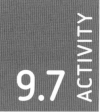

Internet research – Public Health Regulation 2012

View the NSW Health website (**https://www.health.nsw.gov.au**)
and search for 'disposal of the deceased' to find an outline of Public Health Regulation 2012, then answer the following questions:

1   What types of facilities handle deceased people and what transportation methods are used to deliver the deceased people to these facilities?
2   What is your role when transporting a deceased person in your facility?

9.7 ACTIVITY

3   DELIVER THE PERSON

To make the delivery of the person smooth and non-stressful, make sure that the receiving staff are aware of the transport arrangements and that all documentation accompanies the person. This includes request forms, medical records and additional documents such as X-rays or reports. It is your responsibility to make an appropriate entry in the person's notes about the transportation and return the equipment according to organisational protocols.

In the community setting, an independent individual may be dropped off and picked up at a pre-arranged time without the need for a healthcare worker escort. In this case the information and instructions must be relayed by the transport personnel or family members.

Deliver the person and inform relevant personnel of arrival and person's needs

On arrival at the receiving facility, the healthcare worker who delivers the individual has a responsibility to communicate the person's needs so that the receiving staff have a current assessment of the individual. Remember that this reporting is confidential and should only be given to authorised staff. This verbal handover and/or written communication outlines the person's condition so that continuity of care can be maintained.

This includes:

- an update on the person's health condition, including physical limitations and location of any drainage devices or tubing if attached
- communication regarding cognitive needs and/or language barriers
- a handover of documents, scans, X-rays or treatment orders
- any adverse events encountered during transportation – make sure you use objective language that concentrates on facts based on your observations
- clear instructions about pick-up, follow-up arrangements or ongoing appointments.

In some instances, the transport personnel will complete arrival documentation according to organisational policy; for example, ambulance personnel or community transport personnel.

Community transport personnel

People who assist community members with transportation to and from activities, health services, appointments etc.

ACTIVITY 9.8

Community transport personnel

Interview a community transport worker to answer the following questions:

1. How are vehicles booked?
2. What are the regular maintenance and service requirements for vehicles?
3. What are the vehicle logbook departure and arrival requirements?
4. What information is given during handover?
5. What documentation is required for equipment defects?
6. What are the incident/accident reporting requirements?

Return equipment used to deliver the person and accurately complete reporting requirements

Once the person has been delivered safely, the transport equipment needs to be cleaned and returned according to organisational policy. Some equipment may have specific check-in–check-out protocols so that its user and location can be determined. This is also an important inventory control measure and can be used to forecast future equipment needs.

Cleaning of equipment may involve wiping down with appropriate cleaning solutions. Make sure that you read the instructions and wear PPE when undertaking cleaning, and report faults or damage to equipment.

Reporting requirements

When the person returns from their transportation, reports on the outcomes of tests, appointments or alternative therapy need to be communicated to the appropriate personnel so that any new treatments, medications or care can be added to their care plans. Additional reporting requirements may include:

- equipment faults
- travel logbooks
- incidents/accidents
- requests for replacement of equipment.

The completion of the transportation, when performed according to an existing protocol, should be evaluated. The purpose of the evaluation is to identify problems within the system or equipment, deficiencies in training, human errors and risk factors of transportation, and to consider and report on what could have been avoided. After the evaluation, continuous improvements to the protocols are expected. Therefore, the level of the provided care will be continuously upgraded for all people in intra- or interfacility transports.

SUMMARY

Transferring individuals is a multifaceted process requiring preparation of the person for transportation through effective communication and recognition of their needs, coordination of the most appropriate transfer modality and equipment, and care of the person during transportation between or within facilities. This chapter examined the techniques required to safely transport individuals from one site to another while adhering to reporting requirements and organisational policies and procedures.

As an HSA, you are required to provide holistic and continuing care while maintaining the safety and dignity of the person during transportation. This chapter emphasised the knowledge required to identify individual needs and apply appropriate risk-assessment techniques to enable you to deliver a person in a safe and timely manner.

APPLY YOUR KNOWLEDGE

Community transport

Community transport is available to people who have limited transport options and who meet certain eligibility criteria. Jalala was an 83-year-old woman who lived alone and had poor English-speaking skills. She was obese and had arthritis in both knees, which limited her mobility. She relied on a walking frame to mobilise. These health conditions met the criteria for community transport and Jalala used the service for transport to the medical centre for her regular appointments.

This service provides door-to-door transport to and from the destination with trained drivers who can assist persons to and from the vehicle. As an HSA working in home and community care, I was given the opportunity to work alongside the community transport team as part of my training.

1   In preparing Jalala for transport, what information would the community transport personnel need to know to assist her to get into the van?

2   What safety precautions should be considered for this transport?

Jalala found that this service enabled her to maintain her independence and connect with the community. The community transport service provided a multilingual driver who could communicate effectively with Jalala and this gave her peace of mind. During her transport, Jalala confided that she was anxious about the pain in her knees, which was worsening, and she was finding the walking frame difficult to use. The driver and I acknowledged her concern and we organised a wheelchair at the medical centre to get her from the van to reception.

3   What information would need to be communicated to reception staff upon Jalala's arrival?

4   What checks and precautions are required to ensure safe wheelchair transport for Jalala?

5   Using the knowledge learnt in Chapter 8, 'Assist with movement', what planning and body mechanics should be considered when transferring Jalala from the wheelchair to a chair at the medical facility?

6   Why is it important to evaluate the process at the completion of transportation?

Jalala returned home after the appointment with new medication for her arthritis and a referral to the dietitian for a weight loss program. She continued to use the community transport service and her driver, and with her new treatments was able to continue to mobilise with her walking frame and maintain her independence.

7   Understanding the scope of practice as an HSA is essential to working effectively within the healthcare team. How did the HSA demonstrate the scope of their role with the actions in this case study?

◄ REFLECTING ON THE INDUSTRY INSIGHT 💬

1   Why was Mrs Brennan unsuitable for community transport? Because community transport:
   a   is only available to patients who are incontinent
   b   can be used for patients in a stretcher
   c   is used for patients who can walk and live independently
   d   can be used for behaviourally unstable patients requiring restraint.

2   Why was it important for the HSA to take Mrs Brennan's observations prior to transportation?
   a   To ensure that Mrs Brennan's condition was stable prior to transport.
   b   To complete the paperwork for the transport personnel.
   c   So that the correct medication can be given prior to transfer.
   d   Because transport personnel are unqualified to take observations.

3   Why is it important for the transport personnel to know Mrs Brennan's weight and mobility status?
   a   A lightweight patient may not require an escort and only require a driver for the transportation.
   b   To ensure that the correct mobility equipment was available for the transportation.
   c   To allow for family and friends to accompany the patient in the vehicle.
   d   An immobile patent will require an additional payment for the service.

SELF-CHECK QUESTIONS

1   How do you maintain the confidentiality of a patient during transportation?
2   List the type of additional equipment that may be required when transporting individuals.
3   What infection control procedures should be followed when transporting an individual?
4   What are the important safety considerations when transporting a person in a wheelchair?
5   What are the important safety considerations when transporting a person on a trolley?
6   How can the healthcare worker ensure safety with a client receiving oxygen during transportation?
7   Explain why it is necessary to collect feedback from carers about how well the transportation methods used by the organisation are meeting an individual's needs.
8   Describe the reporting procedures that should be followed when an individual is delivered to the designated location.
9   Why would some equipment have specific check-in–check-out protocols?
10 What are your definitions of the following key words and terms that have been used in this chapter?

KEY WORD OR TERM	YOUR DEFINITION
Work role boundaries	
Non-weight-bearing	
Scope of practice	
Clinical constraints	
Interfacility transport	
Risk assessment	
Bariatric person	
N95 mask	

QUESTIONS FOR DISCUSSION

1   Provide examples of any difficulties in transporting people with mental health disorders or dementia and discuss how this is managed in your organisation.

2   Discuss the physical and psychological considerations for ageing individuals when providing transport services.

3   Discuss the differences between metropolitan and remote transport services and when each might be used.

4   Discuss the procedure when transporting an individual who has a critical incident (e.g., seizure) during transportation.

5   Discuss the information required when a person is transferred from acute care to a rehabilitation facility

EXTENSION ACTIVITY

Transporting patients

1   Examine the scenarios outlined in the following table and write how you would prepare the person before, during and after transportation.

SCENARIO	HOW WOULD YOU PREPARE THE PERSON
An elderly person who walks with a frame needs to be transported to the community activities centre in a community bus	
A person who has mild right-sided paralysis and walks with a cane needs to be transported to the nursing home by minivan	
A person with an established tracheostomy needs to be transported in his bed to the dialysis department	
A person with low-flow oxygen therapy via nasal prongs needs to be transported to the respiratory ward on a trolley	
A person with bilateral above-knee amputations needs to be transported to the rehabilitation facility in a wheelchair	
A person with norovirus needs to be transported to an isolation ward in his bed	
A seven-year-old child with bronchitis needs to be transported to the paediatric ward on a trolley	

2   Explain the reasons for your responses to these scenarios.

3   Use the scenarios in the table in a simulated setting by forming groups and practising the clinical skills of transferring and transporting individuals. Remember to use your communication skills in reassurance and empathy when practising the skill.

4   Practise in your groups how you would give a verbal handover report after delivering each person to the receiving facility.

REFERENCES

Acello, B. & Hegner, B. (2016). *Nursing assistant: A nursing process approach* (11th edn). Boston, MA: Cengage. © 2016 Delmar Learning, a part of Cengage, Inc. Reproduced by permission. www.cengage.com/permissions

ACT Health (2021). Canberra Hospital and Health Services: Patient escort and transport within Canberra Hospital campus. Retrieved 17 October 2022 from https://www.health.act.gov.au/sites/default/files/2018-09/Patient%20Escort%20and%20Transport%20within%20Canberra%20Hospital%20campus.docx

Independent Living Centre WA (2015). Transportation of people seated in wheelchairs. Retrieved 20 March 2016 from https://ilc.com.au/wp-content/uploads/2018/05/ILC-Transportation-of-People-Seated-in-Wheelchairs.pdf

NSW Agency for Clinical Innovation (2021). Intrahospital transfer of COVID-19 positive and suspected COVID-19 positive patients from the emergency department. Retrieved 17 October 2022 from https://www.health.nsw.gov.au/Infectious/covid-19/communities-of-practice/Documents/intrahospital-transfer-ed-COVID19-patients.pdf

SA Health (2014) Staff Information on respecting patients' privacy and dignity with patient centred care principles. Retrieved 27 March 2022 from https://www.sahealth.sa.gov.au/wps/wcm/connect/c4293b0045d64eb58290ca574adac1f8/3b_Staff+Info_Respect+patient+privacy_PCC_App2.pdf?MOD=AJPERES&CACHEID=ROOTWORKSPACE-c4293b0045d64eb58290ca574adac1f8-nwMEpMn

Safe Work Australia (2020). Manual handling risks associated with the care, treatment and transportation of bariatric (severely obese) patients in Australia. Retrieved 27 March 2022 from https://www.safeworkaustralia.gov.au/resources-and-publications/reports/manual-handling-risks-associated-care-treatment-and-transportation-bariatric-severely-obese-patients-australia.

Victorian Government (2004). *Occupational Health and Safety Act 2004*. Retrieved 17 October 2022 from http://www.legislation.vic.gov.au/domino/web_notes/ldms/pubstatbook.nsf/f932b66241ecf1b7ca256e92000e23be/750e0d9e0b2b387fca256f71001fa7be/$file/04-107a.pdf

WorkSafe Victoria (2009). A handbook for workplaces. Transferring people safely: Handling clients, residents and clients in health, aged care, rehabilitation and disability services. Retrieved 20 March 2016 from https://content.api.worksafe.vic.gov.au/sites/default/files/2018-06/ISBN-Transferring-people-safely-handbook-2009-07.pdf

PROVIDE NON-CLIENT CONTACT SUPPORT IN AN ACUTE CARE ENVIRONMENT

Learning objectives

By the end of this chapter, you should be able to:

1 comply with the information protocols of an acute care environment

2 collect, process and maintain accurate records in an acute care environment

3 support equipment requirements in an acute care environment.

Introduction

This chapter will provide you with the skills and knowledge to undertake a range of non-client contact support procedures while delivering nursing care in an acute care environment. These non-client contact support procedures include reporting and recording, and the correct use of equipment for patient care.

An understanding of health records, including their processing and storage, form an integral part of patient care. Keeping these documents confidential and secure is a legal and organisational requirement in all acute care facilities. Preparing clear, concise and factual documentation and reports supports continuity of patient care. Additionally, the use of technology to record relevant information is a key skill for a health services assistant (HSA). All of these, along with effective communication, will help support other members of the healthcare team.

The last part of this chapter identifies and describes the equipment required to support patient care, monitoring and ongoing assessment. It also highlights appropriate cleaning, maintenance and storage.

INDUSTRY INSIGHTS

Equipment used in acute care

After completing my Health Services Assistance course, I was given a fob watch as a gift. It was during my first placement that I realised that this was not just a tool used to tell time but an extremely useful and essential item to effectively carry out daily work-related activities. Our hospital also required us to wear this style of watch instead of a wristwatch for hygiene reasons. Also, I was aware that electronic devices could take a pulse, but I learnt that a watch can better evaluate irregularities of beat, and respiration rate can be taken easily with a watch positioned on the chest or waistband.

When I took Mr Sinclair's pulse with my watch I noted that the interval between beats was irregular. I reported this to my RN supervisor and an electrocardiograph (ECG) was taken. I helped to get the equipment for this procedure, including the pre-gelled electrodes and a razor to remove excess chest hair, and watched while it was being done. Mr Sinclair was diagnosed with a sinus arrhythmia with no specific treatment required. We did, however, detail in his progress notes and care plan that his pulse needed to be taken manually for a full minute when monitoring so that irregularities were not missed. I made sure I signed and printed my name and designation in these notes before the RN countersigned. Afterwards, I realised that this small and simple piece of equipment that I use can have a large impact on the nursing care I provide.

1 COMPLY WITH THE WORKPLACE INFORMATION PROTOCOLS OF AN ACUTE CARE ENVIRONMENT

Sources of workplace information in an acute care environment include health records, communication with the healthcare team, and policies and procedures. You will need to comply with protocols by maintaining the information's confidentiality and security in line with both Commonwealth and state or territory legislation and hospital policy. You will also need to use the information to promote patient safety and continuity of care between settings or healthcare personnel.

> **Confidentiality**
> Having another's trust or confidence.

Carry out work with an understanding of the purpose of health records

A healthcare record is the primary source of information about a patient's health and wellbeing. It describes the medical and therapeutic treatment as well as interventions. It also outlines episodes of care and informs care for the future. A healthcare record is a documented account of a patient's health history including investigations, diagnosis, care, treatment and outcomes. You can use the record as a comprehensive communication tool. This helps the entire healthcare team currently caring for the client to share information about treatment. Future providers of care can also use it as a history and to inform future decisions. Health records are not only an account of the patient's past, present and future care but are also used for:

- ensuring patient safety
- investigating complaints
- planning tools
- improving quality of care
- research
- education
- financial reimbursement
- protecting the legal interests of the patient or healthcare personnel.

The healthcare provider needs to develop an appropriate information management system that will ensure the patient's record and health information is uniquely identified. This will help health and community facilities manage the information appropriately. In the acute care environment, the patient is registered and allocated a unit record number. Care providers will use this medical record number or unique patient identifier to identify and link the patient's health information over time.

Health record

A chronological record of interactions, observations and actions relating to a particular patient.

Types of healthcare records

You will encounter several types of healthcare records in your role as an HSA, including:

- integrated progress notes – written when any member of the healthcare team encounters a patient. This includes doctors, nurses, physiotherapists and others involved in patient care. These notes are ongoing records of the person's progress and include interventions, actions taken and responses. They are an important tool for ongoing communication, evaluation and continuous improvement
- admission forms – completed for elective (planned) or non-elective (emergency) patients. They provide detailed information regarding the patient's physical, social and emotional history so that appropriate care can be given. This informs future care and support
- discharge and transfer forms – including a review of the patient that informs communication to other service providers; for example, a general practitioner (GP), rehabilitation or community care service. This ensures continuity of care
- X-rays and other images – photographic or digital records used for diagnostic purposes.
- observation charts – record measurements of vital signs, fluid balance (see Figure 10.1), neurological status, blood glucose level (BGL) and other specific observations. This guides the planning and treatment for individuals.

  Other types of healthcare records include:
- medication charts
- risk assessment charts; for example, falls and pressure areas
- consent forms
- incident/accident forms
- request forms for specimens, blood tests and so on.

The patient's details including name, date of birth and unique patient identifier must appear on each page of these records. Each facility will have their own charts, so it is important for you to become familiar with the online and paper-based records used in your workplace.

FIGURE 10.1 Sample fluid balance chart

THE DUDLEY GROUP OF HOSPITALS NHS FOUNDATION TRUST - FLUID BALANCE CHART

Orders:

Name: _____ Unit No.: _____ Ward: _____ Date: _____

NHS No.:

Time	INTAKE - IV FLUID				INTAKE - ENTERAL							Time	OUTPUT				
	FLUID/DRUGS (e.g. Normal Saline)	Hung Vol Hrs	Actual Vol. Infused	Running Total	Oral Volume	Oral/Tube Food Type	Tube Vol. Hung	Tube Vol. Given	Running Total Enteral				Gastric Aspirate Vomit Volume	Bowel Activity	Other	Urine	Running Total
00.00												00.00					
01.00												01.00					
02.00												02.00					
03.00												03.00					
04.00												04.00					
05.00												05.00					
06.00												06.00					
07.00												07.00					
08.00												08.00					
09.00												09.00					
10.00												10.00					
11.00												11.00					
12.00												12.00					
13.00												13.00					
14.00												14.00					
15.00												15.00					
16.00												16.00					
17.00												17.00					
18.00												18.00					
19.00												19.00					
20.00							If intake is poor, refer to nutrition risk score (MUST)						20.00					
21.00												21.00					
22.00												22.00					
23.00												23.00					
TOTALS	IV: [a]				Oral: [b]	NG Tube pH: Check Length	Tube: [c]						GA [1]	BA [2]	[3]	[4]	[5]	Urine [6]

TODAY'S TOTALS & BALANCE
Signature: _____

Total Intake [a+b+c=d]

Total output [1+2+3+4+5+6=o]

Fluid Balance Today [d–o=x]

Cumulative Balance brought forward from yesterday (v)

Cumulative Balance Today (z) (x+y=z)

Electronic medical records (EMRs) (online records and forms) are used more and more in health care today. These electronic records were developed to standardise documentation, prevent errors and allow ease of access for all healthcare staff. Some of the benefits of EMR include:

- fewer errors with interpreting handwriting
- barcode scanning to correctly identify the patient
- abnormal results flagged to prevent them from being overlooked
- warnings for incomplete data entry or errors
- improved privacy and security, with security access passwords
- quicker access to results; for example, pathology results can be uploaded directly into the patient notes.

> **Electronic medical records (EMRs)**
> Online medical records and forms used to standardise documentation, prevent errors and allow ease of access for all healthcare staff.

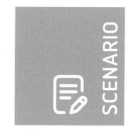

Florence's health information

Florence is admitted to hospital for day surgery. The HSA collects her health information upon admission and this is used by those involved in providing Florence's tests, surgery and post-operative care. This includes anaesthetists, surgeons, radiologists, nurses and pathologists. The entire healthcare team must treat Florence's health information in a confidential manner according to the organisation's guidelines.

1 Florence requests to read her notes. What actions should you take?
2 How are Florence's notes stored confidentially?
3 Florence's medical history can provide valuable health research. Florence consents to de-identified information for this purpose. What is de-identified information?

My Health Record

The My Health Record system is the Australian Government's digital health record system. It contains online summaries of an individual's health information, including medicines, allergies and treatments. It was previously known as an eHealth record. In most parts of Australia, individuals need to actively register for a My Health Record to be able to access their record online.

Access My Health Records from **https://myhealthrecord.gov.au** and answer the following questions:

1 What are the benefits of having a My Health Record?
2 Who can access an individual's health information?
3 What happens to an individual's existing records?
4 How can you ensure that the right information is on your health record?
5 How long do the health summary and documents stay in the health record system?

Organisational security and confidentiality

Health information is one of the most sensitive types of personal information. For this reason, each state and territory has laws regarding its handling, which operate alongside the *Privacy Act 1988*. For example, an organisation generally needs an individual's consent before collecting health information.

Practitioners within the healthcare environment increasingly use paper and electronic information, mail and communication systems as effective ways to maintain and transfer information. Therefore, it is important that healthcare staff fully understand their state or territory's legislation and hospital policy on privacy and confidentiality, as well as on the appropriate, safe and secure use of records and electronic information systems.

Security

Healthcare records must have appropriate security safeguards in place to prevent unauthorised use, disclosure, loss or other misuse. In an acute care setting, all records containing personal health information should be kept in secure access areas when not in use.

Control over the movement of paper-based healthcare records is important. Healthcare providers need a tracking system so that records can be retrieved quickly. This supports patient care and treatment and monitors how efficiently records can be located.

Health record access

Practitioners and healthcare workers should be able to access healthcare records at the site of service delivery. These may be in paper or electronic format, or both – which is known as a **hybrid record**. Records have legal and administrative constraints on their access, with important considerations including:

- access to information may be restricted (full, partial or no access) depending on a person's role – check with your health facility regarding level of access
- accessing electronic data may require staff identification, cards or passwords
- documents are not to be left where members of the general public may access them, as the information within them could be taken out of context or made public
- check with the registered nurse (RN) before allowing family members to access documents. There may be information that the patient does not wish their family, friends or others to know. There may also be medical terminology that will need to be explained
- under the *Privacy Act 1988*, clients can access their own health information.

You will often collaborate with other health professionals and care providers, and this may involve shared documentation, including progress notes, history, tests and so on. This collaboration is documented in the health record and should include information on the nature of the collaboration, the people involved, any outcomes and any possible future collaboration.

You cannot transfer records from one organisation to another unless prior arrangements have been made. This might include home visits or coronial or legal requirements. Practitioners and healthcare providers need to ensure that sensitive or confidential information is not given to anyone who may not treat the information in the same confidential manner as your organisation.

Computer and internet security

Organisations need to ensure that sensitive and confidential information stored on the computer network is secure. Ways to maintain security might include:

- using screensavers and passwords to reduce the chance of casual observation
- considering the location and direction of monitors to protect the confidentiality of information
- changing passwords frequently, particularly if a security risk has been identified
- using passwords that are not easily deciphered
- logging off fully when not using the system or when leaving a terminal

Hybrid record
A health record comprising paper, digitised and electronic formats. A hybrid health record is created and accessed using both manual and electronic processes.

- putting confidentiality statements and warnings on email transmissions
- not sharing passwords or security access cards
- not disclosing patient information on any form of social media; for example, Facebook.

Confidentiality

All of the information in a patient's healthcare record is confidential and subject to privacy laws and policies. Healthcare workers should only access a healthcare record and use or disclose information contained in the record when it is directly related to their duties and is essential for the fulfilment of those duties.

Confidential information may include information relating to:
- patients, family members and advocates (e.g., medical records, conversations)
- employees, volunteers and students (e.g., salaries, employment records, disciplinary actions)
- organisational information (e.g., reports, memos, contracts, technology)
- quality assurance (e.g., reports, presentations, survey results).

Privacy and confidentiality of the patient's details must always be maintained by:
- only discussing personal or sensitive information with the appropriate people, when and where others will not overhear
- being aware and up to date on the relevant legislation for your state or territory, as well as on policies and procedures regarding accessing confidential information
- only reading authorised patient records
- being aware of where you discuss patient or staff information, ensuring it is not in a public place
- discarding information into locked bins for shredding
- signing a confidentiality agreement when you are first employed by an organisation
- obtaining consent before revealing personal information about an individual.

Code of Conduct — privacy and confidentiality

The Code of Conduct for Nurses in Australia is designed for multiple audiences, including nurses, nursing students, people requiring or receiving nursing care, and other health workers. Look up this document at **https://www.nursingmidwiferyboard.gov.au/Codes-Guidelines-Statements/ Professional-standards.aspx**

Answer the following questions about Principle 3.5 — Confidentiality and privacy:

1   What are the ethical and legal obligations that the healthcare worker must comply with to protect the privacy of people requiring and receiving care?

2   When consent is not given by the patient, what must the healthcare worker consider before disclosing information?

3   How can the HSA ensure privacy is maintained when the patient is in a shared room?

Respond to enquiries and requests according to organisational procedures

Enquiries and requests for information are a significant part of communication in health care. Whether it is a patient enquiry or staff member request, healthcare workers need to provide open, accurate and timely information. A key aspect of providing this information involves working within the scope of practice of your role, as well as organisational procedures. It is therefore vital that you understand your job role and policies and know what to do when you are unsure of communication channels.

Enquiries and requests about organisational policies and procedures, such as infection control and work health and safety (WHS), must be dealt with under the relevant legislation. Other issues, such as information processing, may fall within organisational practices and can include responding to enquiries and requests:

- by telephone or email
- in person with staff, patients and others; for example, patient complaints, media requests
- in writing or using workplace forms.

When following up on a patient's request, you may find that you need to refer it to an RN. You may be unable to assist because the request is out of your scope of practice or you cannot leave the unit. It is important, however, to keep the patient informed regarding the progress of their request and double-check the information before passing it on. In acute care facilities, methods of recording and relaying messages may vary, so you need to consult with the RN about the procedures. Regardless of the methods used, reliability and accuracy will help to improve service delivery in the organisation.

Respond to enquiries and requests by telephone

When healthcare workers provide clinical information over the telephone to a patient, or their carer or advocate, they must document their own identification as well as the discussion in the healthcare record. This should include:

- the relationship of the person to the patient
- that the patient, or their carer or advocate, has consented to the caller seeking clinical information about the patient's healthcare record.

Only authorised personnel, such as medical staff, nurses and management, can transfer medical information over the telephone. These personnel will give their details to verify their identity. Do not ever give out any specific patient information when you answer the phone. Instead, refer the enquiry immediately to an RN or member of the medical staff. Inform an RN immediately if you are ever in any doubt as to the caller's identity or suspect that something is not right. Do not comply with any requests from the caller in this instance. Most organisational procedures require that healthcare workers repeat and confirm the order or plan of care prescribed by the doctor. Remember, as an HSA you cannot take telephone orders for medications.

Respond to patient complaints

A patient has a right to complain. Patient concerns should be addressed quickly and efficiently and resolved in a non-confrontational way. Ideally, most complaints should be dealt with directly, with as little formality as possible. You should:

- identify yourself
- listen to the patient's concerns and acknowledge the complaint
- seek assistance from the RN if the complaint is not straightforward.

You can provide the patient with information on the complaints procedures if they wish to escalate their concerns. Patient liaisons or complaint officers may also be available to listen and act on concerns or comments. The Health Care Complaints Commission, Complaints Commissioner or ombudsman are bodies where formal complaints can be lodged. Officers will explain the process of making a complaint and provide assistance if required.

Respond to media requests

Healthcare facilities must respond to appropriate and reasonable media enquiries effectively, accurately and quickly to help promote public understanding of their services and issues. In your role as an HSA, you are not permitted to approach or speak to the media on behalf of the healthcare facility. Instead, you should direct all media enquiries to an RN, who will identify the most appropriate spokesperson. There is always a designated person, such as the communications manager, to speak with the media. Politely decline any requests and refer the person to the RN.

Respond to carer requests

Patients must give permission for a carer to be provided with information and included in care discussions. Once this permission is given, healthcare providers must listen to carers and give them the opportunity to provide and receive information about the patient's condition.

Policy directives

Policies inform staff and guide the direction of the organisation. Read the policy directives from your state or territory health department and identify their relevance to your practice.

POLICY
Communications in healthcare policy
Social media policy
Privacy and confidentiality policy
Electronic information security policy
Complaints handling policy
Infection prevention and control policy

Find where the policy directives are stored in your organisation.

2 COLLECT, PROCESS AND MAINTAIN ACCURATE RECORDS IN AN ACUTE CARE ENVIRONMENT

As a worker in acute care facilities, you will need to become familiar with administrative tasks and protocols relating to record-keeping. This includes how health records and documents are obtained, completed, stored and dispatched in line with government legislation and regulations, and also with organisational policies and procedures. Administrative tasks will involve using business equipment and technology to process this information and you need to understand how to use this to provide holistic care for your patients.

Prepare workplace forms, documents and reports in accordance with legal and organisational requirements

The healthcare team is responsible for producing and maintaining patient healthcare records (paper or electronic), which enables them to provide effective continuing care. The New South Wales Nurses and Midwives' Association guidelines on documentation state that

> … the healthcare record is not a legal document, but a mechanism that allows the healthcare team to communicate effectively; deliver appropriate, individualised care; evaluate the progress and health outcomes of patients/clients; and retain the integrity of health information over time. However, the health care record has the potential to be admitted into evidence, if relevant, in legal proceedings. Producing the health care record requires comprehensive, accurate, high-quality clinical documentation.

NSWNMA, 2018, p. 2

Procedures are normally based on organisational policy, which deals with broad issues relating to a specific task. They provide specific guidelines for completing a task, such as a checklist or submitting a form. This can include administrative forms such as time sheets and leave forms, or patient care forms such as admission and discharge forms and risk assessment reports. These range in complexity, audience and format. The legal and organisational requirements for preparing these forms in an acute care environment include:

- privacy, confidentiality and disclosure
- work role boundaries – responsibilities and limitations
- work health and safety.

If you are unsure of the legal requirements, policies or procedures that apply in your workplace, ask the RN to assist you, or refer to your organisation's manuals.

ACTIVITY 10.4

Incident reporting

A colleague has an accident at work. There is an incident report form and other documents that must be filled out. This ensures that the organisation complies with WHS legislation.

The WHS policy that guides this process is supported by procedures for recording information and processing the necessary forms.

Source an incident/accident report form from your workplace and answer the following questions:

1. List the information that needs to be recorded on an incident/accident form.
2. Which personnel receive this form?
3. How are risk management strategies documented on this form?

Reporting requirements

When reporting, the information must be organised in a logical sequence. Integrated progress notes include entries by all healthcare professionals when the care or treatment occurs. This 24-hour reporting must therefore be prepared in a legible and accurate way. Figure 10.2 summarises the guiding principles for documentation. When developed in line with legal and organisational requirements, these will result in fewer risks and misunderstandings.

FIGURE 10.2 Guiding principles of documentation

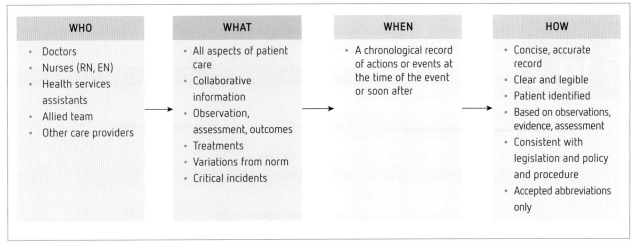

WHO	WHAT	WHEN	HOW
• Doctors • Nurses (RN, EN) • Health services assistants • Allied team • Other care providers	• All aspects of patient care • Collaborative information • Observation, assessment, outcomes • Treatments • Variations from norm • Critical incidents	• A chronological record of actions or events at the time of the event or soon after	• Concise, accurate record • Clear and legible • Patient identified • Based on observations, evidence, assessment • Consistent with legislation and policy and procedure • Accepted abbreviations only

Source: Shutterstock.com/Rawpixel.com

Legal requirements for documentation (NSW Health, 2012, p. 5) include the following:

- correct identification of the patient's name, date of birth and gender
- use of approved abbreviations and symbols
- writing on paper-based forms to be in dark ink that is readily reproducible, legible, and difficult to erase and write over
- document time of entry (using a 24-hour clock – hhmm)
- document date of entry (using ddmmyy or ddmmyyyy)
- identify the author, including their signature, printed name and designation – in a computerised system, this will require an appropriate identification system such as an electronic signature
- entries by students involved in the care and treatment of a patient being co-signed by the RN
- an entry by an HSA should not be the only entry for a shift.
  To be effective, documentation in progress notes must:
- be legible if handwritten and in English so that it can be easily read by others
- be clear and accurate so that other members of the healthcare team can assume care of the patient or provide ongoing service at any time
- be factual and objective in documenting what was observed and measured ('signs') through observation, physical examination and testing; do not include subjective data ('symptoms') such as feelings, perceptions and concerns, which can lead to differing interpretations
- only include relevant and necessary information about the patient's care and treatment
- be sequential – where lines are left between entries, they must be ruled across to indicate they have not been left for later entries
- be timely and record events as soon as possible after they occur.

Objective or subjective data

Indicate whether the information is an example of objective or subjective data. The first answer has been filled in for you as an example.

INFORMATION
Joan looks agitated – subjective
Milos had a BGL reading of 6.7 mmol/L
Chad stated that he felt nauseous
Lucinda's lower arm had a visible rash with weeping pustules
Xavier's urinalysis results indicated the presence of leukocytes
Brian complained of constipation
Mary heard that the new patient had a mental health disorder
Erica was hypotensive, with a blood pressure reading of 95/60 mmHg

Use business equipment and technology to obtain and process information

Business equipment and systems provide a range of tools that can be used to collect and process information. By becoming familiar with these and gaining an understanding of how they work, you can communicate with and support your healthcare team and patients in all areas of the health facility. In health care, using the appropriate technology is critical to ensure patient safety and clinical quality.

Examples and uses of business equipment and technology include:

- photocopier – can be used to copy handouts for educational sessions, minutes of meetings and memos. Many have integrated printing and scanning functions
- printer – allows electronic information to become a paper-based document
- fax/scanning machine – transmits and receives information so that people can check data, read a report or confirm information. Fax machines have been largely superseded by scanners
- telephone/answering machine – used for receiving and sending information quickly or leaving messages. Remember to state your name, designation and time of call when leaving messages, and follow up if the call is not returned
- pager – small, light communication device that allows people who are unable to answer a phone to take short messages. They ensure transmission of messages even in emergencies, with strong signals that do not rely on wireless networks. Recharging requires replacing the batteries. New generation pagers allow two-way communications, where the user can reply to the message alert. Your facility may also have an intranet site that allows paging services to be selected.

Information may be sourced from:

- correspondence – memos, minutes of meetings, letters, email
- computer databases – MIMS, research papers, client activity/transfer system
- computer files – letters and other documents
- charts, forms, progress notes
- laboratory results.

Computers in health care

Hospitals use complex network systems so that all staff can communicate with each other and share data. Through this technology, medical records, X-rays and pathology results are accessible by the healthcare team throughout the hospital, as well as progress notes, diet requirements, discharge summaries, consultations and operation reports. Computers also allow doctors to order pathology tests, medical imaging and allied health consultations.

Computerised technology includes:

- computers on wheels
- laptops or computers at nurse's stations, or point of care solutions
- tablets
- mobile phones.

The availability of patient records in electronic formats (EMRs) means access to information is mobile, so you can have a physiotherapist on an iPad in the ward, an HSA on a computer on wheels in the patient room and a specialist in the consulting rooms all looking at a patient's records.

Point of care solution

A device that is used where direct patient care is delivered.

Telehealth

Telehealth delivers health information, education and consultation through services such as videoconferencing and transmission of voice, data or images to rural and remote communities. It is an effective way to complement local health services. Access Queensland's Health site on telehealth at **https://www.health.qld.gov.au/telehealth** to answer the following questions.

1. What are the benefits of telehealth for patients in regional and rural communities?
2. What are the benefits for health professionals with telehealth?
3. How are telehealth consultations funded?
4. Who can a patient have in the room when they are participating in a video consultation?

10.6 ACTIVITY

Update, modify and file client health records and documentation

Updating health records and documentation makes it easier to share a patient's health history. It also helps a range of healthcare providers to communicate and make decisions about the patient's care. Correct filing maintains the records' security so that any healthcare professional has up-to-date information on the patient.

Updates

Care providers can capture information in the patient's progress notes in 'real time' throughout the shift. This means that updates on the patient's condition can be recorded chronologically. All new entries must include the date and time, and the signature and designation of the person entering the data. In some facilities, notes are documented as a single entry at the end of shift. Charting by exception occurs in care pathways where significant findings outside the norms of the predicted care for the patient are charted.

Charting by exception

Where only significant findings or exceptions to the predefined standards are documented in detail.

When you need to use a new form or write additional notes, you must ensure that the patient's identification and unique identifier is on each page. In acute care facilities, patient identification labels are printed for use on patient forms or are electronically coded into their electronic records.

Modifications and errors

State and territory laws vary on how medical records can be modified when errors occur. In general, the best procedure is for a narrative entry to be placed in the medical record statement indicating that an error has been made and is being corrected, whether it is a paper-based or electronic record. When modifying a record because of an error:

- all errors must be appropriately corrected
- an original incorrect entry must remain readable; that is, do not overwrite incorrect entries, do not use correction fluid
- an accepted method of correction is to draw a line through the incorrect entry or 'strikethrough' text in electronic records; document 'written in error', followed by the author's printed name, signature, designation and date/time of correction.

NSW Health, 2012, p. 6

SCENARIO

Martin — Error correction procedure

Martin, an HSA, is documenting the progress of his post-operative patient today. He has made an error and corrects it according to procedure, as follows:

12/5/18 1300 Nursing: Pt is 4 hrs post-op and resting in bed with no complaints of pain. Dressing site intact. Pt complained of nausea and vomited ~~50 mL~~ (written in error, M. Hennessey HSA) 200 mL clear fluid. Pt attempted to get out of bed to ambulate to bathroom with assistance, but stated he felt dizzy upon standing and was assisted to lie down in bed. Voided 200 mL clear, yellow urine in bedpan. Pt encouraged to deep breathe and cough. Fluid balance chart completed for shift. *M. Hennessey* (Hennessey HSA)/J. Jones RN---------

1 Why is it important to use the 24-hour clock when writing time in a patient's notes?
2 How can Martin maintain confidentiality when entering data in patient notes?

Filing systems (manual or electronic)

Paper-based and electronic filing systems include registers and databases that can be accessed by the entire healthcare team. In many acute healthcare facilities, paper-based files are sent to a medical records/health information department for scanning, collation and storage. You need to follow the correct procedures and be familiar with the way the systems are set up and how to access, retrieve and file information.

Collate and dispatch information according to timeframes and organisational requirements

Information can be collated and dispatched to various departments within healthcare facilities or to alternative locations; for example, a GP, nursing home or allied facility. In an acute care setting, the administrative assistant may be responsible for the collection of healthcare records. You need to be aware of how healthcare providers deliver healthcare records. When a patient is discharged or transferred from an acute care facility, the doctor and discharge planner/RN complete a summary and file it in the patient's medical records where it is available for subsequent reference.

State or organisational health bodies are responsible for ensuring that internal memos, guidelines or directives are distributed appropriately. They are responsible and accountable for ensuring the directives are observed.

Store records and information according to organisation protocols and procedures

As an HSA, you need to understand how records are stored within organisations. This helps ensure that only authorised personnel can access patient information. This includes the destruction of records to maintain patient privacy and confidentiality.

Health record storage

Healthcare providers need to be able to access electronic records 'over time, regardless of software or hardware changes'. They need to able to 'reproduce them on paper where appropriate, and have regular, adequate backups' (NSW Health, 2012, p. 14). The privacy legislation of each state or territory establishes statutory requirements for the storage and security of both paper-based and electronic healthcare records. You should always refer to state/territory legislation and hospital policy about document storage and management, or ask the RN if unsure.

A summary of the NSW Health (2012) policy 'Health care records – Documentation and management' requirements is as follows:

- Documents need to remain private and confidential and must at all times be stored in a secured space for access by authorised personnel only.
- Records must be correctly stored and eventually destroyed by authorised personnel to make sure that information of a sensitive nature is not made public.
- All records must be stored in a secure, safe area where there is no possibility of damage by pests, vermin or environmental factors.
- Records are stored both at internal organisational and registered external storage areas.
- The area must be safeguarded by security, with access determined by an ID system or electronic card recognition system to prevent access from individuals who do not have clearance.
- When stored, there is a system for location of records to allow for ease of access by authorised staff. This may be at the bedside for nursing and medication charts, and at the ward office for progress and historical notes.
- Records must be transported in a safe and confidential manner, ensuring that access is only given to authorised staff.
- 'Entries should not fade, be erased or deleted over time. The use of thermal papers, which fade over time, should be restricted to those clinical documents where no other suitable paper or electronic medium is available; e.g., electrocardiographs.' (p. 14)

Storage of X-rays or diagnostic images

X-rays films cannot be kept in the integrated progress notes because of their size, so they are usually filed separately, according to a unique identifying number that is linked with the patient's

Diagnostic images

Visualisations such as X-ray, CT scans, MRI scans and ultrasounds.

name. Digitised diagnostic images are captured, distributed and stored in a digital format viewable on computer screens around acute care facilities.

Medical record/health information departments in acute care facilities are responsible for the storage of records that are not currently in use. These include:

- scanned medical records
- old paper medical records
- paper and electronic forms.

ACTIVITY 10.7

Health record storage

Robert, an HSA, is admitting Malcom Holland and documenting his personal details, support requirements and lifestyle history. He begins by obtaining the consent for this information and then details the information that will be needed by the healthcare team. On completion of this admission, Robert thanks Mr Holland and checks with the RN that the information is adequate. He stores the admission history in Mr Holland's notes so that all authorised healthcare staff can access the information.

1 Identify where the patient notes are stored in the facility where you work or are undertaking work placement.

2 What other records are stored along with notes for each patient?

Health record disposal

The health facility must maintain the original health record unless it has obtained approval to dispose of it. If the original record needs to be taken out of the health facility – for example, to go to the coroner's court – the owner of the record needs to make a copy before providing the original to the third party. The health facility needs to establish a tracking system to track the location of both the original record and the copy. When records need to be destroyed, this should be done in a way that preserves the privacy and confidentiality of any information they contain. It needs to comply with the following instructions:

Coroner's court

A court that deals with finding out the identity of the deceased person, when and where they died, how they died and the medical cause of death.

- Any confidential paperwork is placed in locked bins and shredded before being sent for recycling. They can also be pulped or burned.
- Disposal of electronic records should make them unreadable and ensure they cannot be reconstructed in any way.
- Health records are kept for as long as they have value. It is generally seven years after the patient's death, but this can vary under certain conditions and cultural considerations.
- Disposal of records needs to comply with state/territory legislation and regulations.

3 SUPPORT EQUIPMENT REQUIREMENTS IN AN ACUTE CARE ENVIRONMENT

To be an effective member of your organisation, you need to know what equipment is appropriate for the task and then follow the instructions for its use. As the first step, you will need to consult with the healthcare team to make sure that the equipment will meet the needs of the patient. To ensure the equipment remains operational, you need to keep it maintained.

Consult with the nursing care team and reference material to determine equipment needs

Nursing care in an acute care environment is planned and organised around specific patient needs. Essential equipment is necessary for meeting patient needs, whether these are for observations, testing or treatment. You must consult with the RN and review the patient's plan of care to determine what equipment is required. This may include:

- positioning and patient mobilisation aids
- personal protective equipment (PPE)
- elimination equipment
- vital signs devices
- monitoring devices
- medical gases/cylinders (fixed and portable) and their accessories
- feeding and hydration equipment
- specimen collection
- wound dressings
- suction units and their accessories
- emergency equipment.

Reviewing the nursing care plan

Keeping the equipment well organised makes it possible to have more timely and efficient care. In reviewing the care plan, you can determine the nursing interventions that require equipment and organise accordingly. For example, a patient whose care plan states that they require a walk belt to mobilise should have the equipment on hand in a convenient location.

Consultation with healthcare team

ACTIVITY 10.8

Who would you consult to determine equipment needs? Match the required patient equipment listed in the table below to the healthcare team member you would consult regarding these needs: physiotherapist, occupational therapist, RN, stomal therapist, team leader or doctor.

EQUIPMENT REQUIRED
Eating and drinking utensils for a patient who has had a right-sided stroke
Ostomy equipment for a patient who has a colostomy
Mobility equipment for a patient who has had an amputation
Drainage devices for a patient who has recently had a catheter inserted
Personal protective equipment for a patient with norovirus
Blood collection equipment for a patient who needs haematology testing

Select and organise equipment appropriate to the task, equipment requirements and guidelines and within agreed timeframes

Equipment requirements in an acute care environment are varied according to the task, as indicated in Figure 10.3. After consulting with the healthcare team and checking the care plan, you should organise the equipment so that the patient can be assessed or treated appropriately. Using unnecessary equipment will increase healthcare costs, so you will need to carefully consider what equipment is needed for the task.

FIGURE 10.3 Equipment requirements in an acute care environment

TASK	EQUIPMENT REQUIRED
Positioning	Slide sheets, standing hoist, hoist
Mobilising	Walk belts, crutches, walking sticks, frames, wheelchairs
Infection control	Sharps container, biohazard bags, PPE – goggles, mask, face shields, gown, gloves, aprons
Elimination	Urinary catheters and drainage bags, uridomes, ostomy appliances, urine testing reagent strips
Vital signs	Electronic devices – BP, pulse oximeter, thermometer
Monitoring	ECG, Doppler, bladder scanner, glucometer, weigh scales
Oxygen therapy	Medical gases/cylinders, oxygen masks, nasal prongs, tubing
Hydration	Intravenous (IV) stand, IV fluids, cannula, syringe pump
Specimen collection	Specimen containers, swabs, spatula, request forms, PPE
Feeding	Nasogastric flow rate device, nasogastric tube, feeding aids
Wound care	Suction units, wound drainage bags, dressing trolley, dressing packs, solutions, gels, wound dressings
Emergency	Resuscitation trolley, tourniquets, IV stands

Biohazard bag
Specialist disposal bag for clinical waste.

Urinary catheter
Drains urine from the bladder into a drainage bag.

Ostomy appliance
Used when a patient has an artificial opening in the colon or ileum due to disease or surgery to the digestive tract.

Positioning

Positioning aids are used to move a bedridden patient either onto their side or further up the bed. They are also used to help a patient sit, stand or move out of a bed or chair. You should review the risk assessment when deciding which positioning aid to use. A patient care plan or notes will have information about this assessment and the type of equipment to use. You will need to ensure that you have had training in the safe use of mechanical aids and assistive devices before you use them. Figure 10.4 lists some of the equipment used for positioning. (For more on this subject, see Chapter 8, 'Assist with movement'.)

FIGURE 10.4 Positioning equipment

MECHANICAL AID OR ASSISTIVE DEVICE	USE IN POSITIONING
Slide sheets	A very smooth piece of strong synthetic material used when manoeuvring a person in a bed
Swivel board (turntable)	A soft pivoting disc for seated transfers, from seated to seated, such as a car to wheelchair for those with rotation difficulties
Standing hoist	A mechanical device with support slings used to help a person stand from a sitting position
Hoist	A mechanical device with slings used to transfer people who cannot weight-bear, from bed to chair or from chair to toilet/commode
Transfer boards	Rigid, smooth boards used when transferring people from one surface to another

Mobilisation

Walking aids support the patient during mobilisation and increase their stability. The patient's condition and the level of support required will determine the type of aid used. For recommendations on the most appropriate equipment, you will need to check with the RN or the physiotherapist. Aids include walk belts, crutches, walking sticks, frames and wheelchairs. (See Chapter 8, 'Assist with movement', for more on these aids.)

Walk belts

These belts can help you stand a patient and assist them to walk. The walking belts come in different designs and sizes, so it is important to use the correct size for your patient.

Crutches and walking sticks

Crutches enable the patient to walk by taking the weight off their body through one or both legs. Underarm crutches can be used by patients with leg injuries (sprains, ligament tears, fractures) and forearm support crutches are commonly used when a patient needs slightly greater support than a walking cane. The user will need to have good upper body strength and stability.

Walking sticks can be used for a person with mild one-sided weakness, and to provide balance and support. When selecting equipment, ensure that rubber tips are in good repair and all screws are tight.

Walking frames and wheelchairs

Walking frames provide greater support and are used when the patient is unsteady or is only partially able to bear weight. There are a number of styles of walking frame, including frames with four, three or two legs, pick-up frames and forearm support frames. The type of walking frame required is specific to each person's walking and balance needs.

Patients for whom walking is difficult or impossible because of illness, injury or disability can use wheelchairs. Manual or electric models are used depending on the patient's needs.

Infection control

You will need to employ both standard and additional precautions to minimise cross-infection and to protect yourself from exposure to bodily fluids. Personal protection is a major step in the prevention of cross-infection. Refer to Chapter 2, 'Comply with infection prevention and control policies and procedures', for more information on equipment requirements.

Elimination

Urinary catheters drain urine from the bladder into a drainage bag. These catheters come in a variety of sizes according to the patient's needs – the size is selected by the EN, RN or doctor. Uridomes are used for male patients. You should consult with the RN for the appropriate drainage bag when assisting with elimination needs (see Figure 10.5). This can include a leg bag, disposable bag or closed system bag with hourly measuring container and sample port. The latter may be required when you need to measure urine output frequently. Attach a drainage bag holder to the bedside or chair to ensure the drainage device is below the level of the bladder, preventing back-flow of urine.

FIGURE 10.5 Urinary drainage bag

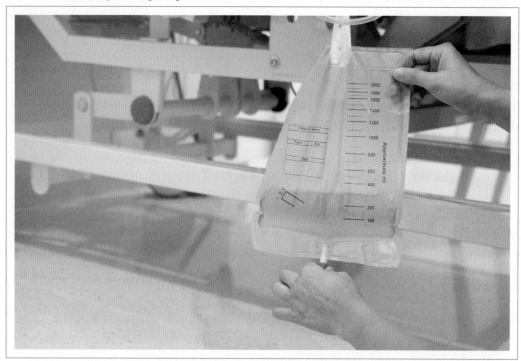

Source: iStock.com / HearttoHeart0225

Urinalysis
Tests the urine for the presence of various substances.

Urinalysis tests the urine for the presence of various substances. Equipment required for this task includes in-date reagent strips, gloves, container and urine sample.

Ostomy appliances are used for patients who have artificial openings in the colon or ileum because of disease or surgery to the digestive tract. The stomal therapist consults with the patient to determine the best appliance to suit their needs. Appliances range from bags with adhesive, attached directly to the stoma site, or bags attached to a base plate that is adhered to the stoma site. When helping a patient change their appliance, you will need gloves, a waste container, swabs to wipe the site and a new appliance.

Vital signs

When measuring a patient's vital signs, you need to determine the observations required from the patient charts and care plans before selecting the appropriate equipment.

Temperature

There are many different types of clinical thermometers that healthcare workers can use to measure a patient's temperature. Tympanic thermometers are most commonly used in acute care facilities. You will need to place a plastic cover over the tip before inserting it into the patient's ear. The reading is determined by heat radiating from the tympanic membrane and the result is displayed on the device's screen. Non-contact infrared thermometers are increasingly being used and can measure body temperature within seconds (see Figure 10.6). Since they do not involve any body surface contact or require probe covers, the risk of cross-infection is reduced.

FIGURE 10.6 Non-contact infrared thermometer

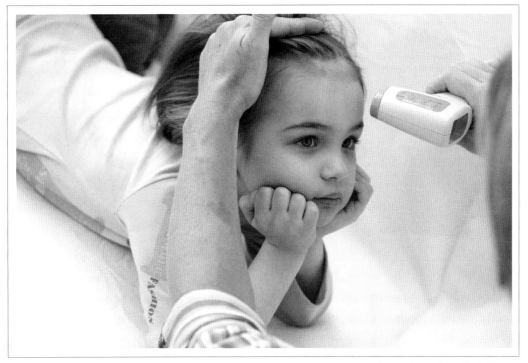

Source: Alamy Stock Photo/Phanie

Electronic thermometers are battery operated with a sleeve placed over the probe, which is disposed of after use. This device emits a signal when the temperature has registered, which is then displayed on its screen. Single-use thermometer strips are often used for newborns.

Pulse oximetry

A pulse oximetry device measures arterial blood oxygen saturation. Healthcare workers place a probe on the patient's finger or toe and LED light waves measure the oxygenated haemoglobin molecules in the blood. The reading is displayed on the oximeter.

Blood pressure

Blood pressure measures the force exerted by the blood on the walls of blood vessels as the heart contracts and relaxes. The device used to measure blood pressure can be manual or electronic and includes:

- a manual mercury sphygmomanometer, which is a pressure manometer and cuff with an inflatable bladder; a bulb is pumped to inflate or deflate the bladder
- aneroid manometers and cuffs that display the reading on a measurement gauge (see Figure 10.7)
- an electronic device in which the cuff is automatically inflated and deflated, and the reading displayed on a screen.

FIGURE 10.7 Manual blood pressure device and stethoscope

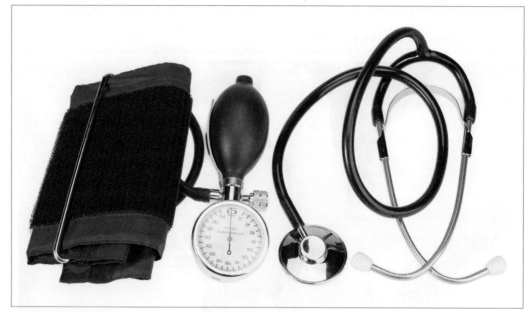

Source: iStock.com / wedmoscow

Many healthcare facilities use portable vital signs machines on wheels (see Figure 10.8), with blood pressure, temperature and pulse oximetry equipment all in the one unit. This is helpful for the nurse, who can wheel the machine from patient to patient or room to room.

Monitoring devices

An **electrocardiogram (ECG)** provides a trace or graphical record of the heart's electrical action. Pre-gelled electrodes, a razor to shave the chest of the patient and the monitoring device are required for this recording (see Figure 10.9).

Doppler ultrasonography involves the transmission of sound waves through the skin. **Transducer gel**, wipes, a probe and Doppler machine are required for this task.

Bladder scanning provides a 3D image of the bladder on a display screen. The scanner is a handheld, wand-like device containing a transducer, which sends out ultrasound waves that bounce off the bladder and are sent back to the computer for interpretation. Additional equipment for this task includes transducer gel and wipes.

Electrocardiogram (ECG)

Provides graphical record (a trace) of the heart's electrical action.

Doppler ultrasonography

Involves the transmission of sound waves through the skin using a Doppler machine.

Transducer gel

Water-based conductive medium that is used in ultrasound, ECG and scanning therapies.

Bladder scanning

Provides a 3D image of the bladder on a display screen.

Glucometers measure the levels of glucose in a patient's blood. There are many types of devices used so check with your facility and become familiar with the instructions for each device. Equipment required includes glucometer, reagent strips, lancet, sharps container and gloves.

Weighing scales are used to determine the patient's weight and can include chair scales or standing scales. The patient's ability to weight-bear will determine which type of scale to use.

Oxygen therapy

Oxygen can be delivered to the patient through several devices (see Figure 10.10). It can be piped through a wall outlet or supplied via a portable cylinder. While an HSA cannot administer oxygen therapy, they can help organise the equipment required for its delivery. Consult with the RN for equipment needs, which can include:

- nasal cannula – two soft plastic prongs that fit into the nostrils
- face masks – available in several styles, flow rates and sizes
- oxygen regulators
- oxygen cylinders (black with white shoulders)
- oxygen tubing.

FIGURE 10.8 Vital signs machine on wheels

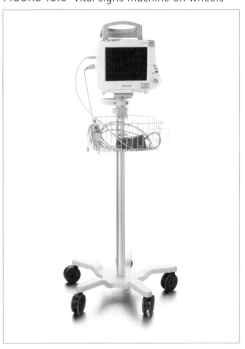

Source: Alamy Stock Photo / Andrew Twort

Glucometer
Measures the levels of glucose in a patient's blood.

Weighing scales
Used to determine the patient's weight; can include chair scales or standing scales.

FIGURE 10.9 Electrocardiogram machine

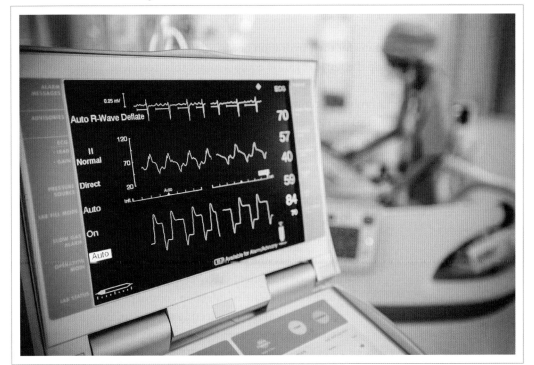

Source: Shutterstock.com / Chaikom

FIGURE 10.10 An oxygen mask in use

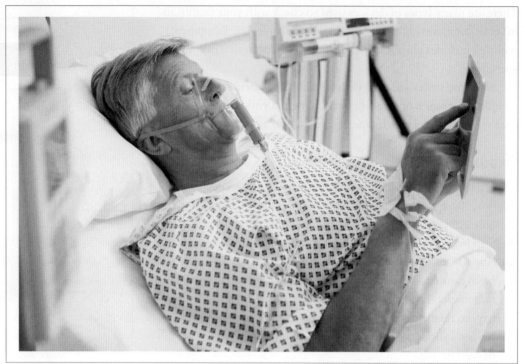

Source: iStock.com/Wavebreakmedia

Hydration

Patients may require IV therapy for their hydration needs when oral intake is inadequate or contraindicated. You can help the nurse organise equipment for this treatment. This can include:

- IV stand
- back slab – to splint the limb if IV cannula site is near a joint
- infusion tubing and burette (see Figure 10.11)
- electronic infusion device
- syringe pump.

FIGURE 10.11 IV infusion device and burette

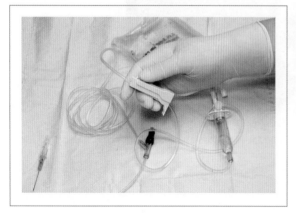

Source: Alamy Stock Photo/MedStockPhotos

Specimen collection

Healthcare teams can learn information about the status of patients by collecting specimens. They can be collected for diagnosis, the presence of disease-causing organisms, monitoring a patient's recovery, or assessment of function. You must be aware of infection control protocols to limit contamination when collecting specimens. Equipment will be dependent on the specimen requested and can include:

- a leak-proof container – 24-hour urine container, stool specimen container, mid-stream urine or biopsy sample container
- a cotton-tipped swab in sterile culture tube for nasal, throat or wound swabs (see Figure 10.12)

FIGURE 10.12 A cotton-tipped swab in a culture tube

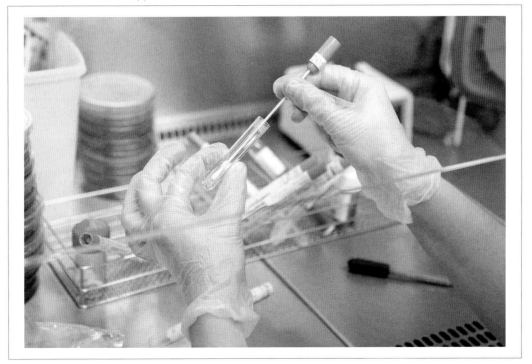

Source: Alamy Stock Photo/BSIP SA

- a spatula to collect stool specimen or help with throat swab
- a syringe to collect catheter specimen of urine
- a biohazard bag to transport specimen
- gloves
- request forms.

Feeding

There are many self-help devices to encourage the patient's independence in feeding themselves (see Figure 10.13). The occupational therapist can help determine the correct devices for the patient. These may include:
- plate guards
- angled cutlery
- cutlery with larger handles
- slip-resistant mats
- cups with two handles
- adult bibs.

Enteral tube feeding administers nutrition to patients who are unable to eat normally. When helping organise equipment for enteral feeding, you must make sure that the flow rate device is working correctly. The RN or doctor will select the correct enteral feeding tube type and size to suit the patient's needs.

Enteral tube feeding

Delivery of nutritionally complete food directly into the gut via a tube.

FIGURE 10.13 Self-help feeding devices

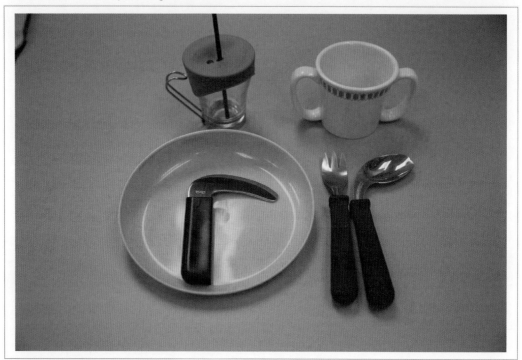

Wound care

When a wound dressing needs to be changed, aseptic technique and infection control guidelines must be followed. Facilities will have their own procedures for wound management and it is up to you to consult with the nursing team and care plan to determine the wound care required. Chapter 11, 'Assist with nursing care in an acute care environment', outlines the wound dressing procedure and equipment requirements. Additional items may include swabs, gauze, scissors or syringes.

Wound dressings, solutions and gels

There are many different types of wound dressings. The type of wound and the mode of action or material will determine the selection. Gels provide additional moisture for wounds and require a secondary dressing to hold the gel in the wound. The care plan, wound care chart, RN or wound consultant can all provide information on the type of dressing, solution or gel required.

Suction and drainage units

Negative pressure wound therapy applies suction to remove fluid, exudate and infectious materials to prepare the wound for healing and closure. It consists of a vacuum pump, drainage tubing, foam or gauze wound dressing, and an adhesive film dressing that covers and seals the wound.

Wound drainage devices collect blood, serum and debris from surgical wounds (see Figure 10.14). These may be free drainage or a self-contained system that provides suction.

FIGURE 10.14 A wound drainage device

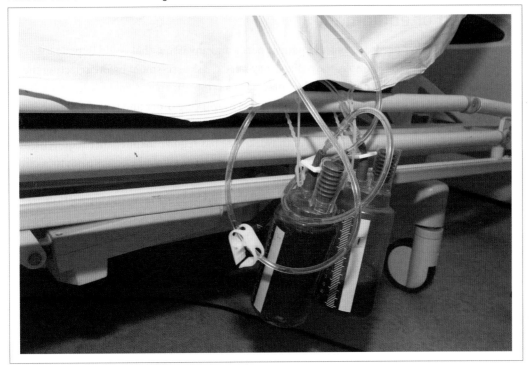

Source: Alamy Stock Photo/CaptureItOne

Emergency equipment

Each clinical area will have an emergency trolley that will have a range of equipment necessary for responding to a medical emergency. The clinical manager should assign responsibility to a relevant RN or EN in each facility to check, maintain and stock resuscitation equipment and drugs. You should participate in any education and training programs about emergency procedures, the use of equipment and your scope of practice in emergency situations.

Emergency trolley

Locate the emergency trolley in the ward where you are working or undertaking work experience and answer the following questions:

1   Familiarise yourself with your scope of practice as an HSA when assisting in emergency situations.

2   Access the emergency trolley checklist and research the name and use of unfamiliar equipment.

3   How often is the emergency trolley checked in your facility?

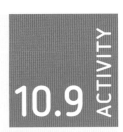

10.9 ACTIVITY

Deal with issues and problems associated with the operation of equipment

The healthcare worker needs to consider patient needs and any issues that could impede the safe use of equipment; for example, the patient may need a risk assessment before selecting the correct manual handling equipment, or they may need a tympanic thermometer when they have had oral surgery. You need to ensure the equipment is in working order and seek assistance if you are uncertain about how to operate it.

Much of the equipment used in the health workplace has regular maintenance requirements or needs repair at some time in order to replace either part of, or all of, the equipment; to rectify malfunctions; or to arrange for external servicing.

Some problems are fairly simple and can often be solved by looking up the instruction manual or troubleshooting tips, but you should consider whether your actions will affect the warranty or pose a danger to you or others. With complex problems, you should advise the RN or the designated person or specialist technician responsible for equipment repair. You also need to be aware of any procedures that relate to usage, repair and maintenance; for example, recording consumables used so that these can be reordered.

ACTIVITY 10.10

Patient considerations

You are preparing to use a hoist to move Mrs Branson, who weighs 134 kilograms and has mild dementia, from the bed to a wheelchair. Before operating the equipment, you:

- check that the battery for the hoist is charged and in good condition
- check the hoist (hooks, wheels) and sling for signs of wear or damage
- make sure you know how to operate all controls of the specific hoist.

1 What additional planning or equipment would you consider before undertaking this task?

2 Find out where spare batteries are kept in your workplace and how often the equipment is maintained.

Clean and store equipment safely and according to organisational procedures and specifications

Equipment should be cleaned and stored according to its type, manufacturer's instructions and local policy. Equipment that cannot be properly cleaned should be discarded. You should consult with the RN about the policy for cleaning, storage or removal of equipment.

Cleaning

Equipment in acute healthcare settings can be used on single or multiple occasions, depending on usage and infection control policies and procedures.

Equipment that has come into contact with mucous membranes or non-intact skin

If the item is single use, it should be disposed of in a sharps container or contaminated waste bin according to organisational policy; for example, nasal prongs, probe covers and spatula.

If the item is to be used on multiple occasions, it should be washed as soon as possible after use and sent to the sterilising unit for further cleaning. Healthcare facilities may use a central sterile supply department, which is a specialised area responsible for collecting, assembling, packing, sterilising, storing and distributing sterile goods and equipment. Examples include respiratory therapy equipment, specula and probes.

Equipment that has come into contact with intact skin

Multi-use equipment should be cleaned as necessary with appropriate solution. This includes stethoscopes, sphygmomanometers, blood pressure cuffs, pulse oximeters, non-invasive ultrasound probes, commodes and intravenous/feeding pumps. If the equipment is single use only, it should be discarded in the appropriate waste container.

Wheelchairs, lifters, hoists, frames, IV poles, monitoring devices and so on should be wiped clean after each use.

Storage

Dry, packaged, sterile equipment should be stored in a clean, dry environment and protected from sharp objects that may damage the packaging; for example, dressing packs, catheter bags, swabs and wound dressings. Non-sterile stock may be stored in the same area as sterile stock but should have clear segregation from the sterile stock by barrier, dividers or partition. Your ward will have a stock storage room (see Figure 10.15) and it is your responsibility to familiarise yourself with its contents, layout and accessibility. Stock replenishment orders are delivered at pre-defined intervals and old stock is placed at the front for first use.

FIGURE 10.15 Stock storage room

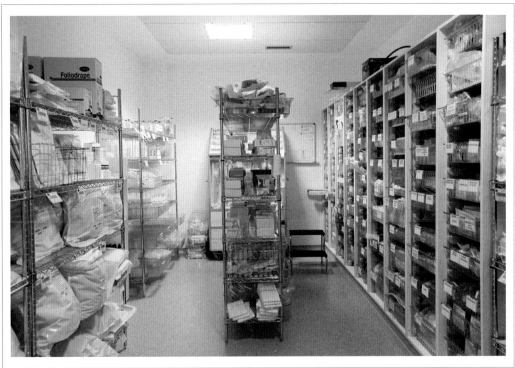

Source: Alamy Stock Photo / age fotostock

Shared equipment (e.g., wheelchairs, lifters, hoists, frames, IV poles, resuscitation trolleys) is located and stored in a way that makes it easy to use. The location of these areas is identified as part of your ward orientation.

ACTIVITY 10.11

Equipment storage

During your work placement or next shift, answer the following questions regarding equipment storage:

1   Where are dressing packs and drainage devices stored in your facility?

2   List the non-disposable items of equipment that are used in your facility.

3   Where is the mobility equipment stored in your health facility?

4   What actions do you take if a patient's bodily fluids contaminate mobility equipment?

5   How often are stores replenished in your ward area?

SUMMARY

Patient care technology has transformed the way nursing care is conceptualised and delivered in acute care facilities. This chapter gave you an understanding of health records in an acute care environment, and the importance of retaining confidentiality and security in line with state/ territory legislation and hospital policy. It also highlighted the processes used to maintain accurate and legal documentation and how to use business technology for effective communication with the healthcare team.

The last part of the chapter outlined the equipment required in acute care environments. Being an informed user of equipment for each task in healthcare means that you can select the appropriate equipment, receive the proper training for its use and support the healthcare team in patient-care procedures. The ongoing monitoring of equipment, along with its cleaning and correct storage, ensures that the best efforts are made to confirm optimum patient safety and care.

APPLY YOUR KNOWLEDGE

Admission protocols in acute care

Angus is a 52-year-old male who presented to his GP with chest pain. He was referred to the heart clinic for an angiogram. This procedure is performed under local anaesthetic and involves the insertion of a plastic tube into an artery in the groin. A catheter is then inserted into the heart and coronary arteries while the heart is monitored by X-ray. Dye is injected and pictures are taken of the arteries and heart chambers. This can detect the presence of coronary artery disease.

As the HSA working in the clinic, my role was to organise Angus's admission paperwork, help him into a hospital gown and take his pre-operative observations, including temperature, pulse, blood pressure and pulse oximetry. An ECG was also performed.

1   Why is it important for the HSA to complete an admission form for this patient?

2   What does pulse oximetry measure and what are the normal values?

3   The HSA is required to assist with the ECG. Using your knowledge gained in Chapter 5, 'Interpret and apply medical terminology appropriately', what is the meaning of the abbreviation 'ECG' and what is the meaning of the root and suffix of this term?

The anaesthetist gained Angus's consent and commenced IV therapy prior to the procedure, and he was given oxygen therapy via nasal prongs. When the procedure was completed, Angus was moved to the recovery ward where he continued to be monitored. The doctor came to see him and reported that his results were clear and that he did not require any further medical treatment.

4   What is the protocol for cleaning or disposal of the equipment that has been used for Angus?

It was recommended that Angus needed to reduce the stress in his life. Later that day he was discharged and his support person was able to take him home and stay with him overnight. The HSA recorded his discharge in the patient notes and had them countersigned by the RN.

5   What is the procedure if errors are made on the patient notes?

6   You were required to re-stock the angiogram room from the storage area in preparation for the next patient. What is the protocol for storage of equipment?

7   Understanding the scope of your role is essential to performing it effectively within the healthcare team. What was the scope of the HSA's involvement in the care for Angus?

◀ REFLECTING ON THE INDUSTRY INSIGHT

1   Why was it important for the HSA to take Mr Sinclair's pulse manually for a full minute?

   a   To detect irregularities in the rate of heartbeat.

   b   Because the electronic BP/pulse monitor cannot be left on for a full minute.

   c   Taking the pulse for a full minute can detect hypotension.

   d   A full minute allows the nurse to talk to the patient during the procedure.

2   What equipment did the HSA organise for the ECG recording?

   a   Doppler machine, tissues, recording paper.

   b   ECG machine, graph paper, IV stand.

   c   ECG machine, razor, pre-gelled electrodes.

   d   Ultrasound machine, request sheet, defibrillation pads.

3   What were the legal requirements for the HSA when writing in Mr Sinclair's progress notes?

   a   Include the time, date and patient's preferences.

   b   Include their signature, printed name and designation.

   c   Write in green ink and include their name and signature.

   d   Ensure it is countersigned by a doctor and include the date and time.

SELF-CHECK QUESTIONS

1   Define the purpose of health records.

2   What does the *Privacy Act 1988* require with regard to the storage and security of personal information?

3   What are examples of legal and administrative restraints on access to health records?

4   What is the role of an HSA when transferring medical information over the telephone?

5   What is the protocol when the original health record needs to be removed from the health facility?

6   List five pieces of equipment/technology used to access information in an acute care setting.

7   List the equipment required when preparing for specimen collection in an acute care environment.

8   How can oxygen be delivered to a patient and what are the contraindications for an HSA regarding oxygen therapy?

9   What actions would you take if the hoist battery expired while the patient was being transferred from bed to chair?

10 What are your definitions of the following key words and terms that have been used in this chapter?

KEY WORD OR TERM	YOUR DEFINITION
Protocols	
Confidentiality	
Health records	
Diagnostic images	
Coroner's court	
Point-of-care solutions	
Charting by exception	
Transducer gel	
Enteral tube feeding	
Biohazard bag	

QUESTIONS FOR DISCUSSION

1   Discuss the critical challenges to successfully implementing new technologies into healthcare environments and nursing practice.

2   Discuss how you would respond to the neighbour of Mrs Baker, while considering the privacy and confidentiality of the patient, when they ask: 'Can you tell me what the doctor said about my neighbour Mrs Baker? What type of treatment did they discuss and why are they changing her medication?'

3   The medical staff in your ward wish to take a photo of a patient's decubitus ulcer. Discuss the protocols and the policy that would support their actions.

4   Discuss the benefits of using electronic medical records in health care.

5   Discuss the benefits of using single use (disposable) devices.

EXTENSION ACTIVITY

Health records and forms

1   Examine the scenarios outlined in the following table and, with the help of your teacher or RN in the workplace, list the health records required.

SCENARIO CASE STUDY	HEALTH RECORDS OR FORMS REQUIRED
The patient is NBM and awaiting a total hip replacement operation this afternoon	
The patient has been seen by the doctor and is commenced on a 1500 mL fluid restriction	
The patient has a surgical wound that requires dressing	
The patient is to be discharged to a rehabilitation facility today via community transport	
The patient has been admitted from a nursing home and is unsteady on his feet	
You are using an electronic blood pressure machine and find that the LED display is faulty	
The patient has been admitted to your ward with unstable diabetes	

2   Look at the different types of charts and forms (both paper-based and online) used in your facility and compare them with other facilities.

3   Can you suggest any improvements or advantages of these forms?

4   Divide into groups and list any secondary uses of the health information noted in the health records described above.

REFERENCES

Australian Government (1988). *Privacy Act 1988*. Retrieved 17 October 2022 from https://www.legislation.gov.au/Details/C2014C00076/Download

New South Wales Nurses and Midwives' Association (NSWNMA) (2018). Guidelines on documentation and electronic documentation. Retrieved 17 October 2022 from https://www.nswnma.asn.au/wp-content/uploads/2018/10/NSWNMA-Guidelines-on-Documentaion-and-Electronic-Documentation.pdf

NSW Health (2012). Health care records – documentation and management. Retrieved 17 October 2022 from https://www1.health.nsw.gov.au/pds/ActivePDSDocuments/PD2012_069.pdf. © State of New South Wales NSW Ministry of Health. For current information go to www.health.nsw.gov.au CC 4.0.

Nursing and Midwifery Board (2019). *Code of conduct for nurses*. Retrieved 21 October 2019 from https://www.nursingmidwiferyboard.gov.au/Codes-Guidelines-Statements/Professional-standards.aspx

ASSIST WITH NURSING CARE IN AN ACUTE CARE ENVIRONMENT

Learning objectives

By the end of this chapter, you should be able to:

1 assist with the delivery of nursing care to clients in an acute care environment
2 support the client to meet their care needs in an acute care environment
3 work in a team environment
4 work effectively under supervision.

Introduction

This chapter provides you with the skills and knowledge required to provide nursing care assistance in an acute care environment. In your role as a health services assistant (HSA), you will:

- plan the patient's care in conjunction with registered nurses (RNs) and enrolled nurses (ENs)
- provide direct care activities to patients according to their nursing care plan under the guidance of an RN
- provide support to the patient.

In planning, the patient's physical, emotional and social needs are considered along with their personal values, such as their cultural, social and spiritual preferences. The care plan can then be determined using a problem-solving approach to achieve functional wellbeing.

This chapter explains the clinical observations, measurements and interventions you will use in the acute care environment, and the supporting actions that enable your patient's daily living needs to be met.

As part of the healthcare team, and working under the direct supervision of an RN, you will share the team's goal of providing nursing care to acute care patients.

INDUSTRY INSIGHTS ➕

Online pre-admission

My first experience with online pre-admission information was when I was working in the day-stay unit. Mrs Korda was being admitted for removal of a skin lesion on her left cheek. She had completed her e-Admission (online pre-admission) form two weeks prior, so the healthcare team was aware of her condition, past history, allergies and medications, and could prepare for her stay.

The staff rang Mrs Korda prior to her admission and informed her to fast from midnight the night before because she was having a morning procedure. In preparation for surgery, she was told to:

- shower on the day of her surgery to minimise infection risk
- brush her teeth but be careful not to swallow any water
- take her regular medications on the day of her surgery with a small sip of water
- remove all nail polish and make-up and not apply any perfume
- leave valuables including jewellery at home
- wear comfortable clothes that were easy to remove and put on
- bring any relevant scans, X-rays or test results, as well health fund cards
- organise an escort to accompany her home and a responsible adult to stay with her overnight.

Mrs Korda came on time to the short-stay unit. We already knew that she would be anxious for this procedure because she had stated this in her pre-admission forms. We also knew that she had a history of hypertension and was allergic to penicillin. I waited until she had settled and took her vital signs. Her anxiety was displayed as symptoms of tachypnoea and diaphoresis. I placed identification and allergy bands on her arm and leg to reinforce her identity to theatre staff. Her procedure went well, and her daughter was waiting for her when she returned. I was glad that I could support Mrs Korda pre-operatively. Knowing some aspects of her physical and emotional state helped me to prepare for her procedure and provide reassurance to allay her anxiety.

1   ASSIST WITH THE DELIVERY OF NURSING CARE TO CLIENTS IN AN ACUTE CARE ENVIRONMENT

An HSA is part of the multidisciplinary team that delivers nursing care to clients. To deliver this care, an initial assessment is made to identify the patient's needs, then the plan is formulated and the nursing interventions implemented and evaluated for effectiveness. This is the nursing process (see Figure 11.1) and it provides the foundations of care. Each plan is individualised and developed through collecting clinical data, identifying client preferences, carrying out procedures safely and reporting back to the team. This collaborative approach ensures that care is tailored to meeting the specific needs and goals of the patient.

FIGURE 11.1 The nursing process

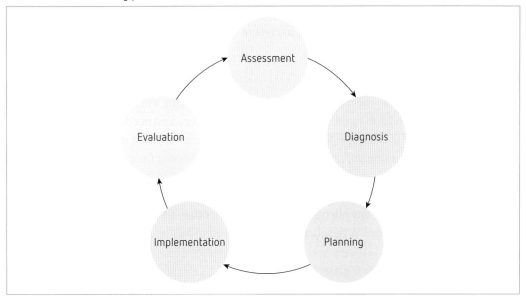

Implement aspects of nursing care to support patient needs according to the nursing care plan

The nursing care plan is a document developed by the healthcare team that records the patient's problems, goals, the nursing actions required and evaluations. They can be paper-based or electronic documents and form part of the patient's health records. It is important that you become familiar with the nursing care plan used in your facility, and the basic principles of assessment, identifying problems, planning, implementation and evaluation.

Assessment

Taking the patient's history is a key component of their assessment and is essential for delivering the correct care. Both subjective and objective data are collected, which provide a holistic assessment of all the factors that could affect a client's health, including information and preferences about personal hygiene, medications, mobility, nutrition, and cultural and social aspects of the patient's life.

Data is collected in the patient's admission interview, by reviewing the patient's nursing history and medical records, and by observing the patient and taking measurements, such as vital signs. During this stage, you should establish a therapeutic relationship with the patient to build trust and mutual understanding. The New South Wales Department of Health (2019) allows an HSA to document all patient responses to the direct care given, including progress notes and clinical records in accordance with the plan of care and organisational protocols. Check with your state or territory and local regulations regarding the scope of practice for an HSA when collecting health information.

Nursing admission interview

As an HSA, you can complete the initial questioning in the nursing admission interview, which will clarify the client's name, address, date of birth, next of kin, emergency contacts, occupation and status. You can also take the required baseline observations of temperature, pulse, respirations, weight and/or urinalysis. By collecting this data, you have an opportunity to introduce yourself to the client, show your interest in them and facilitate discussion regarding care planning.

Nursing history

Nursing history

Data collected about a client's physical, cognitive, social and emotional history.

The RN or the EN will take the nursing history to identify problems and develop the care plan, focusing on questions regarding the client's overall health history and needs, including:

- Language – does the client speak a language other than English? Is an interpreter required? Do they have a condition which makes communication difficult; for example, stroke or dementia?
- Medications – what are their current medications? Have they brought medications with them?
- Allergies – do they have any allergies to drugs, food or other allergens; for example, hand hygiene solutions or tape? A red allergy band will need to be placed on the patient's wrist (see Figure 11.2)
- Sensory aids – do they wear glasses or hearing aids?
- Mobility – are they fully ambulant or do they have difficulty walking? What mobility aids do they require?
- Nutrition – do they have a special diet for health or religious reasons? Do they have any chewing or swallowing problems?
- Elimination – do they have regular bowel habits or take laxatives? How often do they urinate at night? Do they wear incontinence pads?

FIGURE 11.2 Allergy wrist band

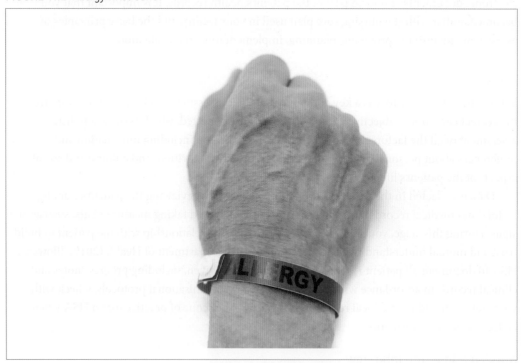

Source: iStock.com / JannHuizenga

- Sleep patterns – what are the client's normal sleeping habits? Do they take any medication to assist with sleep?
- Personal hygiene needs – do they have their own teeth or have dentures? What are their preferences for showering/bathing?
- Smoking, alcohol or recreational drugs – how much do they take and how often? Ask about substance abuse in a straightforward, non-judgemental manner.
- Cultural, spiritual and social needs are also considered and discussed later in this chapter.

Admission history

Provide the rationale for each of the following admission steps:

ASSESSMENT	RATIONALE
Greet the client by name and introduce yourself	
Apply an identification band to the client's wrist and ankle	
Apply a colour-coded band that identifies allergies regarding the client	
Demonstrate the use of the bed controls, buzzer and telephone, and orient the client to the ward	
Explain general routines and schedules that are followed for visiting hours, meals and care	
Take care of the client's clothing and valuables according to organisational policy	
Record vital signs – pulse, temperature, respirations, blood pressure and oxygen saturation, and weight	
Introduce the client to others in the ward and identify the roles of other healthcare workers	

11.1 ACTIVITY

Identify actual and potential problems

Once the history and current health status of the client have been determined, actual and potential problems can be identified. A care plan can now be developed with an overall picture of the client's healthcare needs.

Actual problems are those that the client is currently experiencing; for example, pain in both hips due to arthritis. Potential problems are those that the client may be at risk of developing; for example, their potential for falls due to decreased mobility. Identifying potential problems is important because this allows the nursing team to take preventative actions to reduce the risk of these occurring. In this example, assistive mobility devices may reduce the risk of falls. Once the actual and potential problems are identified, the planning and implementation of nursing interventions can be undertaken to achieve the desired outcomes.

Identifying problems

Phillip Sanderson is a diabetic aged 75 years and he lives alone. He has been transferred to your ward following bilateral knee replacements:

1 What actual and potential problems can be identified for Mr Sanderson?

2 What additional allied healthcare professionals are required to support Mr Sanderson in his recovery and what care would they provide?

Check with your facilitator for any additional problems that could be identified in this case, including potential social considerations.

Plan goals

The next phase is to plan goals in response to the identified problems and needs. These goals can be short or long term. They should be specific, measurable, attainable, realistic and time based (SMART). They can be amended when complications or unexpected events occur. As the client's needs change, so does the care plan. This constant review means that new goals are adapted to suit the client's progress. Discharge planning – anticipating the needs for a client's discharge – is also part of the planning process. This involves ongoing assessment and communication with the entire healthcare team. In some facilities, a discharge planner will undertake these activities and consult with community-based services or a general practitioner for the client's ongoing support.

> **Discharge planning**
> The plan of how the client's medical requirements will be met after he or she is released from treatment.

Implement nursing actions

This involves applying nursing care to achieve the goals outlined using evidence-based practice. It is important to encourage the client to participate actively where possible because this develops independence and confidence. Check if your facility has standardised plans that provide essential interventions for specific groups of clients (see the following 'Clinical pathways' section). Interventions can be direct (e.g., performing active and passive exercises on a client) or indirect (e.g., consulting with the dietitian about food preferences).

Clinical pathways

Clinical pathways are standardised, evidence-based, multidisciplinary plans. They identify an appropriate order of clinical interventions, timeframes and expected outcomes for a common client group. Acute care facilities are increasingly using these documents to reduce variations in care planning. The nursing teams are responsible for implementing and monitoring the client's progress and reporting deviations in the pathway from the norm.

Clinical pathways

Clinical pathways reduce variations and duplication by using a standardised approach to healthcare management. Access or research the clinical pathway for a total knee replacement and answer the following questions:

1 List pre-admission interventions that must be completed.

2 What is the expected length of stay for this procedure?

3   List the nursing care activities that the HSA would assist with for each day.

4   List any special care to be undertaken during the stay.

5   What instructions are given on discharge?

Evaluate results of nursing actions

Once the nursing actions have been implemented, the results must be evaluated for effectiveness. Evaluate the results against the following questions. Have the outcomes been achieved? Was the care effective? Has the client's condition improved? Are new goals and care required? This is a continuous process and shows the extent of the progress towards a given goal.

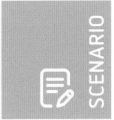

SCENARIO

Implementing the nursing care plan

Mary, an HSA, checks the care plan for her client. One potential problem included is the risk of impaired skin integrity due to immobility, with the goal of preventing pressure ulcers. In implementing the plan, Mary turns the client two-hourly, makes sure that a pressure-reducing mattress is on the bed, ensures the client's skin is clean and dry, and checks the skin on the patient's sacrum, hip and heels for redness. When the client is mobile, she is reassessed and the care plan is re-evaluated.

1   Why would Mary check the sacrum, hip and heels for redness?

2   Why would it be important to keep the client's skin clean and dry?

3   How often are nursing care plans re-evaluated?

Assist to complete assessment tools and collect clinical data using appropriate equipment and procedures as delegated by the RN

The collection of information from assessment tools, notes and charts allows the multidisciplinary team to interpret the client's condition and develop an effective care plan. The effectiveness of this process is dependent on the accurate recording and interpretation of information. If the information collected is abnormal, or outside of normal limits, it must be reported to the RN.

Risk assessment tools

Risk assessment tools are used to measure the levels of risk for specific situations, procedures and outcomes. After identifying the risk, it is evaluated for the likelihood of the risk occurring and its severity, and measures to effectively prevent or control (mitigate) harm are planned. Commonly used risk assessment tools in nursing practice address pressure areas (i.e., Waterlow, Norton and Braden tools) and falls risk assessment tools (i.e., FRAT).

Treatment plans

Treatment plans are frequently used to provide ongoing care and support for a person with a chronic or mental health disorder. It can explain the support provided by each type of professional and when treatment should be provided. In the case of a mental health treatment plan, it may also include what to do in a crisis or to prevent relapse.

Treatment plans are designed for clients who require a structured approach, including those requiring ongoing care from a multidisciplinary team. They ensure that everyone involved in the client's care is working towards planning and coordinating care to achieve the same goals.

Integrated progress notes

Integrated progress notes document a client's status while in hospital or as an outpatient. They form part of the client's medical record. Progress notes serve as a basis for planning care and communicating between health professionals who contribute to this care. Each member of the multidisciplinary team documents information relevant to the client's needs and progress. This can include the dietitian, physiotherapist, nurse consultant and doctors.

Important points for documenting progress notes include:
- sign, date and designate all entries
- avoid leaving blank spaces
- be clear and accurate
- distinguish between what was observed and what was performed.

Flowcharts

Flowcharts show the flow of people, services and information in a hospital; for example, the flow from admission of a client to discharge. They can also list the types of services each unit or person must deliver to meet the client's needs. Examples of common flowcharts used in hospitals include infections control, complaints handling and risk management.

Observation charts

Monitoring and documenting physiological observations are key components of nursing assessment. An observation chart is a document on which client observations are recorded. In some cases, they specify the actions to be taken in response to deterioration from the norm. These charts generally use symbols for vital signs such as pulse, temperature, respirations, blood pressure and oxygen saturation. Some charts also record numerical values or letters for urinalysis, blood glucose level (BGL), weight, bowel movements and pain.

The main types of charts used in Australia are as follows:
- *Colour-coded charts that incorporate a track and trigger system.* The different colours in the charts reflect levels of physiological abnormality. The New South Wales Department of Health standard observation chart is one such example, with colour coding to reflect red and yellow responses and white being within normal limits (Clinical Excellence Commission, 2016).
- *Charts that do not incorporate a track and trigger system.* While these charts sometimes indicate normal values, they do not highlight physiological abnormalities. It is important that you have a sound knowledge of deviations and report these to the RN.

Track and trigger observation charts

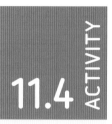

Refer to the Adult Deterioration Detection System (ADDS) observation chart (see Figure 11.3) developed by Queensland Health and the Australian Commission on Safety and Quality in Health Care – available at **https://www.safetyandquality.gov.au/** on the 'Adult Deterioration Detection System (ADDS) chart with blood pressure table' page – and answer the following questions:

1   What is the length of time that this chart can be used?

2   A colour-coded track and trigger system is used to detect a deteriorating client. In this chart, what observations are included in the colour-coded ranges?

3   What does the purple colour represent?

4   What is your responsibility when an observation falls outside the normal ranges?

5   Discuss the advantages and disadvantages of this chart.

6   Discuss how this chart compares to observation charts used in your workplace.

Identify client preferences when collecting information in the development of nursing care plan

As well as collecting information on the client's overall health history and clinical data, cultural, spiritual and social considerations must also be considered when developing the nursing care plan.

Cultural preferences

Rituals or cultural norms have a significant impact on the patient's health and their behaviours. Questioning can identify family dynamics and attitudes towards the healthcare team and this information can be used to provide culturally safe nursing care. Refer to Chapter 6, 'Work with diverse people', for more information on cultural competence.

Spiritual preferences

The spiritual support for a client can come from within the hospital (i.e., pastoral care) or from the community, where a local minister may visit the client. Supporting spiritual needs can provide a sense of hope and strength for the client when they are facing difficult health situations.

Social preferences

Determining the client's relationships, social activities, hobbies and their level of satisfaction with life can give the healthcare team an idea of how engaged the client may be in their self-care. It can also give an indication of the support systems that may be needed on discharge; for example, if they are living alone or with family.

FIGURE 11.3 Adult Deterioration Detection System (ADDS) chart

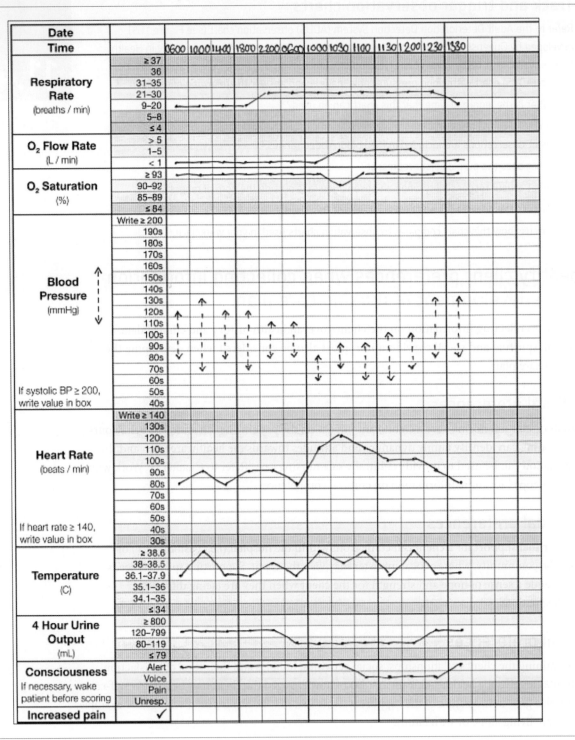

Source: Australian Commission on Safety and Quality in Health Care (2012). Adult Deterioration Detection System (ADDS) chart with blood pressure table. Retrieved 19 October 2022 from https://www.safetyandquality.gov.au/publications-and-resources/resource-library/adds-chart-blood-pressure-table

Social and cultural preferences

Reflect on your own social and cultural perspectives and answer the following questions:

1   How have your values been influenced by your family, friends and life experiences?

2   How has your education and training given you an understanding of diverse cultures?

3   Discuss the different types of social and cultural preferences you have observed in your workplace or class.

4   Why is it important to understand the social and cultural preferences of your patients?

11.5 ACTIVITY

Inform client of purpose of information being sought and the procedure, and gain feedback on patient understanding

When gathering information from a client, you will need to be attentive, patient and thorough so that all information collected is as accurate as possible. An explanation of the purpose of obtaining information should be given so that the client understands why certain questions are being asked.

You can satisfy yourself that the client understands the information presented by doing the following:

*   asking the client to repeat what has been said using their own words, or asking them questions about the information provided
*   providing them with the opportunity to ask questions and ensuring they are answered in a manner the person can understand.

A supportive, non-judgemental attitude may help ease the client's anxiety or possible resentment that you are probing into areas that are too personal. Non-verbal communication is also very important. Maintaining eye contact helps make the interview feel private, and short periods of silence can help the client collect their thoughts before continuing.

Reassure the client that the information collected is part of their medical record and will therefore be kept confidential. It is important to note that if a client is unable to supply all the information needed, it may be obtained from relatives.

Obtain client consent and communicate appropriately before you seek information or provide a procedure or activity

Ethical and legal principles require that health care be provided with consent from an individual who has the capacity to make decisions. This means that when undertaking a procedure or seeking information, you must identify yourself, explain the purpose of the procedure and highlight any issues or risks that may arise. In this way, the client is informed before giving consent. The client has then been provided with sufficient information to make an appropriate decision about the proposed procedure. Consent may be a simple 'yes' or 'no' or could be implied; for example, the client may position their arm so you can measure their blood pressure.

Informed consent is relevant to the entire communication process and ensures that the client fully understands the proposed procedure and has supportive information to make an informed decision about whether or not to agree. Communication should be in a way that is appropriate to the individual's needs and can include diagrams, printed material, video or aural materials. You may have to engage an interpreter if English is an additional language. Give the client time to reflect on and absorb the information and consult their relatives if needed.

By communicating appropriately, you will improve the client's and carer's capacity for involvement, understanding and participation in care. It can also encourage an individual's engagement with the healthcare team.

SCENARIO

Obtaining consent from Ms Hunt

Jonathon, an HSA, is admitting Ms Hunt, who will be having a knee arthroscopy. He explains the need to check her blood pressure, temperature and pulse as preparation for the arthroscopy, before she is seen by the surgeon. He asks if she understands and if she has any further questions. She gives verbal consent for the observations and states that it is her first time in a hospital and she is anxious.

Jonathon describes each step when taking her observations and explains that the readings are within normal limits. He stays with her until the surgeon arrives and passes on the data, including her feelings of anxiety.

1   Why was it important for Jonathon to take observations before surgery?
2   What action would the HSA take if Ms Hunt's temperature was outside of normal limits?
3   Why is it important to pass on Ms Hunt's feelings of anxiety to the surgeon?

Report relevant information, including changes in client condition

Collecting clinical data and observing clients is a vital part of your role as an HSA. Track and trigger charts indicate deviations from the norm, while a sound knowledge of normal and abnormal conditions will assist in identifying client changes.

Observing uses all your senses – smell, sight, hearing, touch. For example, you may smell a strange odour in urine, you may see sweating, you may feel the temperature of the skin, and you may hear laboured breathing. Observation can take place when undertaking basic nursing tasks. Assisting clients with personal hygiene is a good opportunity to observe skin integrity, their communication abilities and any changes in behaviour. Transferring clients from one position to another can provide an opportunity to observe mobility.

When there are changes in the client's condition, the care plan will need to be adjusted accordingly and the healthcare team will need to be made aware of the change. All verbal and written reporting should be:

- clear – neat and easy to understand
- accurate – use exact measurements and terminology
- concise – avoid unnecessary details
- factual – clearly explain what was observed
- objective – what was actually seen and heard, not what was felt or thought.

When documenting on charts, use the correct pen and strike-through and sign errors. Make sure that you report all observations and changes in the client's condition to the RN and re-check observations if unsure. Refer to Chapter 4, 'Communicate and work in health and community services', for more information regarding reporting and recording.

Reporting information

You are currently working in the medical ward of a small country hospital under the supervision of an RN. Mr Lee, 56 years old, has been admitted to the ward with a provisional diagnosis of myocardial infarction (MI). While attending to his needs, he informs you that his left elbow is painful and that he had an episode of chest pain while he was reading the newspaper this morning. His pulse is irregular at 92 bpm and his respirations are 24 breaths per minute; he is sweating and appears anxious.

11.6 ACTIVITY

1 What is the objective data in this case study?

2 What is the subjective data in this case study?

3 What is your responsibility under the scope of your role as an HSA in this situation?

4 Practise giving a verbal report to your teacher/facilitator.

5 Practise writing an accurate, concise and factual nursing report for this client. Note that nursing reports are always countersigned by an RN in the workplace.

Carry out a procedure or activity according to safe work practices

Descriptions of the procedures used to monitor clients and perform nursing activities are outlined in the following section, including:

- checking temperature, pulse, respiration, blood pressure and BGL
- collecting specimens (urine, sputum and faecal)
- measuring and recording weight
- taking neurological observations
- recording food and fluid balance
- application of anti-thrombosis stockings
- assisting with breathing devices under supervision
- performing shallow wound care.

In carrying out these procedures and activities, it is important to follow safe work practices. This includes doing a risk assessment, positioning the client correctly and adhering to the relevant infection control procedures during the task; for example, hand hygiene and the appropriate disposal of waste.

Measure and record a temperature

Body temperature is defined as the level of heat produced and sustained by the body; that is, the balance between heat production and heat loss. Temperatures are taken to assist in determination of general health and more importantly to indicate infection. There are several routes by which a temperature can be obtained – oral, rectal, tympanic and axillary – with tympanic being the most commonly used in the acute care setting.

Normal body temperature ranges from 36.1 to 37.2 degrees Celsius, but this can vary according to where it is measured and the time of day. It can be affected by illness, exercise, hydration, infection, environment or hormonal changes. Figure 11.4 lists some clinical definitions of medical terms relating to temperature.

Body temperature
The level of heat produced and sustained by the body, the measurement of which provides information regarding general health and possible infection. Measured with a thermometer.

FIGURE 11.4 Clinical definitions of medical terms relating to temperature

MEDICAL TERM	CLINICAL DEFINITION
Hyperthermia	Elevated body temperature
Febrile	Relating to fever > 37.8°C
Afebrile	Without fever; temperature within normal limits
Hypothermia	Low body temperature < 35°C

Guidelines to measure temperature

Equipment used to measure temperature includes:

- electronic oral or tympanic (see Figure 11.5) and digital thermometers
- infrared thermometer with a laser pointer and forehead temperature indicators
- vital sign devices that can register temperature, pulse, respiration and blood pressure simultaneously.

FIGURE 11.5 Taking tympanic temperature

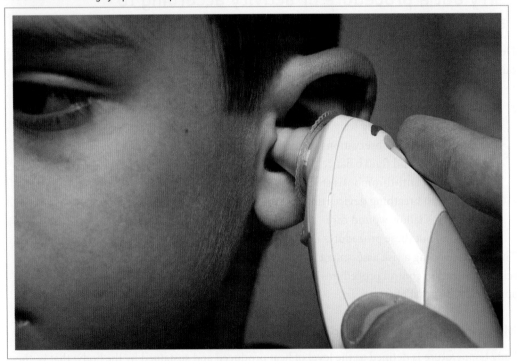

Source: Shutterstock.com/ Dave Clark Digital Photo

Steps to measure temperature are as follows:

1. determine site and choice of thermometer to be used to obtain temperature
2. position the thermometer correctly at the selected site
3. remove the thermometer at appropriate time and read result
4. clean the thermometer/dispose of the probe cover as appropriate
5. perform hand hygiene
6. document observations accurately on observation chart
7. report all findings to an RN.

Figure 11.6 outlines points to remember when measuring temperature.

FIGURE 11.6 Points to remember when measuring temperature

ORAL TEMPERATURE	TYMPANIC TEMPERATURE
Should not be attempted on individuals who: • are dyspnoeic, confused, receiving oxygen therapy, unconscious • have recently had hot or cold food or drink • are under five years of age	• If you are checking a child's temperature, gently pull the child's ear straight back • If you are checking an adult's temperature, gently pull the ear up and then back
Always follow manufacturer's guidelines on the use of thermometers	

Measure and record a pulse rate

A pulse is defined as a wave of distension of an artery following the contraction of the heart. Any artery can be assessed for a pulse rate, but the radial and carotid arteries are easily palpable. The brachial and apical pulses are the best sites for assessing an infant or young child because the other pulses are deeper and therefore difficult to palpate. Figure 11.7 indicates commonly used sites to measure a pulse.

FIGURE 11.7 Commonly used sites to measure a pulse

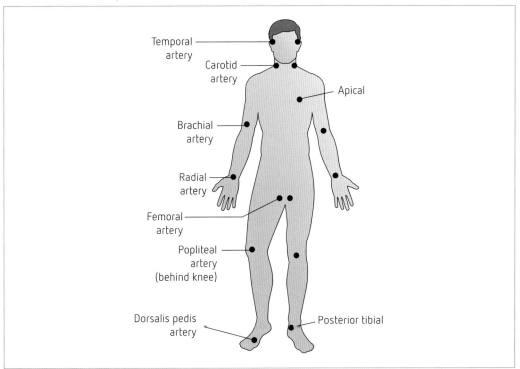

Source: From Hegner/Acello/Caldwell, 3P-EBK: NURSING ASSISTANT A NURSING PROCESS APPROACH, 10E. © 2016 Cengage.

Normal **pulse** rate is 60 to 100 beats per minute (bpm) for an adult and can be affected by exercise, age, emotions, illness and medication. The average pulse rate for an infant is 100 to 160 bpm and for a child it's 70 to 130 bpm. Figure 11.8 lists some clinical definitions related to pulse rates.

Pulse

A wave of distension of an artery following the contraction of the heart.

FIGURE 11.8 Clinical definitions of medical terms relating to pulse rate

MEDICAL TERM	CLINICAL DEFINITION
Bradycardia	Slow pulse: < 60 bpm in adults
Tachycardia	Fast pulse: > 100 bpm in adults
Arrhythmia	Irregular heartbeat

Guidelines to measure a pulse rate

Equipment used to measure a pulse rate includes:

- watch with a second hand
- correct observation chart
- stethoscope if measuring apical pulse
- vital sign devices that can register temperature, pulse (via pulse oximeter), respiration and blood pressure simultaneously.

Steps to measure a pulse rate manually are as follows:

1 Place the tips of the first two fingers of your hand over the groove along the radial or thumb side of the client's inner wrist (do not use the thumb to take a pulse because it has a pulse of its own that can interfere with the measurement).
2 Palpate the pulse.
3 Determine the strength of the pulse (strong, weak or thready).
4 Count the number of beats in 60 seconds (one minute).
5 Assess the pulse rate as either regular or irregular.
6 Perform hand hygiene.
7 Document observations accurately on the correct observation chart.
8 Report all findings to an RN.

Pulse oximetry

Pulse oximeter

Measures heart rate (as bpm) and oxygen saturation (as SpO2) in the blood.

A pulse oximeter (as shown in Figure 11.9) measures heart rate and oxygen saturation in the blood. The oxygen saturation reading is measured as SpO2. Normal oxygen saturation is 95 to 100 per cent, with lower levels indicating hypoxia.

This device is a clip that attaches to a finger, toe or earlobe and records the client's pulse and oxygen saturations on a digital display.

Measure and record respiratory rate

Respiration

The process of inhalation (breathing in) and exhalation (breathing out) to exchange oxygen and carbon dioxide. When measuring, observe the rate, rhythm, volume and symmetry.

Respiration is defined as the process of breathing in and out to exchange oxygen and carbon dioxide. One breath is composed of both an inhalation (breathing in) and an exhalation (breathing out). When measuring the patient's respiratory rate, observe for rate, rhythm, volume and symmetry, which is the ability of the chest to expand equally.

The normal respiratory rate range for an adult is 12 to 16 breaths per minute. However, respiratory rate can be affected by illness, emotion, exercise, age, position and medications. The average respiratory rate for an infant is 30 to 60 breaths per minute and for a child it's 20 to 30 breaths per minute. Figure 11.10 lists some clinical definitions of medical terms relating to respiratory rates.

FIGURE 11.9 Pulse oximeter

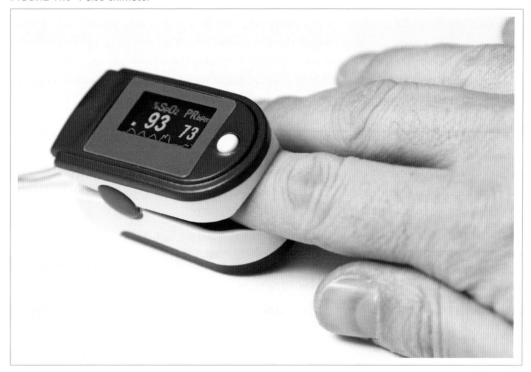

Source: Shutterstock.com / Juan R. Velasco

FIGURE 11.10 Clinical definitions of medical terms relating to respiratory rate

MEDICAL TERM	CLINICAL DEFINITION
Hyperventilation	Rapid breathing
Dyspnoea	Difficult or laboured breathing
Apnoea	Absence of respirations
Wheezing	Difficulty breathing with a whistling sound due to narrowed bronchioles
Stertorous breathing	Snore-like respirations
Cheyne-Stokes respiration	A period of dyspnoea followed by a period of apnoea

Guidelines to measure respiratory rate

Equipment used to measure respiratory rate includes:

- watch with a second hand
- correct observation chart.

Steps to measure respiratory rate are as follows:

1 Count the number of breaths in 60 seconds (one minute).
2 Assess the respiratory rate for rhythm, depth and sound.
3 Perform hand hygiene.
4 Document observations accurately on the observation chart.
5 Report all findings to an RN.

Take and record blood pressure

With each heartbeat, the heart's ventricles push blood into the blood vessels. Since the circulatory system is a closed system, the blood within the walls of the vessels exerts a force against the walls. This is called blood pressure (BP) and it is expressed in millimetres of mercury (mmHg).

Blood pressure is at its highest as blood is forced out of the ventricle during contraction. This is called the systolic pressure. It is at its lowest when the heart is relaxing and filling. This is called the diastolic pressure.

Normal blood pressure guidelines define < 120 mmHg systolic and < 80 mmHg diastolic for an adult; however, this can be affected by illness; shock; medications, such as stimulants, depressants or antihypertensives; age; heredity or weight. The normal range of blood pressure for a child aged between three and six years old is 95–110/60–75 mmHg. Figure 11.11 lists some clinical definitions of medical terms relating to blood pressure.

Systolic

Blood pressure when the heart is contracting – the upper reading.

Diastolic

Blood pressure when the heart is relaxed and refilling with blood – lower reading.

FIGURE 11.11 Clinical definitions of medical terms relating to blood pressure

MEDICAL TERM	CLINICAL DEFINITION
Hypotension	Low blood pressure
Hypertension	High blood pressure
Postural or orthostatic hypotension	Drop in blood pressure that happens when you stand up from sitting or lying down

Guidelines to measure blood pressure

Equipment used to measure blood pressure includes:

- correct observation chart
- sphygmomanometer or electronic device
- stethoscope if measuring blood pressure manually
- some facilities may use disposable cuffs.

Clean the cuff with facility-approved disinfectant between clients. If using a stethoscope, clean the earpieces and bell with alcohol wipes.

Steps to measure blood pressure are as follows:

1   Choose the correct-sized cuff – the length of the bladder should be 80 per cent of the arm circumference.
2   Locate and palpate the brachial pulse.
3   Apply the cuff correctly, with the artery alignment symbol on the cuff over the brachial artery.
4   Electronic blood pressure – turn on the machine and read the results.
5   Manual blood pressure – feel for a radial pulse:
    a   Inflate the bulb until you can no longer feel the radial pulse.
    b   Note the reading, deflate the cuff and add 30 mm.
    c   Place the diaphragm of the stethoscope (ensure it is open) in the correct position over the brachial artery.
    d   Reinflate the cuff to the calculated level (see Figure 11.12).
    e   Release the air and listen for the first beat, then note the position of the needle on the sphygmomanometer (systolic reading).
    f   Continue to release air until the last sound is heard (diastolic reading).
6   Remove the cuff and ensure that the client is comfortable and safe.

7   Clean and return the equipment.
8   Perform hand hygiene.
9   Document observations accurately on the correct observation chart.
10   Report all findings to an RN.

FIGURE 11.12 Measuring blood pressure

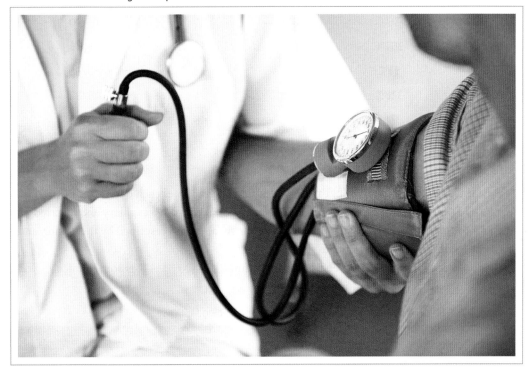

Source: iStock.com/GlobalStock

Figure 11.13 lists some key points to consider when measuring blood pressure.

FIGURE 11.13 Points to remember when taking blood pressure

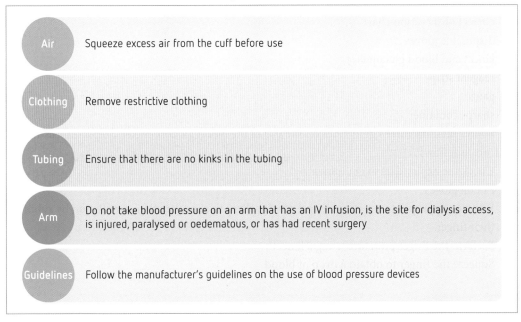

Air	Squeeze excess air from the cuff before use
Clothing	Remove restrictive clothing
Tubing	Ensure that there are no kinks in the tubing
Arm	Do not take blood pressure on an arm that has an IV infusion, is the site for dialysis access, is injured, paralysed or oedematous, or has had recent surgery
Guidelines	Follow the manufacturer's guidelines on the use of blood pressure devices

ACTIVITY 11.7

Documentation of vital signs

Obtain an observation chart from your workplace and enter the following observations.
Which observations are outside their normal range?

TIME	TEMPERATURE	PULSE	RESPIRATION	BLOOD PRESSURE
0200	36°C	80	14	105/70
0600	36.2°C	84	16	115/75
1000	38°C	112	28	150/80
1400	37.8°C	108	24	145/80
2200	37.1°C	80	16	130/70

Measure and record blood glucose level

Blood glucose level (BGL)

Level of glucose present in the blood, the measurement of which is undertaken when a person has or is suspected to have diabetes. Normal BGL is between 4.0 and 8.0 mmol/L.

Measuring blood glucose level (BGL) can be performed several times each day according to the client's condition and care plan orders. A blood sample is taken from a capillary and inserted into a meter for recording. Samples can be collected before meals or as prescribed by the doctor, and treatment is administered according to the results.

The normal BGL range is between 4.0 and 8.0 mmol/L. Figure 11.14 lists some clinical definitions of medical terms relating to BGLs.

FIGURE 11.14 Clinical definitions of medical terms relating to blood glucose

MEDICAL TERM	CLINICAL DEFINITION
Hypoglycaemia	Low blood sugar level: < 4 mmol/L
Hyperglycaemia	High blood sugar level: > 8 mmol/L

Guidelines to measure BGL

Equipment used to measure BGL includes:

* correct observation chart
* disposable gloves
* lancet and blood glucometer
* reagent strip
* gauze
* sharps container.

Follow manufacturer's guidelines on the use of the blood glucose meter. Steps to measure BGL are as follows:

1 Check the expiry date of equipment.
2 Put on gloves.
3 Select an appropriate site (finger) and ask the client to stimulate their circulation by rubbing their finger.
4 Perform the finger puncture using a lancet.
5 Squeeze the finger to obtain a drop of blood.

6   Hold the puncture site over the reagent strip which has been placed in the glucometer and place the drop of blood onto the strip (see Figure 11.15).

7   Read the results after the designated time.

8   Wipe the client's finger with gauze.

9   Dispose of the equipment appropriately.

10   Perform hand hygiene.

11   Document the observations accurately on the correct observation chart.

12   Report all findings to an RN.

FIGURE 11.15 Measuring blood glucose level

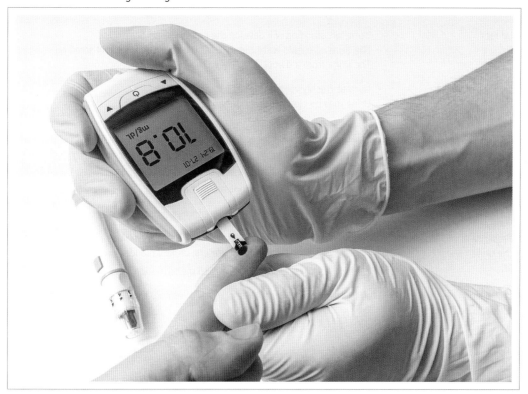

Source: iStock.com/vchal

Collect a urine, sputum or faecal specimen

Specimen collection is the process of obtaining tissue or fluids for analysis. This can carry a risk to staff, so infection control precautions are essential when undertaking these procedures. Check with the RN regarding the storage of specimens. Make sure that the pathology request form is attached, and that the specimen is labelled correctly with the person's details.

Urine

Urine consists of water, salts and urea. Urine is made in the kidneys then excreted through the urethra. The clinical data obtained from a urine specimen is influenced by the collection method, timing and handling. Checking the care plan can determine which of the following methods of collection is required:

* random specimen for analysis (urinalysis)
* 24-hour urine collection
* mid-stream urine (MSU) specimen for microscopic examination.

> **Specimen collection**
>
> The process of obtaining tissue or fluids for analysis; for example, urine for urinalysis, faeces for occult blood testing, or sputum for testing for pathogens.

Urinalysis

This is the physical, chemical and microscopic examination of urine. It involves assessing the urine for its physical appearance and using a reagent strip to test for various substances. Figure 11.16 outlines what the urine should be examined for *prior* to chemical testing. Figure 11.17 outlines some possible clinical abnormalities in urine.

FIGURE 11.16 Urine specimen examination prior to chemical testing

Colour	• Normal urine varies in colour from pale straw to amber • In addition, many compounds may affect the colour; e.g., food pigments, dyes, blood etc. • The colour of urine changes in many disease states
Odour	• Urine left standing will develop the smell of ammonia • The urine of clients with urinary tract infections may be foul smelling • The urine from a diabetic may have the fruity odour of acetone
Clarity (turbidity)	• Normal, freshly voided urine is usually clear • Urine may be cloudy due to urinary tract infections

FIGURE 11.17 Clinical abnormalities in urine

CLINICAL ABNORMALITY	POSSIBLE INDICATION
Presence of glucose in urine	May indicate diabetes
Turbid (cloudy) urine	May be a symptom of a bacterial infection
Presence of red blood cells (erythrocytes) in the urine	May be a sign that there is trauma in the urinary tract (kidneys, ureters, urinary bladder, prostate and urethra) Could be due to menstruation in women
White blood cells (leukocytes) found in addition to red blood cells	May be a signal of urinary tract infection

Guidelines for urinalysis

Equipment used for taking urinalysis includes:

- correct observation chart
- disposable gloves
- receptacle for urine
- reagent strip.

Steps when testing with a reagent strip:

1. Check the expiry date of the strip.
2. Avoid touching the reagent areas of strips.
3. Ensure the bottle cap is replaced tightly, immediately after removing the strip or tablet.
4. Put on gloves and fully submerge the reagent strip into the urine.
5. Wait for the required time and check the results (see Figure 11.18).
6. Record the results.
7. Report all findings to an RN.
8. Store reagents in a cool, dry area, away from sunlight, strong vapours, heat and moisture. Do not remove desiccant pack from bottle, if present.

FIGURE 11.18 Checking reagent strip

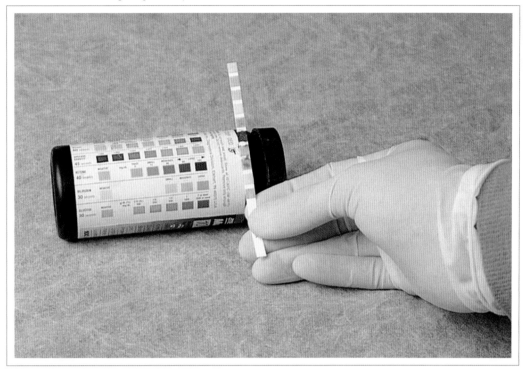

Source: From Hegner/Acello/Caldwell, 3P-EBK:NURSING ASSISTANT A NURSING PROCESS APPROACH, 11E. © 2016 Cengage.

24-hour urine collection

This is performed by collecting a person's urine in a special container over a 24-hour period. It always begins with an empty bladder so that the urine collected is not 'left over' from previous hours. This specimen shows the total amounts of waste the kidneys eliminate over the period.

The test does not require anything other than normal urination. Generally, the client will be given one or more containers to collect and store urine in over the 24-hour time period. Collection is usually commenced in the morning after the first void. The container should be kept refrigerated until collected.

Mid-stream urine sample

An MSU involves taking a 'mid' sample while the urine is being voided, and not taking the initial and end stages of the void. This reduces the risk of contamination from bacteria colonised around the end of the urethra as these bacteria are washed away with the initial urine flow. Always follow standard precautions by using hand hygiene and put on gloves if you are assisting the client with this procedure.

Most clients need education and advice on hygiene before the procedure to prevent contamination from their hands or the genital area. Uncircumcised men should be instructed to retract the foreskin before micturition, and women should be instructed to part the labia. Instruct the client to direct the first part of the urine into the toilet and collect the middle part in a sterile container. The remaining stream of urine can be passed into the toilet.

Faecal specimens

A faecal specimen can be examined for blood, parasites or microorganisms. Steps for taking the faecal specimen are as follows:

1 Provide a bedpan, and if the client wants to urinate first, offer a urinal for a male client or an extra bedpan for a female client. Avoid mixing urine or toilet paper into the sample.
2 Consider standard precautions – perform hand hygiene and wear gloves.
3 With the use of a tongue blade or scoop from the lid of the container, transfer a portion of faeces to the specimen container (see Figure 11.19).
4 Examination for parasites and microorganisms must be made while the stool is warm, so it is essential for the specimen to be sent directly to the laboratory.

FIGURE 11.19 Faecal specimen container

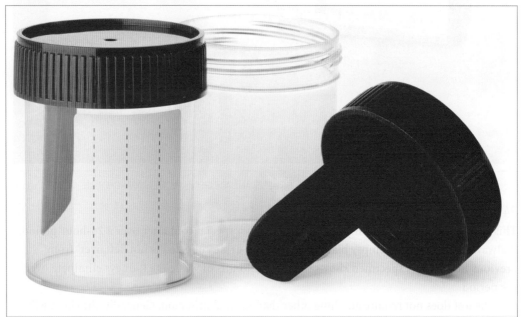

Source: Shutterstock.com / Fotofermer

The faecal occult blood test uses a reagent to detect the presence of occult blood, which is not visible. Follow the manufacturer's guidelines when undertaking this test.

Sputum collection

A sputum specimen is obtained for culture to determine the presence of pathogens. For best results, obtain the sample first thing in the morning before the client eats, brushes their teeth or uses mouthwash.

Steps for taking the sputum specimen are as follows:

1 Consider standard precautions – wear gloves and/or goggles.
2 Assist the client to a sitting position and ask them to cough deeply and spit into the container.
3 Offer the client a tissue to wipe their mouth.

4   Specimens are often taken for three consecutive days because it is difficult for the client to cough up enough sputum at one time, and an organism may be missed if only one culture is done.

5   Record the amount, consistency and colour of the sputum collected, as well as the time and date in the nursing notes.

Matching definitions

Complete the following table by placing each term's number next to the definition in the right-hand column.

11.8 ACTIVITY

1	Melaena	_____ protein in urine
2	Parasites	_____ coughing up blood
3	Polyuria	_____ blood in urine
4	Nocturia	_____ identifies chemical components in substances
5	Anuria	_____ ketones in urine
6	Haemoptysis	_____ substance that lubricates inner surfaces of body
7	Reagent strip	_____ voiding excessive amounts of urine
8	Mucus	_____ glucose in the urine
9	Haematuria	_____ passing urine several times during the night
10	Proteinuria	_____ dark, sticky faeces due to blood in gastrointestinal tract
11	Glycosuria	_____ an organism that lives off or in another organism
12	Ketonuria	_____ kidneys not producing urine

Measure and record weight

Changes in a client's weight can indicate their nutritional and fluid balance status. By taking a baseline weight, these changes can be determined. It is important to weigh the client at the same time of day and with the same type of clothing. Have the client empty their bladder or empty the catheter bag before weighing for an accurate measurement.

Guidelines to measure and record weight

Weighing scales are used to measure weight, and include bed, chair, upright or electronic scales. Steps to measure and record weight are as follows:

1   Assess the client's mobility and ability to weight-bear.
2   Calibrate the scales if required.
3   Place the client on the scales.
4   Ensure the client remains still while on the scales and read the results.
5   Return and clean the equipment appropriately.
6   Perform hand hygiene.
7   Record the results on the appropriate documents.
8   Report all findings to an RN.

Recognise changes in consciousness

You must be able to recognise changes in a client's condition, including their neurological status, which can change rapidly in the deteriorating client. Neurological assessment can detect these changes, including the level of consciousness, motor function, vital signs and pupil reaction.

The Glasgow Coma Scale (GCS) is a tool that is used to assess a patient's level of consciousness (see Figure 11.20), with a score of 15 indicating an alert and orientated person, and a score of < 8 indicating the person is comatose. Acute care facilities may use a combination of the GCS, pupil scale and limb strength when assessing neurological status.

Glasgow Coma Scale (GCS)

A tool that is used to assess a person's level of consciousness. A score of 15 indicates an alert and orientated person, whereas less than 8 indicates they are comatose.

FIGURE 11.20 Glasgow Coma Scale

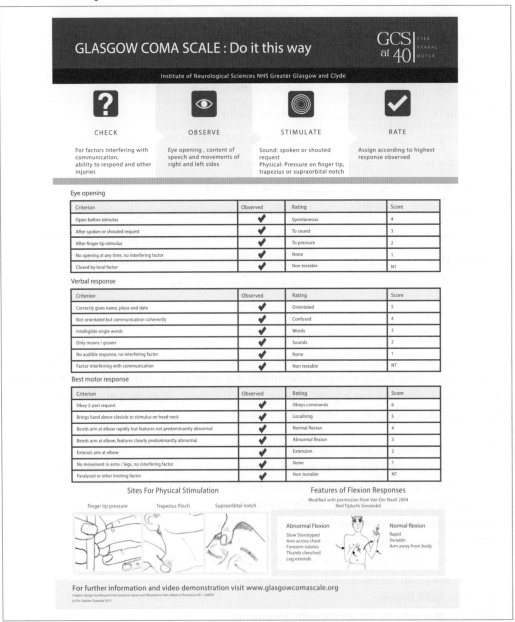

Source: http://www.glasgowcomascale.org/, © Sir Graham Teasdale

Speaking to the client will determine the level of eye opening or motor response. If there is no response, painful stimuli may need to be initiated. The accepted method is the trapezius squeeze, where the trapezius muscle on the upper and back part of the neck and shoulders is squeezed with the thumb and index finger. Check with your facility on the accepted method of painful stimuli.

Questioning the client on person, place and time will determine their awareness, their appropriateness of speech and their best motor response, as follows:

* What is your name?
* Where are you at the moment?
* What day is it today?
* Squeeze my hands.

Evaluating the pupils for size and reactivity will provide information about the brain and intracranial pressure. The size of the pupils should initially be determined before a penlight torch is directed from the outer aspect of the eye towards the pupil to check for reaction.

Guidelines to recognise changes in consciousness

Equipment required to evaluate changes in consciousness includes:

* neurological observation chart
* penlight torch.

    Steps to observe the level of consciousness are as follows:

1 Explain the procedure to the client and determine their comprehension.
2 Assess the patient's verbal response by asking relevant questions about person, place and time.
3 Assess and record:
    * eyes opening response
    * verbal response
    * motor response.
4 Assess and record limb (arm and leg) movement and strength – test right and left sides for power and movement.
5 Assess and record pupil size and reaction using a penlight torch and compare to scale:
    * Are both pupils the same size?
    * Is the reaction brisk or sluggish?
6 Calculate the score.
7 Return and clean all equipment appropriately and perform hand hygiene.
8 Record results in appropriate documents.
9 Report all findings to an RN

Document intake on food record charts

Food record charts play a useful role in the nutritional assessment of clients and inform dietitian treatment plans. They should be started in all situations where there is any concern that a client's nutritional intake might be inadequate. This may be when the body mass index (BMI) of the person is below the normal range, when they have had recent unintentional weight loss, or when they experience poor appetite or physical problems, such as difficulty swallowing.

Food record chart
Used to monitor and assess the nutritional intake of patients where there is concern about their nutrition. Helps to inform dietitian treatment plans.

When documenting food intake, it is important to wait until the client has finished their meal. You should record all intake consumed as accurately as possible, as shown in Figure 11.21. The number of portions and the amount eaten should be documented, as well as any refusal of food.

FIGURE 11.21 Sample food chart

BREAKFAST	MID-MORNING	LUNCH	MID-AFTERNOON	EVENING MEAL	SUPPER
½ bowl porridge Full cup orange juice	1 cup tea 2 × shortbread biscuits	Full bowl soup ½ portion of mince and potatoes Glass milk	Refused tea and biscuit	Refused main meal Ate 1 bowl high-protein custard ¾ glass of milk	½ cup tea 1 slice toast

Record intake on fluid balance charts

Fluid balance chart

Helps to accurately record fluid intake (i.e., oral and IV) and output (i.e., urine, vomitus and drainage).

Accurately recording fluid intake and output on a fluid balance chart is important when a client:

- is at risk of dehydration
- is receiving intravenous (IV) therapy
- has returned from surgery
- has a urinary catheter
- has a disease that requires monitoring of fluid balance; for example, renal failure, congestive heart failure.

Intake and output are calculated by recording the amounts of fluids the client takes in (i.e., oral, IV) and the fluids that the client excretes (i.e., urine, vomitus and drainage). You will need to measure all oral liquids and foods that melt at room temperature (e.g., ice cream), and record any fluids administered through gastric feeding. The RN or the EN will record the amount of IV fluids administered. It is important to learn the fluid content of containers used in your facility. Apply standard precautions and wear gloves when measuring output.

ACTIVITY 11.9

Fluid balance charting

Obtain a fluid balance chart from your workplace. On it, record the 24-hour period intake and output given in the following for an example patient. Determine a negative or positive fluid balance.

1 cup = 150 mL
1 bowl = 200 mL
1 glass = 150 mL

INTAKE	
0700: Breakfast	1 glass apple juice ½ cup tea
1000: Morning tea	1 cup tea Biscuit
1200: Lunch	Bowl of pumpkin soup Chicken and steamed vegetables

INTAKE	
1500: Afternoon tea	Refused liquids
1800: Dinner	½ cup tea Refused dinner
2000: Supper	1 cup of ice to suck

OUTPUT	
0600:	Passed urine × 550 mL
0700:	Vomited undigested breakfast × 200 mL
1200: Lunch	Passed urine 200 mL
1500: Afternoon	Diarrhoea – dark black × 300 mL
1800: Dinner	Passed urine 200 mL Vomited – blood stained × 50 mL

Application of anti-thrombosis stockings

Deep vein thrombosis (DVT) is a blood clot in the deep veins of the leg or groin and a potentially life-threatening complication that can affect any immobilised person. They can be painful and cause swelling in the leg below the clot. Complications can occur when the DVT breaks apart and travels into the blood vessels of the lung, causing pulmonary embolism. The clot blocks off the circulation and prevents oxygen from entering the bloodstream.

> **Embolism**
> The obstruction of a blood vessel by a foreign substance or a blood clot.

To prevent DVT and pulmonary embolism, clients in acute care are often prescribed anticoagulant medication and will also have elastic stockings on their legs. These stockings are called thromboembolic-deterrent stockings or 'TED stockings', and they work by compressing the leg in a graduated fashion to increase the return of blood up the leg veins. Clients are fitted for these calf- or thigh-length stockings to ensure the correct size and length.

Guidelines for application of anti-thrombosis (TED) stockings

Equipment used for the application of anti-thrombosis stockings includes:
- graduated compression stockings
- care plan with order.

Steps for the application of anti-thrombosis stockings are as follows:
1. Assess the relevant documentation and the medical order in relation to size and need to wear stockings.
2. Turn the stocking inside out.
3. Place the client's toes into the foot of stocking, ensuring the stocking is smooth.
4. Slide the remaining portion of the stocking over the client's foot (see Figure 11.22).
5. Ensure the client's foot fits into the toe and heel position.
6. Slide the stocking up over the client's calf until fully extended.
7. Ensure the sock is smooth and has no creases.
8. Assess the client for comfort and re-establish the environment.
9. Perform hand hygiene.
10. Record the application in the appropriate documents.

> **Anti-thrombosis (TED) stockings**
> Calf- or thigh-length elastic stockings that help prevent DVT and pulmonary embolism. Work by compressing the leg in a graduated fashion to increase the return of blood up the leg veins.

FIGURE 11.22 Application of TED stockings

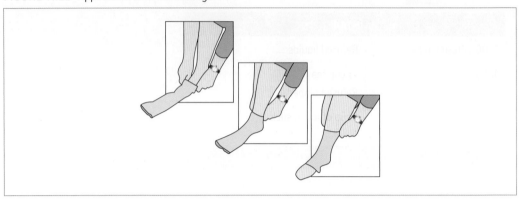

Assistance with breathing devices, under direct supervision

Incentive breathing devices, as shown in Figure 11.23, can help to expand the lungs and prevent potential lung complications. A physiotherapist will initially instruct the client on the correct use of the device and monitor the client for fatigue or dizziness.

FIGURE 11.23 Incentive breathing device

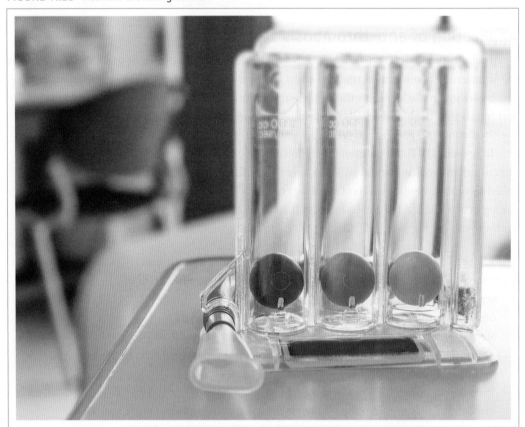

Source: Shutterstock.com/Mathisa

Aerosol therapy (nebulisers) can deliver medication deep into the lungs. Encourage the client to relax while therapy is being delivered. Afterwards, provide mouth care to the client.

Guidelines for assistance with breathing devices

Equipment used when assisting a patient to use a breathing device includes:

- gloves
- sputum cup
- tissues
- incentive breathing device.

    Steps to assist a patient to use a breathing device are as follows:

1 Identify the need for a breathing device by discussing the situation with a health professional and consulting the care plan.
2 Assess the need for pain relief prior to the procedure and report to an RN.
3 Encourage the client to sit or stand erect with their head up and back straight to promote optimal lung expansion.
4 Put on disposable gloves.
5 Instruct the client to take relaxed, normal-sized breaths.
6 Assist the client with the incentive breathing device as directed by the RN.
7 Provide a sputum cup and tissue if the client needs to expectorate.
8 Dispose of the equipment appropriately, wash the mouthpiece and perform hand hygiene.
9 Assess the client for comfort and re-establish the environment.
10 Record the procedure in the appropriate documents.
11 Report all findings to an RN.

Shallow wound care

Wounds occur for a variety of reasons and can be of different levels of severity. Acute wounds occur as a result of injury or surgical intervention; for example, surgical incisions, crushing wounds, shearing wounds and burns. Chronic wounds are the result of an existing condition which impairs the tissue's ability to maintain its integrity or to heal; for example, venous and arterial ulcers, diabetic ulcers and pressure ulcers. Wounds that are necrotic (black in colour) require intervention by the wound care consultant.

Wound healing occurs through primary intention where the wound edges are closed shortly after the primary wound has been created. This usually occurs within 24 to 48 hours to seal the wound from bacterial contamination. Secondary intention healing occurs through the formation of granulation tissue (without surgical intervention). Clean granulation tissue is red/pink in colour. Wound exudate (discharge) has been demonstrated to contain anti-microbial substances that offer protection; however, excessive exudate will macerate the surrounding skin (see Figure 11.24).

FIGURE 11.24 Some classifications of exudate

EXUDATE CLASSIFICATION	MEANING
Serous	Watery and comprised chiefly of serum; clear to slightly brown in colour
Purulent	Thicker due to pus that can have tinges of green or yellow
Sanguineous/haemorrhagic	Consists of large amounts of red blood cells and can be bright to dark red in colour
Haemoserous	Contains both watery serum and red blood cells

Infected wounds present with the following signs and symptoms:

- pus or drainage
- bad smell coming from the wound
- fever, chills
- hot to touch
- redness
- pain or sore to touch.

Wound care promotes healing by providing a warm, moist, non-toxic environment. It should assist the natural healing process and prevent infection. Wound dressings should protect the wound yet provide minimal discomfort.

Types of dressings

The wound care consultant or RN prescribes the most appropriate dressing for the client according to the wound. This is documented in the care plan and should be referred to when performing wound care. Some dressings are waterproof and can be left in place for up to seven days or changed when leakage occurs; others are interactive to promote more effective healing. Other types of dressings (see Figure 11.25) include:

- film dressings – these usually transparent dressings are non-absorbent and permeable and suitable for shallow, lightly exuding wounds or for covering intravenous cannulas
- foam dressings – are absorbent and suitable for heavy exudate. They can fill cavities; for example, pressure ulcers, sinuses
- gels – maintain a moist healing environment and are suitable for necrotic or sloughy wounds.

FIGURE 11.25 Film and foam dressings

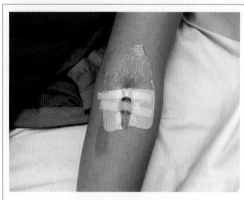
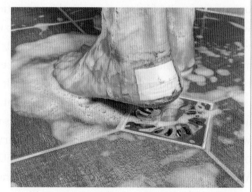

Source: iStock.com/Rosendo Serrano Valera

Source: iStock.com/rdonar

Guidelines for shallow wound care

Equipment used for shallow wound care includes:

- dressing trolley
- disposable gloves
- hand hygiene solution
- contaminated waste container
- dressing pack
- wound cleansing solution (e.g., saline)
- wound dressing.

Steps for shallow wound care are as follows:

1 Adhere to infection control policies and procedures – perform hand hygiene throughout the procedure.

2 Prepare the environment and equipment as stated in the care plan, with the following (if required):

   a   appropriate disposable sheet protector

   b   plastic bag for disposal of all soiled dressings

   c   dressing trolley, equipment, disposable gloves

   d   draw curtains for privacy.

3 Put on disposable gloves.

4 Remove the old dressing using non-touch technique and dispose of it appropriately.

5 Remove disposable gloves and perform hand hygiene.

6 Clean the wound with cleansing solution if required (new gloves are required if any contact is made with the wound).

7 Ensure aseptic technique is used to prevent contamination of the wound and wound care products.

8 Apply a clean dressing and secure it in place.

9 Dispose of equipment appropriately.

10 Assess the client for comfort and re-establish the environment.

11 Perform hand hygiene.

12 Record the procedure in the appropriate documents.

13 Report all findings to an RN.

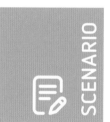

Wound management

Rose, 88 years old, has been living in an aged care facility for five years. She is classified as high care following a series of cerebral vascular accidents (CVA) that left her significantly debilitated. She requires full personal care including feeding, toileting and bathing. Over the years, Rose has suffered considerable weight loss, with a significant loss of adipose tissue, and the bony prominences of her body appear to be covered by a thin layer of skin only.

Rose has now suffered another mild CVA and has been admitted to hospital. She presents with shallow decubitus ulcers on both heels that require cleansing (no packing required).

1 What type of wound is a pressure ulcer?

2 What factors would affect the healing of Rose's ulcers?

3 What are the potential complications of pressure ulcers?

4 How would you position Rose safely for this procedure?

5 How would you relieve Rose's anxiety prior to the procedure?

6 When performing wound care, what observations need to be made?

2 SUPPORT THE CLIENT TO MEET PERSONAL CARE NEEDS IN AN ACUTE CARE ENVIRONMENT

Personal care is attending to the physical needs of clients who are unable to take care of themselves. In an acute care environment, these needs or activities of daily living (ADLs) include personal hygiene, mobility and transfer, continence and nutritional support. You must make every effort to encourage the client's independence in performing these activities and use the appropriate equipment while maintaining confidentiality and privacy. Encouragement not only maintains independence but also aids in maintaining dignity. It is important to report any difficulties when providing personal care because this will impact on the client's ongoing care.

Provide support to meet ADLs using appropriate equipment and aids according to the care plan and protocols

Your client may need your support in performing ADLs involving hygiene and self-care needs. These activities can be very personal, with each person having established practices and preferences as to how they perform their own care. Cultural and religious practices, level of activity and general health and mobility will also have an impact on these self-care practices.

Activities of daily living include:

- personal hygiene – showering or bathing, including bed-making; skin, hair and nail care; oral hygiene; and eye and ear care
- dressing
- eating and drinking
- toileting and continence
- application of a prosthesis
- mobility and transfer.

Showering or bathing

For most people, showering and bathing is an important part of their daily routine. Regular showering and bathing promotes hygiene and comfort, removes bacteria, prevents body odour, stimulates circulation and encourages movement of joints and muscles. Remember that each person will have individual preferences for morning or evening showering or bathing, and these preferences should be accommodated where possible. The level of assistance required with showering or bathing varies between individuals and may range from assisting with preparation only, offering prompts and minimal support, or total care. When giving care, you should use minimal touch at all times to ensure that the client's dignity, self-esteem and independence are maintained.

It is important to remember to:

- follow infection control guidelines
- follow all safety guidelines regarding water temperature, non-slip mats and brakes on commodes
- never leave a client alone unless it is safe to do so
- encourage independence
- not rush the client
- start with the face first and work down the body, leaving the genitals and buttocks till last, when performing a bed bath
- change the washcloths as required
- use the client's preferred cleansing products and if soap is used, rinse well to prevent drying of the skin
- wash all skin surfaces, including natural creases and crevices, when assisting with showering or bathing.

Bed-making

The main purpose of bed-making is to prevent complications by ensuring the comfort and security of the client. Important points to note when making a bed include the following:

- Raise the bed so that you do not have to bend during the procedure and can ensure good body alignment.
- Follow infection control measures, such as:
  - wash hands before and after bed-making
  - keep soiled linen away from your uniform
  - do not shake dirty linen
  - do not mix soiled and clean linen
  - clean soiled areas on mattress with a recommended cleansing agent.
- When making an occupied bed:
  - two staff members need to undertake the procedure to ensure safety
  - remove the pillow unless contraindicated
  - leave one cover over the client and maintain privacy by bedside screening
  - turn the patient on half of the bed and keep the side rails up
  - place a pillow between the client and the bed rail
  - work on the unoccupied side of the bed and roll the dirty sheet towards the client's back
  - place clean and dry linen on the mattress and roll towards the client's back
  - roll the patient to the clean side of the bed, remove the dirty linen and pull through the clean linen
  - replace the top sheet, blanket and quilt if required.
- Ensure the bed linen is free from wrinkles to prevent pressure injuries.
- Some clients may require an absorbent pad near the centre of the bed.

Skin care

When you are providing skin care, it is an opportunity to observe the client's skin condition for bruising, discolouration, texture and skin integrity. Report any abnormalities to the RN. Clients with ageing skin are also at risk of skin tears so it is important to protect their skin by avoiding friction, shearing or pulling the skin. Handle the person with care during transfers and use transfer aids where possible. Padded bed rails and sheepskin can protect the person from rubbing against hard surfaces.

Pressure injuries

Any client who suffers from immobility is at risk of developing a pressure injury. This is also called a pressure ulcer, pressure sore, bed sore or decubitus ulcer, and the unrelieved pressure can damage the underlying tissue by decreasing circulation to the area. Initial skin damage is represented by a reddened area that does not return to normal skin colour after pressure is relieved. In later stages the area looks like an abrasion or blister and can progress to a deep crater with damage to underlying tissue or muscle. Common sites for pressure ulcers are shown in Figure 11.26.

Pressure injury

Also known as a pressure ulcer, pressure sore, bed sore or decubitus ulcer; they are a risk for anyone who is immobile. Unrelieved pressure damages underlying tissue by decreasing circulation. Categorised from Stage I to Stage IV.

FIGURE 11.26 Common sites for pressure ulcers

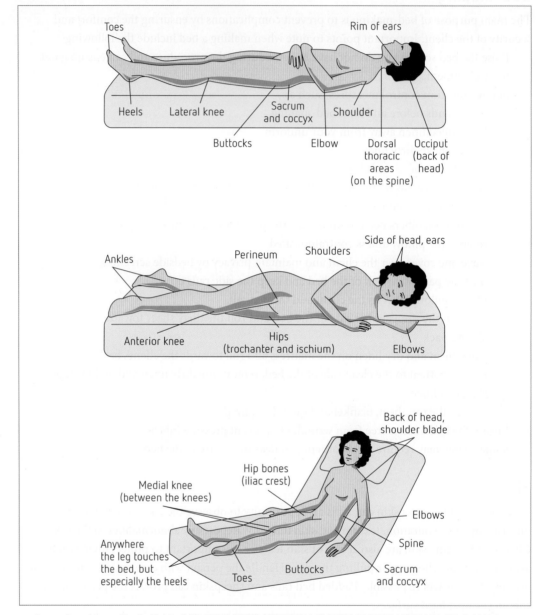

Source: From Hegner/Acello/Caldwell, 3P-EBK:NURSING ASSISTANT A NURSING PROCESS APPROACH, 11E. © 2016 Cengage.

Pressure injuries are categorised into four stages by the European Pressure Ulcer and National Pressure Injury Advisory Panel Classification System (EPUAP, NPUAP and PPPIA, 2021) depending on the level of tissue involvement or depth of the sore:

- Stage I – localised erythema (redness) of intact skin
- Stage II – partial thickness skin loss presenting as a shallow, open ulcer
- Stage III – full thickness skin loss with fat visible in ulcer. Dead tissue may be visible
- Stage IV – full thickness skin and tissue loss with exposed bone, muscle or tendon. Often includes tunnelling.
- Unstageable – Depth unknown because base of ulcer is obscured by exudate or dead (necrotic) tissue.

A risk assessment tool should be used to identify the degree of risk. Figure 11.27 shows the Waterlow pressure ulcer risk assessment tool as an example. When the degree of risk is identified, strategies need to be implemented to prevent breakdown; or if breakdown has occurred, to heal the wound and prevent recurrence. Strategies can include regular changes of position at least every two hours to provide alternative weight-bearing surfaces that relieve pressure, improve circulation and preserve muscle function. Other strategies include protecting the skin with padding or using pressure-relieving devices.

FIGURE 11.27 Waterlow pressure ulcer risk assessment tool

WATERLOW PRESSURE ULCER PREVENTION/TREATMENT POLICY
RING SCORES IN TABLE, ADD TOTAL. MORE THAN 1 SCORE/CATEGORY CAN BE USED

BUILD/WEIGHT FOR HEIGHT	◆	SKIN TYPE VISUAL RISK AREAS	◆	SEX AGE	◆	MALNUTRITION SCREENING TOOL (MST) (Nutrition Vol.15, No.6 1999 - Australia		
AVERAGE BMI = 20-24.9	0	HEALTHY	0	MALE	1	A - HAS PATIENT LOST WEIGHT RECENTLY	B - WEIGHT LOSS SCORE	
		TISSUE PAPER	1	FEMALE	2		0.5 - 5kg = 1	
ABOVE AVERAGE BMI = 25-29.9	1	DRY	1	14 - 49	1	YES - GO TO B	5 - 10kg = 2	
		OEDEMATOUS	1	50 - 64	2	NO - GO TO C	10 - 15kg = 3	
OBESE BMI > 30	2	CLAMMY, PYREXIA	1	65 - 74	3	UNSURE - GO TO C AND SCORE 2	> 15kg = 4	
		DISCOLOURED GRADE 1	2	75 - 80	4		unsure = 2	
BELOW AVERAGE BMI < 20	3	BROKEN/SPOTS GRADE 2-4	3	81 +	5	C - PATIENT EATING POORLY OR LACK OF APPETITE 'NO' = 0; 'YES' SCORE = 1	NUTRITION SCORE If > 2 refer for nutrition assessment / intervention	
BMI=Wt(Kg)/Ht (m)²								
CONTINENCE	◆	MOBILITY	◆	SPECIAL RISKS				
COMPLETE/ CATHETERISED	0	FULLY	0	TISSUE MALNUTRITION	◆	NEUROLOGICAL DEFICIT		◆
URINE INCONT.	1	RESTLESS/FIDGETY	1	TERMINAL CACHEXIA	8	DIABETES, MS, CVA		4-6
FAECAL INCONT.	2	APATHETIC	2	MULTIPLE ORGAN FAILURE	8	MOTOR/SENSORY		4-6
URINARY + FAECAL INCONTINENCE	3	RESTRICTED	3	SINGLE ORGAN FAILURE (RESP, RENAL, CARDIAC,)	5	PARAPLEGIA (MAX OF 6)		4-6
		BEDBOUND e.g. TRACTION	4					
SCORE		CHAIRBOUND e.g. WHEELCHAIR	5	PERIPHERAL VASCULAR DISEASE	5	MAJOR SURGERY or TRAUMA		
10+ AT RISK				ANAEMIA (Hb < 8)	2	ORTHOPAEDIC/SPINAL		5
15+ HIGH RISK				SMOKING	1	ON TABLE > 2 HR#		5
20+ VERY HIGH RISK						ON TABLE > 6 HR#		8
				MEDICATION - CYTOTOXICS, LONG TERM/HIGH DOSE STEROIDS, ANTI-INFLAMMATORY MAX OF 4				

Scores can be discounted after 48 hours provided patient is recovering normally

© J Waterlow 1985 Revised 2005*
Obtainable from the Nook, Stoke Road, Henlade TAUNTON TA3 5LX
* The 2005 revision incorporates the research undertaken by Queensland Health.

www.judy-waterlow.co.uk

Source: Waterlow, J. (2007) Waterlow score card – download. Retrieved from http://www.judy-waterlow.co.uk/the-waterlow-score-card.htm

Pressure-relieving devices

Pressure-relieving devices include special mattress types, such as egg crates, foam, water and gel. These reduce pressure at the 'at risk' sites by distributing an individual's weight more evenly. To be effective, however, all mattresses must be used as per the manufacturer's instructions. Pressure-relieving cushions can be used when the person is sitting in a chair, and other powered devices are available that provide relief on a cyclic basis.

Position the person

Positioning a client correctly maintains body alignment and prevents the complications of pressure ulcers, foot drop and contractures. Several positions should be used to provide comfort, support and good body alignment, with the common positions being:

- semi-upright – Fowlers
- back lying – supine
- side lying – lateral
- front lying – prone.

Pillows can support the client in bed by assisting them to sit up. Positioning a pillow next to the upright bed rails can support the client's back when they are lying on their side, and placing a pillow between the legs can prevent rubbing and pressure. Use the footboards at the base of the bed to help prevent foot drop, or place a folded pillow to support the client's feet to produce the same effect. To facilitate breathing in a client with dyspnoea, position by sitting them up and leaning them forward on an over-bed table, as shown in Figure 11.28. This orthopnoeic position helps to increase lung capacity and reduce the risk of lung congestion.

FIGURE 11.28 Orthopnoeic position

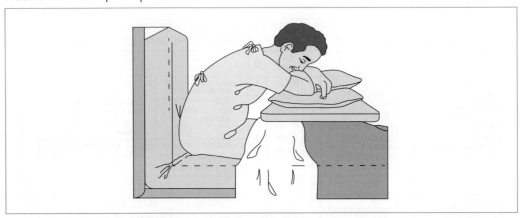

Shaving and hair care

Regular hair care includes brushing, combing and shampooing the hair of the scalp, and the management of facial hair; for example, daily facial shaving for men. Shaving is a personal preference and it is often difficult to shave the face of an elderly male client who has loose skin. Gently stretch the skin to provide a firm surface to manoeuvre the razor. Remember to shave in the direction that the hair is growing and to clean the equipment after the procedure. Check with your organisational policies or RN regarding equipment used in your facility.

A shampoo can be given in the bath, shower or bedside. Always ask the client about their usual hair care routine and preferred products and encourage independence where possible. When assisting with care, it is important to note the condition of the scalp and hair and check for abnormalities, which can be treated with medicated shampoo. Abnormalities include:
- dandruff – itching or flaking of the scalp
- seborrheic dermatitis – scaling and crusty patches on scalp
- pediculosis capitis – head lice.

Nail care

Nail care includes keeping the nails of both the hands and feet clean, shaped and trimmed. Individuals who are particularly prone to infection, such as diabetics, have their nails attended to by an RN or podiatrist. When undertaking care of the hands and feet, you have the chance to observe for health problems including fungal infections, ingrown toenails and poor circulation. Report all abnormalities to the RN and record it in the client's notes.

Oral hygiene

Poor oral hygiene can lead to discomfort, an unpleasant taste in the mouth and disease. If oral hygiene is neglected, further problems can occur including loss of appetite, the inability to eat, infections and low self-esteem. If your client has a sore mouth, it may be due to:

- oral infection or ulceration
- dental caries – holes in teeth
- cracked lips
- malnutrition
- medication
- ill-fitting dentures.

As an HSA, your role is to remind your client to brush their teeth or to help them to perform oral hygiene. This should be carried out after meals with the appropriate solution and a soft toothbrush. It is also a good opportunity to observe for any infection and note whether the mucous membrane in the mouth is intact.

Dentures should be cleaned daily. If you are performing denture care, wear gloves and clean the dentures in a basin that is lined with a washcloth to prevent accidental breakage. Cup dentures in your hand and brush and rinse thoroughly. Provide the client with a mouthwash and determine if cream or adhesive is required before replacing. If a client has ill-fitting dentures, report this to the RN as a new denture may need to be made. Chilled liquids can soothe a sore mouth and artificial saliva can be used if the client has a dry mouth.

Oral swabs are designed for individuals who have difficulty using a toothbrush or who are unconscious (see Figure 11.29). Position the client with their head to the side and chin slightly down, and if the swab is not pre-moistened use minimal amounts of solution. Lanoline or other moisturising treatment can be applied to the lips to reduce cracking.

FIGURE 11.29 Using an oral swab

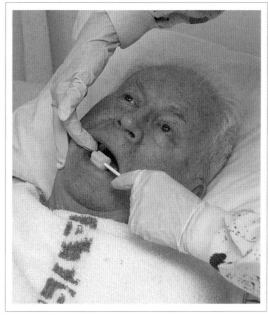

Source: From Hegner / Acello / Caldwell, 3P-EBK:NURSING ASSISTANT A NURSING PROCESS APPROACH, 11E. © 2016 Cengage.

Oral hygiene

Define the following terms that relate to poor oral hygiene:

TERM	DEFINITION
Halitosis	
Sordes	
Gingivitis	
Stomatitis	
Dental plaque	

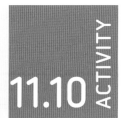

11.10 ACTIVITY

Eye and ear care

The eyes and ears are sensitive and require special attention for cleansing to avoid injury. Care of the eyes and ears is always done as part of the client's personal hygiene requirements.

Eye care

General cleansing of the eye area involves washing with a clean washcloth moistened with water. Do not use soap because it can possibly cause a burning sensation and irritation. When a person has an eye infection, lay the person on the infected side and, using gauze and normal saline, wipe from the inner to the outer canthus of the eye. Use new gauze each time you wipe the eye. Attend the non-infected eye first and never apply direct pressure over the eyeball.

For an unconscious patient, secretions may collect along the margins of the lid and inner canthus when the blink reflex is absent or when the eyes do not completely close. The doctor may order lubricating eye drops to be administered by the RN or EN and in some cases the eyes may be covered to prevent irritation and corneal drying.

Many clients wear glasses, which should be stored in a protective case when not in use. Warm water and a soft, dry cloth may be used for cleaning glasses lens. Plastic glasses require special cleaning solutions and drying tissues. Never place glasses lens side down on any surface.

Most clients prefer to care for their own contact lenses. If the client is unable to remove the lens, you should seek assistance from someone who is familiar with the procedure. The lens should not be reinserted until the client is capable of caring for the lens on their own. Prolonged wearing of contact lenses may cause serious damage to the cornea.

An artificial eye is usually cared for by the client. When assisting you should follow organisational policy, use standard precautions and handle the eye carefully. The eye socket and artificial eye must be cleaned according to the care plan.

When undertaking eye care it is necessary to:
* perform hand hygiene
* observe the eyes for redness, swelling, changes to the size of the pupils, and changes to the conjunctiva (white part of the eye)
* report any changes in vision to the RN.

Ear care

When cleaning the ears, use a clean corner of a moistened washcloth and rotate gently into the ear. A cotton-tipped applicator can be used for cleansing the pinna. Never use sharp objects or cotton-tipped applicators to clean the auditory canal because they may damage the tympanic membrane (eardrum) or cause wax (cerumen) to impact within the canal.

Hearing aids

Hearing loss is a common health problem among the elderly, and hearing aids assist in the ability to communicate and react appropriately in the environment. The care of hearing aids involves routine cleaning with a clean dry cloth, battery care, and proper insertion techniques. The hearing aid should be turned off when not in use to save the battery.

Depending on the type of hearing aid (an example is shown in Figure 11.30), cleaning should follow the manufacturer's instructions. Check with your facility regarding proper cleaning techniques.

FIGURE 11.30 Hearing aids

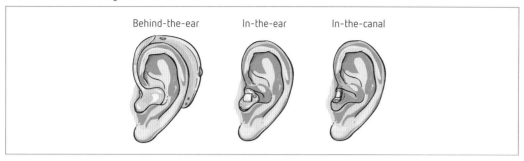

Behind-the-ear   In-the-ear   In-the-canal

Source: Shutterstock.com/corbac40

When reattaching the hearing aid, gently insert the small end of the hearing aid into the client's ear, following its natural contours. Do not pull on the ear, which would distort the shape of the ear canal. If the client has a behind-the-ear unit, make sure it is well anchored. Adjust the volume to suit the client's preference, and if a whistling sound is heard, turn the volume down.

Dressing

The type of clothing worn will differ according to the treatment and abilities of the person. In an acute care setting the client may be wearing a hospital gown. Many of these gowns offer back overlaps or, if not, two gowns can be used for client dignity. In a rehabilitation facility, a person will wear day clothes. It is important to consider cultural preferences when dressing a client.

Some clients will require your assistance with dressing and undressing while others may require minimal assistance (e.g., tying straps at the back of a gown). It is important to consider the condition of the client when assisting them to dress:

- if the client has weakness or paralysis – place the affected arm or leg in the garment first
- if the client has a cast or sling – leave the affected limb outside the clothing
- if the client has tubing in place – ensure that it is hanging freely and not kinked.

Eating and drinking

Some clients may require feeding due to weakness, paralysis, arm casts or confusion. It is important to do so in a relaxed manner so that the client does not feel rushed. Consult the nursing care plan, fluid balance and food charts so that you are aware of feeding requirements.

Before commencing feeding, prepare the client by considering their elimination needs, sitting them up and making sure that their bed table is at the correct height. Place the meal where the client can see and smell it in order to stimulate their appetite and make sure it is the right temperature. Other factors to consider when feeding a client include the following:

- Ask the client about the order in which they would like foods and fluids offered and if they want condiments added.
- Spoons are usually used, as there is less risk of injury. The spoon should be about one-third full because this portion is easily chewed and swallowed.
- Encourage the clients to feed themselves if possible to foster independence and help decrease feelings of helplessness. Family members could also be involved.
- Visually impaired clients require you to describe what you are feeding them. If they are able to feed themselves, describe the foods and fluids and their place on the plate/tray using the numbers of the clock (see Figure 11.31).

- Meals should be a time of social interaction. Sit so that you face the client – this allows you to converse and observe any difficulties swallowing, and conveys that you have time to relax.
- On completion, provide mouth care.

FIGURE 11.31 Describing food's place on the plate using clock numbers

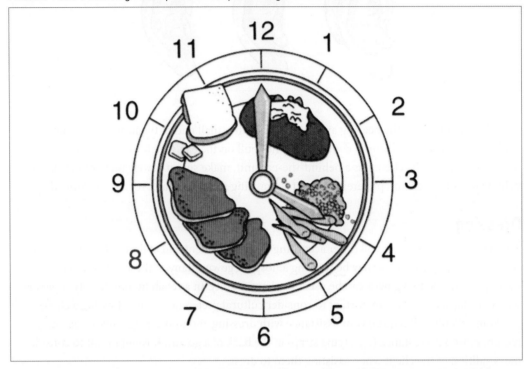

Source: From Hegner/Acello/Caldwell, 3P-EBK:NURSING ASSISTANT A NURSING PROCESS APPROACH, 11E. © 2016 Cengage.

Tube feeding

Clients who are unable to eat or drink fluids may require tube feeding. Tubes can be inserted either through the nasal passageway (nasogastric tube) or surgically/endoscopically inserted into the stomach (i.e., gastrostomy or PEG tube). Blended fluids are passed through the tube to meet nutritional needs. Your involvement will depend on the organisation's policies and procedures. Responsibilities may include observing skin integrity around the tube, preparing feeds, observing the client for any adverse effects, or recording intake in the fluid balance chart.

ACTIVITY 11.11

Therapeutic diets

Complete the following table by describing the rationales for use in an acute care setting.

TYPE OF DIET	EXAMPLE	RATIONALE
Nutrient diets	High fibre	
	High protein	
	Low salt	
	Low kilojoule	
	Low fat	

TYPE OF DIET	EXAMPLE	RATIONALE
Change in consistency	Liquid	
	Thickened fluids	
	Pureed	
	Soft	
	Light	
	Full	
Specific diets	Diabetic	
	Gluten free	

Therapeutic diets

Specific diets may be ordered by a dietitian to improve or maintain the nutrition of hospitalised clients. These are documented in the care plan so that the healthcare team is aware of the specific dietary requirements of the client.

Toileting

You must be aware of the normal patterns of urination and bowel movements for your clients and report any changes to the RN. It is also important to encourage continence in every instance.

Several types of equipment are used when toileting a person:

- Commodes – used for clients with limited mobility; they are a portable chair with an opening that can be placed over a toilet or that can accommodate a pan.
- Bedpans (see Figure 11.32) and urinals – used when clients cannot get out of bed. Males use a bedpan for bowel movements and a urinal for urination.
- A thin bedpan or 'slipper' pan – used for clients who have limited range of motion in their back.

FIGURE 11.32 Bedpan

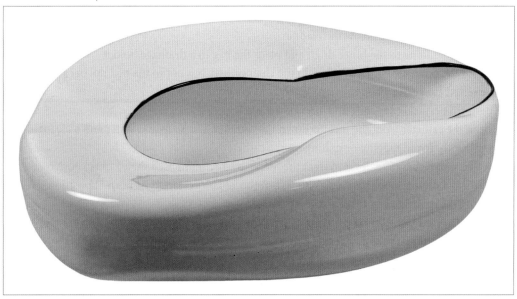

Source: Shutterstock.com/Dani Simmonds

Make sure that clients have easy access to a toilet and have facilities to wash their hands afterwards, and always maintain privacy and dignity.

Bowel care

Normally, faeces are passed easily and without pain or discomfort. They are brown in colour, and formed and excreted in amounts that will vary with each individual. If there are any differences to this, report to the RN and record it in the client notes. To promote regular elimination, the diet should be high in fibre with adequate fluids.

Continence and elimination aids

Normally, urine has a slight odour, is clear and is straw coloured. If the client has difficulty or pain when passing urine or if it is foul smelling, report to the RN and record it in the client notes.

Some clients may have continence problems which may include:

- stress incontinence – loss of urine when the client sneezes, coughs or laughs
- urge incontinence – they experience an urge to go the toilet and must go straight away
- overflow incontinence – loss of urine (dribbling) when the bladder is too full.

Care for these clients includes a continence program that can be facilitated by a consultant nurse. The plan may be in the form of a regular toileting regimen or there are a range of absorbent pads to protect the skin and clothing. It is important for you to check when these pads need to be changed and to ensure that wet clothing is removed, and that the skin is washed and dried to prevent excoriation.

Pelvic floor exercises are isometric exercises whereby the client squeezes and lifts and then relaxes the muscles surrounding the entrances of the vagina, urethra (women) and anus (women and men). This can help with urinary incontinence by strengthening the pelvic floor muscles.

Catheter care

In some instances, an indwelling catheter and drainage device will be required. A catheter can be used before, during and after surgery to drain the bladder, to allow hourly urine drainage when accurate measurement is required, or it may be used as a last resort in incontinence.

When caring for a client with a catheter it is important to:

- check for kinks and leaks
- prevent the client lying on the tubing
- keep the drainage bag below the bladder
- secure the tubing to the inner thigh and place the bag in a drainage holder
- attach the drainage holder and bag to the chair or bed, but not to the bed rail because it may be raised above the bladder when the bed rail is raised
- perform perineal care daily and after bowel movements
- clean the catheter from the meatus down the catheter. Use soap and water and a clean washcloth. Avoid tugging or pulling on the catheter
- separate the labia (female) or retract the foreskin (uncircumcised male); check for crusts, abnormal drainage or secretions; and return the labia/foreskin to its normal position
- empty the drainage bag at regular intervals
- adhere to infection control principles by performing hand hygiene and putting on gloves. Place a jug under the drainage bag and release the valve/clamp to measure the urine. Report and record the results
- report any complaints of burning, urgency, odour or cloudy urine to the RN.

Incontinence
Any accidental or involuntary loss of urine from the bladder or faeces from the bowel.

Pelvic floor exercises
Isometric exercises to strengthen the muscles around your bladder, bottom, and vagina or penis.

Uridomes are used for incontinent males. This rubber sheath slides over the penis and connects to a catheter bag. A new uridome should be applied daily or as required (see Figure 11.33).

FIGURE 11.33 A disposable uridome condom catheter

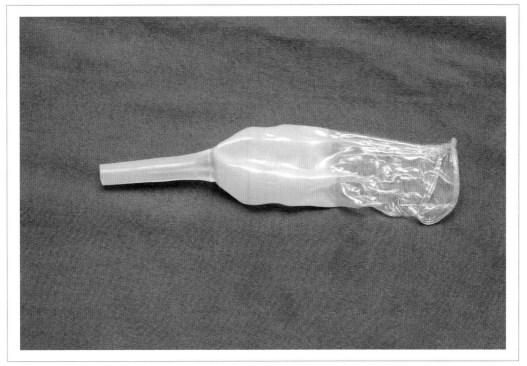

Source: Science Photo Library/Dr P. Marazzi

Ostomy care

An *ostomy* is a surgical opening in the abdomen that collects discharge from the bowel (colostomy) or bladder (urostomy). The client wears a plastic pouch that is attached to the abdominal site and changed or emptied when approximately one-third to half full.

When a new pouch is needed, use standard precautions and assist the client to clean with soap and water before reattaching a new pouch. Each individual may have different appliances and needs, depending on the type of ostomy. It is important to be guided by the RN, ostomy consultant or scope of practice when caring for these clients.

Application of prostheses

Prostheses are artificial devices that replace part or all of a missing extremity (see Figure 11.34). Fitting of a prosthesis is done once the stump is healed and well shaped and is performed by a prosthetist. If your client has a prosthesis, always check the care plan for special instructions for application, removal and care. It is important to remember:

- that the skin under the prosthesis must be kept dry and clean
- to check the skin for ulcers, redness, irritation or blisters
- a stump sock is used to cover the extremity under the prosthesis and protect it from irritation, and this should be washed regularly
- that clients who experience difficulties with the prosthesis should be referred to a specialist for modification.

FIGURE 11.34 Prosthesis

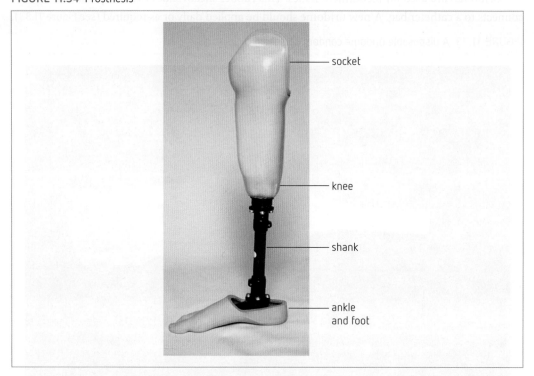

socket

knee

shank

ankle and foot

Source: Alamy Stock Photo / Image Source Plus

Mobility and transfer

It is important for you to use safe manual handling techniques and appropriate equipment to avoid client injuries, such as skin tears or dislocations, and to avoid injuries to yourself. Communicating during the procedure ensures a smooth and coordinated approach for both yourself and the client. Adhering to good body mechanics and undertaking a risk assessment prior to mobilising or transferring a client will maintain maximum comfort and safety. Chapters 8 ('Assist with movement') and 9 ('Transport individuals') outline the procedures for client mobility and transportation.

Report to an RN regarding difficulties in providing client support and assistance

Supporting and assisting a client with illness can be challenging, both physically and emotionally. Clients with cognitive, language or physical barriers can prove difficult if you are unsure of the strategies available to aid you while you provide support.

If you are caring for someone with a cognitive impairment, it is important to understand that if their behaviour changes, it may be due to circumstances outside of their control; for example, they may have a painful urinary tract infection. Aggression, anxiety and confusion can make it difficult for you to undertake the nursing tasks required.

Language barriers make it difficult for the client to understand directions; therefore, non-verbal communication or interpreters may be required. Physical barriers include hearing, visual or mobility limitations, and you must be considerate of the needs of these people. While it is important to be clear in any instructions you give, and to assist the client at every stage of the activity, sometimes you will be unable to provide the support required.

Examples of difficulties in providing support and assistance include:

- performing neurological observations on a confused client
- discussing meal options with a client with hearing or visual impairments
- taking blood pressure on a client with limb injuries or IV tubing
- positioning or bathing a client with contractures
- taking the pulse rate on an elderly client with a weak pulse
- completing the fluid balance chart on a client with incontinence.

When you are unable to support the client, you must report to the RN so that the client's care is not compromised. Report difficulties in an objective manner – not what you *think* and *feel* about a situation. By reporting difficulties, you are carrying out your duty of care and enabling the RN to change the care plan if needed.

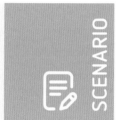

Reporting difficulties for Mr Simbeda

Jocelyn, an HSA, is looking after Mr Simbeda, aged 84 years, who has had bilateral knee replacements. His nursing care plan states that he is to walk with the aid of a frame, but he refuses to use one. You explain the importance of using this support aid for mobilisation and how it provides safety in the event of falls, but Mr Simbeda indicates that he is confident walking unaided. You inform him that you need to obtain advice from the RN. In this way a reassessment may be made to contribute to the changing needs of the client.

1   What are the predisposing factors for Mr Simbeda that make him a falls risk?
2   What alternatives could be used if Mr Simbeda continues to refuse the frame as a support aid?

Provide information to clients to help them meet personal care needs while maintaining confidentiality, privacy and dignity

You must be aware of the need to support and encourage the patient's independence in performing activities. However, clients have the right to make decisions that may include the acceptance of personal risk. This dignity of risk refers to an individual's right to take part in an activity that may entail some element of risk but that has benefits that might include gaining greater self-esteem and independence. Give the client all the information required about the care, procedure or self-care task, and encourage them to use their own abilities and skills whenever possible. Be clear about what the nature of the support is that you are providing and upon which the person is relying. This ensures that you maintain a balance between your duty of care and encouraging the patient to be independent. Make sure that all reasonable care is taken to ensure that the care does not harm or damage the person in any way. Knowing your work–role boundaries, responsibilities and limitations will ensure that you do not undertake tasks that are outside your scope of practice.

> **Dignity of risk**
> A person's right to make their own choices and decisions, even when those decisions could put them at risk, with benefits that might include gaining greater self-esteem and independence.

While allowing clients to maintain their independence and fulfil personal preferences, it is essential that their own safety and the safety of others are taken into consideration. You will need to make sure that wherever the person engages in monitoring their care needs, it is safe for them and the worker. Adhering to work health and safety guidelines, including manual handling and infection control principles, is paramount when you or the client are undertaking tasks.

You also have a responsibility to provide appropriate care in a professional manner to preserve the client's privacy and dignity. Examples include not exposing more of a person than is necessary during a shower and closing the curtains when performing invasive procedures. Confidentiality is maintained by not discussing any information of a personal or sensitive nature where others will overhear the conversation.

ACTIVITY 11.12

Confidentiality, privacy and dignity

Circle true or false for the following statements regarding confidentiality, privacy and dignity:

Discussing a client's nursing care with friends is acceptable at a weekend barbecue	True/false
It is appropriate to leave the curtains open while performing wound care on a person's sacrum	True/false
Every client has the right to respectful care, including consideration of their religious beliefs	True/false
Posting comments on social media about a famous person who is in your care is a breach of confidentiality	True/false
Continuity of care is maintained by discussing care of a client with the physiotherapist during handover	True/false
Informing the client's advocate about the tests that have been ordered for their condition is appropriate	True/false
HSAs have a moral and legal obligation to ensure the safety and wellbeing of others	True/false
You are not overstepping your work–role boundaries if you revisit a client when you are off duty or out of uniform	True/false

3   WORK IN A TEAM ENVIRONMENT

Working effectively in a team environment is fundamental. It requires you to develop skills in effective communication, collaboration, time management and knowledge-sharing. Effective communication requires accurate and efficient reporting of clinical data to the healthcare team and ensures that all members know what is required. Collaboration with others allows problem-solving, and effective time management allows for priorities and schedules to be determined so that the team works smoothly.

Working with a diverse group of people presents many challenges, and learning to work together effectively in a team environment enables everyone involved to achieve their professional and client-centred goals.

Work with colleagues, with consideration of team and group dynamics

Group dynamics
The processes involved when people in a group interact.

Group dynamics are the interpersonal processes that take place in groups. In nursing, groups or teams are consistently the same people with a relevant, shared purpose, common performance goals, complementary and overlapping skills, and a common approach to client care. Most nurses work in groups and are continually interacting with colleagues, clients and the community, so knowledge of group processes is important to facilitate group discussions and to enhance group effectiveness.

The nurse manager is responsible for influencing the group and can act as a facilitator in directing the group to reach goals and work cohesively. The manager's role in group dynamics includes:

- leading by inspiring and motivating staff
- clarifying the roles, responsibilities and accountabilities of team members
- forming effective groups that incorporate HSAs into the acute care clinical skill mix
- collaborating with the team in determining quality improvements that could lead to changes in the delivery of care and client care outcomes
- meeting regularly to share information effectively
- evaluating progress.

It is important to recognise that encouraging open communication with respect for each other and developing team members' ability to constructively discuss differences are important in strengthening group dynamics.

Nursing teams

Nursing care delivered to clients by a team of health workers can include RNs, ENs and HSAs. There is no ideal configuration for these teams because they need to be flexible and responsive to the needs of the client and the healthcare system.

These teams are intended to maximise the skills of all team members, prevent duplication of service delivery and enhance productivity in the workplace. As an HSA, you may be required to undertake specific tasks across a group of clients or work with your healthcare team to perform activities according to your skill level. Total client care involves undertaking all aspects of care for the client and is performed by the entire healthcare team.

Teamwork self-assessment

Complete the following self-assessment by circling the best response for the team in your workplace:

1 How would you rate your team?

2 What strategies could you use to improve the teamwork in your workplace?

WITH REGARD TO OUR TEAM	1	2	3	4	5
	STRONGLY AGREE	AGREE	NEUTRAL	DISAGREE	STRONGLY DISAGREE
1 We support each other	1	2	3	4	5
2 We trust one another	1	2	3	4	5
3 We enjoy working together	1	2	3	4	5
4 Everyone feels accepted	1	2	3	4	5

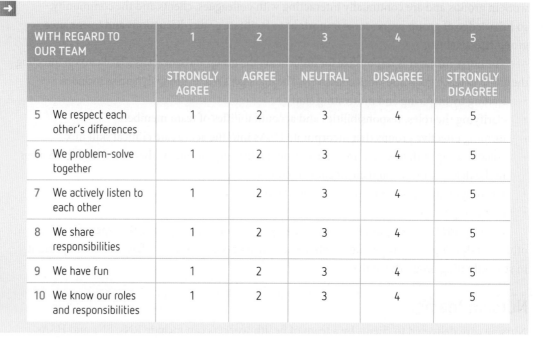

WITH REGARD TO OUR TEAM	1	2	3	4	5
	STRONGLY AGREE	AGREE	NEUTRAL	DISAGREE	STRONGLY DISAGREE
5 We respect each other's differences	1	2	3	4	5
6 We problem-solve together	1	2	3	4	5
7 We actively listen to each other	1	2	3	4	5
8 We share responsibilities	1	2	3	4	5
9 We have fun	1	2	3	4	5
10 We know our roles and responsibilities	1	2	3	4	5

Report clinical data accurately and in a timely fashion to colleagues in the healthcare team

When results or findings are abnormal or deviate from previous results, there is a need to validate and report findings immediately. When validating results, you should:

- visually and verbally assess the client
- check with baseline observations
- check equipment for reliability
- repeat investigations
- report to the RN.

Reporting data accurately and efficiently is a professional responsibility. Accurate and timely documentation ensures that information is available to all members of the healthcare team and contributes to enhancing efficient, individualised client care. Continuity of care and the pursuit of common objectives depend upon the accurate and precise reporting and recording of information.

SCENARIO

The importance of reporting clinical data

Theo Blair is 62 years old and presented to the accident and emergency centre with a headache that would not go away. A week ago, he was changing a light globe and fell off the chair and struck his head on the table. Mr Blair thinks the headache started either at that time or shortly after. Mr Blair has a past history of mild hypertension, which is controlled by medications. He stated that he hasn't been sleeping well.

Mr Blair described his headache as continuous, all over his head, extending into his posterior neck muscles, which were tight. The HSA took neurological observations, which were normal, and

→

Mr Blair did not have any nausea. He was given pain-relieving medication by the RN and admitted for observation. The HSA took his vital signs and reported to the RN that Mr Blair had hypertension – 140/90 and tachycardia – 102 bpm.

The next day, Mr Blair's appearance and manner had changed markedly. He seemed drowsy, and his headache was worse. He described it as a throbbing pain that increased if he lay down, pressed against his head or flexed his neck. His vision was still normal. Although he was not vomiting, he did not want to eat. When obtaining clinical data, the HSA noted that Mr Blair had no fever; however, his blood pressure was 165/95, up from 140/90 the day before. His skull remained tender to the touch. His neurological observations indicated that his level of consciousness appeared to be altered. The HSA reported this data immediately to the RN.

This change in condition alerted the healthcare team and the doctor sent Mr Blair for a CT scan of the head and a series of blood tests. The radiologist reported that the CT scan showed a large subdural haematoma. Further testing revealed raised intracranial pressure.

Mr Blair was taken to theatre to release the pressure in his skull from the subdural haematoma. Mr Blair recovered well post-operatively and was discharged later that week. The importance of efficiently reporting changes in Mr Blair's condition and accurately recording the altered clinical data had ensured that the appropriate treatment was given to Mr Blair before further complications could arise.

1   Why is it important to report objective rather than subjective data?
2   Why was it important to report the changes in Mr Blair's condition immediately to the RN?
3   How did the HSA demonstrate the scope of their role in the care of Mr Blair?

4   WORK EFFECTIVELY UNDER SUPERVISION

Supervision can vary in terms of what it covers. It may incorporate direction, guidance, observation, teamwork, exchange of ideas and coordination of activities. It may be direct or indirect according to the nature of the work being delegated. Supervision plays a key role in providing support to the individual by validating their work, providing clarity regarding roles and expectations, providing feedback on performance tasks and quality of care, and opportunities for reflection. As an HSA, you may be supervised by an EN or RN and should always seek clarification from them if unsure when carrying out nursing care.

Carry out work instructions within agreed timeframe and seek clarification to complete work instructions

When working in a team, the need to communicate clear instructions in both written and verbal forms is critical. From time to time the instructions that you need to follow may not be clear and you may have some concerns about what action to take. If at any time you do not understand an instruction, you need to ask the speaker to repeat or clarify the information in the instruction or ask questions of that person to gain clarity. If you choose to seek clarification from another staff member, it is very important that the person you ask is in a position to give you accurate information.

It is extremely important to clarify any unclear instructions because the health and safety of patients may depend on their implementation. By not clarifying instructions so that you understand them, you may breach your duty of care, responsibilities and obligations.

Some examples of clarification-seeking questions are:

- 'I'm not quite sure I understand what you are saying.'
- 'I don't feel clear about the task I have to perform here.'
- 'When you said ... what did you mean?'
- 'Could you repeat that again for me please?'

Sometimes, it is the written policy or procedure itself that is not clear, in which case it is your responsibility to report your concern about the lack of clarity in the instruction. It is important for you to be committed to giving ongoing feedback to the RN about these and other issues so that policies and procedures can be reviewed and changed as necessary.

Refer any difficulties experienced carrying out work instructions to an RN

At times you may experience difficulties carrying out work instructions (either verbal or written) due to:

- lack of physical resources
- insufficient training – for example, using new equipment
- uncertainty about what action to take – for example, doing a new task
- conflict with your personal philosophy/belief system.

By seeking advice and referring these difficulties to the RN, the best outcome can be achieved for the client and yourself. As an employee, you need to support the organisation's policies by following its procedures and sticking within the limits of your roles and responsibilities when carrying out work instructions.

Always try to:

- be mindful of your job description and scope of practice, and focus on completing tasks that are clearly defined as your responsibility
- be honest and direct when discussing your difficulties so that positive outcomes can be achieved.

ACTIVITY 11.14

Referring difficulties

Identify the actions that you should take as an HSA in the following situations:

1. The EN asks you to help with a lift and states that there is no need to use a lifting device.
2. The client's relatives become argumentative when you are trying to reposition the client in the bed.
3. You do not understand your work limitations when working in the radiology ward.
4. You notice that your co-worker does not perform hand hygiene when attending a client's dressing.

SUMMARY

The essential core of practice for you, as an HSA, is to deliver client-focused care under the supervision of a registered professional. By using the nursing processes of assessment, planning, intervention and evaluation, the quality of client care is ensured. This chapter emphasised these processes and the procedures used to provide optimum client care, including determining client needs and preferences and using assessment tools to collect data. The procedures and activities used to collect information and techniques used to support a client with activities of daily living were also highlighted, along with the safe use of equipment required for this support.

The last part of the chapter outlined the importance of providing clear instructions to clients when undertaking procedures, while maintaining confidentiality, privacy and dignity. The significance of reporting accurate data and relevant information to the team, including changes in the client's condition so that amendments could be made to the care plan, was emphasised. By working effectively as a team member, holistic care can be delivered to the client and effective outcomes can be achieved.

APPLY YOUR KNOWLEDGE

Acute care observations

Samuel, aged 57 years, is admitted to your ward for a partial bowel resection following the detection of colon cancer. Pre-operative observations need to be recorded and as the HSA looking after Samuel, you are required to take his blood pressure, temperature, pulse, respirations and oxygen saturations and report any deviations.

1 What are the normal readings for Samuel's blood pressure, temperature, pulse, respirations and oxygen saturations?

2 What situations could affect the normal readings for temperature and pulse?

The following day, Samuel undergoes the resection with no complications, although he feels nauseous. You are assigned on the morning shift and are looking after him post-operatively. He has an IV for fluids and pain relief, an IDC on hourly measures, and a wound with a transparent dressing and drainage system which has drained 200 mL. He has oxygen therapy at 6 L/min and is on hourly observations. You are required to record his intake and output on a fluid balance chart.

3 What fluids are measured for Samuel's intake and output on the fluid balance chart?

4 Using the knowledge you gained in Chapter 7, 'Organise personal work priorities and development', how would you prioritise your workload to ensure tasks for Samuel are completed?

5 Providing personal care to Samuel includes catheter care. What are the important considerations when caring for a patient with an indwelling catheter?

Samuel is prescribed TED stockings post-operatively by the surgeon and his wound site is to remain intact. He has not complained of excessive pain and appears to be progressing well, and you inform him that his wife will be coming in to visit later in the afternoon.

6 What are TED stockings and what is their purpose?

7 Understanding the HSA scope of practice is essential when caring for acute patients. How did the HSA demonstrate the scope of their role in this case study?

Samuel is discharged five days later. He is given instructions on his diet and medications and told to avoid strenuous activities, but with walking each day recommended.

◄ REFLECTING ON THE INDUSTRY INSIGHT 💬

1 Why was Mrs Korda told to shower on the morning of her surgery?
   a To allow the Betadine skin preparation solution to adhere to the skin more effectively.
   b For the staff to identify any skin conditions pre-operatively.
   c To minimise the risk of infection.
   d Because moist skin assists with the surgical procedure.

2 What physical signs indicated Mrs Korda's anxiety pre-operatively?
   a Hypotension, tachycardia and arrhythmia.
   b Hypertension, tachypnoea and diaphoresis.
   c Bradycardia, hypertension and pyrexia.
   d Arrhythmia, tachycardia and hypoglycaemia.

3 Why were two identification bands placed on Mrs Korda pre-operatively?
   a Two patient identifiers improve the reliability of the patient identification process.
   b Each band holds different information that in combination provides all necessary patient data.
   c Illegible information on one band can be clarified on the other.
   d One band needs to be removed during the operation.

SELF-CHECK QUESTIONS

1 Describe each stage of the nursing process.
2 What is the difference between actual and potential problems?
3 What are integrated progress notes?
4 Explain how orthostatic blood pressure is measured.
5 Explain the reasons why a patient may be required to use an incentive breathing device and who is responsible for instructing in its use.
6 List the factors that may influence an individual's ability to maintain personal hygiene independently.
7 What conditions might a client have that requires them to have their nails attended to by a podiatrist?
8 What is the HSA's responsibility when validating results?
9 What are some potential difficulties faced by an HSA in carrying out work instructions?
10 What are your definitions of the following key words and terms that have been used in this chapter?

KEY WORD OR TERM	YOUR DEFINITION
Nursing history	
Discharge planning	

KEY WORD OR TERM	YOUR DEFINITION
Informed consent	
Systolic	
Diastolic	
Embolism	
Diarrhoea	
Group dynamics	
Prosthesis	
Clarification	

QUESTIONS FOR DISCUSSION

1   Person-centred practice is crucial in reducing functional decline in older people in hospital. Discuss what this means and how the HSA can implement strategies to lead to better outcomes for these individuals.

2   Discuss the ways in which clinical pathways can reduce the variance of care for a post-operative patient

3   Discuss the importance of taking a 'mid stream' sample of urine and the standard precautions used in its collection.

4   Discuss the care of an unconscious client under the following headings:
    a   positioning
    b   skin
    c   mouth care
    d   eye care
    e   nutritional needs
    f   elimination needs.

5   Discuss how positive group dynamics can play an important role in working effectively in an acute care team environment

EXTENSION ACTIVITY

Planning care

Raymond Nguyen, 74 years of age, has been admitted to your ward with a diagnosis of pneumonia. He appears anxious and weak and is using his accessory muscles to breathe. He has limited English and has his son with him for support. His observations are:

Temperature	38.9°C
Pulse	132 bpm
Respirations	38 breaths per minute
Blood pressure	125/80 mmHg

1   Document these observations on a 'between the flags' chart and identify which readings are outside normal limits. From the case history, prepare a nursing care plan for Mr Nguyen.

2   Identify Mr Nguyen's actual and potential problems.

3   Identify the personal support assistance that Mr Nguyen may require.

4   Plan the goals in response to the identified problems and needs.

5   Document the nursing care needed to achieve the goals identified.

6   How would you decide whether the nursing care has achieved the goals identified?

7   Raymond is required to provide a sputum specimen. What equipment and standard precautions do you need to consider?

8   Team up with your colleagues and practise the following:
    a   positioning a patient to optimise their breathing
    b   performing deep breathing and coughing exercises in order to collect a sputum specimen
    c   giving oral handover for Mr Nguyen, with your colleagues taking handover notes.

REFERENCES

Clinical Excellence Commission (2016). Between the flags, keeping clients safe. Retrieved 28 May 2016 from http://www.cec.health.nsw.gov.au/programs/between-the-flags

European Pressure Ulcer Advisory Panel (EPUAP), National Pressure Ulcer Advisory Panel (NPUAP) and Pan Pacific Pressure Injury Alliance (PPPIA) (2021). Prevention and treatment of pressure ulcers. Retrieved 17 October 2022 from https://clinicalexcellence.qld.gov.au/resources/pressure-injury-guidelines

NSW Health (2019). Assistants in nursing working in the acute care environment. Retrieved 17 October 2022 from https://www.health.nsw.gov.au/workforce/Publications/ain-acute-care.pdf

RESPOND EFFECTIVELY TO BEHAVIOURS OF CONCERN

Learning objectives

By the end of this chapter, you should be able to:

1 identify behaviours of concern in line with your work role and plan appropriate responses

2 apply appropriate response in line with organisation policies and procedures, seeking assistance as required

3 report and review incidents according to organisational policies and procedures and access support from legitimate sources when appropriate.

Introduction

This chapter will provide you with the knowledge required to respond effectively to behaviours of concern by patients. Skills learnt are associated with handling difficult incidents rather than managing ongoing behaviour difficulties.

Behaviours of concern can arise in a patient due to multiple complex causes and the triggers can be traced back by looking at the medical state or the context and what happened just before the reaction. This chapter will provide you with a thorough understanding of behaviours of concern as well as the responses required that can either minimise or halt these behaviours. By recognising these behaviours, responding appropriately and reporting and reviewing incidents, you will be able to comply with organisational policies and procedures and sustain continuous improvement. This will help patient interaction and provide vital information for the revision of care plans to accommodate the ongoing needs and management of the patient.

INDUSTRY INSIGHTS 💬

Acquired brain injury services

After working in a hospital for some years as a health services assistant (HSA), I started a new job in a community centre that assists clients with acquired brain injuries (ABI). These are the result of external forces applied to the head from accidents. The role of the centre was to plan and establish community support systems for people with ABI. Many of the clients displayed behaviours of concern including irritability, aggression, frustration, lack of social judgement, lack of motivation and emotional lability. These behaviours had a significant impact on their work, family, friends and relationships.

My role included administration and assisting the healthcare team. The services on offer included:

- behaviour consultancy and advice to assist ABI people and their families to understand and manage their challenging behaviour
- behavioural intervention such as counselling, education, anger management and training to give the person skills to proactively manage and live with their behaviour.

I learnt that irritability and anger were common issues for these people and that understanding the cause was important in deciding on management strategies. Alcohol, drugs, stress and fatigue could be triggers for the frustration and anger they displayed, so it was important to recognise these and develop coping strategies to help. I sat in on a training session with a client which focused on relaxation and breathing techniques and talking through feelings to calm down. The psychologist also got the client to write down their specific triggers, strategies to de-stress and contacts because they had difficulty remembering and concentrating. This could help the individual to identify feelings, calm down and to have a list of who they could talk to next time they experienced these emotions.

I felt fortunate to be working for this community service and could see that people with acquired brain injury could have an improved quality of life and optimal independence through community integration and through access to these appropriate services.

1 IDENTIFY BEHAVIOURS OF CONCERN AND PLAN RESPONSE

Behaviours of concern are sometimes called challenging behaviours. They are any behaviours that cause stress, risk of or actual harm to the individual, staff or those around them. As an HSA, you will need to identify the reason for these behaviours so that an appropriate response can be implemented. This will decrease or eliminate the behaviour and prioritise safety for the individual and staff. Your roles and responsibilities will be governed by your scope of practice and the organisation's policies and procedures. You need to understand these boundaries to ensure there are no misunderstandings or unsafe practices when caring for individuals with behaviours of concern.

Identify behaviours of concern in line with work role and organisational policies and procedures

The management of behaviours of concern involves both an immediate response and the need to examine the underlying causes or triggers. The triggers can be environmental, psychological or medical and should be noted in the care plan, patient history and progress notes, along with strategies to reduce their impact. Once the trigger is identified, the appropriate health professional can be referred, and management of the trigger commenced. The health professional may be the doctor, nurse, psychologist, counsellor, psychiatrist, pharmacist or physiotherapist.

Environmental causes of behaviours of concern

Maslow's hierarchy of needs, shown in Figure 12.1, identifies the physiological needs of survival as being the foundation for higher order needs. A person may exhibit behaviours of concern when their physiological, safety or social needs are not met; for example, hunger, thirst, elimination, pain, fatigue, temperature, over/under stimulation and social engagement.

FIGURE 12.1 Maslow's hierarchy of needs

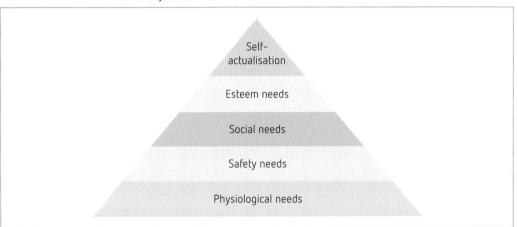

Source: Based on Maslow, A. H. (1943). A theory of human motivation. *Psychological Review*, 50(4), 370 – 96.

Accumulated stressors such as noise, temperature and light can also contribute to behaviours of concern because they lower the threshold for stress tolerance. Additionally, a behaviour of concern, such as dementia, can lower a person's ability to deal with daily stress and increases the susceptibility to environmental stressors.

Psychological causes of behaviours of concern

Individuals often resort to challenging behaviour as a means of communication, especially if the person has limited ability to express themselves clearly or to understand others. This may be due to the following conditions:

- mental illness
- feelings of frustration
- poor self-esteem
- confusion
- loss/grief

Dementia

A progressive state of confusion and deterioration of intellectual and physical ability, resulting in eventual death.

387

- experience of abuse
- short-term memory loss
- dementia.

Medical causes of behaviours of concern

When examining the cause of behaviours of concern, it is important to first determine if there are any medical triggers. Once these are eliminated, the behaviour may cease. Figure 12.2 outlines some possible medical causes of behaviours of concern.

FIGURE 12.2 Medical causes of behaviours of concern

MEDICAL CAUSE OF BEHAVIOUR OF CONCERN	EXAMPLES
Impaction	Faecal impaction
Medication	Sedatives, alcohol, polypharmacy
Systemic	Hypoglycaemia, vitamin B12 deficiency, dehydration
Trauma	Chronic pain, head trauma, fractures such as hip and rib
Infection	Urinary tract infection, pneumonia, septicaemia
Metabolic	Hypothyroidism / hyperthyroidism
Degenerative	Chronic illness

Source: Heerema, E. (2019). Physical causes of challenging behaviours in dementia. *Very Well*. Retrieved from https://www.verywellhealth.com/physical-causes-of-challenging-behaviors-in-dementia-97618

SCENARIO

Mrs Beaumont – responding to behaviours of concern

Mrs Beaumont, 78 years old, was admitted to the hospital from the local nursing home for a complete hip replacement following a fractured femur. Since the operation, she has displayed behaviours of concern. This morning she refused to eat her porridge for breakfast, became quite abusive and threw the bowl back at the nurse. When the nurse reminded Mrs Beaumont that this was not appropriate behaviour, Mrs Beaumont slapped her face. Mrs Beaumont's husband tried to help her with her breakfast, but she continued to be verbally aggressive and shouted at him to leave.

Later that morning, the nurse took Mrs Beaumont's bedpan away and noticed that her urine was cloudy and smelled offensive. The nurse tested the urine and the test results indicated an increased level of leukocytes. This was reported to the healthcare team and a provisional diagnosis of urinary tract infection was made. Mrs Beaumont commenced a course of antibiotics. She responded well and within two days had ceased being agitated. Her husband noted that she was behaving normally again.

1 As well as the medical cause of Mrs Beaumont's behaviours of concern, what environmental impact may have caused her to become agitated?

2 Why is it important for the health professionals to rule out medical causes before determining a management plan?

Symptoms of behaviours of concern

Because behaviours of concern can vary, staff must become familiar with the causes of the person's behaviour through their symptoms and current medical conditions in order to recognise the early warning signs. Assessing a client's presentation over a period of days can determine patterns of behaviour. Once you have identified these signs, you and the healthcare team can determine strategies to prevent the behaviour from escalating.

Anxiety

Anxiety is a feeling of worry, nervousness and apprehension caused by stressful events. For example, a person may become anxious in unfamiliar surroundings or after a traumatic incident. The anxiety can develop into hostility or aggression if not managed effectively. For many patients, a hospital is an unfamiliar environment and combined with poor health can increase their vulnerability to developing symptoms of anxiety.

Although the experience of anxiety will vary between people, feeling stressed and worried are common symptoms. Other symptoms of anxiety include:

* restlessness
* avoidant behaviour
* rapid heartbeat
* trembling or shaking
* feeling light-headed
* numbness or tingling sensations
* nausea
* sweating.

Anxiety
Feelings and experiences that occur at times of stress. Symptoms include nervousness, fear, worry, excessive sweating, irritability, breathlessness, palpitations and racing pulse.

Confusion or cognitive impairment

Confusion, often associated with anxiety, is when a person is unable to think rationally or to understand their situation. Confusion can be linked to dementia but can also be caused by medical conditions such as dehydration, hypoglycaemia, infection or medication. If the behaviour is caused by a medical condition, the confusion should be resolved once the cause is treated. Confused or cognitively impaired patients may struggle with orientation and may fail to identify where they are and/or where they are going.

In an acute care setting, a confused patient may pull at tubes and intravenous lines or try to climb out of bed. Trying to prevent this can result in injury because the confused patient may retaliate when physically restrained.

Symptoms of confusion may include:

* disorganised thoughts
* disorientation
* impaired ability to make decisions
* decreased alertness.

Orientation
A person's ability to identify their position in the environment relative to known landmarks (i.e., knowing where they are and where they are going).

Aggression and anger

Aggression and anger are common behaviours of concern and can be expressed both physically and verbally. Anger can also be part of a grieving process and is often misdirected and unreasonable. When assessing behaviours of concern, remember that people grieve in different ways influenced by their culture, behavioural patterns and social norms. While anger may present as a feeling of annoyance, it can quickly develop into hostility and aggression. Patients with dementia may behave aggressively if they feel frustrated, frightened or threatened. The acute care environment can be frightening for patients who have difficulty coping with changed situations.

Physical signs of aggression and anger include:

- pacing or agitation
- threatening body language; for example, clenched fists or finger pointing
- breathlessness
- dilated pupils
- flushed face.

Verbal signs of aggression and anger include:

- noisy agitation such as shouting, yelling or screaming
- abusive or derogatory remarks
- threats of 'losing control' and harming self or others.

Intoxication

Intoxication is the term used to describe any change in perception, mood, thinking processes and motor skills as a result of the effect of drugs or alcohol. It may present as anger and aggression, which can harm the intoxicated patient or others. Withdrawal from alcohol can cause anxiety and, in severe instances, seizures and delirium. Other signs of intoxication may include:

- slurred speech
- lack of balance and coordination
- confusion
- rudeness.

Intrusive behaviour

Intrusive behaviour presents as an invasion of another's privacy or personal space. It may be an attempt to attract your attention. Examples include:

- uninvited presence in other patients' rooms or conversations
- looking through other patients' belongings
- being overfamiliar.

Manipulation

Manipulation occurs when one person exploits another by deliberately creating an imbalance of power to serve his or her agenda. The manipulator may use verbally offensive and threatening language to control others. Other examples include:

- behaving differently in front of different people in different situations
- distorting facts
- seeking opportunities to exploit weaknesses
- imposing unreasonable demands on others
- bullying behaviour.

Self-destructive behaviour

This is behaviour that can cause harm to the patient. Self-destructive behaviour is often associated with guilt, shame and a need for self-punishment. The patient experiences a real or perceived personal failure that motivates a need to self-harm to justify feeling bad. Examples include:

- self-harm through cutting and/or suicide attempts
- substance abuse
- lack of self-care
- eating disorders.

Wandering

This is when a patient, usually with dementia, wanders away from their caregiver or controlled environment, such as a healthcare facility. This is common at sundown and increases the risk of harm to the individual, who is often confused.

Warning signs

With each condition listed, indicate whether it is an environmental, psychological or medical cause of behaviours of concern:

- loss/grief
- hunger
- anxiety
- infection
- pain

- impaction
- dehydration
- fatigue
- confusion.

Identify and ensure appropriate and planned responses to maximise the availability of staff and resources

Challenging behaviour can be distressing not only for the person affected but also for the patient's family and friends and the healthcare worker. The management of and interventions for these behaviours will require an initial assessment to identify triggers that may contribute to them. It will then require the use of a range of resources, environmental adaptations or diversional strategies. A satisfactory outcome can be achieved by identifying triggers and responding with the appropriate staff and resources.

Plan responses

When planning responses, information can be gathered from the patient, their family, staff and health professionals. The patient's medical records, including care plans or progress notes, can identify significant information that can assist the healthcare team to plan responses to behaviours of concern. Care plans provide information about the patient's needs, preferences and history. Progress notes document changes in the patient's condition, past behaviours and significant medical conditions. Psychologists may have conducted behavioural assessments that can provide a background to any potential triggers or causes for concern.

As an HSA, you can prepare so that you respond quickly and appropriately to behaviours of concern. Read the patient's documentation and use your skills to anticipate and assess situations and prevent potential escalations of behaviour. Additional skills include:

- knowledge of your scope of practice and organisational policies and procedures, including safe work practices
- knowledge of available resources such as staffing and supervisory support, alarms, phones and security equipment
- identification of triggers that may cause concern
- remaining alert, and observing and monitoring patients closely
- knowledge of the individual and their underlying causes of behaviour of concern
- awareness of cultural sensitivity and treating the patient with respect
- knowledge of what to report and record
- communication techniques to calm the patient and prevent escalation of behaviour.

If you have been assigned to a new patient, read their notes and/or behaviour plan and seek advice on preventative strategies from your co-workers. If you have had minimal experience with patients who have the potential for behaviours of concern, it is your responsibility to ask your supervisor for training.

Preventative strategies

If you are familiar with the patient's history and causes of their challenging behaviour, you have a greater chance of preventing the behaviours of concern. Allowing the patient to make choices, treating them with respect and validating their feelings can reduce frustrations and help calm an anxious patient.

Environmental adaptations can assist in the reduction of potential stressors; for example, removing disturbing sensory stimuli, and providing a schedule for the patient and a quiet place for them to feel relaxed. Music or personal photos can sometimes distract a person and calm them before the behaviour escalates.

SCENARIO

Appropriate resources for Audrey

Audrey, a 78-year-old, has been admitted to the local hospital after experiencing a cerebrovascular accident (CVA), otherwise known as a stroke. She is cognitively impaired and agitated. The entire healthcare team becomes involved when planning the appropriate strategies to treat Audrey. Doctors, psychologists, dietitians, occupational therapists and social workers will contribute their specific professional expertise to Audrey's care plan.

As an HSA, you read Audrey's physical, social and emotional history to gain an awareness of her preferences. You discuss with your co-workers the planned responses to minimise her agitation and report and record any changes. You carefully observe Audrey and attend to her needs. In this way, all healthcare team members are working together to respond to her behaviours of concern.

1 Why is it important for the healthcare team to become aware of Audrey's preferences?
2 Why is it important to be aware of Audrey's social history?
3 What strategies could the HSA use to prevent further agitation in Audrey?

Give priority to the safety of yourself and others in responding to behaviours of concern

Your organisation will have policies and procedures for dealing with behaviours of concern. These may form part of the organisation's mandatory training and/or emergency response procedures. Procedures for dealing with behaviours of concern address workers' safety; for example, in some high-risk facilities, staff must work in pairs and carry duress alarms.

Check on your scope of practice and responsibilities for safely managing patients who display challenging behaviours.

The first step when a patient demonstrates behaviours of concern is to prevent further conflict. You may need to remove the person or other people in the room or the conflict trigger while monitoring the environment and the person involved. Remain alert and be aware of what is going on around you. If the person becomes violent:

- do not isolate yourself from other staff
- do not allow the potentially violent person to block your access to an exit
- call for assistance; for example, from other staff, supervisors, security or police
- activate the duress alarm
- escape is always the preferred option, but if this is not possible, you can reasonably protect yourself to prevent the assault from happening or continuing.
  Indicators that may be associated with impending violence include:
- agitated body language
- threatening and/or intimidating gestures; for example, a raised fist or a face red in colour
- noisy agitation such as yelling or screaming
- verbal expressions of anger and frustration
- physical behaviour such as slamming doors or throwing objects
- signs the patient may use an object as a weapon or has a weapon.

Restraints (restrictive practice)

Restraints (now referred as restrictive practice) interfere with the individual's ability to have free movement. Restrictive practices should only be used as a last resort – alternative restraint-free strategies should be used to manage the patient first. Types include:

- chemical restraints – e.g., medications
- environmental restraints
- mechanical restraints – e.g., bed rails, tray tables, lap belts, vests
- seclusion
- physical restraint – using force to subdue movement of a person.

When using restrictive practices, always maintain the safety, wellbeing and dignity of the patient and staff. Refer to Chapter 14, 'Provide support to people living with dementia', which describes restraints in more detail.

Legal and ethical considerations

If you adhere to your organisation's policies, you are fulfilling your duty of care. Alert your team if a situation may be potentially harmful. Report changes in the patient's behaviour so they can be monitored and changes can be made to the care plan.

Human rights
The basic freedoms and protections that belong to every single human.

You can recognise the patient's human rights (including religion, culture and beliefs) by treating them equally, with respect, and giving them choices. This can reduce anxiety and stress in a patient and therefore reduce or eliminate behaviours of concern.

ACTIVITY 12.2

Human rights

The basic human rights enshrined in Victoria's Charter of Human Rights and Responsibilities are outlined in the following table. Refer to these when reading the case study and answer the questions that follow.

Sophia, a 27-year-old with aggression, is restrained with Velcro straps on her arms. The nurses have restrained Sophia because she spits, scratches and attempts to harm herself and staff when they are trying to treat her. The physical restraint was used as a last resort where less restrictive interventions were insufficient to protect Sophia.

FREEDOM	EQUALITY
Freedom of movement, assembly, expression and association	Equal recognition before the law
Rights to liberty and security	Enjoy rights without discrimination
Contact with the legal system	Equality in law without discrimination
Freedom of thought, conscience, religion and belief	Entitlement to participate in public life
Property rights	Dignity
Respect	Prohibition on torture and cruel, inhuman or degrading treatment
Right to life	Prohibition on forced work
Protection of families	Protection of privacy and reputation
Protection of children	Humane treatment when deprived of liberty
Cultural rights	Appropriate treatment of children in the criminal process

1. Which human right is limited in Sophia's case?
2. Is the limitation likely to achieve the intended purpose?
3. Is the limitation excessive or out of proportion to its purpose?
4. Are there any less restrictive means reasonably available to achieve restraint?

2 APPLY RESPONSE

When you respond to behaviours of concern, follow your organisation's policies and procedures and seek assistance if required. Responses need to be planned to take the individual's needs into account. Responses need to use the appropriate staff and physical resources, recognise the environment and consider the patient's history. You should use preventative skills where possible when responding to behaviours of concern.

Ensure responses to instances of behaviours of concern reflect organisational policy and procedures

Information is vital when you respond to behaviours of concern. When an incident occurs, you may have limited information about the patient. It is essential that you respond using the organisation's policies and procedures and work health and safety (WHS) guidelines. Maintain the patient's confidentiality and privacy when accessing information and be non-judgemental in your approach. Different types of challenging behaviour require different responses. Your response will vary depending on the triggers, the nature and severity of the incident, and its potential effect on the patient, staff and those around them.

ABC model

When developing a suitable response to behaviours of concern, the ABC model shown in Figure 12.3 is a method for understanding what happened before the behaviour (antecedents), what the behaviour was (behaviour), and what happened after the behaviour (consequences) (Ellis, 1957). Identifying the ABCs can help to develop strategies aimed at reducing the antecedents or modifying the consequences.

FIGURE 12.3 ABC model

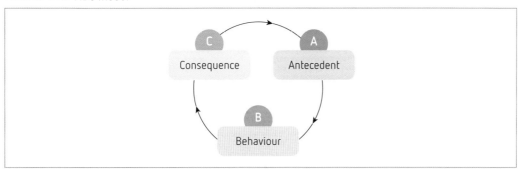

Source: Based on Ellis, A. (1957). Rational psychotherapy and individual psychology. *Journal of Individual Psychology*, 13, 38–44.

Antecedents

These are factors that occurred before the behaviour. For example:
* What did people around the patient say or do?
* Was the patient tired, stressed or in pain?
* Was the environment around the patient busy, bright or noisy?

By recognising these factors, you may be able to avoid triggering the behaviour. In an acute care setting, you can prepare the patient for the antecedent:
* During admission, explain that the ward is busy, bright and noisy. You can help the patient by talking about their expected reactions and ways they can cope with the environment.
* Ask the patient if they are in pain and refer them to the registered nurse (RN) for treatment.
* Distract the patient or redirect them away from the factors that may trigger the behaviour.
* Build a relationship with the patient so that they are comfortable talking about their concerns.
* Minimise lighting and draw the curtains to avoid the triggering factors.

Behaviour

You need to describe and report the specific observable actions that occurred because this can help with planning; for example, 'Mrs Baker was shouting at the physiotherapist when they were adjusting the sling on her wrist.'

Consequences

Before you respond to the behaviour, you need to understand its purpose or what it is expressing about the patient and his or her unmet needs. In some cases, the behaviour may be displayed to gain attention, and ignoring the behaviour is the best response.

Consequences can either increase or decrease the likelihood of the behaviour occurring again. By helping a patient understand the consequences of his or her behaviour, the healthcare team can support the patient to change their behaviour. For example, if the patient makes inappropriate comments and the staff laugh, the patient is likely to continue with the behaviour. The consequence of this inappropriately managed situation can cause escalation and in turn

FIGURE 12.4 24-hour behaviour monitoring record

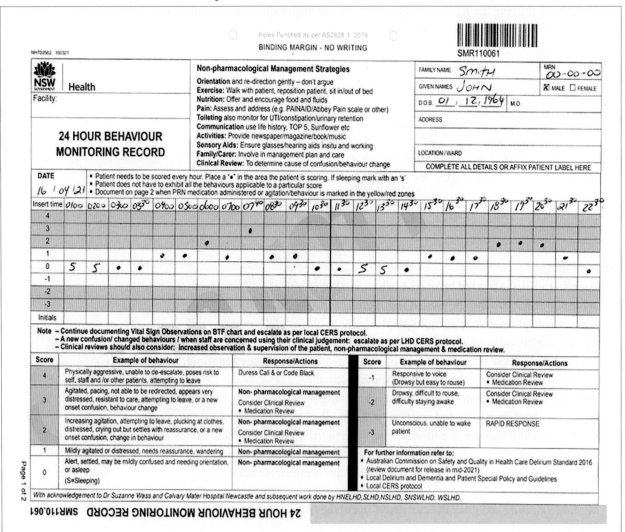

Source: 24-hour behaviour monitoring record, Product code: NH700562, https://aci.health.nsw.gov.au/__data/assets/pdf_file/0007/656809/ACI-24-hour-behaviour-monitoring-record-guide.pdf, © State of New South Wales (Agency for Clinical Innovation) 2020.

become another antecedent. If, however, the staff ignore the comments, the person is likely to cease the behaviour. To be effective, the reactions to the behaviour must be consistent from all staff. Information gained from the ABC approach can then be assessed by the team to make informed decisions about further management strategies.

NSW Health utilises a 24-hour behaviour monitoring record that provides an overview of a patient's behavioural fluctuations or changes (see Figure 12.4). This record monitors the antecedents or triggers for behaviours, a description for the behaviour and the interventions or strategies.

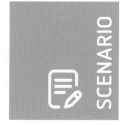

ABC model for Marta

Marta Brennon is 91 years old and has mild dementia. She has been admitted, confused, to the local rural hospital. Last night she wandered and was found in another patient's room. When the HSA tried to take her back to her bed, Mrs Brennon became angry and shouted at her. Mrs Brennon said that she was looking for her husband, who had passed away five years ago.

The healthcare team uses the ABC approach to document Mrs Brennon's behaviour and to help target interventions aimed at modifying the consequences.

ANTECEDENT	BEHAVIOUR	CONSEQUENCE
Marta has not been sleeping well and is in an unfamiliar environment	When found wandering, the healthcare worker respects Marta's personal space and uses a calm tone when speaking to her, while redirecting her back to bed	Marta continues to wander but can be easily redirected without expressing anger

1 What other strategies could the healthcare team use to minimise Mrs Brennon's behaviour?
2 Why is it important to clearly document the behaviour of and interventions for Marta?

Seek assistance and deal with behaviours promptly, firmly and diplomatically in accordance with policy and procedure

Many state/territory health networks have policy frameworks and guidelines that support healthcare workers in responding appropriately to challenging behaviours. These follow the principles of hazard identification and risk management as outlined in Chapter 1 ('Participate in workplace health and safety') and in SafeWork Australia codes of practice. Some have mandatory training that must be undertaken upon employment with a health service.

You should seek assistance from your supervisor or other staff members if you are unsure of the technique required to manage behaviours of concern. To learn these techniques, you should attend the relevant debriefing session or workshop, or research behaviour management.

Always respond in a way that helps to diffuse anger and frustration. Stay composed and give the patient time to calm down. Deal with the behaviour promptly and escalation of the behaviour may be minimised. If you are diplomatic, the patient will be able to maintain their dignity and self-respect. Other techniques include the following:

* Do not become anxious as this may increase the patient's agitation.
* Do not command or argue with the patient.

- Be polite, tolerant and respectful.
- Give the patient physical space.
- Speak slowly to reassure and validate the patient while maintaining eye contact; for example, 'I sense you are frustrated or angry.'
- Avoid behaviour that may be seen as aggressive; for example, moving rapidly, getting too close, touching or yelling at the patient.
- Distract the patient by redirecting them to another activity; for example, looking at photos, listening to preferred music, having cups of tea and snacks.
- After the incident, debrief, report and record the details.

Use communication effectively to achieve the desired outcomes in responding to behaviours of concern

Empathy
The ability to understand and share the feelings of another.

It is vital that you convey a message of empathy and reassurance to the person concerned. By using both non-verbal communication and verbal communication, you can allay anxiety to minimise concerning behaviours.

Non-verbal communication

Non-verbal communication includes posture, gestures and facial expressions. When talking to a patient, make non-threatening eye contact. Be mindful of how close you position yourself, especially with people from different cultural backgrounds. Try to adopt a posture which is open and non-threatening. Face the person and keep your expression calm and your hands open. All these strategies communicate that you mean no harm, are prepared to listen and are willing to help.

You can determine if your actions are impacting the other person by observing their body language. You are having a positive impact if the person maintains eye contact, relaxes their gestures and/or sits down. However, you will need to re-evaluate your communication if they continue to display behaviours of concern.

Verbal communication

You will convey you are in control by speaking in a calm and positive way. Use short instructions so the patient will understand what is expected. Explain that their behaviour is inappropriate. Modify your language to suit the patient's needs; for example, patients from a non-English-speaking background may need simple words or the assistance of an interpreter, while patients with hearing difficulties may need a combination of verbal and non-verbal cues. You can avoid misunderstandings by using active listening and questioning.

Active listening

Use active listening to focus attention on the speaker. You must then interpret what you think the speaker has said, in your own words. By interpreting the speaker's message in your own words, you are able to clarify any information that you do not understand; for example, 'My understanding of what you have just said is …' You (the listener) do not have to agree with the speaker but simply translate what you think the speaker meant. This allows the speaker to determine whether you understood their message. Use encouraging words (e.g., 'Go on …') or nod to keep the patient talking. By using active listening, you can:

- encourage other people to listen attentively
- avoid misunderstandings
- encourage patients to share more of their thoughts
- prove to the speaker that they are being heard.

Questioning

This can be a tool to gain information and better understand the behaviours of concern. Keep your questions brief and clear. If you require a simple 'yes' or 'no' answer, use closed questioning; for example, 'Do you need to go to the bathroom?' If you want the patient to give as much information as possible, use open questioning. For example, 'I sense that you are feeling anxious about your operation. Can you tell me what is concerning you?' Avoid arguments or judgemental responses because this may agitate the patient more.

Open questioning

Change the closed questions below to open questions. This technique helps to gain additional information from the patient.

ACTIVITY 12.3

CLOSED QUESTION
Do you feel anxious?
Did you throw that bowl across the room?
Are you responsible for the errors in the written report?
Are you wandering again?
Are you in pain?
Can you remember what your medications are?
Mr Smith seems very confused, don't you think?

Select appropriate strategies to suit instances of behaviours of concern

When considering a patient's care plan, their background, needs and circumstances must be examined within the environment in which the behaviours of concern are occurring. Select strategies and interventions based on the patient's presentation.

All interventions should be based on:
- a comprehensive assessment of the challenging behaviours
- strategies that alleviate or address the triggering factors (antecedents)
- evaluating the effectiveness of the strategy
- preventing recurrence of the behaviour
- improving the quality of care.

Anxiety

Anxiety may present as panic attacks, compulsive disorders or phobias (e.g., phobias about needles, surgery or being in confined spaces, such as MRI scanner tunnels). Symptoms of anxiety can be physical or psychological.

When working with an anxious patient, remain calm, try to identify what is triggering the anxiety, and reassure and empathise with them. If you cannot help, communicate with the appropriate staff and assure the anxious patient that their concerns are being addressed. Other strategies include:

- giving the person physical space – an anxious person may feel more threatened if there are too many people in a room or space
- diversional activities, which can help to relax the anxious person – for example, change the focus of conversation, offer them a book to read or a cup of tea
- not arguing with the person as this can turn to anger – speak calmly and try to ease the mood
- ensuring you have clear access to an exit should the situation get out of control.

Confusion

Confusion may cause patients to react in a violent or withdrawn way. By communicating the details of an incident of a person who is chronically confused (e.g., those suffering from dementia) to the healthcare team, the information can help establish patterns that can be useful in behaviour modification programs. Responsive strategies for a confused person include:

- staying calm and trying to reassure the person
- not challenging or arguing with the person
- avoiding rushing or grabbing a patient unless they are about to harm either themselves or someone else because this will frighten them and may put you at greater risk
- avoiding crowding or threatening the person
- prioritising your safety – ensure you maintain clear access to an exit and get help.

Aggression and anger

If you are confronted by an angry or aggressive person, remain calm and appease the person if possible. Often, aggression is based on fear or arises from feelings of grief. Try to find out what has triggered the anger and acknowledge the trigger. Try to address the cause of the person's anger or refer the person to another staff member. If the person appears to be irrational or under the effects of drugs or alcohol, be aware that violence is more likely. Additional strategies include:

- keeping distance between yourself and the person and not crowding them
- providing opportunities for the person to talk – this provides an outlet for their feelings
- trying to listen and empathising with what they have to say – do not argue
- not turning your back on the person
- if the person is being verbally aggressive, prioritising your safety – verbal aggression can precede a physical assault. Do not attempt to handle the situation alone
- if a colleague is being confronted by an aggressive person, calling for help before attempting to intervene
- if your colleague is being physically assaulted or you feel assault is imminent, calling for help – do not attempt to intervene.

If you are dealing with a grieving person, acknowledge their grief. It can be unhelpful to give personal examples of similar losses. The person's grief is unique to them and should not be compared to that of others. Allow the person to grieve in their own way and use active listening. Let the person know that you will listen in a non-judgemental way if they wish to talk.

Intoxication

An intoxicated person's behaviour can be unpredictable. To ensure that minimal harm comes to the person, consider their immediate physical and psychological wellbeing. Strategies to deal with intoxicated patients (SA Health, 2022) include:

- treating them with respect
- speaking slowly and giving clear and simple information
- being accepting and non-judgemental to engage with the person
- developing a relationship based on empathy and trust
- watching for signs of worsening intoxication or withdrawal. Health care incorporates appropriate screening tools and withdrawal scales to monitor the person
- moving the person to a quiet place if possible
- once the behaviour subsides, referring the person to an appropriate drug and alcohol or mental health service
- ensuring the safety of yourself and those around you.

Intrusive behaviour

Intrusive behaviour can cause offence, but the offender may not be aware that their behaviour is offensive. Strategies to manage the behaviour include:

- remaining calm and professional – avoid escalating the problem
- diverting attention away from the intrusive behaviour or guiding the offending person away
- explaining to the offending person that their behaviour can cause offence to those around them.

Manipulation

Determining the root cause of manipulation is complex. However, it is important that you recognise when your rights and the rights of those around you are being violated. When you intervene, explain to the patient why their behaviour is inappropriate. Being diplomatic but firm allows you to maintain a workable relationship with the patient. By asking probing questions, you put the focus back on the manipulator and may help them recognise the inequity of their behaviour. For example, by asking 'Does this seem reasonable to you?' the manipulator may become self-aware and cease the behaviour.

Self-harming behaviour

Depression, attention-seeking or feelings of hopelessness can all trigger self-harm. When a patient is at risk of self-harm, it is important to recognise the triggers for this behaviour. You must remain calm and reassure the patient. Remove any items that could be used for self-harming, especially sharp objects. If the patient is in crisis, do not leave them alone. Seek support from your supervisors or, if necessary, obtain emergency help.

Wandering

Wandering can be caused by a loss in short-term memory but is also common in patients with dementia. If a patient is in an unfamiliar environment, such as an acute care facility, wandering can be dangerous. To prevent wandering, there are locked codes on exits and entrances in aged and (some) hospital settings.

To minimise the risk of wandering, ensure that the patient is wearing an identification label, that their room is clearly labelled, and that staff are aware of the potential for the patient to wander. You will need to monitor these patients closely and use diversional activities to keep them occupied. If a patient has wandered, you must notify staff immediately and search for the patient. When they are found, speak calmly and guide them back to a safe environment.

Diversional activities

Diversional activities can engage a wandering patient and distract them by calming them. Diversional therapists can recommend activities to minimise behaviours of concern. These activities can include:

* music therapy
* games, cards, painting, singing or jigsaws
* talking with relatives or friends
* gardening or walking
* a cup of tea or juice.

Strategies for positive relationships

Hamish Johnson is a war veteran and gets scared if he hears someone yelling. He often misinterprets the tone of voice and body language as a potential threat and becomes fearful. He responds automatically by aggressively lashing out to keep himself safe.

1 Identify strategies to put in place to help Mr Johnson establish positive relationships with those around him.
2 Why is empathy important when responding to behaviours of concern?

3 REPORT AND REVIEW INCIDENTS

Follow your organisation's legal and professional requirements for documenting procedures undertaken when the patient is displaying behaviours of concern. These procedures may include completing an incident report, updating the patient's progress notes and giving a verbal handover to the healthcare team. Check your policy and procedure manual or ask your supervisor if you are not sure how to complete these procedures. By reporting and reviewing incidents, risks of or triggers for behaviours of concern are identified and staff can implement appropriate defusing techniques while continuously improving protocols.

Report incidents according to organisational policies and procedures

To ensure accuracy, incidents or near misses should be reported as soon as possible after they occur. All staff involved in the incident should be asked to participate so that a complete account can be documented.

Most institutions have incident report forms (many in electronic format) that will include:

- date and time
- location of incident
- nature of incident
- objective information describing what occurred
- identity of witnesses
- description of action taken after incident.

Write the facts of the incident, not your opinion or why you think it occurred. Your professional accountability requires you to be fair and objective. When objectively reporting the incident, the following behavioural information is required:

- observed triggers that caused the incident
- the duration of the behaviour
- the verbal and physical reactions of the patient
- changes that occurred in the patient's appearance during the behaviour
- strategies used to minimise or stop the behaviour
- how the patient reacted after the incident – what they told you, if they were making sense, if they were speaking clearly, if they knew where they were and what time it was.

Incident reporting

Conduct some research into incident reporting and answer the following questions:

1. Incidents can be classified as clinical, behavioural, environmental or medication. Give examples of the types of incidents under these categories.
2. Who completes the incident report form if the incident was not seen but discovered?
3. Why is it important to report and record near misses on an incident form?
4. Can a patient report an incident? If so, how is this processed?
5. What is a sentinel event?
6. Research safety measures that have been implemented in acute care facilities following incident reporting.

Review incidents with staff and offer suggestions appropriate to your area of responsibility

After the incident report form has been completed, it should be distributed to the appropriate department for examination. All staff directly involved in the incident, and all those with an indirect responsibility, such as managers and supervisors, should participate in the review. Involving family members in the review process can improve the individual's care plan. By including both the healthcare team and family, new behavioural goals or measures for intervention can be agreed on to prevent similar incidents recurring. When reviewing, ask the following questions:

1. What were the causes or triggers for the incident? Was there an environmental, behavioural or medical trigger?
2. Was the incident preventable?

3 Was the incident managed promptly and effectively? Did the strategies minimise or stop the behaviour? If not, why?

4 Can anything be done to prevent similar incidents happening in the future?

5 Does any action have to be taken regarding this incident?

Reviewing the incident ensures that accountability, safety, improved patient care and strategies can be developed to reduce the risk of future incidents.

SCENARIO

Mr Tupu – reviewing an incident

John Tupu, 67 years old, was admitted to the haemodialysis unit for his regular session of dialysis. A new graduate nurse was allocated to Mr Tupu and she was hesitant about setting up the dialysis machine and cannulating him. The experienced staff members were on leave, the nurse manager was at a meeting and the agency nurses were attending to their own patients. The graduate nurse rang the clinical nurse educator who said he could assist in one hour. Mr Tupu became frustrated and aggressive as a result of the delay in attending to his needs.

As part of the healthcare team, you are reviewing this incident to develop strategies to prevent recurrences.

Suggestions for improvement include:

* training staff in effective communication techniques to minimise aggressive behaviours
* ensuring that an experienced staff member is on shift at all times by reorganising rosters
* ensuring that the nurse manager is not away at critical times of the day (e.g., when patients first need to be set up on dialysis machines) by reorganising meeting times
* making sure that new graduate nurses are not allocated complex patients
* making sure that graduate nurses who start work in the haemodialysis unit are competent and confident in machine set-up and cannulation techniques
* documenting who to contact if there is a delay in booking the clinical nurse educators; for example, doctors or other nurse educators in the hospital.

1 Why is it important to review incidents with the entire healthcare team?

2 What strategies could the healthcare team implement to reduce Mr Tupu's frustrations and aggression as a result of the delay?

Access and participate in debriefing mechanisms and associated support, and access support from legitimate sources when appropriate

Debriefing
Providing a summary update of a condition or situation to the affected or concerned people.

Critical incident
Any situation that creates a significant risk of substantial or serious harm to the physical or mental health, safety or wellbeing of another.

Staff can be impacted by behaviours of concern that lead to injury or high levels of stress. Individual reactions to these stressful situations can vary from short-term trauma to long-term psychological reactions. Your own stress must be acknowledged and addressed following an incident. Debriefing after an incident helps you care for your psychological safety.

Critical incidents

Critical incidents are events, such as death or serious injury, that cause a strong emotional reaction and may overwhelm a healthcare worker's usual coping skills. These events are significantly distressing and, as Figure 12.5 demonstrates, can spiral into acute distress or even post-traumatic stress disorder (PTSD), which 'is a severe reaction to an extreme and frightening traumatic event' (Phoenix Australia, 2019). The severity of the distress is heightened if the person has not developed a stable set of strategies for coping with stressors.

FIGURE 12.5 Spiralling effects of critical incidents

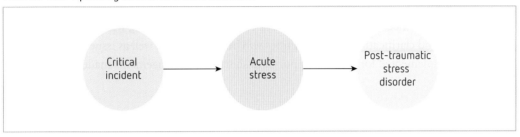

Post-traumatic stress disorder (PTSD)

A disorder that develops in some people who have seen or lived through a shocking, frightening or dangerous event. Main symptoms are re-experiencing the trauma (memories, nightmares or flashbacks), avoiding reminders of the trauma, and negative thoughts and mood.

Typically, there is an initial sense of shock and disbelief. The individual is protected from the full impact of the incident by this emotional numbing. After the initial period, the individual is likely to experience a variety of effects, such as:

- a reduction in work performance
- poor sleeping habits
- inability to concentrate
- substance abuse
- withdrawal
- poor diet
- physical symptoms; for example, breathlessness, headaches, fatigue, nausea or dizziness.

Management

Critical incident stress management provides support to staff who experience distress following an abnormal event. It may be carried out by a supervisor or qualified professional and the goal is to minimise any adverse emotional reactions for the staff member. You should make sure that you are familiar with all strategies, procedures and critical incident stress management plans.

Usually, management includes:

- preparation
- demobilisation
- debriefing
- follow-up support.

Preparation

Preparation includes assessing the work environment and developing procedures for responding appropriately to critical incidents. Strategies include training in mental health first aid, being aware of the contact details for emergency personnel, having an emergency procedures chart with instructions, having extra staff available at certain times of the day and pairing less experienced staff with those who are more experienced.

Demobilisation

Critical incidents can trigger a wide range of symptoms, including increased heart rate, nausea and anxiety. Demobilisation manages symptoms in staff affected by a critical incident. This means rest, providing information and time out, and ensuring that the healthcare workers' needs are met and that they are not alone while dealing with their stress.

Demobilisation is actioned by a supervisor or manager who was not involved in the incident. They will convene a meeting of those involved as soon as possible, during which a summary of the incident and clarification of uncertainties will be discussed, as well as issues of concern. Plans will be implemented for further support and short-term arrangements made for work responsibilities.

Debriefing

Acute stress felt by staff involved in a critical incident can be alleviated by debriefing. This is usually carried out within three to seven days of the critical incident because the incident is still fresh in the minds of the staff and distortion of the facts is minimised. The structured debriefing discussion aims to put the critical incident into perspective and offers clarity about the incident as well as assisting to establish a process for recovery. It also allows anyone to voice concerns or complaints and make suggestions for continuous improvement.

When providing support, it is important to:

* establish empathetic communication
* commence support as soon as possible after the incident
* respect the affected staff members' needs
* define boundaries for what is expected
* validate the reactions of the staff.

During the debriefing sessions, trained professionals help affected staff to explore and understand the incident. Each person's experience is discussed as well as the methods to manage the emotional responses resulting from the incident. It is important to gain closure on the experience and also to remind people that talking about the incident is healthy.

Follow-up support

Follow-up support may be required because the perspective of the affected staff may change after the first debriefing session. Additional sessions may need to focus on new aspects of the incident or stress reactions. If counselling is required, the staff members can be referred to an appropriate service for additional support.

Places where you can seek follow-up support include:

* your supervisor or manager
* other experienced workers in your team
* a counsellor
* employment assistance program (EAP)
* WHS officer
* health and safety representative
* your doctor.

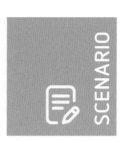

The debriefing process

Consider the following scenarios and describe the debriefing process for each.

Scenario 1: Mr Lu, a 34-year-old man, did not recover from a cardiac arrest. You had looked after him for the last three weeks and formed a special bond with him because of your shared interest in Asian cooking. You experience shock and disbelief and are visibly shaken after this incident.

Scenario 2: Mrs Farugia, 87 years old, was admitted to the ward with pneumonia. She became confused and fell from the bed and fractured her hip. You are frustrated with the staff for not making sure that the bed sides were raised and shout out your frustrations during the handover.

Scenario 3: Ms Whitten, 18 years old, has just been diagnosed with leukaemia. She and her family are in disbelief and become hysterical. You are very upset because of this diagnosis and their reactions.

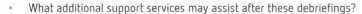

*   What additional support services may assist after these debriefings?

SUMMARY

In this chapter, you have learnt to identify and implement strategies that minimise the impact of behaviours of concern. You have seen that these behaviours can arise in many acute care patients and the triggers for these behaviours can usually be traced back by looking at the patient's environment, medical or psychological history.

This chapter highlighted that by collecting this information, a pattern will emerge which will help the nurse–patient interaction and provide vital information for the revision of care plans to accommodate patient needs. Selection of appropriate strategies can then be made to minimise or resolve the behaviour of concern.

The last part of the chapter emphasised the importance of reporting and reviewing incidents according to organisational policies and procedures. Debriefing was then discussed as a way of understanding the incident and managing the resulting emotional responses.

APPLY YOUR KNOWLEDGE

Alcohol withdrawal

Danil was admitted to the emergency department with symptoms of alcohol withdrawal. He presented with vomiting, tremors, sweating and confusion. After having IV fluids and medications in the emergency department for the symptoms, he was transferred to the ward. You were the HSA on the ward and were assigned to his care along with the registered nurse. As you were unfamiliar with the care of a patient with alcohol withdrawal, you asked the RN to assist you with his nursing care planning.

Danil was placed in a single room with the bed rails raised. You were required to take his vital signs fourth hourly and report to the RN any increased heart rate, blood pressure or confusion.

1   What is the purpose of nursing Danil in a single room?

2   Using your knowledge learnt in Chapter 11, 'Assist with nursing care in an acute care environment', define the normal limits for pulse and blood pressure in an adult.

3   What is the procedure if Danil's behaviour becomes increasingly confused?

After five days, Danil recovered from his symptoms. He spoke about his depression and years of homelessness and feelings of despair, which have resulted in his alcohol abuse and aggression towards those around him. You understand that you must use empathy and reassurance to minimise Danil's concerning behaviours.

4   What is the antecedent for Danil's aggression and why is it important for the healthcare team to recognise this factor?

5   What active listening techniques can the HSA use to encourage Danil to fully express his feelings?

Danil was referred to a social worker, counselling and a drug and alcohol program. You feel these support services could really help Danil to achieve his goals and prevent further escalations of his behaviours of concern.

6   How did the HSA demonstrate an understanding of the scope of their role when providing nursing care to Danil?

◄ REFLECTING ON THE INDUSTRY INSIGHT ➕

1 The industry insight described a community centre focusing on acquired brain injury. What could cause an acquired brain injury?
   a Genetic malformation of the brain during its development.
   b Lack of oxygen to the brain at birth.
   c An external force applied to the head from an accident.
   d Degenerative diseases such as Alzheimer's.

2 Why would the psychologist get the client to write down triggers, strategies and contacts as part of their management plan? Because people with acquired brain injury:
   a have difficulty remembering, concentrating or paying attention
   b cannot understand spoken words
   c have better visual capacity than hearing capacity
   d cannot understand directions.

3 Why is it important to maximise community integration for people with acquired brain injury?
   a To restore full functionality in these people.
   b So that they can return to optimal independence
   c So that they do not need further healthcare support.
   d To reduce the amount of medications taken.

SELF-CHECK QUESTIONS

1 What medical factors can contribute to behaviours of concern?
2 Identify ways to reduce the risk of harm to staff in a situation where the patient may become violent.
3 What are your obligations under your duty of care when dealing with patients who display behaviours of concern?
4 Describe the ABC model for developing a suitable response to behaviours of concern.
5 How can you, as a health services assistant, minimise the risk of wandering?
6 What are the benefit of diversional activities for behaviours of concern. Give examples.
7 What are some examples of objective data that can be used when reporting behaviours of concern?
8 Explain the benefits of debriefing.
9 List sources of advice and assistance that you could access after dealing with a critical incident.
10 What are your definitions of the following key words and terms that have been used in this chapter?

KEY WORD OR TERM	YOUR DEFINITION
Orientation	
Anxiety	
Antecedent	
Human rights	
Empathy	
Critical incident	
Post-traumatic stress disorder	
Restrictive practice	

QUESTIONS FOR DISCUSSION

1   Patients with an existing cognitive impairment, such as dementia, are at the greatest risk of developing delirium during their hospital stay. Discuss the factors that may contribute to this occurring.

2   Discuss how you would maximise resources and the abilities of staff when you are responding to behaviours of concern in an intoxicated and aggressive patient.

3   'Behaviours of concern do not just belong to the individuals. They belong to the entire environment of which the person is the focal point.' What do you think this statement means?

4   Discuss how the healthcare team's responses to behaviours of concern reflect organisational policies and procedures.

5   Discuss how supporting and debriefing with the client post-incident is crucial to their recovery and helps to decrease the chances of behaviours of concern escalating in the future.

EXTENSION ACTIVITY

Recognising effective and ineffective healthcare strategies

Rajesh Patel, 89 years old, presented to the emergency department with a suspected fractured humerus following a fall on his balcony steps at home. He informed the doctors that he was trying to get back inside his home to avoid the rain and slipped on the stairs. He told them that he lived alone and did his own cooking and personal care but had home support for the shopping and gardening. He appeared unkempt, but the doctors thought this may be because he had been outside in the rain. His daughter lived two hours away and his son lived interstate.

Upon questioning, he could not remember what day it was or when he last went to the general practitioner (GP) for a check-up. His daughter was contacted and she informed the healthcare team that her father had been living alone for 10 years since his wife had died. She said that he wanted to live alone rather than intrude on his family. His daughter would not be able to come to the hospital until the next day. The GP was then contacted and the healthcare team were informed that Mr Patel was on thyroid and antihypertensive medications.

On examination, Mr Patel appeared dehydrated and in pain. Intravenous (IV) therapy was commenced, pain relief was given, and an X-ray confirmed a fracture of the humerus. The doctors decided to treat the fracture conservatively with a sling for support. Mr Patel was admitted to the general medical ward in a four-bed room for treatment and follow-up. He told the nurses that he had never been in hospital before and that he was scared.

That evening, Mr Patel's confusion escalated and he became distressed. He kept calling out, but the ward was very busy. He tried to get out of bed and fell, causing a head injury which required suturing.

1   Review this scenario and discuss the effective and ineffective strategies that were used by the healthcare team.

EFFECTIVE STRATEGIES	INEFFECTIVE STRATEGIES

2   Form three groups and identify:
   a   what happened before the behaviour (antecedents)
   b   what the behaviour was (behaviour)
   c   what happened after the behaviour (consequences).
3   In groups, write up a nursing care plan in the following table to identify and minimise the behaviours of concern.

ASSESSMENT	PLANNING	IMPLEMENTATION	EVALUATION

4   In groups, practise appropriate communication strategies that could decrease Mr Patel's distress.

REFERENCES

Australian Commission on Safety and Quality in Health Care (ACSQHC) (2021). Incident management guide. Retrieved 10 April 2022 from https://www.safetyandquality.gov.au/publications-and-resources/resource-library/incident-management-guide

Ellis, A. (1957). Rational psychotherapy and individual psychology. *Journal of Individual Psychology*, 13, 38−44.

Phoenix Australia (2019). *What is trauma?* Melbourne: Phoenix Australia. Retrieved 10 April 2022 from https://www.phoenixaustralia.org/recovery/fact-sheets-and-booklets/

SA Health (2022). Alcohol withdrawal management. Retrieved 10 April 2022 from https://www.sahealth.sa.gov.au/wps/wcm/connect/public+content/sa+health+internet/clinical+resources/clinical+programs+and+practice+guidelines/substance+misuse+and+dependence/substance+withdrawal+management/alcohol+withdrawal+management

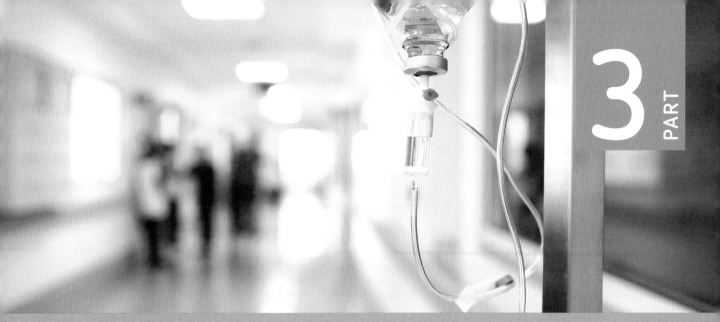

ALTERNATIVE ELECTIVE UNITS

In the acute care environment, patients' needs vary depending on their culture, condition and progression of illness. Using a client-centred approach will help you understand these diverse needs.

Chapters 13, 14 and 15 provide information to help you work effectively with clients who have mental health issues, dementia or life-limiting illness. The client-centred approach incorporates strategies to empower individuals, respect their rights and promote dignity, so that care providers can address their holistic needs.

Chapter 16 applies to all of the care that a health services assistant provides and emphasises the need to provide quality patient care reflective of the National Safety and Quality Health Service (NSQHS) Standards, and to strive to deliver excellent service at all times.

Chapter 17, the final chapter, describes the skills and knowledge required to provide basic assistance to an allied health professional in a range of settings, including acute and primary care, aged care and rehabilitation. This new chapter expands the field of delivery for a Certificate III worker as a health services or allied health assistant with a focus on promoting and enabling clients to have a healthy lifestyle and gaining or maintaining independence.

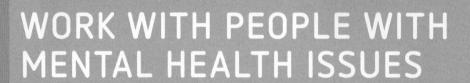

CHAPTER 13

WORK WITH PEOPLE WITH MENTAL HEALTH ISSUES

Learning objectives

By the end of this chapter, you should be able to:

1 establish respectful relationships with people with mental health issues
2 determine the needs of people with mental health issues
3 work with people with mental health issues to meet aspirations and needs.

Introduction

As a health services assistant (HSA) in an acute care setting, you may come into contact with people with mental health issues. This chapter will provide you with the skills and knowledge required to clarify the needs of, and establish relationships and work collaboratively with, people who are living with mental health issues.

By creating a dialogue with a client who has a mental illness, you can foster a therapeutic relationship that can promote recovery. The patient's recovery should be self-directed where possible, with you supporting their needs, preferences and rights. This chapter emphasises that you should recognise that dignity of risk is important when the individual makes decisions regarding their care.

The last part of the chapter highlights the networks and service organisations that support and encourage the independence of the person, including the importance of accurate service delivery plans that address management and/or referral in crisis situations. Your role boundaries are also emphasised so that your care for a person with a mental illness is within the limits of your knowledge and abilities.

INDUSTRY INSIGHTS ➕

Mental health day programs

Part of my workplace experience as an HSA involved placement in a mental health facility. One of the areas that I worked in was the day clinic for anxiety. The clinic ran group therapy programs especially designed to help people with anxiety disorders. The clients were of various ages and came from many cultures, and the programs focused on providing them with the appropriate skills and support to help improve their quality of life and break the cycle of relapse. The goal of the programs was to help people respond positively to their negative thoughts by promoting the use of effective coping strategies. Psychiatrists, psychologists, occupational therapists, social workers and specialist nurses were involved. The main treatment modes were cognitive behaviour therapy, acceptance of anxiety, assertiveness and mindfulness. The therapists responded to the clients by acknowledging their feelings and asking them to elaborate.

This was so different from my acute care clinical placement. There were no observations to take and no personal care tasks, just a focus on therapeutic communication and observation, and this was done predominantly by sitting attentively in silence until the person in the group chose to speak.

Over the four weeks that I attended my placement, I saw real changes in these anxious people. The group therapy allowed them to discuss their difficulties in a safe and supportive environment and the psychologists gave them helpful feedback. Goals were set and problem-solving was used. While I didn't see a wound heal or a cardiac arrhythmia resolve, I did see emotional healing. This gave me an understanding of the challenges faced by people with mental health disorders who don't have the physical characteristics of an illness to help people accept them or understand their behaviour.

1 ESTABLISH RESPECTFUL RELATIONSHIPS WITH PEOPLE WITH MENTAL HEALTH ISSUES

Embrace Multicultural Mental Health (2021) defines a mental illness as 'a health problem that significantly affects how a person feels, thinks, behaves and interacts with other people. It is diagnosed according to standardised criteria'. Mental health problems can be 'experienced temporarily as a reaction to the stresses of life' and result in a great deal of suffering for individuals, as well as their families and friends. It is essential that you establish respectful relationships through effective communication with people suffering mental illnesses, as well as respecting their cultural, spiritual and social differences, and supporting their rights, confidentiality and privacy. When a person feels respected, they are more willing to reveal their thoughts and work collaboratively towards recovery.

Mental illness
Conditions that significantly affect how a person feels, thinks, behaves and interacts with others.

Communicate to develop and maintain respect, hope, trust and self-direction

Communication with people with mental health issues is an essential component of all therapeutic interventions. As an HSA, you should use interpersonal skills to nurture the development of a therapeutic relationship based on respect, trust and hope. The same skills are essential in helping the person suffering mental illness to open up. Use of these skills requires knowledge of the barriers to communication, as well as knowledge of the use of communication techniques when working with individuals, their carers and others involved in their care.

Barriers to communication

Developing a respectful relationship means understanding the misconceptions that cause discrimination and prejudice for people with mental health issues. These barriers, in the form of attitudes, stigma and myths, often mean that the person with mental illness faces isolation and discrimination just for having an illness. These barriers need to be kept in mind and dealt with in a sensitive manner when dealing with mental health issues, and once they are removed, a positive relationship can be established, and the person can feel comfortable in expressing their concerns and needs.

Attitudes

The existence of negative attitudes towards mental illness has an impact on people who have mental health issues. Regardless of the reason for the negative attitude (which may be a lack of knowledge or pre-existing beliefs), the impact can mean social exclusion in employment, accommodation and relationships. The development of positive attitudes of family, significant others, healthcare workers and members of the community towards people with mental illness is critical to ensuring quality of life for the individual and supports their recovery. As an HSA, you can help by:

* considering mental illnesses like any other illness or health condition
* talking about mental illness openly
* educating yourself so you can overcome negative attitudes based on misinformation.

Respectful communication

Felicity is an HSA who likes to treat everyone with the same respect, regardless of their mental health condition. She has completed some online learning modules on mental health disorders to inform herself of common symptoms and nursing management. No matter what the task, who the person is or their condition, Felicity always uses effective communication strategies that best suit the person's needs; for example, speaking clearly to people from different cultural backgrounds and paraphrasing to check and clarify understanding. Felicity always greets the person by name, explains what she plans to do for the day and checks that the individual agrees with the plan or thinks it needs any changes. By being informed and communicating with respect, she has negated any pre-existing beliefs and developed positive relationships with the people in her care.

1 What impact does Felicity's display of respect and person-centred communication have on the individual and their recovery?

2 Why is it important for Felicity to make sure that the individual agrees with the plan?

Stigma

Stigma is a mark or label that sets a person apart. The World Health Organization (WHO) describes stigma as:

> … a major cause of discrimination and exclusion: it affects people's self-esteem, helps disrupt their family relationships and limits their ability to socialise and obtain housing and jobs. It hampers the prevention of mental health disorders, the promotion of mental well-being and the provision of effective treatment and care. It also contributes to the abuse of human rights.

WHO, 2013

Stigma about mental illness discourages people from seeking treatment. People may be 'reluctant to seek help because they do not understand what the symptoms mean, or they associate mental illness with negative stereotypes' (SANE Australia, 2014, p. 13). Stigma can erode a person's self-confidence and cause them to withdraw from society because they may fear ridicule. This social isolation and loneliness 'make it harder for people to cope with the symptoms of mental illness, or seek help to treat their illness' (p. 15). 'Fear and ignorance about mental illness [also] contribute to discrimination, making it harder for people with a mental illness to find work and/or a place to live, and to be accepted as valued members of the community' (p. 14).

Myths about mental illness

Some people believe mental illness is caused by a range of factors, including biological, psychological, social, spiritual and cultural ones. These beliefs hold varying degrees of negative association for those living with a mental illness and can prevent acceptance of the mentally ill. Figure 13.1 dispels commonly held myths about mental illness.

FIGURE 13.1 Dispelling common myths about mental illness

MYTH	FACT
Mental illness is incurable and lifelong	Most people with a mental illness recover well with appropriate, ongoing treatment and support
People are born with a mental illness	Some families may be more genetically predisposed to mental illnesses than others; e.g., bipolar disorder. However, many people develop mental illness with no family history
Only certain types of people develop a mental illness	Mental health problems can affect anyone. They affect people regardless of age, education, income or culture
People with a mental illness are violent	People being treated for a mental illness are no more violent or dangerous than the general population
People with a mental illness should be isolated from the community	With appropriate treatment and support, people with mental illness can live successfully in the community

Adapted from: SA Health (2022). Myths and facts about mental illness. Retrieved 24 October 2022 from https://www.sahealth.sa.gov.au/wps/wcm/connect/public+content/sa+health+internet/healthy+living/healthy+mind/myths+and+-facts+about+mental+illness#:~:text=Fact%3A%20A%20mental%20illness%20is%20not%20caused%20by,recover%20quickly%20and%20do%20not%20need%20hospital%20care

Stigma

A mark or label that sets a person apart. It can create negative attitudes and prejudice.

Bipolar disorder

Extremes of mood, between manic and depressive, that interfere with everyday life.

Effective communication techniques

Communication skills form the basis of every intervention. Maintaining an effective relationship with the person who has a mental illness and their family involves interpersonal skills that display empathy, engagement and being non-judgemental (see Figure 13.2). Communication starts with listening and can be enhanced by non-verbal communication, paraphrasing/ rephrasing, summarising and questioning. Non-verbal communication demonstrates respect by showing that you are listening to the person.

FIGURE 13.2 Communication skills form the basis of every intervention

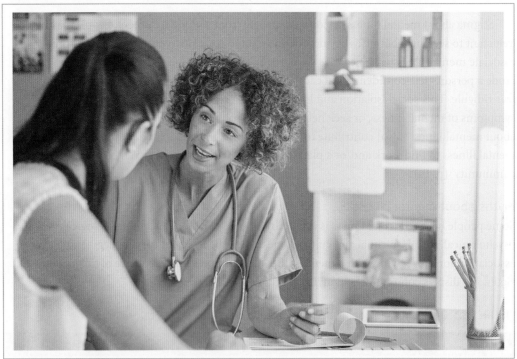

Source: iStock.com/sturti

Listening

Listening means that you are allowing a space for the person to talk. This is different from listening actively, where you are giving your full attention to the person who is talking. Listening actively involves:
- offering time and a quiet and private space, free from distractions, to listen to the person
- listening with the purpose of understanding the person's message
- giving full attention by focusing on what the person is saying
- tuning out external and internal distractions, such as background noises and thoughts about what to say next
- using prompts to encourage the person to elaborate; for example, 'Go on', 'Please continue', 'I see'.

Non-verbal communication

Non-verbal communication can be modelled by looking interested and concerned and maintaining good eye contact. It can also be demonstrated by an attentive posture; that is, leaning forward and nodding your head in acknowledgement. When working with people from different cultural backgrounds, be mindful of and sensitive to different practices concerning the use of eye contact, and gender, and modify your body language accordingly. Effective non-verbal communication can confirm and emphasise what is being said.

Paraphrasing

This involves expressing the person's core message in a different way, using your own words. Paraphrasing is a valuable tool because it demonstrates that you are listening and have heard what has been said. This realisation can make the person feel very supported and therefore has a therapeutic effect. Paraphrasing can also be used to check clarity and understanding; for example:

* 'It makes me so annoyed when the doctors don't listen to me. I think that they aren't interested in my concerns' can be paraphrased as 'You get annoyed when you are not being listened to?'
* 'I feel apprehensive about my group therapy session tomorrow' can be paraphrased as 'You feel apprehensive?'

Summarising

This involves offering the person a summary of the information that they have shared. For the person, hearing a summary of what they have said can help to confirm to and reassure them that you have heard and interpreted their words correctly. It also gives the person the opportunity to hear the main points of their discussion, to elaborate further and to correct any misinterpretations. For example, 'Let me check what I think you have said so far ...' or 'If I have heard correctly, what you have said is ...'

Questioning

Probing skills involve the use of different styles of questioning. The most useful questions are open-ended and begin with the words 'why', 'what' or 'how'. Asking an open-ended question invites a full and descriptive reply. Probing questions push the person to think more about the subject. Reflective questions highlight the theme of what the person has said. Encouraging questioning invites the person to add more to the conversation (see Chapter 4, 'Communicate and work in health and community services', for more on effective questioning). Examples are as follows:

* Open question – 'What made you decide to come to the counselling sessions?'
* Probing question – 'Tell me about your concerns.'
* Reflective question – 'So you feel that ...'
* Encouraging question – 'That sounds interesting. Can you say some more about that?'

Promote the person's right to define and direct their recovery

For a person with mental illness to recover, they must be empowered to live a self-determined life. This means having power over their own lives – having choice, individual responsibility and the right to make decisions about their health and recovery. Active involvement in the community in meaningful and interesting activities helps to develop social and support networks; for example, informal community resources, such as local cafés, sports teams, social groups, book clubs, churches and cultural groups. These are particularly important because they provide social relationships, material items and the experiences that give rise to a sense of belonging, community attachment, hope and self-confidence.

To achieve these goals, the healthcare team and the patient must communicate effectively to allow them to plan for the services that are required. Communication strategies for this planning can include:

- offering information about treatments, advocacy support, education and training
- fostering collaborative partnerships between services, people accessing services and their significant others
- focusing on the person's strengths and promoting a culture of hope
- being responsive to diversity by viewing people in the context of their whole selves, lives and wellbeing, including their cultural values and relationships.

Victorian Department of Health, 2015

ACTIVITY 13.1

Contexts in mental health

Describe how approaches to working with people with mental health issues have changed over the past 40 years in regard to:

1   attitudes towards mental health

2   society's views of mental health

3   treatments for mental health

4   political contexts; for example, government policies and initiatives that affect the mental health sector.

Recognise and respect the person's social, cultural and spiritual differences

A person's culture plays a very important role in the way they understand health and ill health and it influences how they seek help from healthcare professionals. When assisting someone from culturally and linguistically diverse (CALD) or Aboriginal and Torres Strait Islander backgrounds, it is important that you take into consideration the spiritual and cultural context of the person's behaviours.

Culturally and linguistically diverse (CALD)
People born in a country where English is not the main spoken language.

Being culturally competent when providing care to people with mental health issues involves being:
- person centred and family centred
- respectful and non-judgemental
- curious about cultures
- able to seek cultural knowledge appropriately
- able to change approaches in response to different cultural situations.

It also means understanding how people's cultural and individual beliefs and values affect their perceptions and understanding of their mental illness.

Victorian Department of Health, 2015

Culturally and linguistically diverse groups

The cultural variety of CALD groups is broad and so are the definitions of mental health disorders among them. You need to consider what mental illness means for these groups before providing support. When approaching someone outside your own culture or community to discuss their mental health, be aware that what is considered respectful communication (including body language, seating position and use of certain words) may differ from community to community. For example, some communities perceive making eye contact as staring and it may make people from those communities feel as though they are being judged (Mental Health First Aid, 2008).

Many people from different cultures have experienced stress due to separation from their country of origin, their families and their communities. In these situations, you must ensure that you understand and use culturally appropriate communication, be respectful of values and customs and use appropriate body language. You also need to consider food, religious and spiritual preferences.

When you are communicating with people from a CALD background, use simple language and gestures or, if needed, make use of interpreters. Do not use family members or non-professional interpreters unless in an emergency situation. Interpreters are an important resource in providing a voice for patients whose English is not fluent.

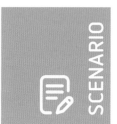

Culturally appropriate communication with Mrs Wei

Mrs Wei, a recent Chinese immigrant, has a history of restlessness and feeling on edge. These episodes occur without warning and last a few minutes. Through a translator, she describes symptoms of being easily fatigued, having difficulty concentrating, and muscle tension and sleep disturbance. In recognising Mrs Wei's cultural background, the mental health worker asks if she is using any herbs or alternative medicines. This is important because some herbs or alternative medicines may contain stimulants or ginseng that can cause or exacerbate anxiety. By being culturally competent, the mental health worker can assist the team to accurately diagnose Mrs Wei's disorder and provide appropriate treatment.

1   What does cultural competence mean in this scenario?
2   What other reasons make it important for the healthcare team to know if Mrs Wei is taking alternative medicines?

Aboriginal and Torres Strait Islander cultures

Aboriginal and Torres Strait Islander people understand mental health within a broad context of health and wellbeing. Sometimes, symptoms of mental illness are understood as part of a person's spirit or personality and not seen as a form of treatable mental illness. It is common for the experiences of Aboriginal and Torres Strait Islander peoples (seeing spirits or hearing the voices of deceased ones) to be misdiagnosed as mental illness, and fear of this misdiagnosis can be a strong barrier to seeking help. When help is sought, some Aboriginal and Torres Strait Islander communities will involve a senior female family member rather than a parent. The healthcare team needs to ensure that they involve families, Aboriginal and Torres Strait Islander mental health workers, a respected Elder or community liaison officer to help build trusting relationships so that the affected individual can develop feelings of purpose, belonging and achievement.

Muslim culture

Muslims believe that mental illness can develop either from natural causes or spiritual illness and that both traditional and Western methods of treatment can be used together because they complement each other. However, members of the Muslim community are often reluctant to access mental health services. This can be due to negative experiences in their country of origin, where they have witnessed or experienced the stigma and discrimination that results from a lack of awareness and understanding of mental illness. The healthcare team can access imams and other religious scholars as the first point of contact for members of the Muslim community who are seeking support with mental health issues (eCALD, 2012).

ACTIVITY 13.2

Multicultural youth

Young people from different ethnic backgrounds, whether they were born in Australia or overseas, can feel caught between two sets of cultural standards and values.

1   Discuss this statement in relation to the mental health challenges that these people face.

2   How can schools and teachers support these young people?

3   How has society in general embraced multiculturalism?

4   Identify online support services that can assist youth with mental health issues.

Support the person to understand and exercise their rights

A person with mental health issues has a right to direct their own recovery. They have rights to social inclusion, equity and access to services, and information that enables them to accept and understand their health condition. This information needs to support them to effectively manage their mental health condition, make healthcare choices and interact with a variety of services. The healthcare team empowers the individual to determine their self-care needs by giving them the autonomy to make these decisions.

Autonomy

This is the right of patients to make choices about their medical care without their healthcare provider trying to influence the decision. For the healthcare team, this means providing information about options, benefits and risks of treatments. The person with mental illness (or their advocate) should be encouraged to ask clarifying questions.

The healthcare team may need to choose between actions that support autonomy (freedom) and those that support safety. In legally defined situations that apply to mental health crises and emergencies, the healthcare team can select safety and make use of the legal options of restraints, medications or seclusion. Otherwise, autonomy means that the healthcare team should:

* inform patients about their care options and associated risks
* provide care in consultation with the person
* respect and accept decisions made by patients about their personal care
* maintain privacy and confidentiality of information.

Empowerment

Empowerment
Defined by the WHO as the 'process of taking control and responsibility for actions that have the intent and potential to lead to fulfilment of capacity'.

Empowerment has been defined by the WHO as the 'process of taking control and responsibility for actions that have the intent and potential to lead to fulfilment of capacity' (WHO, 2010). For individuals with a mental health issue, this means that they are entitled to participate in activities to support their wellbeing. To empower people with mental health issues who are receiving treatment or services, the healthcare team should:

* provide them with all healthcare options and give them the right to choose
* provide them with information regarding their rights

- allow them to participate jointly in their care planning
- maintain safety, dignity and respect for the patient when delivering services
- offer information regarding community-based services that minimise isolation; for example, self-help groups or a community recreation centre program.

Access and equity

All mental health services should aim to be accessible and responsive, with outcomes that are transparent for both the person and their carer/s. Health equity is achieved by removing unfair barriers that compromise a person's health. Health access focuses on fair resource distribution and availability. By working with other organisations, an equitable approach can be achieved for people with mental health issues. This includes:

- prioritising those in need to ensure access to services
- focusing health promotion initiatives on those with mental health issues
- using community initiatives to strengthen all aspects of the mental health community
- advocating to reduce social inequities.

Citizenship

Building a meaningful life through connections, care, work and security is a core part of an individual's recovery journey. It is also something that individuals with mental health issues are entitled to and strive for (see Figure 13.3). A person with a mental illness may have their rights affected by the degree to which they have been subject to stigma, discrimination and prejudice, and how this has affected them emotionally. Pursuing their rights as part of reclaiming citizenship is important for a person with mental health issues, as is their therapeutic relationship with the healthcare team.

FIGURE 13.3 Citizenship rights

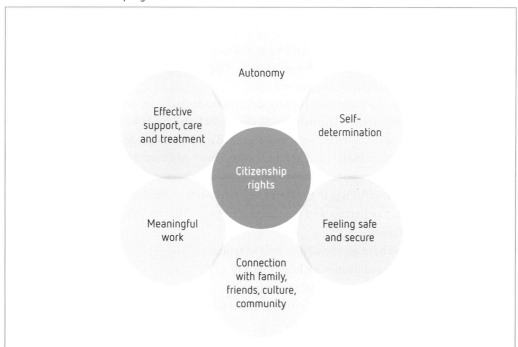

ACTIVITY 13.3

Strengthening patients' rights

Read Queensland Health's 2016 report *Connecting care to recovery 2016–2021* on the Queensland Health website (**https://www.health.qld.gov.au**).

Priority 5, strengthening patient's rights, has a focus on:
- contemporary mental health legislation
- supporting recovery of people with mental illness
- promoting and protecting the rights of people with mental illness.

Queensland Health, 2016, p. 24

1   What actions support this focus?

2   How is this being implemented?

Maintaining confidentiality and privacy

Normally, information about a person's care and treatment is confidential and requires consent before it is discussed. However, there are exceptional circumstances that do enable you to disclose private information, but this is generally only when you become aware that someone may be harmed. For example, if there are concerns that a person with mental health problems might hurt themselves, or pose a threat to another individual or group, confidentiality might need to be broken to ensure the safety of those concerned. Confidentiality might also need to be broken for the organisation to comply with its legal obligations. It is important for you to demonstrate respect for confidentiality and privacy while ensuring that risks are properly addressed and managed.

The Australian Department of Health (2010, p. 20) provides the following criteria that can be met to ensure privacy and confidentiality:

- service provider facilities having private interview rooms
- residents having space for personal possessions including a lockable wardrobe or drawers (accommodation services)
- patients being given information on admission about confidentiality and its limits
- confidentiality and its limits being covered during orientation for new staff, volunteers, contractors and students
- expectations of organisational behaviour being made clear – for example, workplace signs reminding staff that files must not be left on desks, that computer screens are to be turned off when not in use and not be visible to the public
- material such as posters and brochures on privacy and confidentiality should be displayed.

The various mental health Acts in the states and territories of Australia also allow for certain information to be given to a person who is a designated carer. This includes disclosing if the person with a mental illness:

- leaves the facility without permission or fails to return
- is transferred/discharged to another health facility
- is reclassified as a voluntary/involuntary patient
- is having an emergency surgical operation without their consent (under the *Mental Health Act 2007* [NSW]).

Informed consent

Informed consent means that the person understands the information and its consequences and is capable of making a decision without influence from others. An individual cannot give valid consent if they lack the capacity to make an informed decision. For a person with a mental health issue, their capacity to provide informed consent may fluctuate. When the healthcare team requires consent from a person with mental health issues, the following should be considered:

- information might need to be provided in different ways, depending on the individual's needs and mental state at the time
- what the consent applies to should also be made very clear – what information will be shared, with whom and how
- the need to avoid assumptions that consent provides a blanket approval for sharing information
- [individuals] have the right to change or retract their consent.

Consideration should also be given to the [individual] having the opportunity to nominate someone they trust to make decisions on their behalf if they are unable to give informed consent.

Australian Department of Health, 2010, p. 18

Informed consent
A person's voluntary decision to agree to healthcare intervention after accurate information has been given regarding choices.

Mental health legislation

There are a number of laws covering the whole of Australia that are of particular interest to people with mental health conditions. These include human rights, disability discrimination and privacy legislation. With regard to mental health legislation, there is a general lack of clarity in the various definitions of mental illness, resulting in every Australian state and territory having their own mental health Acts. However, the basic criteria for the admission and detention of voluntary and involuntary patients reflect the human rights principles set out by the United Nations in 1948 and are present in all legislation. Overall, mental health laws are intended to protect individuals and others from the consequences of mental illness, and to provide a framework for the provision of services and practice.

United Nations Principles for the Protection of Persons with Mental Illness and the Improvement of Mental Health Care

These principles, adopted by the United Nations in 1991, identify the rights of people with mental illness in health care. There are sections on informed consent, confidentiality, standard of care and treatment, and the rights available to people in mental health and disability facilities.

Mental health Acts – Australia and New Zealand

The main purpose of these Acts is to define the circumstances in which compulsory measures can be taken by mental health services to treat a person where illness has impaired their capacity to direct their care.

The principles that underpin these Acts (RANZCP, 2017) include:

- a commitment to recovery-oriented practice
- responding to the culture of patients and providing culturally-informed care
- Utilising supported decision-making through involvement and assistance from people close to the individual

- Applying the least restrictive alternative by placing a duty on health members to seek effective treatment in the community, and to do everything practicable to provide treatment on a voluntary basis.
- ensuring that treatments are appropriate and the autonomy and dignity of patients is respected.

Australian Human Rights Commission Act 1986

The *Australian Human Rights Commission Act 1986* promotes an understanding and acceptance of human rights in Australia. The commission is empowered to handle discrimination complaints covered by Commonwealth anti-discrimination legislation. These include discrimination on the basis of age; race, colour or nationality; religion; sex; pregnancy; marital status; national extraction or social origin; medical or criminal record; physical, mental, intellectual or psychiatric disability or impairment; sexual preference; political opinion; or trade union activity.

Disability Discrimination Act 1992

The *Disability Discrimination Act 1992* provides protection for everyone in Australia against discrimination based on disability. 'Disability' under this Act includes mental illness. The Act makes it unlawful to discriminate against a person because they have a disability in areas of public life including 'work; accommodation; education; access to premises, clubs and sport; the provision of goods, services, facilities and land; and the administration of Commonwealth law and programs' (Part 1.3) subject to certain exceptions and defences.

Privacy Act 1988

The *Privacy Act 1988* sets out the privacy principles that apply to the collection, retention, use and disclosure of personal information and access to personal information held by the Commonwealth public sector and the private sector. This includes health information and records that may be collected as part of an individual's admission into a health facility.

Records management

The Australian Privacy Principles (APP) are contained in the *Privacy Act 1988* and outline how organisations must handle, use and manage personal information that is collected from and about a patient. This can include:

Individual service plans

Plans that set out goals and strategies and explain the support provided by each member of the healthcare team, as well as who is responsible for what and when.

- individual service plans
- assessment records
- personal records
- referrals.

The following principles are relevant to health record management:

- APP 11 – Security of personal information – reasonable steps must be taken to protect personal information from misuse, interference and loss, and from unauthorised access, modification or disclosure. An entity has obligations to destroy or de-identify personal information in certain circumstances (Office of the Australian Information Commissioner, 2019a).

- APP 12 – Access to personal information – this outlines obligations for when an individual requests to be given access to personal information held about them by the entity. This includes a requirement to provide access unless a specific exception applies (Office of the Australian Information Commissioner, 2019b).

Individuals are granted access to their own records in accordance with Commonwealth, state and territory legislation. Access can be restricted in some circumstances and is only permitted after careful consideration. Denial of access should be explained to the person in a way that is appropriate to their personal circumstances.

Legal orders – Community Treatment Orders

A **Community Treatment Order (CTO)** is a legal order made by the Mental Health Review Tribunal or by a magistrate. It sets out the terms under which a person must accept medication and therapy, counselling, management, rehabilitation and other services while living in the community. It is implemented by a mental health facility that has developed an appropriate treatment plan for the individual person.

Mental Health Review Tribunal, 2018

13.4 ACTIVITY

Research CTOs and answer the following questions:

1   What happens when a person breaches a CTO?
2   Who can apply for a CTO?
3   How does the tribunal decide on a CTO application?
4   When does a CTO come to an end?

2   DETERMINE THE NEEDS OF PEOPLE WITH MENTAL HEALTH ISSUES

Once a supportive relationship is developed with the client, it is easier to work with them in determining their needs. An understanding of mental health disorders will assist in determining these needs so that strategies to support empowerment with recovery-orientated practice can be made in a safe and dignified manner. When you are gathering information, it is important to maintain privacy and confidentiality and to ensure that consent has been given.

Gather and interpret information

To fully determine the needs of the person with a mental health condition, the healthcare team must first gather information so that they gain a clearer understanding of the issues. Accuracy in obtaining and interpreting the information assists with assessing the situation, the level of immediacy and the interventions. This can be achieved by:

- observing and documenting the person's mental and emotional state
- responding appropriately to signs of distress
- actively listening and questioning – this can determine personal circumstances and support networks
- obtaining and documenting information from other sources; for example, family, friends and/or a general practitioner (GP) can identify strengths and weaknesses in the person and their ability to cope with their own needs.

Community Treatment Order

Sets out the terms under which a person must accept medication and therapy, counselling, management, rehabilitation and other services while living in the community.

Recovery-orientated practice

Sets of capabilities that support people to recognise and take responsibility for their own recovery and wellbeing and to define their goals, wishes and aspirations.

The patient's needs can range from activities of daily living (ADLs) to participation in self-help groups. Questioning the patient and their family can determine if they can manage shopping, meals, finances, medication and appointments. By interpreting the symptoms displayed by the patient, and collecting information from a variety of sources, a picture of their mental state is revealed and will guide the support required.

Signs and symptoms of common mental health disorders

Mental health disorders include conditions such as anxiety, depressive disorders and substance misuse disorders, as well as more severe conditions such as schizophrenia, personality and bipolar disorders. Mental illnesses vary in severity, with some being transitory and some requiring long-term support. The following section describes signs and symptoms of common mental health disorders. An understanding of these symptoms can assist in determining support needs and the development of a mental health recovery plan for the individual.

Anxiety disorders

'An anxiety disorder is a medical condition characterised by persistent, excessive worry' (SANE Australia, 2018). This can be so distressing that it interferes with a person's ability to carry out daily activities. A person with an anxiety disorder will feel distressed a lot of the time for no apparent reason. Symptoms may include:

- persistent, excessive or unrealistic worries (generalised anxiety disorder)
- compulsions and obsessions which they can't control (obsessive compulsive disorder)
- intense and excessive worry about social situations (social anxiety disorder)
- panic attacks (panic disorder)
- an intense, irrational fear of everyday objects and situations (phobia).

Other symptoms of anxiety disorders may include: a pounding heart, difficulty breathing, upset stomach, muscle tension, sweating or choking, feeling faint or shaky.

SANE Australia, 2018

Depressive disorders

Depressive disorders significantly affect the way someone feels, causing a persistent lowering of mood. Depression is more than just feeling sad. It lasts longer than a bout of sadness, causes more distress and disruption to life, and is less likely to go away without treatment. Symptoms (Reach Out, 2019c) include:

- low moods
- loss of interest and motivation
- loss of pleasure in activities
- negative thoughts
- changes to sleep patterns, appetite and energy levels.

Bipolar disorder

Individuals with bipolar disorder 'experience serious extremes of mood, to the point where the moods interfere with everyday life'. Someone with bipolar disorder will experience mood changes between manic and depressed episodes. They can become high, over-excited and reckless; or extremely low, feeling helpless and depressed, and have difficulty making decisions or concentrating (Reach Out, 2019b).

When experiencing a manic episode, it is common to feel or experience:
- extreme happiness
- increased energy
- racing thoughts
- irritability
- reduced need to sleep
- increased sexual activity.

When experiencing a depressed episode, it is common to feel or experience:
- lack of interest in all activities
- changes in appetite
- weight loss or gain
- changes in sleeping patterns
- loss of energy
- inability to concentrate.

Schizophrenia

Schizophrenia is a mental illness that affects the way the brain functions by interfering with a person's ability to think, feel and act. Psychotic symptoms (Lifepath Psychology, 2017) may include:
- confused thinking; difficulty concentrating or remembering
- delusions – thinking things are happening that are not
- hallucinations – seeing, hearing, feeling, smelling or tasting things that are not real
- mood swings or changes in feelings (may be sudden)
- abnormal motor behaviour – it affects some individuals by making them more agitated, or by making them withdraw or become childlike, or by making it hard to do everyday tasks and live their life effectively.

Personality disorder

People affected by borderline personality disorder frequently experience distressing emotional states. This causes them to have intense emotions, and they find it difficult to relate and interact with other people and their environment, making everyday life difficult and distressing for them. Symptoms (Reach Out, 2019a) may include:
- deep feelings of insecurity
- unstable relationships
- continually seeking reassurance, even for small things
- difficulty coping with fear of abandonment and loss
- impulsiveness resulting in self-harm (e.g., cutting, burning, or abuse of alcohol or drugs) or attempts at suicide
- confused, contradictory feelings.

Treatments

Treatment includes all the different ways in which someone with a mental illness can get help to minimise the effects of the illness and promote recovery. Treatment for the milder forms of depression involves a combination of medication and psychological treatments, such as cognitive behaviour therapy and interpersonal psychotherapy. Treatment for other disorders includes a combination of psychological therapy, medication and community support.

The doctor and caseworker work with the patient, their family and advocates to determine their physical, pharmacological, psychological and social needs. Planning is then done to provide appropriate treatment for realistic outcomes.

ACTIVITY 13.5

Cognitive behaviour therapy

Cognitive behaviour therapy (CBT) is a type of psychotherapy that can help the person to change unhelpful or unhealthy habits of thinking, feeling and behaving.

Research CBT and answer the following questions:

1 What types of conditions can CBT treat?

2 What strategies does CBT utilise?

3 What complementary treatments can be used alongside CBT?

4 What are the benefits of CBT?

5 How long does CBT take?

6 Who can provide CBT?

Strategies and services that support recovery

Recognising that self-determination and empowerment are vital parts of successful treatment and recovery is important for a person with mental illness. To ensure that a program is developed with goals that assist the patient to recover, it must identify their strengths and weaknesses and their ability to address their own needs. It must also utilise family and community mental health services as support networks. Recovery-orientated practice, early intervention and a holistic approach are strategies that support this empowerment and recovery.

Community mental health services
Services and teams that deliver care outside of inpatient settings.

Early intervention
Responding early in the course of a mental health disorder or illness, and early in an episode of illness, to reduce the risk of escalation.

Recovery-orientated practice

Recovery-orientated mental health practice means supporting patients to recognise and take responsibility for their own recovery and wellbeing, and to define their goals, wishes and aspirations. The Department of Health defines *recovery-orientated practice* as mental health care that:

- recognises and embraces the possibilities for recovery and wellbeing created by the inherent strength and capacity of all people experiencing mental health issues
- maximises self-determination and self-management of mental health and wellbeing
- assists families to understand the challenges and opportunities arising from their family member's experiences.

Australian Health Ministers Advisory Council, 2013, p. 3

Staff who work in multidisciplinary teams providing recovery-orientated practice have the positive expectation and commitment that patients will move to less restrictive environments along their pathway to recovery. Through the combination of services, treatments and supports, awareness of trauma-informed care and the elimination of discrimination, a recovery-orientated culture within mental health services can be achieved. This is supported by the practice domains of the 2013 National Mental Health Strategy (see Figure 13.4).

FIGURE 13.4 Recovery-orientated practice domains

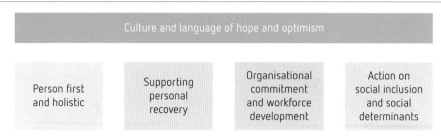

Domain 1: Promoting a culture and language of hope and optimism
* A service culture and language that makes a person feel valued, important, welcome and safe, communicates positive expectations and promotes hope and optimism – this is central to recovery-orientated practice and service delivery

Domain 2: Person first and holistic
* Putting people who experience mental health issues first and at the centre of practice and service delivery; viewing a person's life situation holistically

Domain 3: Supporting personal recovery
* Personally defined and led recovery at the heart of practice rather than an additional task

Domain 4: Organisational commitment and workforce development
* Service and work environments and an organisational culture that are conducive to recovery and to building a workforce that is appropriately skilled, equipped, supported and resourced for recovery-orientated practice

Domain 5: Action on social inclusion and the social determinants of health, mental health and wellbeing
* Upholding the human rights of people experiencing mental health issues and challenging stigma and discrimination; advocating to address the poor and unequal living circumstances that adversely impact on recovery

Source: A national framework for recovery-oriented mental health services – Guide for practitioners and providers, © Commonwealth of Australia 2013, pp. 4, 10, Reproduced with permission.

Recovery-orientated mental health practice (see Figure 13.5) is achieved by the following:

1   Uniqueness of the individual:
* recognising that recovery is not necessarily about cure but is about having opportunities for choices and living a meaningful, satisfying and purposeful life, and being a valued member of the community
* accepting that recovery outcomes are personal and unique for each individual and go beyond an exclusive health focus to include an emphasis on social inclusion and quality of life
* empowering individuals so they recognise that they are at the centre of the care they receive.

2   Real choices:
* supporting and empowering individuals to make their own choices about how they want to lead their lives and acknowledges choices need to be meaningful and creatively explored
* supporting individuals to build on their strengths and take as much responsibility for their lives as they can

FIGURE 13.5 Recovery-orientated practice

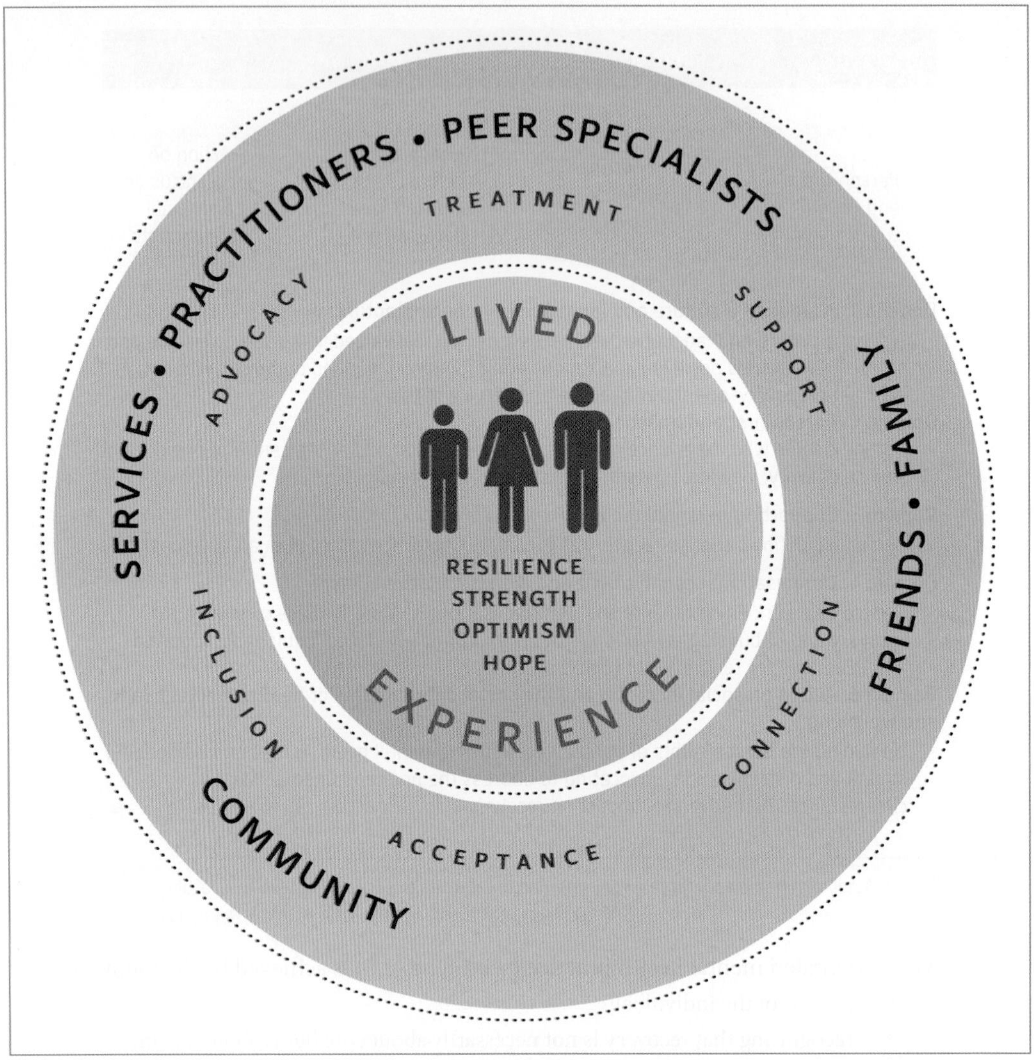

Source: A national framework for recovery-oriented mental health services – Guide for practitioners and providers, © Commonwealth of Australia 2013, p. 12. Reproduced with permission.

- • ensuring that there is a balance between duty of care and support for individuals to take positive risks and make the most of new opportunities.
3 Attitudes and rights:
  - • listening to, learning from and acting upon communications from the individual and their carers about what is important to the individual
  - • promoting and protecting an individual's legal, citizenship and human rights
  - • supporting individuals to maintain and develop social, recreational, occupational and vocational activities which are meaningful to them
  - • instilling hope in an individual about their future and ability to live a meaningful life.
4 Dignity and respect:
  - • being courteous, respectful and honest in all interactions
  - • displaying sensitivity and respect for each individual, especially for their values, beliefs and culture

- challenging discrimination wherever it exists within our own services or the broader community.

5 Partnership and communication:
- acknowledging that each individual is an expert on their own life and that recovery involves working in partnership with individuals and their carers to provide support in a way that makes sense to them
- sharing relevant information and the need to communicate clearly
- working in positive and realistic ways with individuals and their carers to help them realise their own hopes, goals and aspirations.

6 Evaluating recovery:
- ensuring and enabling continuous evaluation at several levels
- ensuring individuals and their carers can track their own progress
- services demonstrating that they use the individual's experiences of care to inform quality improvement activities
- reporting on key outcomes that indicate recovery. These outcomes include housing, employment, education, social and family relationships, health and wellbeing.

Australian Department of Health, 2010, pp. 8–9

Trauma-informed recovery-orientated approach

An understanding of trauma is part of a recovery-orientated approach. Many people living with mental health conditions have experienced trauma in their lives and it may be a factor in their emotions and relationships with others. A trauma-informed recovery-orientated approach is person-centred and involves being sensitive to individuals' particular needs, preferences, safety and wellbeing.

Early intervention

Early intervention is the process of providing intervention and support to a person who is experiencing any of the early symptoms of mental illness. It can help in preventing or reducing the progress of a mental illness and improving a person's community participation and outcomes into the future. Prompt diagnosis of the mental illness in its initial stages and implementing treatment can lead to:
- improved diagnosis and treatment
- more timely and targeted referrals to specialist services
- improved confidence and engagement of primary care providers.

The primary healthcare sector is ideally placed to identify mental health problems at their early stages. There are well-known risk factors, predispositions, assessments and screening programs for mental health that can be used to identify people who require early intervention.

Holistic approach

A holistic approach addresses all parts of the individual, not just the physical aspect of a person where displayed illnesses are most apparent. Utilising psychological, pharmacological and community supports, and ensuring the individual maintains a healthy lifestyle, contribute to a person's recovery goals and aspirations.

Psychological

Psychotherapy can help many people affected by mental illnesses, especially anxiety disorders, depression and personality disorders. A doctor, psychologist or other health professional talks with the person about their symptoms and concerns, and discusses new ways of thinking about managing them. These treatments help by giving the person an opportunity to talk about their thoughts and feelings, in order to understand why they think and feel in that way, and to adapt these feelings to bring about helpful and positive results.

Pharmacological

Some people with mental illness are helped by taking medication over a short term; others may need it on an ongoing basis. Medications help the brain to restore its usual chemical balance, so that the symptoms are reduced or even eliminated. It is important that the particular medication and dose is suited to help the person most effectively, and that side effects are monitored and minimised.

Community

Community development and education provides support for the person with a mental illness through social inclusion and access to resources. Community programs offer a broad range of activities to help the person identify and build on internal strengths and skills. These include a healthy lifestyle, skills development, culturally appropriate support services, employment and emotional support.

Healthy lifestyle

People who experience mental health problems frequently have poorer physical health outcomes than the general population. By improving physical health, recovery from mental illness can be enhanced. This can be achieved by working collaboratively with primary care providers to improve physical health outcomes. A healthy lifestyle includes:

* ensuring the person gets adequate sleep and eats a healthy diet
* reducing stress
* using physical activity to relax
* reducing alcohol consumption
* maintaining relationships with family and friends.

ACTIVITY 13.6

Health promotion and prevention

Treatment interventions alone cannot reduce the burden of mental disorder, so the implementation of promotion and preventative strategies are important in reducing the impact of mental illness on a person.

1 Identify initiatives that have been taken to progress mental health promotion.

2 Identify early intervention strategies that aim to reduce or prevent the long-term impact of mental health disorders.

3 What benefits can early intervention have on the affected person and significant others?

Avoid imposing your values and attitudes

All individuals should be treated with respect and have the right to hold values and beliefs. A person's wellbeing is related to their ability to express their identity and preferences. Once these are determined, it then becomes possible to provide the necessary support and assistance. This can be in the form of treatment options, social engagement or services. This may be delivered by your facility or another provider who can best accommodate the person's needs.

You can support expression of identity and preferences by:

- providing options so that the person can choose what is best for their needs
- actively encouraging the person in their own care
- respecting alternative viewpoints
- working ethically and professionally at all times
- encouraging activities to support expression of identity; for example, music and art.

It is important not to impose your own values or attitudes because this can negatively affect the working relationship and outcomes for the person. Try to understand the person's perspective without being judgemental. By responding with sensitivity, you demonstrate respect for their needs. Mental health practitioners are expected to understand, reflect on and use their own values and beliefs in a positive way at work.

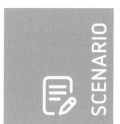

Supporting Mary's identity and values

Mary, aged 55 years, has been admitted with a diagnosis of depression. She is teary and has not been sleeping well. Her notes describe a loss of interest in work and leisure activities and she has been unable to function at work.

As the HSA assigned to her today, you begin your shift by introducing yourself and encouraging Mary to attend to her personal hygiene. You ask her preferences for when she would like to shower and what clothes she would like to wear. You take time and do not rush Mary when interacting with her; instead you are patient and show a sense of empathy. You encourage her to understand that feeling good often starts with caring about yourself.

By praising her strengths and recognising the accomplishment of her ability to attend to her personal hygiene, you can help her to improve her feelings about herself. By using open-ended questions, you can also encourage her to verbalise her feelings and worries. In this way you are developing trust and a therapeutic relationship with Mary.

1   How can giving Mary personal autonomy and a positive sense of self impact on other areas of her life?
2   Why is forming a therapeutic relationship important for Mary and the HSA?

Identify duty of care and dignity of risk

You have a duty of care to those you support by not being negligent in exposing them to avoidable risk. You have an obligation to report work health and safety concerns that could affect yourself, your colleagues or the person you are providing care for. Any hazard that can affect a person's health and safety should be identified and assessed for risk so it can be addressed. Strategies must take into account duty of care and maximising choice with dignity of risk.

Duty of care

The concept of duty of care ensures that you do not perform any acts that could harm others, or that your own inactions do not result in harm. If there is a belief that the person with a mental health disorder poses a health and safety concern, you have a duty of care to respond and take action to prevent and/or minimise any risk. Failure to do so can result in negligence. It is important that you know what your scope of practice is, so that you can provide a reasonable standard of care to protect the patient.

SCENARIO

Implementing duty of care

Jonathan, aged 35 years, was diagnosed with schizophrenia 10 years ago. He has been admitted to the mental health facility after an episode of unusual behaviour. While you are looking after him today, he confides that he does not want to take his medication any more because he does not like the side effects. He tells you that as soon as he is discharged, he will stop taking the tablets.

As the HSA, you have a duty of care to inform your supervisor of these comments. In this way you are taking action to prevent or minimise risk to Jonathan's health and safety because his decision may lead to further harm.

1   What actions might the mental health team take to educate Jonathan about the importance of taking his medication regularly?
2   What does 'duty of care' mean in this scenario?

Risk assessment versus dignity of risk

When caring for a person with a mental health issue, there may be some degree of risk; however, this should be measured against dignity of risk. This means respecting each individual's autonomy and self-determination (or 'dignity') to make choices for themselves, even though they may contain some degree of risk. As long as precautions are taken to assess and minimise the risk, it may be acceptable to allow the individual to make a choice. In a mental health context, risk assessment means:

1   identify the risk – identify internal and external clinical risks that may pose a threat to the facility, team and/or patient
2   analyse and evaluate the risk – undertake a systematic analysis to understand the nature of risk and to identify any further action
3   treat the risks – identify the range of options to treat risks, assess the options, prepare risk treatment plans and implement them using available resources
4   review the measures.
    Communication and consultation are vital throughout all of these stages.

In considering dignity of risk, use common sense and respect the individual's rights. The person with mental health issues needs to be able to understand the risks and accept responsibility for the risks, as long as they will not result in harm or injury. By utilising family, community and professionals to give the person information regarding their choices, they can make an informed decision about their health and wellbeing. In supporting dignity of risk, consider that the decision:

*   respects the person's values and preferences
*   maximises the person's connection with family, support networks and community
*   enhances the person's self-esteem
*   offers opportunities for a person to learn new skills and maximise their potential.

Managing risk in community integration

The process of managing risk must promote an environment of safety and support for individuals while advocating independence and self-direction.

Twenty-four-year-old Joseph suffers from anxiety disorder. His goal is to take basic computer classes at the local community college. Joseph completed Year 10 at school but did not pass his exams because he had difficulty concentrating. He has been unemployed since leaving school and is on social security benefits. He lives at home with his parents and occasionally goes to a club with his father to play snooker. The community college is four blocks from his home.

Complete the risk assessment tool for Joseph, using the above information:

13.7 ACTIVITY

SKILLS REQUIRED	GETTING TO CLASS ON TIME	ABILITY TO USE COMPUTER	SUPPORT FROM FAMILY TO GET TO CLASS	APPROPRIATE CONVERSATION SKILLS	ABILITY TO COMPLETE HOMEWORK
Identified risks					
Likelihood and frequency of risk					
Severity of risk					
Is the risk worth taking?					

3 WORK WITH PEOPLE WITH MENTAL HEALTH ISSUES TO MEET THEIR NEEDS AND GOALS

When working to meet a person's needs and goals, it is important to collaborate with the entire healthcare team, the person and their support network. By using a person-centred approach, you will reinforce the person's rights and empower them to assist in their self-direction. A case manager can assist to develop a service delivery plan to outline the person's needs and goals. This includes community support programs to integrate the person back to society. This can be amended as the support needs change and particularly if the person experiences a crisis situation. As an HSA, it is important to refer any unusual behaviour to your supervisor or to the care network.

Provide support while upholding the person's rights

Providing ongoing care and support for someone who is living with a mental illness can involve many different support organisations. These may include psychologists, GPs, psychiatrists, psychiatric nurses or other community care providers. They are all part of the healthcare team, who work together to provide the person with mental illness with the best level of care possible.

Person-centred approach

Collaboration is a vital component of a person-centred approach. It empowers the person by encouraging them to develop an understanding of what they want and need, and supports them to make decisions and choices to control all aspects of their lives. A person-centred approach shifts the balance of power to give people with mental illness, their families and carers greater control over the supports and services they access.

A person may not be able to make informed life choices during a period of acute illness; however, during recovery, opportunities exist to shape decisions, often with guidance from family members and carers. People discharged from hospital after a period of severe mental illness are likely to need a range of supports and services. In addition to needing clinical treatment, a person may face challenges including eviction, loss of job, a lack of money to pay bills or child-related issues at school. A person-centred approach to planning at discharge ensures that these challenges are identified and a range of supports and services are put in place to address such needs.

Case management

Case management is a type of community mental health service that is used to provide ongoing management for people with mental health issues. The role of the case manager is to undertake assessment, monitoring, planning, advocacy and linking of the individual with rehabilitation and support services. This can assist with illness management and relapse prevention. Case meetings are convened during the management process whereby key decisions are made relating to the individual's needs. This ensures that everyone is clear about the purpose, intent and direction of the intervention. Principles of effective case management include the following:

- Case managers should deliver as much of the 'help' or service as possible.
- Landlords, employers, teachers, art clubs and so on are primary partners in care solutions.
- When individuals are working in the community, case managers should ensure that all parties are aware of the patient's care plan.
- Both individual and team case management can be used.
- Case managers have primary responsibility for a person's services.
- Case managers should be experienced and fully accredited.
- Case load size should be small enough to allow for a relatively high frequency of contact.
- Case management service should not be time limited.
- Access to familiar people should be available around the clock, every day.
- Case managers should foster choice.

SCENARIO

Case management for Martin

Martin is a 27-year-old who has recently been discharged from the army on medical grounds. During his service, Martin experienced high levels of stress and anxiety. He has coped with this by drinking heavily and has been diagnosed with post-traumatic stress disorder (PTSD) and alcohol dependency.

The case manager develops an understanding of Martin and his condition and helps him to develop a plan with goals to enable him to build strategies and a resource network to access for support. This includes behavioural therapy to teach him to tolerate stress and medication to alleviate anxiety. The case manager provides contacts for an alcohol rehabilitation (Alcoholics Anonymous; AA) program, which includes counselling. Ongoing support is provided through regular sessions and referral to a local community health clinic.

Over a number of months, Martin achieves progress with his AA group and starts to use the behavioural strategies effectively. He realises that his improvement will have its ups and downs, but that with assistance from the support networks he can make progress towards tolerating stress without having to escape through the use of alcohol.

1 Why is it important for Martin to maintain a relationship with his case manager in the early stages of his road to recovery?
2 What is the benefit of referring Martin to a local community health clinic?
3 Why is it important for Martin to attend regular sessions of AA?

Community support programs

Support programs are important for people with mental health conditions, and they must be combined with understanding and acceptance by the community. Community support programs include:

- peer support
- family and carer respite and supported accommodation services
- harm reduction and personalised support programs
- supported employment programs
- clubhouses.

The support these provide may include health information; accommodation; help with finding suitable work, training and education; psychosocial rehabilitation; and mutual support groups.

Peer support

Peer support refers to support from a person who has knowledge of a particular condition from their own experiences. Social isolation is a concern for people with mental health conditions and this support can allow the person to form trusting relationships to overcome this seclusion. It supplements and enhances other healthcare services by providing emotional, social and practical assistance to manage a person's illness so that they stay healthy.

Respite and supported accommodation services

Planned respite services provide a short-term change in environment for a person with a mental illness, and a break for carers. Supported accommodation services provide long-term psychosocial rehabilitation support in a residential setting to people with psychiatric disability.

Harm reduction and personalised support programs

Harm reduction programs include needle and syringe provision and safe places for intoxicated people. Personalised support programs help people to identify and meet their personal goals; for example, housing, employment and education. Through building the capacity of these programs and improving coordination, individuals will be supported to remain at lower risk of harm in an environment that is best suited to their needs.

Supported employment programs

These programs help people with mental illness to locate jobs that match their strengths and interests. Once employment is found, these programs provide continuous support to overcome obstacles and succeed in the workplace. A partnership is developed between the employer, mental healthcare providers and the person with mental illness. This team then helps individuals identify goals and work towards achieving them.

Clubhouse

These are local community centres that provide individuals with opportunities to build long-term relationships that, in turn, support them in obtaining employment, education and housing (see Figure 13.6). This gives the individual hope and opportunities to achieve their full potential.

FIGURE 13.6 Clubhouse

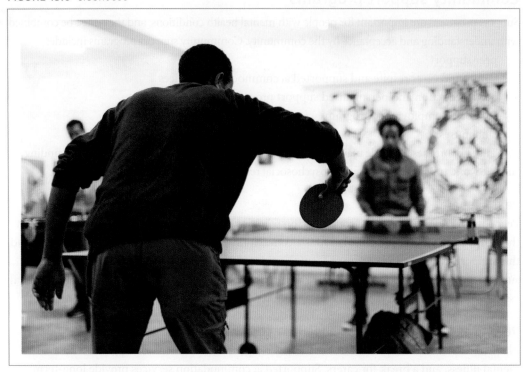

Source: Alamy Stock Photo/Chris Bull

The staff have generalist roles and are involved in activities including daily work duties, social and recreational programs, employment programs, outreach, supported education and community support programs. The staff engage with individuals and encourage them so that they can sufficiently recover from the effects of mental illness to become integrated into society.

ACTIVITY 13.8

Psychosocial rehabilitation

Psychosocial rehabilitation services provide structured activities ranging from specific skill development to creative pursuits. These facilitate the optimal recovery of the individual in the community.

1   Complete the following table to identify the benefits of undertaking these activities:

ACTIVITY	BENEFITS
Financial counselling	
Fitness and exercise regimens	
Recreational activities	
Parenting support	
Stress management	
Basic life skills training	
Drug and alcohol management programs	
Relationship counselling	

2   Discuss why the following criteria are considered to be important when a person with a mental illness undertakes these programs:

    a   include the objective of increased responsibility on the part of the individual

    b   be structured, with clearly defined goals and outcomes

    c   be closely monitored, with regular reporting

    d   be implemented over a short period.

Adapt services to meet specific needs and requirements

Service delivery needs for a person with mental health issues vary according to the individual. As such, planning should indicate the level of support and the responsibilities expected from each member of the healthcare team. The unique strengths and needs of the person experiencing mental health problems are the key focus of individualised planning, support and services. Documenting protocols and procedures can vary between organisations; however, each interaction with an individual should be documented so that care improvements can be discussed and legal requirements met.

Individual service plans

Individual service plans are a written summary of the goals and strategies for an individual with mental health issues and are compiled by the person and the healthcare team. The plan explains the support provided by each member of the healthcare team and their responsibilities. It may also include what to do in the event of a crisis or to prevent relapse. The healthcare team, person and family work together to identify recovery options that best support the person's needs. This involves the coordination of services, including referrals, community support and any other service that can assist the person in their recovery, such as:

- inpatient or community care
- crisis treatment
- residential rehabilitation
- disability support.

Individual service plans should be reviewed regularly to make sure they continue to meet the person's needs. Significant changes will require a new service plan. A date for review should also be written into the service plan. Goals identified in service plans should be realistic enough to enable the individual to achieve them, but also be challenging. Loss of motivation can occur if the goals are unrealistic. When considering recovery strategies, the healthcare team must ensure that resources and support are available as required by the person. Some examples of recovery strategies include exercising, group therapy, professional services, nutrition and medication.

Goal-setting

Collaborative goal-setting can maximise the person's focus to achieve their potential. These goals should have objectives related to enhancing quality of life. The objectives can be broken down into a series of steps to make the goals more achievable.

Arnold Baker is 55 years old and suffers from depression. Since the loss of his wife two years ago he has had severe episodes where he has withdrawn from society. He lives in a hostel and has lost contact with his immediate family.

1   Identify realistic goals that Mr Baker may wish to achieve so that he can improve his quality of life.

2   Consider the skills and steps required to achieve each goal.

3   Consider the resources and support required for Mr Baker to reach his goals.

4   What challenges may Mr Baker face in attempting to reach his goals?

Respond to people experiencing distress or crisis

Crises are acute, time-limited events experienced as overwhelming emotional reactions to one's perception of an event. A mental health crisis is a behavioural, emotional or psychiatric response triggered by an event. If left untreated, it could result in an emergency situation, self-harm or significantly reduced levels of functioning in the person's ADLs.

When caring for someone with a mental illness, there may be times when crisis causes their health to deteriorate to a point where immediate support is required. This situation may be because they have developed suicidal thoughts or are perhaps so agitated that they may be a risk to others. In these emergency cases, the person must be removed from the situation. Physical restraint is a final response to an immediate danger situation when less restrictive measures fail. The challenge is to implement safety measures while maintaining the dignity of the individual.

Considerations when caring for people in crisis include:

- always seek help from your supervisor if you have concerns or if the management of the person is outside your scope of practice
- introduce yourself to the person and explain why you are present
- remain courteous and non-threatening, but be honest and direct
- listen to the person in a non-judgemental way
- avoid confrontation
- do not attempt to manhandle the person, except to prevent serious assault or suicide attempts
- if the incident was traumatic for you, or you feel anxious or distressed, debrief these issues at work, or seek professional help.

Western Australia Department of Health, 2009, p. 2

Your organisation should provide you with the training required to enable you to determine the degree of urgency and to take appropriate action to prevent escalation of the situation.

Self-harm

This may occur as 'an extreme way of trying to cope with distressing or painful feelings. Self-harm includes cutting, burning or hitting oneself, binge-eating or starvation, or putting oneself in dangerous situations. It can also involve abuse of drugs or alcohol' (SANE Australia, 2019). In many cases, self-harm is not intended to be fatal, but it should be taken seriously. In an acute care setting the healthcare team must provide constant supervision through close observation and document any changes clearly in the care plan. Care for these individuals includes:

- teaching them coping techniques that might help them to feel better
- providing positive distractions
- building a therapeutic relationship
- using professionals or agencies that can help the individual
- making the environment safe.

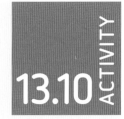

Signs of binge eating disorder

Binge eating disorder is a serious mental illness whereby the person eats large quantities of food rapidly and often when not hungry (Eating Disorders Victoria, 2016).

1   Research this disorder and list the psychological and physical signs that someone may be binge eating, apart from those that are obvious.

2   What treatment options are available for a person with this disorder?

Work within your limits making referrals

When you require assistance beyond your scope of practice, you must refer to your supervisor for support. This is also true when a facility cannot provide adequate services for the person with mental health needs. They can be referred to another agency. In some instances, external service providers are sourced because the facility does not have the necessary expertise to manage the person, or they do not have adequate resources to meet the needs of the person.

Specialist mental health services provide a high level of care for a particular field. Examples include:

- eating disorder clinics
- acute mental health wards
- specialist homelessness services
- psychiatric disability support services
- child and adolescent services
- allied psychological services.

As an HSA, you will not refer directly to external organisations; however, you can clarify that the person understands the reason for the referral and/or seek assistance from supervisors if the person needs more information. Give them as much information as possible about the referring service. This may be in the form of brochures or websites. Check with your facility's protocols regarding what documentation should accompany the person to their referring service.

ACTIVITY 13.11

Referrals

1 Develop a directory of referral services and/or organisations in your local area that could assist a person with a mental illness who is:

a homeless

b unemployed

c suicidal

d an Aboriginal or Torres Strait Islander

e a young person

f pregnant.

2 Provide details of the services provided and outline the referral criteria for individuals in these categories.

3 What is the referral protocol for someone who is an immediate threat to themselves, a family member or someone else's safety?

SUMMARY

In this chapter, you have learnt how to establish respectful relationships with people who have mental health issues. Communication plays a significant part in your development of this relationship. You will establish rapport to show respect, which gives the individual hope, trust and self-direction. As well as encouraging the individual to exercise their rights and express their own identity, your respect enhances the road to empowerment and recovery.

This chapter emphasised that by understanding mental health conditions and identifying the needs of people with mental health issues, supportive care strategies can be developed. Understanding that each individual has cultural, social and emotional differences assists with the development of care strategies. By collaborating with the individual, their family and their support networks, progress towards the person's goals is facilitated.

The last part of the chapter emphasised the importance of meeting the needs and aspirations of these individuals and, in particular, responding to people experiencing distress or crisis. By understanding your own abilities and limits, you can work as an integral member of your healthcare team to provide effective care, support and dignity to those who are experiencing mental health issues.

APPLY YOUR KNOWLEDGE

Recovery-orientated practice

As the HSA working in a community mental health centre, you have been assigned to Adrian, aged 43 years, who voluntarily visits the centre each six weeks to see the psychiatrist. Adrian was diagnosed with bipolar affective disorder when he was 22. He was hospitalised many times during his twenties, mostly when he was manic and became dangerous to himself and others.

Adrian married at age 31 and has two small children. He is generally well, although he has had two significant episodes of depression in the last few years, when he had to have time away from work. Adrian confides to you that prior to today's session, he has been having trouble sleeping and has had no energy or interest in spending time with his children or friends.

1   What is your duty of care when you hear this response from Adrian?

2   The HSA reports to the supervisor and in the patient notes in 'real time' during this shift. Using the knowledge you gained in Chapter 10, 'Provide non-client contact support in an acute care environment', what are the advantages of reporting in real time?

The psychiatrist will be using the recovery-orientated practice approach during the sessions with Adrian.

3   What is your understanding of recovery-orientated practice?

4   Why is it important to use a holistic approach regarding Adrian?

After the session, Adrian lets you know that he will be coming back in six weeks. He finds the sessions helpful in that they allow him to determine his pathway to recovery. This empowerment makes him feel valued and gives him optimism. He understands that it is a long process, but with continued support from the mental health team and the healthy lifestyle strategies he feels he may be able to have a meaningful and satisfying life with his family.

5   Discuss the importance of empowerment for Adrian and how the healthcare team can support this right.

6   What healthy lifestyle strategies could Adrian work on to improve his recovery goals?

7   Understanding the scope of your role as an HSA is essential to performing your role effectively within the healthcare team. How did the HSA demonstrate the scope of their role when working in the community mental health centre?

◄ REFLECTING ON THE INDUSTRY INSIGHT

1 The case study highlighted the importance of forming therapeutic relationships with clinic patients. Which action best describes a therapeutic relationship?
   a Giving the patient advice on how to cope with depression.
   b Commencing communication by selecting topics for discussion.
   c Sitting attentively in silence until the patient chooses to speak.
   d Halting the conversation when confronting issues come up.

2 How would you demonstrate cultural competence when looking after clients in an anxiety clinic?
   a Providing culturally appropriate activities.
   b Advising a client to visit with the social worker.
   c Giving the client a Bible to read.
   d Ordering standard meals to be delivered during the lunch break.

3 During the group therapy session, one client was very anxious. What would be the most appropriate response from the therapist?
   a Deny that the anxiety exists.
   b Recognise the anxiety and ask the client to elaborate.
   c Tell the client to ignore the anxious feelings and be stronger.
   d Accept that the client is anxious and prescribe medication.

SELF-CHECK QUESTIONS

1 Why is non-verbal communication important when developing a therapeutic relationship with a person who has mental health issues?

2 What are the best ways to communicate with people from a non-English-speaking background with mental health issues?

3 What does autonomy mean in the treatment of or services for people with mental health issues?

4 How does the *Disability Discrimination Act 1992* protect everyone against discrimination based on disability (including mental illness)?

5 During a manic episode, what feelings are commonly felt or experienced?

6 What is the difference between a delusion and a hallucination?

7 Describe examples of community support programs for people with mental health issues.

8 How can individual service plans assist with the treatment of a person with a mental health disorder?

9 What do you need to consider when caring for people who display signs of self-harm?

10 What are your definitions of the following key words and terms that have been used in this chapter?

KEY WORD OR TERM	YOUR DEFINITION
Stigma	
Self-determination	
Early intervention	
Personality disorder	
Individual service plans	
Bipolar disorder	
Community treatment order	
Community mental health services	

QUESTIONS FOR DISCUSSION

1   Why it is necessary to be aware of your own attitudes and beliefs when caring for a person with a mental health issue?

2   What do you think can be done to reduce the stigma and myths about mental illness?

3   Why is it important for the person with mental health issues to actively participate in their own recovery?

4   Read the Australian Government's *Vision 2030; Blueprint for Mental Health and Suicide Prevention* at the National Mental Health Commission website (**https://www.mentalhealthcommission.gov.au/**). Discuss the three focus areas for development at the local level that will make a difference to the effectiveness and sustainability of the mental health system.

5   The therapeutic community has been described as 'one of the most significant innovations in the history of psychiatry' (Mills & Harrison, 2007). Discuss.

EXTENSION ACTIVITY

Providing care for a person with a mental health disorder

Brian, an 85-year-old man, was admitted to the acute care facility with a medical diagnosis of congestive cardiac failure. His psychiatric diagnosis was paranoid schizophrenia and he has had numerous mental health admissions for this condition in the past.

The staff at the facility were inexperienced with psychiatric disorders and complained when Brian made inappropriate comments and had verbal outbursts. He demanded constant attention and screamed until someone came to see him. This made the other patients uncomfortable. Staff were unhappy because they did not have the time to spend with Brian and asked not to be assigned to him.

After a few days, Brian refused to get out of bed and stated that he wanted to go home. He became more withdrawn and uncooperative. The mental health assessment team was asked to assess Brian and suggest strategies to manage his behaviour. Their assessment recommended:

- staff education regarding mental health disorders and conflict resolution
- reassuring Brian and communicating so that his needs were met
- removing Brian from situations where he was disruptive to other patients
- rewarding Brian for good behaviour
- distracting Brian with diversional activities.

Cognitive behaviour therapy and person-centred care was initiated. As staff learnt more about Brian's condition and care, they responded more appropriately to him, and his inappropriate behaviour diminished.

Answer the following questions related to the strategies suggested by the mental health assessment team:

1 How could education and conflict resolution assist staff in caring for Brian?

2 Why is reassurance important for Brian?

3 How would you reward Brian's good behaviour?

4 What diversional activities would be appropriate for Brian?

5 How could you help the other staff to understand Brian's behaviour?

6 What discharge planning should be considered for Brian?

7 Form groups to practise your communication techniques for Brian, including reassurance, positive encouragement and conflict resolution.

8 Develop a care plan that outlines the strategies you have considered and present these to your colleagues.

REFERENCES

Australian Department of Health (2010). Implementation guidelines for non-government community services. Retrieved 17 October 2022 from https://www.health.gov.au/sites/default/files/documents/2021/04/national-standards-for-mental-health-services-2010-and-implementation-guidelines-implementation-guidelines-for-non-government-community-services.pdf

Australian Government (2019). *Disability Discrimination Act 1992*. Retrieved 17 October 2022 from https://www.legislation.gov.au/Series/C2004A04426

Australian Government, National Mental health Commission (2020). *Vision 2030; Blueprint for Mental Health and Suicide Prevention*. Retrieved 17 October 2022 from https://www.mentalhealthcommission.gov.au/getmedia/28fe94a6-ae18-47d3-bd62-ad8a048b8582/NMHC_Vision2030_ConsultationReport_March2020.pdf

Australian Health Ministers Advisory Council (2013). A national framework for recovery-oriented mental health services: Guide for practitioners and providers. https://www.health.gov.au/sites/default/files/documents/2021/04/a-national-framework-for-recovery-oriented-mental-health-services-guide-for-practitioners-and-providers.pdf

Department of Health, Victoria (2015) Culturally competent mental health care. Retrieved 4 June 2022 from https://www.health.vic.gov.au/rights-and-advocacy/culturally-competent-mental-health-care

Eating Disorders Victoria (2016). Binge-eating disorder. Retrieved 10 March 2019 from https://www.eatingdisorders.org.au/eating-disorders/binge-eating-disorder

eCALD (2012). Practical tips for working with Muslim mental health clients. Retrieved 17 October 2022 from https://www.ecald.com/assets/Resources/Assets/Toolkit-Muslim-MH-Clients.pdf

Embrace Multicultural Mental Health (2021). What is mental illness? Retrieved 24 October 2022 from https://www.embracementalhealth.org.au/sites/default/files/2021-04/English_mental.pdf

Lifepath Psychology (2017, 11 May). What is schizophrenia? Retrieved 17 October 2022 from https://lifepathpsychology.com.au/what-is-schizophrenia/

Mental Health Coordinating Council (2018). Recovery Oriented Language Guide 2E. Retrieved 5 June 2022 from http://www.mhcc.org.au/wp-content/uploads/2019/08/Recovery-Oriented-Language-Guide_2019ed_v1_20190809-Web.pdf

Mental Health First Aid (2008). Cultural considerations & communication techniques: Guidelines for providing mental health first aid to an Aboriginal or Torres Strait Islander person. Melbourne, VIC: Mental Health First Aid Australia and beyondblue, pp. 2–3. Retrieved 17 October 2022 from https://mhfa.com.au/sites/default/files/AMHFA_Cultural_guidelines_email_2012.pdf

Mental Health Review Tribunal (2018). Community Treatment Orders: Section 51, *Mental Health Act 2007*: What is a Community Treatment Order (CTO)? Retrieved 17 October 2022 from https://www.mhrt.nsw.gov.au/civil-patients/community-treatment-orders.html

Mills, J. & Harrison, T. (2007). John Rickman, Wilfred Ruprecht Bion, and the origins of the therapeutic community. *History of psychology*, 10(1), 22–43. Doi: 10.1037/1093-4510.10.1.22

New South Wales Government (2018). *Mental Health Act 2007 (NSW)*. Retrieved from https://www.legislation.nsw.gov.au/#/view/act/2007/8

Office of the Australian Information Commissioner (2019a). APP Guidelines Australian Privacy Principle 11 – Security of personal information. Retrieved 17 October 2022 from https://www.oaic.gov.au/privacy/australian-privacy-principles/read-the-australian-privacy-principles

Office of the Australian Information Commissioner (2019b). APP Guidelines Australian Privacy Principle 12 – Access to personal information. Retrieved from https://www.oaic.gov.au/privacy/australian-privacy-principles/read-the-australian-privacy-principles

Queensland Health (2016). Connecting care to recovery 2016–2021: A plan for Queensland's State-funded mental health, alcohol and other drug services. Retrieved 28 January 2019 from https://cabinet.qld.gov.au/documents/2016/Aug/CareRec/Attachments/Plan.PDF

Royal Australian and New Zealand College of Psychiatrists (RANZCP) (2017). Mental health legislation and psychiatrists: Putting the principles into practice. Retrieved 17 October 2022 from https://www.ranzcp.org/news-policy/policy-and-advocacy/position-statements/mental-health-legislation-and-psychiatrists-putti

Reach Out. (2019a). Borderline personality disorder. Retrieved 17 October 2022 from https://au.reachout.com/articles/borderline-personality-disorder

Reach Out (2019b). What is Bipolar disorder? Retrieved 17 October 2022 from https://au.reachout.com/articles/what-is-bipolar-disorder

Reach Out (2019c). What is depression? Retrieved 17 October 2022 from https://au.reachout.com/articles/what-is-depression

SA Health (2022). Myths and facts about mental illness. Retrieved 24 October 2022 from https://www.sahealth.sa.gov.au/wps/wcm/connect/public+content/sa+health+internet/healthy+living/healthy+mind/myths+and+facts+about+mental+illness#:~:text=Fact%3A%20A%20mental%20illness%20is%20not%20caused%20by,recover%20quickly%20and%20do%20not%20need%20-hospital%20care

SANE Australia (2014). *The SANE guide to reducing stigma: A guide to reducing stigma against mental illness and suicide in the media* (2nd edn). Retrieved 17 October 2022 from https://www.sane.org/images/PDFs/SANE-Guide-to-Reducing-Stigma.pdf

SANE Australia (2018). Anxiety disorder. Retrieved 16 June 2016 from https://www.sane.org/information-stories/facts-and-guides/anxiety-disorder

SANE Australia (2019). Self-harm. Retrieved 17 October 2022 from https://www.sane.org/information-and-resources/facts-and-guides/self-harm

Victorian Department of Health (2015). Recovery-oriented practice in mental health. Retrieved 24 October 2022 from https://www.health.vic.gov.au/practice-and-service-quality/recovery-oriented-practice-in-mental-health

Western Australia Department of Health (2009). Mental health first aid. https://www.health.wa.gov.au/

World Health Organization (WHO) (2010). User empowerment in mental health: A statement by the WHO Regional Office for Europe, p. 1. Retrieved 17 October 2022 from http://www.euro.who.int/__data/assets/pdf_file/0020/113834/E93430.pdf

World Health Organization (WHO) (2013). Stigma and discrimination. Retrieved 17 October 2022 from http://www.euro.who.int/en/health-topics/noncommunicable-diseases/mental-health/priority-areas/stigma-and-discrimination

PROVIDE SUPPORT TO PEOPLE LIVING WITH DEMENTIA

Learning objectives

By the end of this chapter, you should be able to:

1 provide support to those affected by dementia

2 use appropriate communication strategies

3 provide activities for maintenance of dignity, skills and health

4 implement strategies to minimise the impact of behaviours of concern

5 complete documentation

6 implement self-care strategies.

Introduction

This chapter describes the skills and knowledge required to provide person-centred care and support to those living with dementia. This involves following and contributing to an individual plan.

Supporting a person with dementia includes interpreting the individual plan and communicating appropriately by using verbal and non-verbal strategies to reassure and relieve distress. By providing activities that maintain the dignity and independence of the person, the health services assistant (HSA) can minimise the impact of behaviours of concern while ensuring the safety and comfort of the person balanced with autonomy and risk-taking. These strategies can minimise the impact of these behaviours and support the team in planning effective care.

Through effective reporting, recording and evaluation, the healthcare team can successfully manage and support the person with dementia as well as their family, carers and significant others.

This chapter will also inform you how to monitor your stress levels and use self-care strategies so that you can contribute effectively to maximise engagement of the person with dementia.

A person-centred approach for Dr Catherine

Today I am looking after Dr Catherine Croxton, who has moderate dementia. Dr Catherine was a specialist paediatrician and worked in one of the major city hospitals in the state.

I wake Dr Catherine up in the morning, introduce myself and help her to get everything ready for her wash and a change of clothes. I assist her and give her time to dress because she tends to become focused on the buttons, the fabric and the colours of the clothes that she wishes to wear, and she repeatedly folds and refolds the clothes. Distraction helps so I enquire about what she would like to eat. We eventually make our way to the breakfast table and greet the other residents. Dr Catherine likes to sit with others, but she has difficulty holding a conversation and is confused at times. I ask her simple questions, always refer to her as Dr Catherine and do not contradict her.

I have been able to gather quite a bit of information from Dr Catherine. Using a person-centred care approach I ask her questions about her working and home life. Sometimes she talks about caring for children and 'giving them medicines to make them better' and other times she talks about her late husband. Throughout the day Dr Catherine takes naps, looks at books or the television, or walks around the facility.

Sometimes I find the work of caring for people with dementia difficult and physically and emotionally tiring, but when I connect with Dr Catherine and get glimpses of her life by making her the focus of attention, I feel enormously satisfied and that I am making her life more enjoyable.

1 PROVIDE SUPPORT TO THOSE AFFECTED BY DEMENTIA

As our population ages, with more people living over the age of 85, the incidence of dementia increases. This disorder affects areas of the brain which control memory, recognition, communicating and behaviour. The common symptoms are progressive and can worsen over time and can also result in behaviours of concern. In supporting a person with dementia it is important to remember that these changes can cause anxiety and distress in the person, which is why a person-centred approach is needed to manage not just the physical but also the psychological needs of the person. This should be planned with the family and significant others in a stable and familiar environment that focuses on the person's specific needs and wants, while recognising and reporting if there are any signs of neglect or abuse.

Apply a person-centred care approach to the person living with dementia

A **person-centred approach** recognises that dementia is only one part of the person and helps to move the focus from the disease to the person's psychological and emotional needs. It aims to

> **Person-centred approach**
>
> Caring holistically for the person, which includes their preferences, needs and values, and those of their carers.

provide an environment that is both safe and supportive, and that affords high levels of dignity and respect for those living with dementia. By using the person-centred approach to dementia, you can ensure that the person living with dementia remains the focus rather than the illness, and that you are always treating each client as an individual and with respect. It is important to understand dementia and its signs and symptoms in order to develop a person-centred plan and deliver appropriate care (Alzheimer's WA, 2018).

By collecting as much information as possible, a care plan can be individualised to focus on the person. This includes:

- interviewing the family and significant others
- obtaining a physical, psychological and social history
- reviewing the medical history with the registered nurse (RN)
- observing the individual and their behaviours.

Person-centred care checklist

Think of an aged person that you know or have cared for and answer the following questions:

1   Are they being treated with dignity and respect?

2   Do staff/you know their likes and dislikes – their favourite music or hobbies?

3   Is their opinion and personality understood and taken into account?

4   Do they seem valued as a human being, regardless of their age or how advanced their illness is?

These answers assist in developing a person-centred care plan for the individual, one that considers their needs and wants.

14.1 ACTIVITY

What is dementia?

Dementia Australia (n.d.) refers to dementia as 'a collection of symptoms that are caused by disorders affecting the brain. Dementia affects thinking, behaviour and the ability to perform everyday tasks'. It is a disease symptom and not a normal part of ageing, and it occurs in both men and women, although there are more women with dementia due to them living longer than men.

The brain and dementia

The brain is a central component of the nervous system; nerve cells transmit signals to and from different parts of the body and regulate involuntary and voluntary actions. The cerebrum is the largest part of the brain and is associated with functions such as thought and action. It is divided into four sections, called lobes: the frontal lobe, parietal lobe, occipital lobe and temporal lobe (see Figure 14.1). Damage to these lobes results in many of the symptoms of dementia.

The functions of each lobe and how it relates to symptoms of dementia are as follows (University of Queensland, 2018):

- Frontal lobe – controls emotions, planning, reasoning and problem-solving. In frontotemporal dementia, personality changes are often the first signs of the disease.
- Parietal lobe – behind the frontal lobe. Areas in this lobe control sensory information, including touch, temperature, pressure and pain, as well as space, perception and size. Damage to this part of the brain can result in problems with reading and writing, recognising faces and apraxia (inability to perform tasks or movements).

FIGURE 14.1 Lobes of the brain

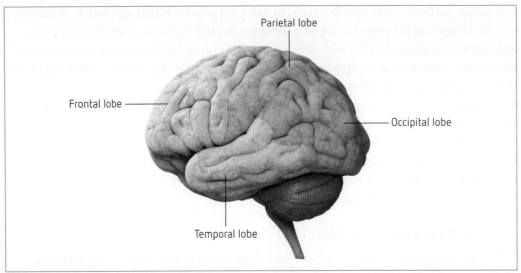

- Temporal lobe – controls processing sensory information, hearing, recognising language and forming memories. Dementia affecting this part of the brain can be recognised by memory loss.
- Occipital lobe – the major visual processing centre in the brain. Damage to this lobe can cause difficulty in recognising objects or words.

Early signs and symptoms

The symptoms of dementia can be very subtle in the early stages, which makes dementia difficult to diagnose. It also depends on which part of the brain is damaged. Early signs include:

- personality changes
- recent and frequent memory loss
- getting lost in familiar places
- misplacing things
- difficulties with common tasks
- poor judgement
- forgetting simple words.

Diagnosis

There is no one test to determine if someone has dementia. Diagnosis is based on a medical history, a physical examination, laboratory tests, and the characteristic changes in thinking, everyday function and behaviour.

Medical, physical and psychological history

The general practitioner (GP) or aged care assessment team (ACAT) is usually the first point of contact when concerns about cognition arise. The GP can take a medical history and may carry out a test of memory and concentration. A physical examination includes blood and urine testing and these tests can rule out other causes including infection, vitamin deficiency, thyroid or liver problems or anaemia. Additional information is gathered from the person as well as family and significant others, and if there are concerns, the GP may refer the person to a specialist.

Specialists may perform neuro-psychological tests to evaluate concentration, problem-solving, memory cognition and awareness. Testing may include copying a diagram, learning a short list of words or naming common objects. Other assessment tools include the Mini-Mental State Examination (MMSE), the Brief Cognitive Rating Scale and the Alzheimer's Disease Assessment Scale – Cognitive (ADAS-Cog). They may also perform brain scans to detect reduction in brain size, blood flow through the brain or areas of the brain that are damaged.

Memory clinics are also used which incorporate a range of specialists involved in the diagnosis of dementia. Memory clinics are known as Cognitive Dementia and Memory Services (CDAMS) in Victoria.

Behavioural and psychological symptoms

Most people who suffer from dementia have some behavioural and psychological symptoms. Non-pharmacological strategies are used as the first line of action, with family and carers included in the development of a person-centred care plan. Figure 14.2 lists and describes some of the common symptoms of dementia.

FIGURE 14.2 Symptoms of dementia

SYMPTOM	DESCRIPTION
Hallucinations	Distorted sensory experiences that appear to be real for the person. They can be heard, seen, smelt or felt; e.g., seeing insects crawling over your dinner
Delusions	A belief in something that is untrue; e.g., a belief that the carer is stealing your money
Wandering	The aimless or random movement that can occur when the person with dementia does not know where they are
Sundowning	A behaviour that occurs in the late afternoon or evening and is associated with increased confusion, restlessness and wandering
Repetitive behaviour	Repeating the same question, performing the same movement, or carrying out the same activity over and over again; e.g., repeatedly asking what day it is
Agitation	Excessive physical movement or verbal activity. This can include calling out, crying, pacing and wandering
Aggression	Behaviours that are challenging; e.g., verbal – swearing, screaming, shouting or making threats; or physical – hitting, pinching, scratching or biting
Depression	A feeling of extreme sadness and loss of interest in previously enjoyed activities. Can include poor sleep, loss of appetite and lack of energy
Withdrawal	Loss of motivation and social engagement – can be a coping mechanism to avoid anxiety resulting from dementia
Sleep problems	Some people sleep during the day and are awake and restless at night, and others need less sleep

Adapted from: Better Health Victoria (2014). Dementia – Behaviour changes. Retrieved 24 December 2018 from https://www.betterhealth.vic.gov.au/health/conditionsandtreatments/dementia-behaviour-changes

Treatment of dementia

Treatment of dementia depends on its cause. In the case of most dementias, including Alzheimer's disease, there is no cure and no treatment that stops its progression. Psychological therapies involve activities to stimulate the mind – these are discussed later in the chapter. Medications can temporarily improve functioning and alertness and reduce the impact of the symptoms. It must be remembered that there are side effects with medications and a healthcare professional should prescribe the medication that best suits an individual's condition and situation.

Types of dementia

The most common types of dementia are Alzheimer's disease, which accounts for two-thirds of dementia cases, followed by vascular dementia and dementia with Lewy bodies. A number of different illnesses can also result in dementia and each has its own features. Figure 14.3 outlines the main types of dementia and their causes.

FIGURE 14.3 Types of dementia

TYPE OF DEMENTIA	CAUSES
Alzheimer's disease	Amyloid plaques and neurofibrillary tangles. The plaques and tangles can damage the nerve cells, causing a progressive decrease in memory and thinking
Vascular dementia	Associated with disease in the blood vessels in the brain. The blood vessels can leak or become blocked and blood cannot reach the brain cells, which can eventually die
Lewy body dementia	Associated with abnormal deposits of a protein called alpha-synuclein (Lewy bodies) in the brain. These deposits affect chemicals which can lead to problems with thinking, movement, behaviour and mood
AIDS-related dementia	A complication that affects some people with HIV and acquired immune deficiency syndrome (AIDS) where the virus damages brain cells
Alcohol-related dementia	Brain damage associated with excessive alcohol intake, particularly if associated with a diet deficient in thiamine (vitamin B1). Wernicke / Korsakoff syndrome is a particular form of alcohol-related brain injury
Frontotemporal dementia (Pick's disease)	Damage to the frontal and temporal lobes of the brain causing behavioural, personality and / or speech problems
Parkinson's disease	Deficiency of dopamine causing progressive mental decline including memory loss, confusion and slowed thinking. Occurs in approximately 20 per cent of people with Parkinson's disease
Huntington's disease	A progressive genetic disorder that causes the brain to lose nerve cells. This affects the part of the brain that regulates mood, movement and cognitive skills
Younger onset dementia	Any form of dementia diagnosed in people under the age of 65. This can result from a head injury, Down syndrome or alcohol abuse

Adapted from: Better Health Victoria (2018). Dementia – Different types. Retrieved 22 December 2018 from https://www.betterhealth.vic.gov.au/health/conditionsandtreatments/dementia-different-types

Alzheimer's disease

Alzheimer's disease is the most common form of dementia and one that worsens over time. Each stage presents different symptoms and challenges that the HSA must be aware of in order to care for the person appropriately. Figure 14.4 describes the three stages of Alzheimer's disease and its common symptoms.

FIGURE 14.4 Stages of Alzheimer's disease

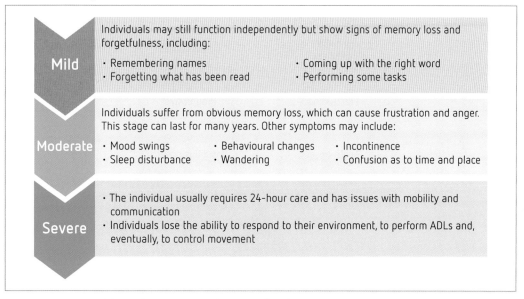

Adapted from: Alzheimer's Association (2018). Stages of Alzheimer's. Retrieved 18 October 2022 from
https://www.alz.org/alzheimers-dementia/stages

The rate of progression of Alzheimer's disease varies, with the average person living between three to eleven years after diagnosis. People with severe dementia may still be able to hear and respond to emotion and you must take this into account when caring for the person. The most common cause of death for someone with Alzheimer's is pneumonia due to impaired swallowing.

Conditions with similar symptoms to dementia

There are some conditions that closely resemble dementia, including:

- delirium (see Figure 14.5)
- depression
- vitamin deficiencies
- medication irregularities
- infections
- brain tumours.

However, all of these are reversible or can be treated in some manner. Correct diagnosis by the medical team and monitoring and reporting on what is observed can also assist to develop strategies to manage these disorders.

Delirium

An acute confusional state that can be caused by acute illness or drug toxicity. It is often reversible.

FIGURE 14.5 Delirium versus dementia

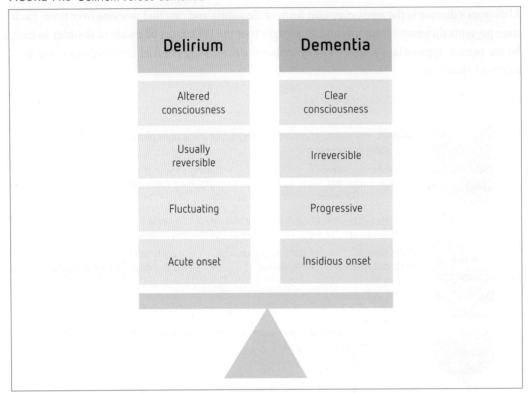

Interpret the person's individualised plan and familiarise self with their needs and wants including a familiar environment

The individualised care plan is based on the person's needs and wants so it is important to collect as much information as possible about the person and the disease. By understanding the stages of dementia you will be able to determine how the symptoms will impact on the person and plan accordingly. Planning should be reviewed as the disease progresses and the person becomes more dependent, and their levels of ability and support change.

The person's needs and wants will change regarding their ability to communicate and perform activities of daily living (ADLs), requiring regular planning and review as the disease progresses. Remember to always promote self-care and include the individual and family as much as possible when familiarising yourself with the needs and wants of the person.

ACTIVITY 14.2

Individualised planning

Mr Park is 85 years old and has moderate dementia with occasional confusion, memory loss and wandering. He and his family emigrated from Korea 60 years ago and he worked as a civil engineer during his adult life. He enjoyed playing cards and listening to music and always followed a routine of both rising early and going to bed early. He is a widower and was living with his daughter before his condition deteriorated.

Complete the following questions regarding individualised planning for Mr Park:

1   Develop a daily plan (morning, afternoon and evening) for Mr Park that considers the following:
    a   his cultural likes, dislikes, strengths, abilities and interests
    b   how he used to structure his day
    c   what times of day he functions best
    d   ample time for meals, bathing and dressing
    e   regular times for waking up and going to bed.

2   What would you do if Mr Park displayed irritability with your afternoon's planned activities?

3   What strategies could you use to minimise any risk with Mr Park's wandering?

Familiar environment

By being provided with a familiar, comfortable and inviting environment, the person with dementia can reach their full potential. Even if their perception of time and space has changed, relationships, objects and situations still matter. The environment should be in line with the person's social and cultural norms, and their needs and capabilities, and comply with organisational policies and procedures (Victorian Department of Health and Human Services, n.d.).

A familiar and stable environment includes:
- pictures of family and significant friends to give the person a sense of identity
- friendly and approachable staff
- choice in communications, activities and involvement to give them a sense of inclusion
- music appropriate for their age group
- respecting privacy, dignity and personal possessions
- adequate lighting.

Recognise and report signs consistent with financial, physical or emotional abuse or neglect

People with dementia can be vulnerable to financial, physical or emotional abuse or neglect. It is important that you recognise the signs consistent with abuse so that you can report to your supervisor and contribute to the planning of preventative strategies. Behavioural changes due to abuse can include but are not limited to:
- sudden changes in behaviour
- depression
- confusion
- changes in sleeping or eating patterns
- fear of a person
- shaking and trembling
- anxiety and avoidance of eye contact
- defensive postures.

It must be noted that some of these changes may also be associated with dementia so it is important to determine the context in when they occur. Figure 14.6 lists examples of these types of abuse and some of the signs to look for.

FIGURE 14.6 Signs of abuse

Financial abuse	• Sale of property without approval • Money for activities of daily living not provided • Items of value disappearing • Bills not being paid
Physical abuse	• Unexplained pain or bruises • Burns or repeated injuries • Over-sedation • Person left in wet continence pads • Inadequate nutrition or hydration
Emotional abuse	• Time not being spent with the person • Inadequate clothing or personal items provided • Carer or family scolding or rude towards the person • The person being restrained

2 USE APPROPRIATE COMMUNICATION STRATEGIES

Communicating with a person who has dementia can be challenging, and it is essential to understand that every person is an individual. Being patient, calm and using effective verbal and non-verbal strategies will maximise engagement, and reassuring the person will help gain their cooperation. The use of validation strategies, reality orientation, distraction and reminiscence can relieve distress and agitation in the person, and an appropriate environment will allow them to remain calm and relaxed.

Use verbal and non-verbal communication strategies to maximise engagement

In following the principles of person-centred care, you should empathise with the client and consider how they are trying to communicate. Patience and displaying positive non-verbal communication are important to encourage and allow the person to respond. Many people with dementia may not understand your words but can understand your gestures. Non-verbal strategies can include:

* maintaining eye contact
* not encroaching on the person's personal space
* using gestures instead of words
* spending time with the person
* maintaining a pleasant facial expression
* being attentive.

Environmental cues can also be used to communicate and support the person with dementia. For example, using signs, labels and nametags to identify time, objects and people (i.e. calendar, clock) will help to orientate the person, and using a communication board to outline activities will give them information about the day.

Reality orientation

Attempts to orientate the person with the present using reminders of the time (clocks), the day (calendars) and current surroundings (signage).

Distraction

Used to refocus the attention of a person with dementia from a negative behaviour to a positive one.

Reminiscence

Using written, pictorial or oral life histories to enhance the psychological wellbeing of a person with cognitive impairment.

Communication techniques

Francis, the HSA, worked last night and is now on the early shift. She is looking after Joseph, who has moderate dementia and tends to hoard magazines and newspapers.

She rushes into Joseph's room, turns on the lights and says, 'Hi Joseph, how are you today? Wow, this room really needs a clean-up. I'll stack all these old newspapers away so that the room looks cleaner.'

She then opens the curtains and says, 'It's a beautiful day today. Are you ready for breakfast? Have you had a shower already? 'We need to hurry up because I've got a busy day ahead.'

Joseph does not cooperate with Francis, and she then complains to the RN that he is a cranky old man.

Answer the following questions regarding Francis's communication techniques:

1   What communication techniques would have been more beneficial for Joseph?

2   Consider alternative questions that would allow Joseph to have choice in his care?

3   What strategies are effective for a person who displays hoarding behaviours?

Gain cooperation and provide reassurance by using reality orientation

A person with dementia may not remember that you looked after them before due to their memory loss. Therefore, it is important that you use reassurance to put them at ease. Your body language can convey reassurance through smiling, eye contact and giving the person your full attention. Phrases like 'It's OK' and 'You're doing well' can provide encouragement if they are confused or agitated.

Reality orientation

Reality orientation therapy was originally developed for war veterans who had post-traumatic stress disorder (PTSD) with flashbacks and an inability to differentiate between reality and war memories. Reality orientation attempts to orientate the person with the present. This can be done by providing reminders of the time (using clocks), the day (using calendars) and current surroundings (using signage) and can be integrated into a reality orientation board (see Figure 14.7). In verbal communications, you can integrate reality orientation into conversations with the client by (Heerema, 2019):

* talking about orientation, including the time of day, the date and season
* using the person's name frequently
* discussing current events
* referring to clocks and calendars
* placing signs and labels on doors, cupboards and other objects
* asking questions about photos or other decorations
* wearing your name badge.

FIGURE 14.7 Reality orientation board

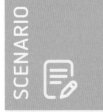

Source: CDS Boutique

Reality orientation for Mrs Chapman

Colin is looking after Mary Chapman, who suffers from Alzheimer's disease and has been a long-term resident at Bundalong Nursing Home. He tries to use reality orientation in his conversations with Mrs Chapman to help clear up her confusion and ease her anxiety: 'Hi Mrs Chapman. I'm Colin, your carer for today. It's a beautiful sunny day this morning and today is Melbourne Cup Day. That's the first Tuesday in November.'

Colin helps Mrs Chapman to wash and get ready for breakfast and walks her to the dining room. He says: 'Mrs Chapman, let's look at the board for today. You can see that it's Tuesday and we are at Bundalong Nursing Home. I'll help you sit down. What would you like for breakfast this morning?'

1   How did Colin use reality orientation effectively?
2   What reality techniques did Colin use to orientate Mrs Chapman?

Cautions about reality orientation

In many situations, such as casual conversations, reality orientation can be used to help remind the person where they are. However, as dementia progresses, reality orientation becomes counterproductive and should be avoided. This is because in later stages of the disease, any attempt to orientate can result in further anxiety or confusion. In this case it may be more appropriate to use validation strategies, which we will now explore.

Use validation strategies to relieve distress and agitation in the person

When a person is anxious or distressed, the use of validation therapy can build a sense of trust and security in the person with dementia. Validation therapy teaches that, rather than trying to bring the person with dementia back to reality, it is more positive to enter their reality. In this way you can develop empathy with the person, reduce their anxiety, embrace what is important to them and help maintain their dignity and self-esteem.

Validation therapy
A communication technique that focuses on the individual's emotions, rather than reality. Its primary goal is to try to see the world from the individual's point of view.

Validation techniques

Remember that maintaining trust and letting individuals express themselves is a core component of validation therapy. Maintaining a patient's mental wellbeing is equally as important as maintaining their physical health. By offering validation, you are not only building a relationship with the individual but also improving their level of care. Include verbal and non-verbal cues to reassure the person while rephrasing what they say and allowing the expression of feeling.

Rephrase

Rephrasing the person's feelings back to them provides reassurance. This also shows that you understand them. For example, saying 'You must really miss your mother' can decrease anxiety because the person hears you expressing what they are feeling.

Allow expression of feeling

Join the person in their feelings. After acknowledging the feeling, communicate what it may have meant for them in an empathetic, non-judgemental way. For example, you could say, 'You must miss your mother. You must have had a special relationship with her.'

Using these techniques encourages reminiscing and gives the person with dementia an opportunity to explore their past through describing memories, which can be comforting for them.

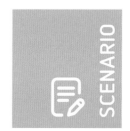

Validation techniques for Mrs Dimitrio

You are looking after 90-year-old Maria Dimitrio, who has dementia. When you are helping her with a change of clothes, she starts calling you Angelo (her late husband) and demands that you take her home.

You understand that Maria has dementia and has lost the ability to think logically, and that she needs to mentally return to the past when she felt loved and needed. You use validation techniques to connect with Maria to maintain her mental wellbeing.

Rephrase

'You miss your husband and want to be at home with him.'

Allow expression of feeling

'What do you miss the most about your husband?' or 'What would you do at home with your husband?'

Maria starts to talk about her husband and how much he meant to her and how they used to do the gardening together. She seems to calm down and after a while she is ready to go into the sitting room for morning tea.

1 Validation is a useful technique to allow Maria to express her feelings. What non-verbal cues can you also use to reassure and connect with Maria?

ACTIVITY 14.4

Validation strategies for Mrs Volparto

You are a new HSA in the Sands Aged Care Facility. You are looking after Connie Volparto who is 92 years old. She appears agitated and pushes you away and keeps saying, 'I have to get home. Momma is expecting me and I get into trouble if I am late.'

1   What validation strategies could you use to de-escalate the situation?

2   Identify appropriate questioning to build a positive relationship with Mrs Volparto.

3   How does validation maintain Connie's dignity and self-esteem?

3   PROVIDE ACTIVITIES FOR MAINTENANCE OF DIGNITY, SKILLS AND HEALTH

Understanding the person with dementia will help you to plan appropriate activities for them. Activities should be directed at maintaining the person's independence by using familiar routines and existing skills. This information can be obtained from the person and with the help of family and significant others and should balance safety with autonomy. For the person with dementia, this means that they have the right to determine if they want to participate in activities or not. For staff, this means that they should respect dignity and promote the person's sense of self.

Autonomy

Having control and choice over one's life.

Organise activities to maintain independence, using familiar routines and existing skills

When organising activities, you should encourage the person with dementia to be as independent as possible and to use familiar and existing skills. If the person is able, you can have one-on-one discussions with them to find out their likes and dislikes. The family can also play a part by providing information about the person's social history and memorable times. Once this information is obtained, it can be incorporated into their individual care plan.

Building a rapport with the individual can enable you to access information about their reminiscences and routines from the present as well as the past in order to structure activities which will have a familiarity to them. Activities such as watering the garden, sweeping, drying dishes or helping in the kitchen can enable the person with dementia to feel useful and give them a sense of responsibility. Remember that a person with dementia can have fluctuating mood and ability, and the activities should be adapted or ceased if they are not successful and causing distress.

Personal care activities

When undertaking personal hygiene tasks, the person should be encouraged to do as much for themselves as possible. You may need to assist with the task by reminding them, giving them a toothbrush or appropriate clothing, or starting the task for them and then encouraging them to take over.

Giving choice is important because each person has personal likes and dislikes and cultural considerations. The person may also need prompts regarding the most appropriate clothing; for example, 'It's a cold day today, we may need a cardigan to keep warm.' They may also need prompting regarding personal grooming; for example, 'Your whiskers are growing. Would you like to shave?'

Familiar activities

A person with dementia can often undertake familiar activities more easily than new tasks. It is important to ask the person or their family what activities they enjoyed (see Figure 14.8). Not only will the individual be more successful at the task, but they will also find it more enjoyable and they may seem more relaxed. Activities can include:

- arts and crafts
- listening to music
- watching television
- dancing
- looking through books or magazines
- walking
- card or board games.

FIGURE 14.8 Familiar activities can have a relaxing effect

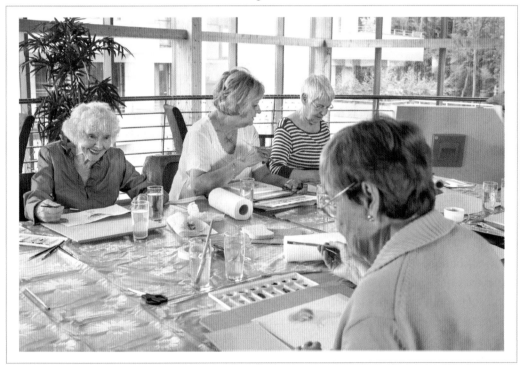

Source: Shutterstock.com/belushi

Considerations when planning activities

Activities for a person with dementia should be developed in collaboration with the person, eliminate boredom, maintain safety and security, and increase the person's self-esteem. They should:

- incorporate existing skills only, not new learning
- encourage independence
- not be overstimulating – e.g., noise, crowds

- provide enjoyment and social contact
- be sensitive to the person's culture
- be simple and unhurried, with tasks communicated in easy, manageable steps
- be planned for a time that suits the person's best level of functioning.

ACTIVITY 14.5

Activities for dementia

It is important to set up an environment that allows independence for the person with dementia. A creative environment will maximise the person's ability to be involved.

Answer the following questions regarding activities for dementia:

1   What are examples of structured activities (i.e., that require staff involvement) that could be organised?

2   What are examples of unstructured activities (i.e., that the person can participate in independently) that could be organised?

3   How would you ensure safety for the person with these activities?

Organise activities appropriate to the individual, reflecting their cultural likes and dislikes, to bring back pleasurable memories

When organising activities, you must ensure that they are appropriate for the individual's cultural requirements. Customs and beliefs regarding religion, food and language should be incorporated into all activities. If the person is from a non-English-speaking background, they may revert to their native language as dementia progresses, so the family or interpreters can assist; however, when the person with dementia cannot be understood, non-verbal communication should reflect warmth and calmness.

Examples of activities are outings that can provide enjoyment or looking through old photos to help the person recall times past. The celebration of cultural events (e.g., Greek Easter) can also be considered. Sensory activities can also bring back pleasurable memories by engaging the senses. They can trigger emotions and memories for the confused person who has lost their ability to connect with the world and can be linked to the interests the person had prior to dementia. Complementary or alternative therapies can also improve someone's functioning and quality of life and bring back pleasurable memories.

Massage

Massage involves hands-on manipulation of the body's soft tissue. There is often a lack of human touch in caring for the elderly, which can lead them to feel isolated. Massage therapy can help ease the effects of isolation, loneliness and anxiety while encouraging feelings of wellbeing.

Music therapy

Using music can improve the wellbeing of people with dementia. This can include listening or singing to music, playing instruments or interacting with the beat. Using familiar and favourite music can reduce behaviours of concern, so it is important to determine likes and dislikes before choosing the most appropriate music.

Pet therapy

Animals or pets can also improve the behaviour of people with dementia (see Figure 14.9). Visiting pet services or family member's pets can reduce anxiety and stress and divert attention in an agitated person. This should always be done under supervision because animals can be unpredictable.

FIGURE 14.9 Therapy pets can have a positive impact

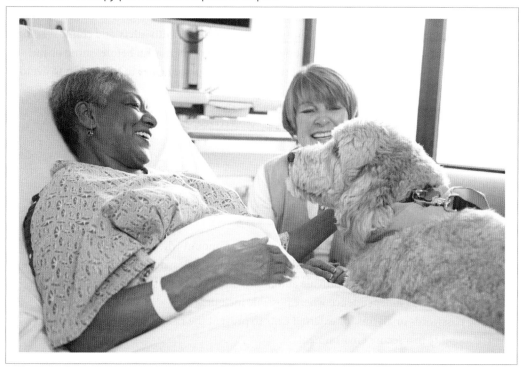

Source: Shutterstock.com/Monkey Business Images

Dementia in the Aboriginal and Torres Strait Islander context

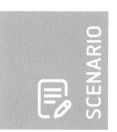

SCENARIO

The prevalence of dementia in Aboriginal and Torres Strait Islander people is between three and five times higher than that in the non-Indigenous Australian population (Dementia Training Australia, 2017).

When an elderly Aboriginal person moves into a facility, the HSA needs to take a culturally safe and competent approach to optimise the quality of care and improve the impact of the placement on the person and their family or carers.

Acknowledge to the Aboriginal or Torres Strait Islander person with dementia and their family or carer that there may be a lot that you don't know about their culture. Ask them to tell you if you say something that they find culturally offensive; this will help you to improve your communication style. Involve carers and other key family members as partners in providing appropriate care and communication.

1 How can you provide a culturally sensitive environment for Aboriginal and Torres Strait Islander patients with dementia?

2 What are the benefits of providing culturally sensitive care to Aboriginal and Torres Strait Islander patients with dementia?

3 What other key family or community members may be beneficial in providing culturally appropriate care or communication?

Ensure the person's safety and comfort is balanced with autonomy and risk-taking

When planning activities for a person with dementia, safety must be considered. The physical spaces and social approaches must support freedom of movement and choice while providing safety and security. Autonomy is the right to make choices, and although the individual with dementia may be confused at times, you can encourage choice in clothing, activities and meals.

Your duty of care for the individual must also be considered, with safety and comfort being paramount. An example could be to check the temperature of their meal before eating or the shower before washing or making sure that the cup of tea is placed close to the person to avoid spillage.

Safety and comfort for the individual with dementia will depend on:

* the person's level of dementia
* workplace policies and procedures
* the individual's care plan
* the level of risk for that person.

Risk management

Reducing or eliminating the risks to ensure safety is paramount when undertaking activities or personal care tasks. Organisations have risk management policies, documentation and programs that can both promote safety and provide autonomy. Strategies for risk management that can maintain the person's independence where possible include:

* using passwords or alarms for external exits to prevent the risk of wandering, yet allowing free mobility in a secure environment
* adopting a falls risk assessment and prevention program to identify the person's risk of falling and help to identify what interventions to implement. This also includes active and passive exercises to build the person's strength and mobility
* promoting regular oral hygiene to prevent the risk of dental/oral problems and to also maintain nutrition
* ensuring regular toileting and implementing continence programs for those at risk of incontinence. This can also include making sure that the person is dressed for comfort while allowing easy undressing to prevent incontinence
* regularly checking skin integrity and using risk prevention methods to prevent pressure areas
* ensuring the person has adequate rest and sleep so that they can participate in activities to maintain their self-worth
* meeting the person's nutritional needs balanced with a diet that allows independence of feeding for as long as possible.

Safety versus autonomy

Mrs Christie needs to have a shower. She is very unsteady on her feet and slightly confused but wishes to have her privacy maintained and refuses your assistance.

Answer the following questions regarding safety and autonomy:

1 What steps would you take to provide a safe environment for Mrs Christie?

2 What suggestions would you make to Mrs Christie to ensure that she independently maintains her hygiene?

3 How would you maintain autonomy for Mrs Christie with her personal care?

Access information about the person's reminiscences and routines with family and carers

'*Reminiscence* refers to the act of recalling memories from the past.' In a care facility, relatives or friends can provide photographs, CDs or information about significant events and memorable occasions. This can engage the attention of a person with dementia more fully (see Figure 14.10). Conversely, relatives or friends can provide information on anything that may distress the person. Using the person's different senses can assist the act of remembering (Kennard, 2019). These include:

* visual – looking at photographs, pictures, memory albums or objects that have a special meaning
* aural – listening to familiar music from the radio or CDs
* smell or taste – eating familiar or culturally specific foods
* tactile – touching objects or feeling textures.

FIGURE 14.10 Reminiscence helps to engage the attention of a person with dementia

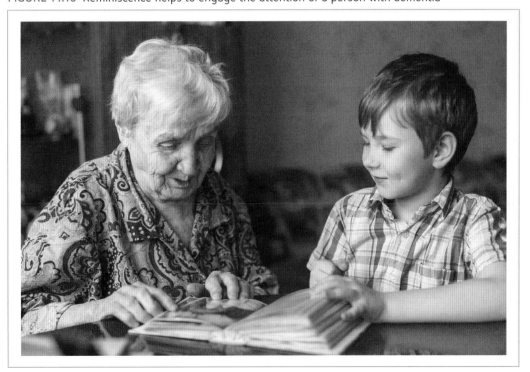

Source: Shutterstock.com/De Visu

SCENARIO

Reminiscing with Mr Furlong

Brian Furlong was a 94-year-old who was new to the aged care facility. He had mild dementia and was sometimes agitated in the afternoon. Cora, the HSA, noticed a photograph of a young Brian standing next to a car and asked him about the car. Brian described the car, an old 1953 Morris Minor, in great detail – the leather seats and the split windscreen and how it was difficult to start in the cold weather. He went on to say how much he enjoyed driving it and going on road trips. Cora asked him questions about the road trips and Brian elaborated. Afterwards he appeared much more relaxed and Cora felt that their bond had grown.

1 What are the benefits of reminiscence for a person with dementia?
2 How can the nurse use the information from Brian's reminiscence to enhance his mood and stimulate wider communication?

ACTIVITY 14.7

Memory album

Think of an aged relative or friend that you have and answer the following questions regarding their memories:

1 What information would you collect to include in a memory album?
2 How could you put this information together to aid reminiscence?
3 What signs may indicate that the person is engaging in the reminiscence activity?

Provide support and guidance to family, carers and significant others

As dementia progresses, so too does the amount of care that is needed. This can take a toll on the physical and emotional wellbeing of the family, carers and significant others of the person with dementia. You can assist by providing support and guidance, especially if there is a lack of understanding from the family or others. Strategies include:

* talking with relatives to get to know them
* asking visitors to come for short times and not too many at once
* suggest activities for the visit, such as going for a walk or bringing something to do together
* communicating changes in condition.
  Support for families and carers can also be sourced through organisations, including the following:
* Dementia Australia – a part of their website contains carefully selected content that is relevant and useful to families, friends and carers (https://www.dementia.org.au/information/about-you/i-am-a-carer-family-member-or-friend). This is available in different languages as well
* carer support groups – bring families and friends together with the assistance of a facilitator
* carer advisory and counselling services – provide carers with information and advice about services and entitlements
* My Aged Care (https://myagedcare.gov.au) – a government website that provides information on aged care for older people, their families and carers as well as service providers, and offers help in finding local providers, such as aged care homes
* Aged Care Assessment Teams (ACAT) – provide information on suitable care options or arrange referral to appropriate services
* Commonwealth Respite and Carelink Centres – provide information about the range of community-care programs and services available.

Support services

Read the Dementia Support Australia services overview (**https://www.dementia.com.au/**) and answer the following questions:

1   How does the Dementia Behaviour Management Advisory Service support carers?

2   What are Severe Behaviour Response Teams?

3   Who is eligible for help from this service?

14.8 ACTIVITY

4   IMPLEMENT STRATEGIES TO MINIMISE THE IMPACT OF BEHAVIOURS OF CONCERN

People with dementia often misinterpret the stimuli around them. This can result in altered behaviour that can be concerning. The behaviour is usually out of the person's control and they may be quite frightened by it and need reassurance. It is important for the care worker to identify the triggers for these behaviours and to take action to minimise their likelihood. Evaluation of the strategies with the team is also important so that everyone can contribute to whether or not they were effective in reducing the behaviours and their impact on the person and others.

Identify behaviours of concern and potential triggers and contribute to team discussions on support planning and review

Some people with dementia can exhibit behaviours of concern. These can occur in isolation or be combined with other behaviours. These behaviours may be related to changes taking place in the brain or changes in the environment or medication. Remember that the behaviour is not deliberate and anger or aggression can often be directed against family members and carers because they are closest. The behaviours may resolve on their own or escalate as the disease progresses. Refer to Chapter 12, 'Respond effectively to behaviours of concern', which describes behaviours of concern in more detail.

Examples of behaviours of concern in dementia include wandering, hallucinations, delusions, hoarding, aggression, sundowning, repetition, inappropriate sexual behaviour and catastrophic reactions.

Triggers

People who suffer from dementia have difficulty communicating what they want, which can cause them to become overwhelmed and frustrated. This can be displayed by combative behaviour, verbal aggression or resistance. Trigger types are as follows:

*   *Physical triggers* – unmet needs, such as thirst or hunger; pain; feeling hot, cold or tired; or having sensory impairments. For example, the person may need to use the bathroom or have wet incontinence pads. Also, a bladder infection can dramatically affect behaviour, so it is important to monitor and report cloudy, offensive smelling urine and frequency.

*   *Emotional triggers* – emotions may become overwhelming when people expect the person to do things they cannot. They may not understand what is happening or may be responding to the emotions of the caregivers or other individuals who are displaying confusion or other negative emotions.

- *Environmental triggers* – the environment may be noisy or too bright, or there may be too many people speaking at once or rushing the person. This can cause stress because they are unable to process everything. Changes in routine and changes in staff also fall under this category. People with dementia can become upset if they find themselves in a strange situation or among a group of unfamiliar people where they feel confused and unable to cope.

Support planning and review

As an HSA, your role is to contribute to team discussions on planning and reviewing once strategies are implemented. Once assessment of the behaviour is identified, planning can be done to help identify strategies on how to manage the behaviour. Strategies include:

- looking for possible causes and minimising them if it is within your scope of practice
- satisfying any physical or emotional needs
- checking and reporting to a supervisor if the person is in pain or unwell
- checking if your responses are contributing to the behaviour.

The decision-making flowchart in Figure 14.11 is sourced from Dementia Support Australia. It provides a comprehensive overview of how to respond to changed behaviour by identifying the behaviour, assessing the behaviour and any causes, and responding to the behaviour with appropriate strategies.

FIGURE 14.11 Behaviour support process flowchart

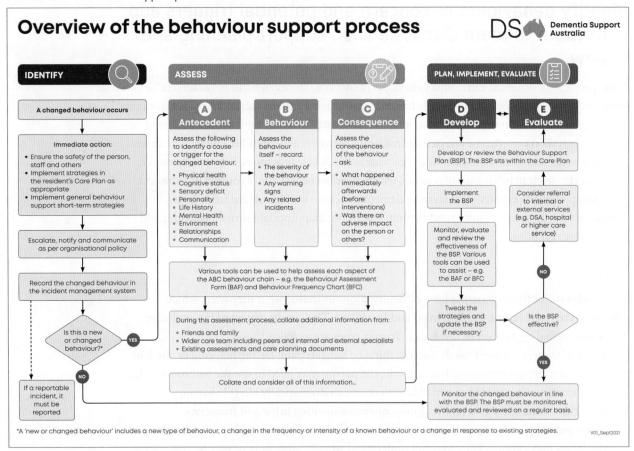

Source: Dementia Support Australia, https://www.dementia.com.au/resource-hub/behaviour-support-plan-resources

Take action to minimise likelihood and reduce impact of behaviours on the person and others

Some behavioural problems in people with dementia are controllable without having to seek medication. This can be done by identifying the triggers and then resolving problems through words and actions. A calm, unstressed and familiar environment can help to avoid many difficult behaviours, as can the use of distraction. This redirection to another task or thought can relieve distress and potential behaviours of concern. Figure 14.12 lists identified behaviours of concern and actions to reduce the impact on the person and others.

FIGURE 14.12 Actions to minimise impact for behaviours of concern

BEHAVIOUR	ACTIONS TO REDUCE IMPACT
Wandering	• Provide a safe area for walking • Ensure the person has identification • Exits should be secured
Hallucinations	• Remain quiet or neutral because the person may be frightened by the hallucination • Distract the person to refocus their attention • Maintain a consistent routine • Ensure the individual is wearing their hearing aids or glasses
Delusions	• Do not question or argue • Provide distractions; e.g., music, exercise, activities • Record to establish whether these behaviours occur at particular times of the day or with particular people so that planning can be considered
Hoarding	• Provide an area to keep items of interest so that the person can sort them out and be kept busy • Learn the person's usual hiding places
Aggression	• Look for triggers – the aggression may be due to frustration • Redirect, distract – activity and exercise may help prevent outbursts • Speak slowly, calmly and clearly
Sundowning	• Encourage exercise throughout the day • Provide a calm environment in the afternoon and evening • Monitor diet and restrict sweets and caffeine consumption to the morning • Consider the effect of bright lights and noise from TVs and radios
Repetitive behaviour	• Provide distractions; e.g., a walk or cup of tea • Give the individual tasks with repetition; e.g., clothes to fold
Inappropriate sexual behaviour	• Take the individual to a private room • Do not overreact
Catastrophic reactions	• Look for triggers • Record to identify the circumstances under which they occur • Redirect and distract • Speak slowly, calmly and clearly

Remember, if behaviour becomes difficult, do not attempt any form of physical contact such as restraint, leading them away or approaching from behind. It may be better to leave the person alone until they have recovered or call for support.

Restraint-free environment

A person-centred approach is a restraint-free approach. There are many different options to provide for client safety other than restraints, which should be used as a last option:

- *Activities and programs* can provide distraction and engage the client in meaningful activities
- *Physical strategies* include a comprehensive medical check-up, and medication management including preventing pain and infections
- *Psychological therapies* include companionship through visitors or staff, touch and sensory stimulation
- *Nursing care actions* include treating clients as individuals, supervision, routines and risk management
- *Environmental strategies* include adequate lighting, non-slip flooring, removal of obstructions, mobility aids, signage, protected outdoor areas for wandering, quiet areas and lowered beds.

Restrictive practice

Restrictive practice
An intervention that restricts the rights or freedom of movement of an individual.

Restraints interfere with the individual's ability to have free movement, and a restraint-free environment is the recommended standard of care (Australian Department of Health, 2012). The Australian Department of Health initiated legislation changes effective from 2021 using the term restrictive practice instead of 'restraint'. Restrictive practices include chemical, environmental, mechanical and physical restraint as well as seclusion:

- *Chemical restraints* include the use of medication to influence a person's behaviour; e.g., psychotropic medications.
- *Environmental restraints* restrict the person from having free access in their environment; e.g., locking away phones, tea or coffee, TV.
- *Mechanical restraints* can include bed rails, tray tables, lap belts and vests. They can cause physical and psychological harm and, contrary to belief, do not prevent falls or fall-related injuries.
- *Physical restraint* is the use of force to subdue movement of a person; e.g., pushing or pulling a person or holding them down to receive medication.
- *Seclusion* involves solitary confinement in a room; e.g., locking a client in their room.

The care team should identify issues that may lead to harm for the individual and those around them, and include a behaviour support plan in the existing care plans that outlines the behaviour, the assessment and the restrictive practice being used. Restrictive practices should only be used as a last resort – alternative restraint-free strategies should be used to manage the patient first.

ACTIVITY 14.9

Restrictive practice

Restrictive practice requirements must be met before they can be used in residential aged care facilities. The Australian Department of Health (2021a) has a fact sheet which provides an overview of restrictive practice. Look up 'Restrictive practice use in aged care facilities' at **https://www.health.gov.au/** to answer the following questions:

1   What requirements must be met before restrictive practice can be implemented?

2   What are emergency use restrictive practices?

Evaluate implemented strategies with your team to ensure effectiveness in minimising behaviours

Regularly reviewing strategies can help you evaluate what is working best and what needs to be improved. It must be remembered that the person with dementia experiences a progressive decline in symptoms, and so strategies that were effective previously may not be effective in the future. Review of the strategies should be done regularly or if the person's condition changes, or if the strategies used are no longer meeting the person's needs. Documentation and observation are two important methods for evaluating whether a plan is working or not; for example, noting weight loss, altered sleep patterns or changes in behaviour. The entire team and family should be included in reviewing because some people may notice subtle changes that others may not.

5 COMPLETE DOCUMENTATION

Documentation of behaviours is an important part of your role. You will be required to provide hands-on care as well as perform administrative tasks, such as filling in forms, writing reports on the support and care given, evaluating the effectiveness of the interventions and giving verbal reports. The documentation needs constant review as the individual with dementia has changing needs and support requirements according to the progression of their illness.

Comply with the organisation's reporting requirements

Early identification and close observation can prevent more serious problems occurring. When observing behaviour, it is important to consider:
* *What* was the behaviour and were there any triggers?
* *Where* did the behaviour occur – was it in the dining room or bedroom? Was the environment noisy, bright or cold?
* *When* did the behaviour occur – does the behaviour occur at a specific time of day or with a specific person?

Always report abnormal or changed behaviour to your supervisor. When documenting, ensure that it occurs at the time of, or as soon as practicable following, the event. Reportable observations to make for a person with dementia include changes in the following:
* level of consciousness – increase in sleeping or drowsiness, inability to follow instructions
* mood – onset of agitation, resistance to care, destructive behaviours, increased confusion
* memory or communication – difficulty remembering person, place, time or responding
* observations – increased temperature, changed breathing patterns
* ADLs – new incontinence, decline in ability to perform personal hygiene needs, refusal to eat or drink.

Types of documentation

An understanding of the correct documentation is vital. You will find that each organisation has its own documents, either paper based or electronic; however, the primary purpose for each is the same. Figure 14.13 outlines common documents and their purpose.

FIGURE 14.13 Types of documentation

DOCUMENT	PURPOSE
Nursing care plans	To assess the needs and record information about individuals to help plan, implement and evaluate care
Behaviour charts	To track events leading up to the incident and help to understand what may have caused it. This should include events leading up to the disturbance, what behaviour occurred, and what was the response (see Figure 14.14)
Bowel chart	Monitors bowel function and allows for consistent recording and evaluation of interventions; e.g., Bristol stool chart (see Figure 14.15)
Medication chart	Communication tool shared between doctors, nurses, pharmacists and other health professionals regarding an individual's medication. It is used to direct and record how and when drugs are to be administered
Food chart	To assess a person's nutritional intake and help to determine subsequent treatment plans; e.g., sample food chart (see Figure 14.16)
Continence chart	To record the times of passing urine, the amount of urine passed and incidents of incontinence
Progress notes	Facilitates communication between healthcare workers and identifies care, treatments and planning

FIGURE 14.14 Behaviour chart

ANTECEDENT – BEHAVIOUR – CONSEQUENCE (A-B-C) CHART				
NAME:				
DATE: / /				
Time	Frequency	Activities prior to behaviour	Behaviour of concern	What was your reaction?

FIGURE 14.15 Bristol stool chart

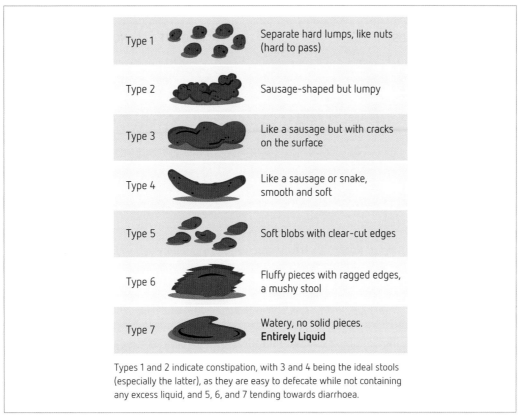

Type 1		Separate hard lumps, like nuts (hard to pass)
Type 2		Sausage-shaped but lumpy
Type 3		Like a sausage but with cracks on the surface
Type 4		Like a sausage or snake, smooth and soft
Type 5		Soft blobs with clear-cut edges
Type 6		Fluffy pieces with ragged edges, a mushy stool
Type 7		Watery, no solid pieces. **Entirely Liquid**

Types 1 and 2 indicate constipation, with 3 and 4 being the ideal stools (especially the latter), as they are easy to defecate while not containing any excess liquid, and 5, 6, and 7 tending towards diarrhoea.

Source: Heaton, K. W. & Lewis, S. J. (1997), Stool form scale as a useful guide to intestinal transit time. *Scandinavian Journal of Gastroenterology*, 32(9), pp. 920–4 Reprinted by permission of the publisher (Taylor & Francis Ltd, http://www.tandfonline.com)..

Australian National Aged Care Classification (AN–ACC) Assessment Tool

The Australian National Aged Care Classification assessment tool has replaced the Aged Care Funding Instrument (ACFI). Since October 2022, aged care providers have received funding according to the care needs assessed for each of their permanent residents. Download the 2021 reference manual and assessment tool from the Australian Department of Health (2021c) website (**https://www.health.gov.au/**) and answer the following questions:

1   What are the four main areas that the assessment tool considers for each resident?
2   What are the qualification requirements for independent assessors?
3   What are the 13 classes of care funding?

AN-ACC reappraisals can be undertaken where the aged care resident's care needs have changed significantly or 6–12 months have elapsed since the last assessment for specific classes.

14.10 ACTIVITY

FIGURE 14.16 Sample food chart

DATE	TIME	FOODS		AMOUNT	NOTES

Grains	Fruit	Vegetable	Dairy	Protein	Fat	Sweets	Non-calorie fluids
☐☐☐☐☐☐ ☐☐☐☐☐☐	☐☐☐☐☐☐ ☐☐☐☐☐☐	☐☐☐☐☐☐	☐☐☐☐☐☐	☐☐☐☐☐☐	☐☐☐☐☐☐	☐☐☐☐☐☐	☐☐☐☐☐☐ ☐☐☐☐☐☐
6–11 Servings	2–4 Servings	3–5 Servings	2–3 Servings	2–3 Servings	In moderation	In moderation	☐ = 1 cup

Exercise:

Comments:

Complete, maintain and store documentation according to organisation policy and protocols

Information regarding the individual must be accurate and factual, and be signed and designated by yourself, with a countersignature according to organisational requirements. Individuals' files are subject to privacy and confidentiality and only authorised people caring for the person can have access to the files. The information written in these files is regularly monitored and evaluated. Chapter 10, 'Provide non-client contact support in an acute care environment', describes the collection, processing and maintenance of records in more detail.

All records must be accessible to authorised healthcare workers when required for the care and management of the individual. Each facility will have specific policies and procedures, documents and forms, and requirements for maintenance and storage. It is your responsibility to make sure that you are familiar with these upon employment.

6 IMPLEMENT SELF-CARE STRATEGIES

Caring for a person with dementia can be challenging and stressful. How you cope plays a significant part in how you interact with individuals and their families. It is important to monitor your own stress levels and use appropriate strategies to maintain wellbeing and to seek support if required. This also relates to the primary caregiver, who also needs support to ensure that their stress levels do not escalate to the point of being unable to provide adequate care for their loved one.

Monitor own stress level in relation to working with people with dementia and use self-care strategies and support if required

Caring for someone with dementia can be physically and emotionally challenging. You may find that there are some aspects of caring you can manage easily, while others prove more difficult. Two of the main challenges of working with a person with dementia are that as the person's condition progresses, their needs and abilities will change; and that people with dementia often display a range of emotions. These challenges can cause anxiety, which makes it important to monitor your stress levels so that your wellbeing and that of the person you are caring for is not affected. Stress can result in absences from work, physical signs and symptoms, substance abuse, conflict or accidents. Chapter 1, 'Participate in workplace health and safety', describes stress in more detail, including physical and psychological signs and the importance of reflection as a tool to monitor your stress levels.

Self-care strategies

Taking care of yourself can keep you in good shape both physically and mentally for managing stress. You can become more resilient towards the unexpected, use the resources you have to their fullest, and become less reactive towards the stress you face. Self-care strategies to reduce stress include:

- looking after yourself by watching your diet, getting regular exercise and maintaining your social contacts and lifestyle
- educating yourself about dementia
- reflecting on what you enjoy about caring and supporting someone with dementia
- prioritising your tasks to determine which things you really need to do and which things are less important, and do the most important things first
- focusing on what the person with dementia can still do and supporting them to do these things. Try not to focus on what they cannot do
- knowing your limits and remembering that there is only so much that you can do. Try to focus on this and accept what you cannot change
- being aware of your feelings to make it easier to deal with them
- talking with friends and family. This can make you feel less isolated and stressed, and can help to put things in perspective

- talking to colleagues to share advice and discuss your experiences. Sometimes this is easier because they understand what you are going through
- asking for help and support if you need it. Your GP can assist with referrals to appropriate support networks
- taking breaks away to find time for yourself to relax.

Self-care activities for families

Maintaining your health and wellbeing provides you with the best frame of mind when caring for individuals with dementia. Answer the following questions, then share your answers with your class:

1   What strategies would you suggest for the family who is caring for someone with dementia so that they have the energy and capacity to cope with the challenges faced in their role?

2   What support groups are available for families of those caring for people with dementia?

SUMMARY

This chapter described the support required for those affected by dementia. It outlined the importance of using a person-centred approach in all interactions while familiarising yourself with the person's needs and wants in collaboration with family and significant others.

The use of appropriate verbal and non-verbal communication strategies was shown to maximise engagement, while reassurance, reality orientation and validation could assist in relieving distress and agitation and calming the person with dementia.

The importance of providing activities for maintenance of dignity, skills and health was outlined, with the emphasis on using familiar routines, reflecting on the person's likes and dislikes and integrating culture into care. The significance of ensuring safety and comfort in activities while balancing with autonomy and risk-taking was also highlighted. Minimising the impact of behaviours of concern was described through identification of triggers and implementing strategies and evaluating their effectiveness.

The last part of the chapter highlighted the importance of documentation and reporting and how to monitor your own stress levels by implementing self-care strategies. By using these strategies, you will be able to manage the person with dementia in a calm and measured way, reduce the person's anxiety, embrace what is important to them, and maintain their dignity and self-esteem.

APPLY YOUR KNOWLEDGE

Parkinson's dementia

Morris, a 72-year-old widower, has been living with Parkinson's disease for over 15 years. His family have noticed that, along with the symptoms of shakiness, muscle stiffness, a shuffling step and difficulty initiating movement, he has trouble remembering, paying attention and forgets how to do tasks. They made the difficult decision of moving him to a low-care aged facility.

1   What is the physiological cause of Parkinson's dementia?

2   Why is it preferable to promote independence in the low-care facility for Morris?

Morris settled in well in the facility and was able to attend to most of his hygiene needs; however, his shakiness made preparing meals, dressing himself and doing his laundry difficult. The facility was able to accommodate these needs so that he could maintain some degree of independence.

3   How could the staff encourage Morris to do as much for himself as possible with his personal care?

4   How can you promote autonomy for Morris whilst maintaining safety and security?

Morris's dementia progressed and he was eventually transferred to the high-care section of the aged facility. He became aggressive at times and had occasional hallucinations. This took its toll on the emotional wellbeing of Morris's family.

5   Using the knowledge you learnt in Chapter 12, 'Respond effectively to behaviours of concern', what potential triggers could cause Morris's behaviours?

6   What strategies can the HSA implement to provide support for the family?

Morris continued to deteriorate and passed away peacefully 14 months later. As the HSA looking after him during this time, you reflected that this was challenging and stressful but rewarding in that Morris's care was tailored to his needs throughout the progress of his disease.

7   Understanding the scope of your role is essential in performing it effectively within the healthcare team. What was the scope of the HSA's involvement in the care for Morris and his family whilst he was in care?

◄ REFLECTING ON THE INDUSTRY INSIGHT ✚

1   What is the main goal of therapy for a person with dementia, and how does the HSA demonstrate this with Dr Catherine in the 'Industry insight' box?
   a   By treating the symptoms.
   b   Maintaining Dr Catherine's independence by allowing her time to utilise existing skills.
   c   Reversing the cognitive decline.
   d   Treating the behavioural complications.

2   Dr Catherine spends much time folding and refolding clothes. What strategies did the HSA use to calm Dr Catherine during this repetitive act?
   a   Turned the action into an alternative activity by using distraction.
   b   Asked her to stop.
   c   Took the item away from her or stopped the activity.
   d   Ignored the behaviour in order to allow it to stop.

3   How did the HSA provide person-centred care for Dr Catherine, who has moderate dementia?
   a   Chose the clothing that they would like Dr Catherine to wear.
   b   Gave Dr Catherine multiple tasks to do.
   c   Used medication to treat the agitation and aggression.
   d   Made Dr Catherine the focus of attention, not the illness.

SELF-CHECK QUESTIONS

1   Identify the most common symptoms and causes of dementia.
2   What is the difference between delirium and dementia?
3   What is a person-centred approach to persons living with dementia?
4   What are the benefits and risks of reality orientation for the person with dementia?
5   What is validation therapy and how can it reduce distress in the person with dementia?
6   Identify risk management strategies that can maintain a person's independence and wellbeing?
7   How can the HSA access information about a person's reminiscence and routines?
8   List the documents required to maintain the safety and comfort of an individual with dementia.
9   Describe self-care strategies that can be used by the HSA to minimise the stress associated with caring for someone with dementia.
10 What are your definitions of the following key words and terms that have been used in this chapter?

KEY WORD OR TERM	YOUR DEFINITION
Sundowning	
Alzheimer's disease	
Reality orientation	
Delirium	
Validation therapy	
Autonomy	
Reminiscence	
Distraction	

QUESTIONS FOR DISCUSSION

1   Paulo is from Argentina and is displaying behaviours of concern. Discuss how the HSA could use his culture to de-escalate his behaviours.

2   Rina has Alzheimer's disease and is from a non-English-speaking background. She is agitated because she cannot understand you. Discuss the communication strategies to de-escalate this situation.

3   John Farris has early signs of memory loss and confusion and often removes his clothing in public. Discuss appropriate strategies for maintenance of dignity for John.

4   Roland has advancing dementia and is swearing and hitting his carers. Discuss the impact of these behaviours of concern on his family.

5   Felicity is wandering in the open areas of the aged care facility and tries to leave every time the external doors are opened. Discuss appropriate strategies to distract Felicity.

EXTENSION ACTIVITY

Providing care for a person with dementia

Agnes is 87 years old and has been living with dementia for the last five years. Before her diagnosis, Agnes was very involved with the local bowls club, her church and her grandchildren. Since her husband died two years ago, Agnes has struggled and has had increasing memory loss. Her two sons live nearby but work full-time and cannot manage Agnes's need for care, so it was decided to move Agnes to a local residential care facility. Agnes was very opposed to this, but her GP encouraged the move because she was mismanaging her medication, had fallen a few times and was malnourished.

Her family spent time making the room in her care facility familiar and brought her favourite pictures, armchair and bed cover. The family discussed her social history, her preferences and her habits; however, after moving into the facility, Agnes's condition deteriorated. Her interest in food and socialising declined, and she had a number of skin tears. She now walks with a frame and spends much of her time sleeping. The care staff have noticed that she seems more confused and becomes agitated when they attend to her personal care.

The class should split up into three groups to plan the care for Agnes.

- Group 1 – Discuss the ways a person-centred approach could be used to enhance Agnes's wellbeing.
- Group 2 – Describe appropriate communication strategies that staff can use when attending to Agnes's care.
- Group 3 – Develop appropriate activities to ensure Agnes's dignity, skills and independence are maintained.

Once completed, present your findings and ask for contributions from others in your class.

REFERENCES

Alzheimer's WA (2018). Person centred approach. Retrieved 22 December 2018 from https://www.alzheimerswa.org.au/about-dementia/understanding-dementia-care/person-centered-approach/

Australian Department of Health (2012). Decision-making tool: Handbook – supporting a restraint free environment in residential aged care. Retrieved 28 December 2018 from https://agedcare.health.gov.au/sites/default/files/documents/09_2014/residential_aged_care_internals_fa3-web.pdf

Australian Department of Health (2021a). Restrictive practice use in aged care facilities – Overview. Retrieved 23 March 2022 from https://www.health.gov.au/resources/publications/restrictive-practice-use-in-aged-care-facilities-overview

Australian Department of Health (2021b). Types of restrictive practices. Retrieved 23 March 2022 from https://www.health.gov.au/resources/publications/types-of-restrictive-practices

Australian Department of Health (2021c). AN-ACC Reference Manual and AN-ACC Assessment Tool. Retrieved 23 March 2022 from https://www.health.gov.au/resources/publications/an-acc-reference-manual-and-an-acc-assessment-tool

Dementia Australia (n.d.). What is dementia? Retrieved 22 December 2018 from https://www.dementia.org.au/about-dementia/what-is-dementia

Dementia Training Australia (2017). Cultural assessment for Aboriginal and Torres Strait Islander people with dementia – Resource pack. Retrieved 28 December 2018 from https://www.dementiatrainingaustralia.com.au/resources/cultural-assessment-atsi-resource/

Heerema, E. (2019, 18 September). Using reality orientation in Alzheimer's and dementia: Strategies and cautions in its use. *Very Well Heath*. Retrieved 22 December 2018 from https://www.verywellhealth.com/treating-alzheimers-disease-with-reality-orientation-98682

Kennard, C. (2019, 31 July). Reminiscence therapy for Alzheimer's disease: The benefits of recalling memories. *Very Well Health*. Retrieved 23 December 2018 from https://www.verywellhealth.com/reminiscence-as-activity-and-therapy-97499

University of Queensland (2018). Lobes of the brain. Retrieved 30 December 2018 from https://qbi.uq.edu.au/brain/brain-anatomy/lobes-brain

Victorian Department of Health and Human Services (n.d.). Designing for people with dementia. Retrieved 27 December 2018 from https://www2.health.vic.gov.au/ageing-and-aged-care/dementia-friendly-environments/designing-for-dementia

DELIVER CARE SERVICES USING A PALLIATIVE APPROACH

Learning objectives

By the end of this chapter, you should be able to:

1 apply principles and aims of a palliative approach when supporting individuals
2 respect the individual's preferences for quality-of-life decisions
3 follow the individual's advance care directives in the care plan
4 respond to signs of pain and other symptoms
5 follow end-of-life care strategies
6 manage your own emotional responses and ethical issues.

Introduction

This chapter identifies the skills and knowledge required to care for people with life-threatening or life-limiting illness or normal ageing process within a palliative approach. A person's quality of life can be enhanced by using a palliative approach through reducing suffering and treating pain, as well as attending to their holistic needs.

Quality of life
Includes a person's physical, social, psychological and spiritual needs and can only be determined by each individual.

This chapter will highlight the importance of respecting the person's preferences for their quality of life, including following the person's advance care directives in the care plan. The chapter will emphasise thinking about, communicating and documenting wishes for future care and medical treatment, and responding to signs of pain and other symptoms.

The last part of the chapter will focus on following end-of-life care strategies to meet the person's immediate physical, emotional and spiritual comfort needs and support the person's family. How carers manage emotional responses and ethical issues is also considered, so you can develop self-care strategies to meet your own physical and emotional wellbeing during times of grief and loss.

INDUSTRY INSIGHTS 💬

Palliative day care

Before I started my health services assistance course, I worked as a trained volunteer in the palliative day care unit that was attached to our local hospital. The unit offered programs that allowed respite during the day for people who had life-threatening illness but were well enough to participate in activities away from home. This also gave families a break from their role as carers and relieved their stress and exhaustion from looking after a loved one at home. Most of the clients attended the day unit once a week and accessed the multidisciplinary palliative care team during that time. They were able to share their fears and anxieties with experienced palliative day care staff. My duties included helping in art classes, gardening, games and providing gentle massage for comfort and relaxation. Other programs included discussion groups, guest speakers and physiotherapy sessions. Many of the clients participated in the activities while others sat in the reclining chairs and rested.

I found that the sense of community and relationships allowed the palliative clients to relax in a warm, homely environment, and they seemed comforted by the fact that they could then remain in their home for as long as possible and give a well-earned break to their carers. My volunteer work really confirmed my passion for nursing because I could see the difference that the staff and I made to the clients. Not only did we provide social interaction and psychological support, but the therapeutic relationships formed by the staff through their use of open questioning and clarifying concerns helped them to better understand the client's needs while monitoring their symptoms.

1   APPLY PRINCIPLES AND AIMS OF A PALLIATIVE APPROACH WHEN SUPPORTING INDIVIDUALS

Palliative care is care that relieves the physical and mental distress of the dying person. The World Health Assembly recognises that:

> … palliative care, when indicated, is fundamental to improving the quality of life, well-being, comfort and human dignity for individuals, being an effective person-centred health service that values patients' need to receive adequate, personally and culturally sensitive information on their health status, and their central role in making decisions about the treatment received.
>
> World Health Assembly, 2014, p. 1

Palliative care is not simply confined to the final stages of an illness. It acknowledges that the quality of life of a person with a life-limiting illness can be maintained by early identification, assessment and treatment of pain, and by meeting the person's physical, cultural, social, psychological and spiritual needs. It is adopted when a person is moving towards the end of their life and there is no likelihood of extending their life by curative means.

Palliative care places the person at the centre of their care (see Figure 15.1). The person's needs and preferences are assessed regularly, and the services are able to adapt accordingly.

Palliative care

Care that improves the quality of life of a person and their family through the prevention and relief of suffering by assessment and treatment of pain and other problems – physical, psychosocial and spiritual.

It is important to apply the principles of a person-centred approach when supporting people with life-limiting conditions so that their holistic needs are met, including their pain and comfort levels. This will enable them to experience the best quality of life until their death. Consideration must also be shown for families and carers to ensure that they have the information and help needed to support the palliative patient and their wishes.

FIGURE 15.1 A person-centred approach

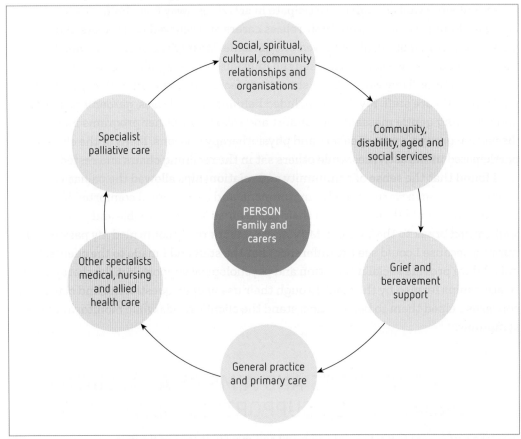

Source: Australian Department of Health (2018). National Palliative Care Strategy 2018, p. 6. Retrieved from https://www.health.gov.au/resources/publications/the-national-palliative-care-strategy-2018

Curative and palliative care

When referring to a palliative approach, it is important to be aware of the differences between curative and palliative care. Curative care is the treatment of symptoms with the use of medications and therapies to cure the person's problem. Palliative care is when cure-orientated goals are replaced by comfort-orientated goals.

Curative care
Healthcare practices using medication and therapies that treat patients with the intent of curing them.

Aims of palliative care in Australia

Palliative care is offered in almost all settings where health care is provided, including in the home, community-based settings, palliative care units and hospitals. In 2010, Australian health ministers, palliative care service providers and community-based organisations met to develop a coordinated and consistent approach to the delivery of high-quality palliative care policies, strategies and services across Australia. This involved the implementation of the National Palliative Care Strategy to enhance the quality of care for palliative patients, which was updated in 2018.

The guiding principles of the 2018 strategy (Australian Department of Health, 2018, p. 5) are identified as fundamental to ensure that all people experience the palliative care they need. They are as follows:

- Palliative care is person-centred care.
- Death is a part of life.
- Carers are valued and receive the care they need.
- Care is accessible.
- Everyone has a role to play in palliative care.
- Care is high-quality and evidence-based.

National Palliative Care Strategy

The updated National Palliative Care Strategy provides a further road map for the future of palliative care services across Australia. This strategy, *Palliative Care 2030: Working towards the future of quality palliative care for all*, highlights Australia's changing demographics and the need to plan for persons living longer, requiring an improved quality of life and need to access high-quality palliative care. It also has a focus on people living with dementia, with a projected increase of almost 1.1 million by 2058, generating in turn an increasing demand for palliative care services.

The strategy's guiding principles will help policy planners to prepare for the future and work towards ensuring Australians have access to high-quality palliative care in the future (see Figure 15.2).

Recognise the holistic needs of the person

People approaching the end of their life frequently have complex, wide-ranging and changing needs. Recognising these needs requires effective communication between the different teams involved in providing care. By using a palliative approach and recognising the patient's holistic needs, their physical, psychological and social requirements are met. These needs include:

- physical needs:
  - pain relief
  - oral care
  - nutrition
  - positioning
  - bowel and bladder care
  - hygiene
- psychological needs:
  - counselling and grief support
  - emotional support for families
- social needs:
  - resources such as home care help and equipment
  - referrals to respite care services
  - spiritual support
  - cultural support
  - services such as financial support.

FIGURE 15.2 Guiding principles for palliative care

Whole of government
Palliative care is now a national health priority. There is a whole-of-government approach to needs-based planning and adequate funding of palliative care and specialist palliative care services.

Workforce
Health professionals providing palliative care are supported by a specialist palliative care workforce, information sharing, remuneration, referral pathways and education and training options.

Community awareness and mobilisation
Individuals and their families have access to the required information at the right time to enable informed decision-making.

Advance care directives now ensure people can clearly express their individualised preferences and choices.

Research, data and advances in technology
Investment into future funds for palliative care will be focused on research and increased use of new and adaptive technologies, resulting in care being more agile, predictive and proactive.

Best practice and innovation models
Involves an agreed set of criteria for earlier identification of when palliative care would be beneficial for an individual, and appropriate referral to specialist palliative care, particularly when there are complex and persistent care needs.

Funding models
Funding item numbers are more suited to provide for palliative care and specialist palliative care needs across the health sector, including tertiary and 24-hour community-based care.

Grief and bereavement
Grief and bereavement support is not just an integral component of specialist palliative care but of all health care.

Access to medications
The introduction of new collaborative, funded models to support community pharmacy, general practice and other practitioners to safely provide opioids and other medicines, including off-label indications.

Source: Palliative Care Australia 2018, Palliative Care 2030 – working towards the future of quality palliative care for all, PCA, Canberra.

Once the holistic needs are recognised, actions can be developed. There should be a strong focus on supporting the patient's choices and decision-making, and on helping the patient, their carers and family to identify and achieve the outcomes they want wherever possible.

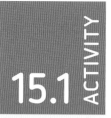

Holistic care for Gina

Gina is a 78-year-old who has been a patient in the palliative care unit for two weeks with a life-limiting illness. The palliative care team, including the social worker and chaplain, met with Gina and her family to consider how to achieve the best quality during her final stages of life.

They discussed Gina's personal values and goals of care while she was still able to communicate and were able to learn what quality of life meant to her. She stated that she did not want cardiopulmonary resuscitation or to remain ventilated. She wanted to be kept comfortable and as pain-free as possible, and if she could not return home with an acceptable quality of life, she wanted to be able to say goodbye to her children and grandchildren and to be blessed by her parish priest. Although her family were distressed, they agreed with these goals and asked if they could seek grief counselling during this difficult time.

1   Outline how Gina's physical, psychological and social needs have been met.

2   What palliative care principles (refer to Figure 15.2) are identified in this scenario?

3   How can grief counselling assist Gina's family?

Support the person, carers and family to express needs and preferences, including quality of life, pain and comfort

The palliative approach encompasses the needs of the person, their carers and family, all of whom have needs that must be addressed. This approach can provide comfort by the management of symptoms; by discussing death and dying openly with the person, their carers and family; and by knowing and following the person's wishes. While some people may want to know every piece of information about their condition and its likely course, some may not want any information at all. An individual approach is needed and must be supported by the healthcare team. As a health services assistant (HSA), you should be guided by the registered nurse (RN), and when unsure of how to communicate, seek their assistance. The person, family and carers and the multidisciplinary team are all essential for discussions and decision-making at the end of life.

Quality of life

Quality of life includes physical, social, psychological and spiritual needs and can only be determined by each individual. It also changes over time and varies according to the stage of disease and also by the stage of life. Symptoms, mood states, roles and sense of self all have an impact on quality of life. Figure 15.3 represents the multifaceted components that comprise quality of life.

FIGURE 15.3 Facets of quality of life

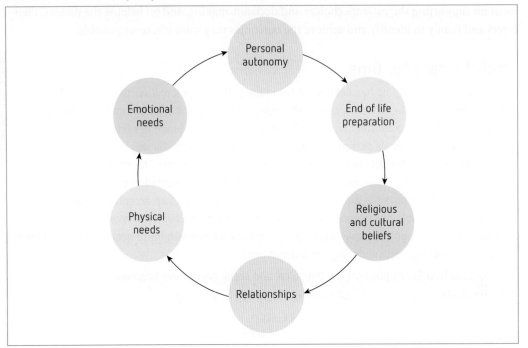

15.2

Quality of life

Answer the following questions relating to quality of life in a palliative patient:

1   How would you define quality of life?
2   Why is it important for the multidisciplinary team to understand a person's individual needs?
3   How might a person's physical, psychological and social needs change as an illness progresses?

Respect the family and carers as an integral part of the care team and ensure they have the information and support needed

Care that is focused on the patient, family and carers as a unit is essential for a palliative approach. Show respect for their needs by being inclusive, open, honest and available for them, when they need you.

Meetings may be organised to facilitate communication and decision-making, and to support families and carers to identify realistic care goals, while also assisting them to deal with their own distress (see Figure 15.4). Meetings also ensure that important information is relayed regarding the ongoing care of their loved ones. This information may include:

- referral to a palliative care unit
- discussion of disease progression
- discussion of the patient's wishes for treatment
- changes in the patient's condition with reassessment of goals.

FIGURE 15.4 A family meeting with the healthcare team

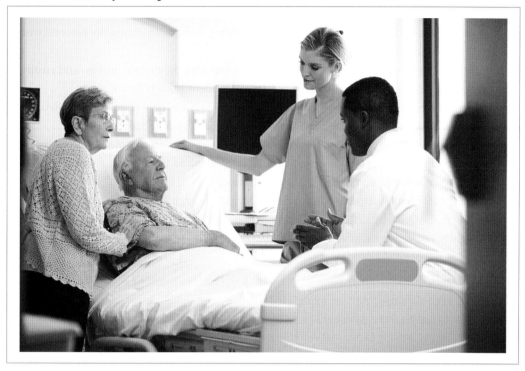

Source: Alamy Stock Photo / MBI

It is important to get to know family members and carers and include them in all communications and care decisions. By making them an integral part of the team and forming a relationship, you are more able to provide emotional and spiritual support, ongoing education about care and management, support during decision-making on end-of-life issues, as well as support after the person's death. As an HSA, your role is to recognise and refer to the RN, supervisors or other members of the multidisciplinary team if any additional support and information for families and carers is needed.

Multidisciplinary team

The family and carers form part of the multidisciplinary team, with each having a role in providing holistic support for the palliative patient. The members of the multidisciplinary team include:

- doctors or specialist physicians; for example, oncologist
- RNs and enrolled nurses (ENs)
- HSAs
- chaplains or other culturally appropriate people
- social workers
- physiotherapists
- dietitians
- pharmacists
- psychologists/counsellors.
  Responsibilities of the team include the following:
- pain management and management of other symptoms such as depression and anxiety

- management of issues relating to nutrition and hydration, as the person may stop eating and drinking towards the end of life
- support regarding advance care planning; i.e., planning and documenting the person's wishes for their end-of-life care
- education of the person and significant others in relation to the disease process and ensuring that they are fully informed about the likely path that the disease will take
- support for increasing disability; e.g., providing additional personal hygiene and toileting support, and the use of mobility aids when the person is no longer able to walk
- spiritual support for the person, carers and family as the person proceeds towards the end of life
- support to ensure the person, carers and family have access to bereavement care, and referrals to community resources and support services
- providing information about medications or alternative medication
- assisting in dealing with death and offering help in talking about emotions and thoughts, and finding ways to manage concerns.

ACTIVITY 15.3

The multidisciplinary team

James has been diagnosed with an aggressive form of cancer and has been told that he has less than a year to live. He lives alone but has a son and daughter-in-law and two grandchildren who live nearby. James and his family met with the palliative specialist who asked him about his goals for the next year. He was clear that he did not want heroic measures to extend his life when the time came, wanted to be pain-free as much as possible, and wanted to spend quality time with his family, in particular his grandchildren.

The specialist organised for these directives to be noted and introduced a medication regimen that would ease James's physical pain. It was arranged that the local pharmacist would regularly drop off the medications and that a community nurse would check up on James as his disease progressed. A counsellor was organised to help support James and his family through the emotional challenges of his life-ending illness. It was also arranged that when James required additional support, palliative care at home could assist with personal hygiene, medication and any additional care needs. Although religion had not been part of his life for a number of years, James asked for spiritual guidance because he felt that this may comfort him as the disease progressed.

1 Identify the members of the multidisciplinary team that will provide James and his family with the information and support required during his end of life.

2 Can you think of additional support services that may assist James and his family?

3 At what stage would palliative care at home not be recommended for James?

2 RESPECT THE PERSON'S PREFERENCES FOR QUALITY-OF-LIFE DECISIONS

Every person has their own preferences for the place and manner in which they would like to die. By creating a supportive environment, the patient and their family and carers are encouraged to share information regarding needs and preferences. In supporting the palliative patient, you should use a non-judgemental approach and communicate with empathy. This will enable the person to express their physical, emotional, social, spiritual and cultural needs in a safe environment.

Create a supportive environment and use a non-judgemental approach that encourages everyone to share information regarding changing needs and preferences

Open communication about the changing condition of the palliative patient is the key to providing ongoing care that supports both the person, their family and/or significant others. When providing support, it is important to listen without judgement and allow the person to feel and express themselves in any way that they need to. Remember that each person has unique needs and may make individual choices. Using a non-judgemental approach includes:

* listening and allowing the person to express their feelings
* using the non-verbal communication skills of touch and silence appropriately
* accepting the person the way he or she is
* maintaining a safe environment where emotions can be freely expressed
* observing the person's body language and maintaining an open posture to allow for open communication
* listening to the tone of voice.

Having as much information as possible about the patient regarding their lifestyle and social, spiritual and cultural choices is vital to ensure any plans and decisions are inclusive and that staff are advocating appropriately for them. Active listening is a skill that can enhance this important process.

Encourage the person and significant others to discuss spiritual and cultural issues

When someone is nearing the end of their life, they may start to question their beliefs, reflect on their life or wonder about the meaning of life. To ensure a holistic approach to care, it is important to address these spiritual and cultural issues. Strategies can include:

* asking the family/person to explain their rituals and beliefs
* asking the question 'Are you at peace?' or 'Where do you find strength in difficult times?' or 'Are there ways we might help with your spiritual needs or concerns?'
* making sure that the person is not alone; being supportive and listening can help
* referral to a member of the team trained specifically in spiritual or cultural care at the end of life, or someone from the person's own spiritual community or tradition.

Spiritual needs

Spiritual support is essential to a palliative approach and may help give access to rites and rituals that offer symbolic meaning to the palliative patient. This will vary depending on ethnicity, gender, social class and the personal experiences of each individual. While spiritual support may be provided by a healthcare worker, specific religious care is best provided by a person from the same faith community. You can provide spiritual support by encouraging the person to reflect on parts of their life that are meaningful and allowing expression through prayer, meditation, rituals or any other activities that provide spiritual or religious connectedness. Spiritual and religious needs are an important part of the care plan and should be reviewed regularly so that preferences and goals are met.

Cultural needs

Culture refers to the particular customs and way of life of a society or group. The palliative patient's cultural needs must be recognised and addressed. Culture can determine a person's view of the nature and meaning of illness and death, of how bad news should be communicated and of how end-of-life decisions can be made. People may have specific needs regarding end-of-life care and it is important to allow them to openly discuss their cultural needs so that you are able to deliver appropriate care. To provide culturally appropriate palliative care requires that a person's culture is understood and that assumptions are not made about the patient's needs.

ACTIVITY 15.4

Spiritual issues

Beryl's condition was deteriorating, and the palliative care nurse visited her at home to review what support was needed in preparation for end of life. The nurse asked her, 'Where do you find strength in difficult times?' and found out that Beryl found inner peace with the Catholic faith. She arranged for the priest from Beryl's local Catholic church to visit and Beryl received Holy Communion each week.

1 How can the identification of spirituality assist a person during their end of life?

2 Why is it important to consider spiritual needs for the palliative patient before, during and after life?

3 What type of spiritual care workers are available for palliative patients?

Communicate with empathy and provide emotional support and refer issues outside of your role

It is important that the palliative patient has the information that they need to enable informed decision-making, and that the healthcare team clearly understands the person's and family's emotions and preferences when developing care goals. It is important for you to refer issues outside your scope of practice to the RN.

Empathy is defined as the action of understanding, being aware of and being sensitive to another's feelings. Expressing empathy is part of establishing a therapeutic relationship with the person and their family and is crucial to understanding their illness and needs. Providing empathy and emotional support is essential because each individual's experiences and responses to end-of-life issues are varied. This may be due to fear, uncertainty about the future, loss of control or challenges to relationships. People may respond to these responses in different ways, so it is important to identify the emotions of sadness, withdrawal, anger or depression and to use empathy to communicate in an open and sensitive way.

By preparing for conversations and using empathy, you can understand what a person is feeling and why their decisions have made sense to them. This can be achieved by:
- watching and listening for cues that the person wants to talk
- ensuring privacy and uninterrupted time for discussion

- making eye contact (if culturally appropriate), sitting close to the person, using appropriate body language, and allowing silence and time for the person to express their feelings
- asking open-ended questions to determine how the person is feeling; for example, 'Tell me about …'
- using clear, jargon-free, understandable language
- giving the person the option not to discuss issues if they feel uncomfortable
- considering that cultural and contextual factors may influence their conversation
- being open and honest – if you are concerned about the questions being asked or you are unable to answer, refer to the RN or supervisor.
  Unhelpful statements that should be avoided include:
- 'Be brave.'
- 'Let's not talk about this now.'
- 'Just remember the good times.'
- 'Why don't you try …'
- 'I know just how you feel.'

You may feel uncomfortable about how to respond to the palliative patient and their family. However, using appropriate listening skills and being empathetic regarding their situation and feelings can often be enough.

Effective communication with Colin

Colin, a 75-year-old war veteran, has just been diagnosed with advanced cancer and has opted to end treatment. Last night he went to the nurse's station and talked with his favourite nurse about his life worries, the break-up of his relationship with his ex-wife, and his fear of dying. The nurse used her empathetic listening skills by stopping her work, making eye contact with Colin and listening without interrupting. She clarified what he was saying and feeling and watched his body language. She did not say too much, instead allowing Colin to talk.

1 What questions could be asked to allow Colin to further explore his feelings?

2 What questions could be used to determine if additional support is needed for Colin at his end of life?

3 Why was it important for the carer to watch Colin's body language when actively listening?

4 Consider any additional communication skills or questioning that may be of benefit in this scenario.

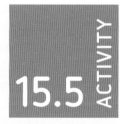

3 FOLLOW THE PERSON'S ADVANCE CARE DIRECTIVES IN THE CARE PLAN

When people know that they are approaching the end of their lives, there is an expectation that their wishes for medical care will be respected, even if disease takes away their decision-making capacity. An advance care directive (ACD), sometimes called a 'living will', is a document that describes the future preferences for medical treatment in anticipation of a time when the person is unable to express those preferences because of illness or injury.

Advance care directive (ACD)

Sometimes called a 'living will', this is an outline of your preferences for your future care along with your beliefs, values and goals when you can no longer make these decisions yourself.

Other ways of documenting end-of-life wishes include appointing a trusted person as an enduring guardian. This person is authorised to make treatment decisions when the person is no longer able to do so for themselves. It is important for the entire healthcare team to be aware of and follow ACDs. Services need to be delivered that support the right of individuals, including the location of their end-of-life care.

Interpret and follow advance care directives in the care plan

Often, when a person becomes ill and is unable to make decisions about their own treatment, family members or significant others have to decide what the person would have wanted, without really knowing the person's wishes. Advance care planning allows for treatments that are consistent with the person's preferences at the end of life. In almost all hospitals, they prevent the implementation of measures such as cardiopulmonary resuscitation, which may not be what the person would have wished.

Advance care directives

An ACD (see Figure 15.5) allows a person to write down their goals and preferences for end of life, or any treatments that they would refuse. States and territories have different legislation regarding ACDs, so it is important to know what applies in each jurisdiction as well as your own organisational policies or procedures that relate to ACDs.

The following points should be considered when following advance care planning and directives:

- An ACD can be updated as long as the person has the capacity.
- An enduring guardian can refer to an ACD before making any health decisions but cannot contradict what is documented.
- If a health professional gives treatment against what is in the ACD, the health professional can incur criminal or civil liability for providing that treatment.
- The person has the right to make their own decisions regarding medical care and treatment and should be supported in doing so.
- The person with decision-making capacity has the right to refuse any and all life-sustaining treatments at end of life.
- If a person lacks decision-making capacity and has no directive, clinicians must consult the family member or person responsible for treatment and care decisions.
- A power of attorney does not allow someone to make healthcare decisions.
- If an ACD is valid, then it is enforceable under law and should be followed.
- In an ACD, specific treatment preferences may be mentioned; for example, 'I do not want cardiopulmonary resuscitation' or 'I want to be pain-free and comfortable'.

Some people may not want to plan for end of life or discuss their care choices in the event of their deterioration. They may prefer to leave the decision-making in the hands of their family. Their right to do this must be respected.

Power of attorney

Gives an assigned third party the power to make decisions on a person's behalf regarding managing assets and financial affairs in the event that they are unable to do so when the need arises.

FIGURE 15.5 An example of an advance care directive form

Advance Care Directive Form

By completing this Advance Care Directive you can choose to:

1. Appoint one or more Substitute Decision-Makers and/or

2. Write down your values and wishes to guide decisions about your future health care, end of life, living arrangements and other personal matters and/or

3. Write down health care you do not want in particular circumstances.

Government of South Australia

Part 1

You must fill in this Part.

Part 1: Personal details

Name: _____
(Full name of person giving Advance Care Directive)

Address: _____

Ph:_____ ☎ Date of birth: ___/___/_____

Part 2a

Your Substitute Decision-Maker fills in this section and must sign before you do.

You must provide the Substitute Decision-Maker with the Substitute Decision-Maker Guidelines prior to completing this section.

Your Substitute Decision-Maker fills in this section. →

If you did not fill in any of this Part please draw a large "Z" across the blank section.

Only fill in Part 2a if you want to appoint one or more Substitute Decision-Makers.

Part 2a: Appointing Substitute Decision-Makers

I appoint: _____
(Name of appointed Substitute Decision-Maker)

Address: _____

Ph:_____ ☎ Date of birth: ___/___/_____

I,_____
(Name of appointed Substitute Decision-Maker)

am over 18 years old, and I understand and accept my role and the responsibilities of being a Substitute Decision-Maker as set out in the Substitute Decision-Maker Guidelines.

Signed: _____ Date: ___/___/_____
(Signature of appointed Substitute Decision-Maker)

Part 2a
(continued over page)

Your initial:_____		See page 15 for suggested certification statement
Witness initial:_____	Certification statement or JP stamp	1 of 6 Advance Care Directive Form
Date:___/___/___		

Source: South Australia Heath, reproduced with permission. https://advancecaredirectives.sa.gov.au/upload/home/ACDFormSecure.pdf

ACTIVITY 15.6

Advance care directives

Download an advance care directive form for your state or territory by visiting **https://www.advancecareplanning.org.au/** and answer the following questions:

1 What are the options for cardiopulmonary resuscitation?
2 Why is it important to consider personal values as part of advance care planning?
3 What are the options for where you would like to die?
4 Why is it important to consider specific requests with regard to medical care?
5 Consider any specific treatment limitations that could be included in the advance care plan.

Comply with end-of-life decisions and in keeping with legal requirements

End-of-life care can result in issues regarding symptom management, pain control, comfort and psychosocial treatment. This makes it important for you to practise within legal requirements and adhere to your scope of practice. The person's care plan should be maintained so that it is always up to date, reflecting changes in condition and care as they occur. The care plan may also indicate formal ACDs or less formal wishes, such as whether the person wants to see particular family members or friends before death.

End-of-life issues that may have legal implications you need to be aware of include the following:

* pain management – this is a fundamental part of palliative care and a human right. People administering medications must comply with the *Therapeutic Goods Act 1989* and the Poisons Standard
* documentation – this must be accurate and comply with legal requirements
* duty of care – you have an obligation to ensure that duty of care is carried out when caring for the palliative patient. This includes using the correct equipment and avoiding harm to the patient when carrying out procedures and minimising risk
* ACDs – failure to comply with ACDs may result in the health professional incurring criminal or civil liability.

Patient rights

Everyone who is seeking or receiving care in the Australian health system has certain rights regarding the nature of that care. These are described in the Australian Charter of Healthcare Rights (Victorian Department of Health). The rights included in the charter relate to:

* access – to adequate and timely health care
* safety – to safe and high-quality care
* respect – to receive care in a way that is respectful of your culture, beliefs, values and characteristics like age and gender
* communication – to be informed about services, treatment, options and costs in a clear and open way
* participation – to be included in decisions and choices about care

- privacy – to ensure privacy and confidentiality of information
- comment – to be able to comment on care and have concerns addressed.

You must ensure that the person's rights are upheld and refer any concerns to the RN or supervisor.

Enduring power of attorney

When someone is appointed an enduring power of attorney, they are given the power to make decisions on a person's behalf regarding managing assets and financial affairs in the event that the person is unable to do so when the need arises. A person can only appoint an attorney if they are over 18 years of age and able to demonstrate capacity to make the appointment. If a family member has been granted a power of attorney to make decisions for the person, then the legal document stating this must be sighted by a member of the palliative care team and its powers and limitations noted on the person's record. Only in Victoria, the ACT and Queensland can an enduring power of attorney also be used to authorise medical and health decisions.

Enduring guardianship

In some states, a power of attorney only grants authority to handle property and financial matters, not medical and health decisions. An enduring guardianship is the additional document that allows a person to legally appoint a decision-maker of their choice to make those medical and healthcare decisions should they lose the capacity to make their own decisions. It is important for these legal documents to be included in the person's medical records and that the healthcare team is informed regarding the person's end-of-life decisions.

Do not resuscitate orders

A DNR order (do not resuscitate) is a medical order to withhold cardiopulmonary resuscitation (CPR) techniques (see Figure 15.6). The law in Australia regarding DNR orders is found in both common law and various legislation in states and territories. Under common law, any competent adult can complete an ACD, which can extend to refusing CPR. As an HSA, it is important to understand the legislation in your state/territory. When unsure, you should refer to the RN for advice.

Consent

In Australia, medical services cannot be provided without the consent of the person concerned. Consent is considered to be informed when the person voluntarily agrees to a treatment without duress and after they have been provided with adequate information. The only exception is when the person's capacity to consent is impaired; for example, because of a serious illness or cognitive condition.

Enduring guardianship

Allows you to legally appoint a decision-maker of your choice to make lifestyle and healthcare decisions should you lose the capacity to do so.

DNR order (do not resuscitate)

A medical order to withhold cardiopulmonary resuscitation (CPR) techniques.

FIGURE 15.6 An example of a do not resuscitate (DNR) order

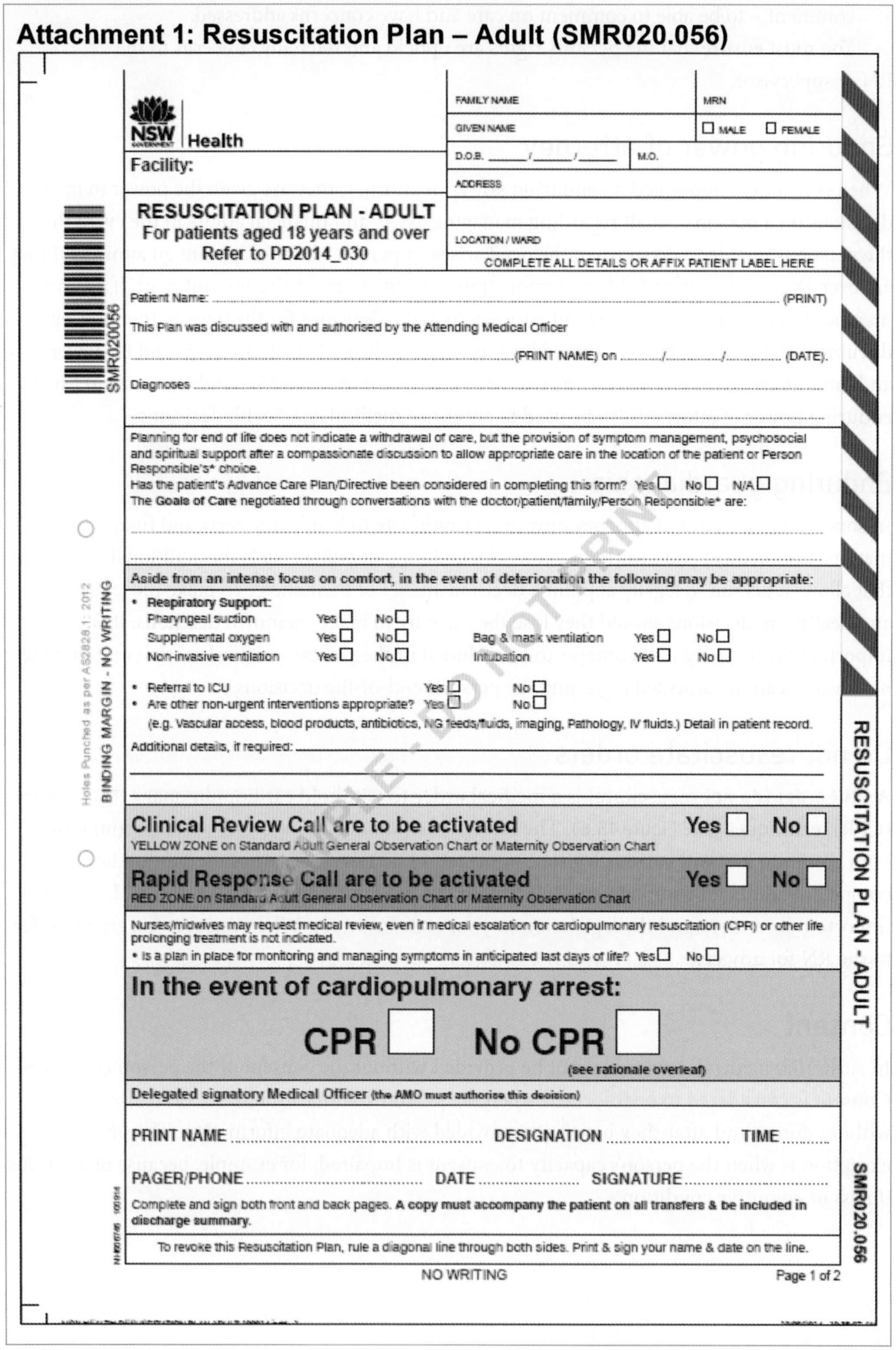

Attachment 1: Resuscitation Plan – Adult (SMR020.056)

NSW Health

Facility:

FAMILY NAME		MRN
GIVEN NAME		☐ MALE ☐ FEMALE
D.O.B. ____/____/____	M.O.	
ADDRESS		

RESUSCITATION PLAN - ADULT
For patients aged 18 years and over
Refer to PD2014_030

LOCATION / WARD

COMPLETE ALL DETAILS OR AFFIX PATIENT LABEL HERE

SMR020.056

Patient Name: .... (PRINT)

This Plan was discussed with and authorised by the Attending Medical Officer

....(PRINT NAME) on ..../............../............... (DATE).

Diagnoses ....

Planning for end of life does not indicate a withdrawal of care, but the provision of symptom management, psychosocial and spiritual support after a compassionate discussion to allow appropriate care in the location of the patient or Person Responsible's* choice.

Has the patient's Advance Care Plan/Directive been considered in completing this form? Yes ☐ No ☐ N/A ☐

The **Goals of Care** negotiated through conversations with the doctor/patient/family/Person Responsible* are:

....
....
....

Aside from an intense focus on comfort, in the event of deterioration the following may be appropriate:

- **Respiratory Support:**
  Pharyngeal suction   Yes ☐ No ☐
  Supplemental oxygen   Yes ☐ No ☐   Bag & mask ventilation   Yes ☐ No ☐
  Non-invasive ventilation   Yes ☐ No ☐   Intubation   Yes ☐ No ☐

- Referral to ICU   Yes ☐ No ☐
- Are other non-urgent interventions appropriate?   Yes ☐ No ☐
  (e.g. Vascular access, blood products, antibiotics, NG feeds/fluids, imaging, Pathology, IV fluids.) Detail in patient record.

Additional details, if required: _____
_____
_____

Clinical Review Call are to be activated   Yes ☐ No ☐
YELLOW ZONE on Standard Adult General Observation Chart or Maternity Observation Chart

Rapid Response Call are to be activated   Yes ☐ No ☐
RED ZONE on Standard Adult General Observation Chart or Maternity Observation Chart

Nurses/midwives may request medical review, even if medical escalation for cardiopulmonary resuscitation (CPR) or other life prolonging treatment is not indicated.

- Is a plan in place for monitoring and managing symptoms in anticipated last days of life?   Yes ☐ No ☐

In the event of cardiopulmonary arrest:

CPR ☐   No CPR ☐
(see rationale overleaf)

Delegated signatory Medical Officer (the AMO must authorise this decision)

PRINT NAME ....   DESIGNATION ....   TIME ....

PAGER/PHONE ....   DATE ....   SIGNATURE ....

Complete and sign both front and back pages. A copy must accompany the patient on all transfers & be included in discharge summary.

To revoke this Resuscitation Plan, rule a diagonal line through both sides. Print & sign your name & date on the line.

NO WRITING   Page 1 of 2

Holes Punched as per AS2828.1 : 2012 — BINDING MARGIN - NO WRITING

RESUSCITATION PLAN - ADULT   SMR020.056

Legal requirements

Research power of attorney and guardianship on your state/territory government websites and indicate whether the following statements are true or false:

	TRUE	FALSE
A guardian or power of attorney must be 18 years of age or older		
A power of attorney can refuse emergency lifesaving treatment for the person who is dying		
A power of attorney must be signed in the presence of two witnesses		
Family or relatives are only able to be guardians		
An enduring power of attorney ceases when the patient dies		
You can appoint more than one enduring guardian as joint enduring guardians		

15.7 ACTIVITY

Report the person's changing needs in relation to end of life and refer impact on families, carers and/or significant others

As the person's needs change, the care plan needs to be regularly updated to reflect the ongoing care. Changes in mobility, self-care, pain and elimination and mental status need to be noted in the care plan and communicated to the healthcare team. As a person's life is ending, their condition will deteriorate progressively and their care needs will change accordingly. Physical comfort will be most important as well as emotional and spiritual support. As an HSA, your responsibility is to report any changes to the patient's physical or cognitive state, as well as reactions from family or significant others.

Changing needs of Jose

Eighty-nine-year-old Jose has pancreatic cancer and has been cared for by his wife for the last three years. He has now been admitted to hospital as his deterioration has been such that his wife is no longer able to care for him. Soon after admission, the multidisciplinary team has a meeting with his wife and informs her that Jose's condition will become worse: he will gradually become weaker, his appetite will decrease and his breathing will change. But they assure her that staff will care for him as his needs change. As he also has a heart condition, Jose may die suddenly. While Jose's wife is visibly upset, she appreciates the opportunity to plan preferences with her husband.

1   When reporting the reactions of Jose's wife, what support services are available to assist with her emotions?

2   As Jose becomes weaker and is unable to mobilise, what strategies would maintain skin integrity and prevent decubitus ulcers?

3   What strategies would the nurse use to maintain oral care as Jose's breathing changes?

15.8 ACTIVITY

Deliver services to support the right of individuals to choose the location of their end-of-life care

Good quality end-of-life care can be provided in a hospital, residential aged care facility or in the person's home if staff and/or family are provided with the necessary resources. This will mean that the person remains in appropriate or familiar surroundings and can be cared for by people who understand their needs.

If a person decides to remain at home, strong family and health support is required because caring is a 24-hour undertaking. Some people decide to die in hospital and their families are relieved of the burden of home care. Ultimately it is an individual choice; however, as people approach death, their care needs become increasingly complex, and they need pain and other symptom management including personal care assistance. Supporting the person and their significant others in wherever they choose for their end-of-life care is a priority to achieve dignity and respect for all.

Hospice care

Hospice care represents a compassionate approach to palliative care while enhancing the quality of remaining life. Hospice care involves palliative care (pain and symptom relief) rather than ongoing curative care and enables the person to spend their end of life with dignity and support. Some hospitals and nursing homes provide hospice care on-site and hospice care can also be achieved in the home. This enables the person to spend their final days in a familiar, comfortable environment with their loved ones and with the help of hospice staff.

If a person decides to spend their end of life at home, the palliative care team develop a care plan that is individualised for the needs of the person and provide all the medication, medical supplies and equipment needed. Typically, a family member acts as a primary caregiver with supervision from medical staff who make regular visits to assess the person and provide additional care and services as needed. This can reduce the anxiety of both the palliative patient and their family who can then spend quality time together.

Source: Adapted from Segal, J. & Robinson, L. (2019) Hospice and palliative care. Helpguide. Retrieved 2 November 2016 from http://www.helpguide.org/articles/caregiving/hospice-and-palliative-care.htm

ACTIVITY 15.9

Location for end-of-life care

Anne is 91 years old and has been admitted to hospital with a fractured hip. She has been a widow for the last 12 years and lives two hours' drive away from her daughter, Francie. Her other two children live interstate. As Francie is the person that Anne relies on the most, the healthcare team asks if Anne has made any ACDs such as power of attorney to formalise future care-management arrangements.

It is arranged that Francie is appointed power of attorney and enduring guardian. Anne lets Francie know that she does not want any further medical intervention if she suffers a stroke or heart attack, and that she would prefer hospital to home care at the end of her life. This is documented in an advance care plan.

1 What are the advantages and disadvantages of hospital or home care for the palliative patient?

2 Why do you think Anne chose hospital care for her end-of-life location?

3 Who should copies of the ACD be given to?

4 RESPOND TO SIGNS OF PAIN AND OTHER SYMPTOMS

When a person is at the end of their life, the healthcare team can offer treatments that will promote comfort by minimising pain and other symptoms, such as anxiety, constipation, dyspnoea and restlessness. The assessment and management of pain and other symptoms and the explanation of misconceptions regarding pain relief will enable the palliative patient to be as comfortable as possible.

Observe and report the person's pain and symptoms and implement and evaluate strategies to promote comfort

The palliative care approach to symptom management is based on a thorough assessment of current symptoms and planning ahead for common problems. The common physical problems which need to be assessed and planned for include:

- pain
- inadequate nutrition and hydration
- nausea and vomiting
- bladder and bowel problems
- breathing difficulties.

Pain

Pain is the most common symptom of a person who is in the terminal phase of life. Pain that is not well controlled causes significant distress and disability; therefore, the effective management of pain is a vital part of palliative care practice. Pain is managed best by a process of assessment, intervention using a range of drug and non-drug therapies, and evaluation of their effectiveness.

Types of pain

Understanding how pain is defined is important in order to learn how to better control it. Acute pain is defined as pain lasting less than three to six months, or pain that is directly related to tissue damage, such as post-operatively. Acute pain disappears when the underlying cause of pain has been treated or has healed. Clinical signs of acute pain are increased blood pressure and heart rate, sweating, pallor and anxiety. Chronic pain results from chronic pathological processes, often has a gradual onset and becomes progressively worse. The person may appear depressed, withdrawn and lethargic. Treatment for chronic pain requires determining the underlying cause and providing pharmacological or non-pharmacological management.

Because pain is a subjective symptom, the most accurate evidence of pain is based on the person's description, which may include aching, burning, heaviness, sharpness, 'pins and needles', tingling or tightness. Non-verbal responses to pain may be agitation, restlessness, and changes in facial expressions such as frowning or grimacing, or making noises such as crying, groaning and moaning. The person may also experience nausea, vomiting, anorexia or dyspnoea due to pain.

Pain assessment tools

Effective pain management requires careful assessment and regular review of pain. Since pain is a subjective symptom, pain assessment tools are based on the person's own perception of their pain and its severity. A pain assessment tool gives a baseline from which to evaluate treatment interventions. It also gives the person a more active role in describing and dealing with their pain.

Pain assessment tools include the following:

- Numerical Rating Scales (NRS; see Figure 15.7) – where numbers are used to represent the strength of the pain, with 0 representing no pain and 10 representing unbearable pain.
- Abbey Pain Scale – an Australian-developed tool for people with dementia. Scores are totalled for vocalisations, facial expressions, and physical and psychological changes, with a score nearing 7 to 10 being assessed as severe pain.
- Wong-Baker FACES Scale – a number of faces are shown on a scale from a smiley face to a crying face (see Figure 15.7). This is useful for people who cannot verbalise their pain, and in particular younger people.
- Pain Assessment in Advanced Dementia (PAINAD) Scale – this pain behaviour tool is used to assess pain in older adults who have dementia or other cognitive impairment and are unable to reliably communicate their pain.
- Brief Pain Inventory (BPI) – this is a nine-item, self-administered questionnaire used to evaluate the severity of a person's pain and the impact of this pain on the person's daily functioning.

FIGURE 15.7 Numerical Rating Scale (NRS) and Wong-Baker FACES Scale

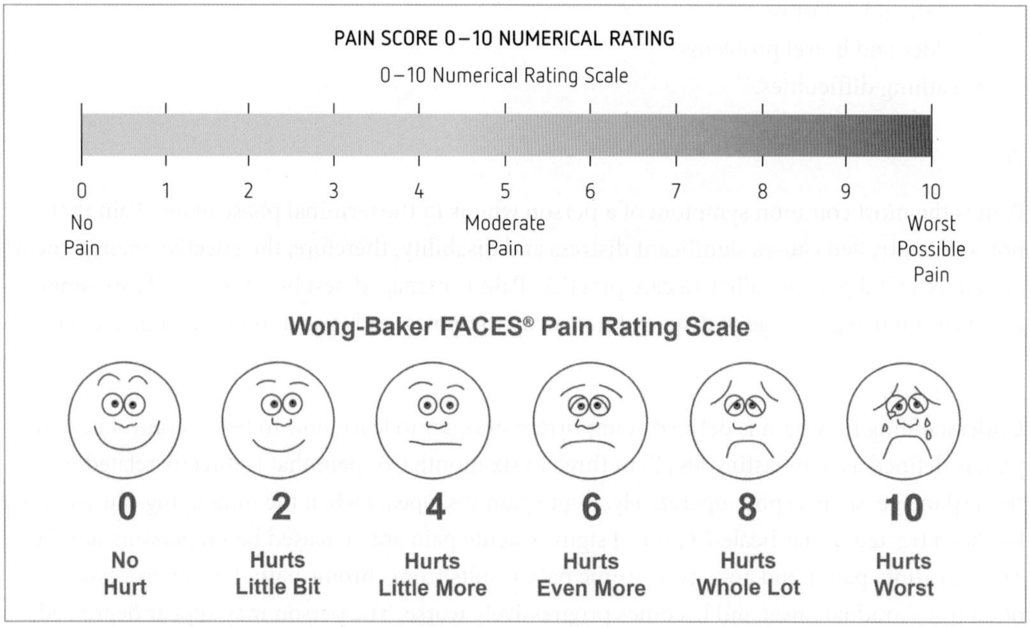

Source: © 1983 Wong-Baker FACES Foundation. www.WongBakerFACES.org. Used with permission. Originally published in Whaley & Wong's Nursing Care of Infants and Children. © Elsevier Inc.

Pharmacological management

The most common medications in palliative care are opioids, such as morphine, and lesser-strength drugs including codeine and paracetamol for mild pain. One of the major considerations when opioids are used is that in the elderly, liver and kidney function is reduced, causing opioids to accumulate in the body with a higher chance of side effects. The use of multiple drugs in the elderly can also interact with opioids, causing adverse reactions; therefore, the use of opioids in the elderly requires caution and review.

Morphine can be given in a number of forms including tablets and liquid, injection and via patches on the skin. When the person is approaching death and is unable to swallow, morphine and other drugs may be given via a syringe driver (see Figure 15.8). This is a battery-operated pump that provides a prescribed amount of medication continuously via a needle that is placed under the skin. As an HSA, you cannot dispense medications, but you can report on pain and the effectiveness of medication.

FIGURE 15.8 A syringe driver

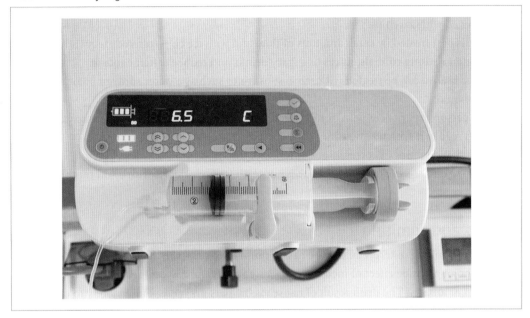

Source: Shutterstock.com/Yuriy Bartenev

Non-pharmacological management

Non-pharmacological approaches, including complementary therapies for pain management, have an increasingly important contribution to make to the holistic care of the person alongside analgesics. Management (CareSearch, 2017) may include:

- counselling
- positioning
- massage/relaxation techniques
- aromatherapy
- naturopathy
- therapeutic touch/reiki/reflexology
- herbal/traditional Chinese medicines
- music therapy
- meditation/hypnotherapy
- acupressure/acupuncture.

Inadequate nutrition and hydration

When a person is at the end of life, they experience loss of appetite and dehydration. This is a normal part of the dying process because metabolism is slowing down and the body requires less nutrition. The person becomes increasingly weak and drowsy, and swallowing and digesting food and fluids often becomes harder and can place strain upon the body. Nevertheless, although the person may have a reduced oral intake, it is important to maintain good oral care.

Comfort strategies for the person experiencing loss of appetite and dehydration are as follows (adapted from CareSearch, 2017):

- If a person is still capable of eating, they can be offered food that they enjoy. Ice-cream and ice blocks soothe a sore mouth and are easily swallowed.
- Encourage the person to drink water after meals and medications.
- Keeping the mouth clean and moist is essential. Lanolin can be applied. Lips can also be moistened with ice chips.
- Thirst is best treated by small amounts of fluid and with ice chips offered frequently.
- Discourage strong cordials, juices or sugary drinks and reduce caffeine intake.
- Reduced saliva can be treated with saliva substitutes such as a water spray or an oral balance gel or liquid.
- If the person experiences pain or ulceration in the mouth, help them to rinse or swab their mouth regularly with warm saline.
- Check that dentures fit correctly and offer cold, soft food.
- If the person has a coated tongue, mucosa or teeth, remove debris with a soft toothbrush or mouth swab.

Nausea and vomiting

Nausea and vomiting in terminal disease have a number of causes including dehydration and constipation or as a side effect of medication. Nausea and vomiting can be triggered by smells, tastes, pain or anxiety. The main result of nausea is the person's increasing inability to eat well. Vomiting can cause exhaustion as well as potentially serious effects of dehydration and lack of absorption of medications.

Comfort strategies for the person experiencing nausea and vomiting are as follows:

- When vomiting ceases, rinse the mouth, clean the teeth and offer small sips of water or ice cubes.
- Manage constipation if this is a causative factor.
- Keep food smells or other unpleasant smells to a minimum.
- Manage posture and avoid lying down immediately after eating.
- Appropriate medication can be given by a registered professional.

Bladder and bowel problems

Bowel symptoms such as constipation or faecal incontinence can have a negative effect on a person's quality of life. Bowel care is an important part of a palliative approach as the person may be taking opioids, which are a major cause of constipation. Loss of sphincter control can also cause urinary incontinence.

Comfort strategies for the person experiencing constipation or urinary incontinence are as follows:

- Record daily the patient's bowel habits.
- Administer medication to prevent constipation if fibre or fluid cannot be maintained.
- Use protective continence pads, or external or internal urinary drainage devices to prevent discomfort and skin breakdown from urinary incontinence.
- Maintain skin integrity and provide clean and dry sheets.

Breathing difficulties

Dyspnoea (shortness of breath) can be due to pain, psychological issues such as anxiety, or poor lung function from the disease process. The person may be unable to cough or expectorate to clear their airway.

Comfort strategies for the person experiencing breathing difficulties are as follows:

* Providing oxygen (administered by a registered professional) can take away the feeling of suffocation.
* Sitting the patient upright supported by pillows can help with breathing, and if this is not possible, position on the side to prevent aspiration of secretions.
* Give verbal reassurance.
* Avoid lying the patient flat before and after meals.
* Maintain good mouth care for the patient.

Evaluation

It is important to constantly evaluate strategies of symptom relief for a palliative patient. This can be achieved by communicating verbally with the person, observing facial expressions, movement, respirations etc., as well as asking family members for their observations. Pain and observation charts, as well as progress notes and reporting at handover, inform the healthcare team so that new strategies can be put in place if required.

Care planning for comfort

15.10 ACTIVITY

Eighty-four-year-old Melanie's terminal condition has deteriorated and she is now semi-conscious and appears restless. Her fragile skin is becoming reddened on her bony prominences and she has urinary incontinence. She is unable to tolerate food and fluids and her breathing patterns alternate between fast and slow, with her open-mouthed breathing causing her to have a dry mouth and lips. Her family is openly distressed and wishes to remain with her, along with the pastoral care minister.

Answer the following questions regarding care planning for comfort:

1 What comfort measures will assist Melanie during her last stages of life?

2 How can the healthcare team support Melanie's family in their grief?

3 How can the family assist the healthcare team during Melanie's final stages of life?

Refer misconceptions surrounding the use of pain-relieving medication to the appropriate staff member

One barrier to good pain management at the end of life occurs when there are misconceptions about the use of opiates (the morphine group of drugs). Some people worry that using pain-relieving medicines will cause addiction or that overuse will hasten death. Other misconceptions include that overuse will cause tolerance or that injections are the only method of treatment. Figure 15.9 lists common misconceptions and facts regarding pain relief.

FIGURE 15.9 Misconceptions and facts regarding pain relief

MISCONCEPTION	FACT
Opioid medicines cause addiction or dependence	Opioid medicines are not addictive when used for pain
	Addiction only occurs when people have no pain and they abuse opioid medicines
Opioid medicines hasten death	Opioid medicines are for improving life, not hastening death. Relieving pain changes the quality of life, not its duration
Opioid medicines cause terrible side effects	All medicines can have side effects. The side effects of opioid medicines (constipation, drowsiness, nausea, dry mouth) are usually manageable
Medicines will 'cover up' the progression of the illness so you won't know how you are going	Pain medication will not stop the healthcare team monitoring the progress of the illness – they have health assessment tools for monitoring illness
The most effective way to take medication is by injection	Opioid medications can also be effectively taken by a skin patch, liquid, spray or a tablet
Over time the pain medicines will become less effective	Tolerance can develop as a normal result of opioid use. A dose escalation is all that is usually required for additional pain control

Adapted from: Palliative Care Australia (n.d.). Facts about morphine and other opioid medicines in palliative care. Retrieved from https://palliativecare.org.au/resources/facts-about-morphine-and-other-opioid-medicines-in-palliative-care

When health professionals administer pain medications for the dying patient, the intent is to relieve symptoms, even if the possibility exists that such treatment might hasten death. Communication with the family must stress this goal. Communication and teamwork between health professionals, patients and their care workers are crucial to the successful management of pain.

5 FOLLOW END-OF-LIFE CARE STRATEGIES

When following end-of-life care strategies, ongoing discussions with the person and significant others should be held often and include the entire multidisciplinary team. Aspects of care such as setting and reviewing goals, supporting preferences including spirituality and culture, and maintaining dignity as death approaches and occurs must be maintained. The loss and grief following death must also be acknowledged so that comfort and support strategies can be implemented.

Check for changes of care plan that indicate decisions made by the person have been reviewed

The person's care plan should be regularly updated and should reflect discussions with the healthcare team, family and carers. The person may develop new health problems or there may be worsening of a current health issue. There may also be changes to goals in collaboration with the family. Reviewing and documenting changes in the care plan ensure that all staff caring for the person are aware of the current care goals and the person's wishes. Additional decisions that may be made by the person who is nearing end of life and their significant others include:

- changes to the ACD, enduring power of attorney and/or guardianship
- a preferred funeral director
- preference to die at home rather than in a hospital
- preference for cremation or burial
- specific religious and/or cultural preferences
- special wishes; for example, see a person or place before death.

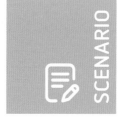

End-of-life care for George

George, aged 72 years, completed an ACD three years ago when he developed lymphoma. He also took the opportunity to appoint his wife as his power of attorney and enduring guardian. He is now in palliative care and has decided to review the plan as his wife has early dementia. He wishes to appoint his daughter as his substitute decision-maker rather than his wife. He also wishes to change his ACD, as he no longer wants to be resuscitated and only wants comfort treatment. In consultation with George's daughter and the doctor, a new form is signed with George's wishes. A copy is placed in George's medical records and the healthcare team is notified of the changes.

1 What is the difference between a power of attorney and enduring guardianship?
2 Why was it important for George to change his ACD?
3 Why is it essential to have a copy of George's directive in the medical records?
4 Search for 'Planning your palliative care' at **https://www.health.gov.au/** for more information on advanced care directives.

Support the person's significant others, preferences and culture and maintain dignity when providing end-of-life care and care following death

Palliative care involves assisting the person and their families to communicate those things that are important to them about end-of-life issues and preferences. An important aspect of maintaining dignity when providing end-of-life care is to accommodate these preferences and promote individualised care that benefits everyone's wellbeing. Understanding practices, attitudes and beliefs, including religious and cultural preferences, assists in meeting the care needs at end of life.

Maintain dignity in death

Shared decision-making between the healthcare team, the person and their families is possible when everyone has an awareness of the person's approaching death. Clear information should be given to them about the dying process and what to expect, as this will ensure that the person's preferences can be addressed. By listening and respecting the choices made by the palliative patient and their family, a dignified death can be achieved. Some suggestions for achieving a dignified death include:

- maintaining open communication with the person, family and carers and being prepared to change care as required

- adhering to spiritual and cultural preferences
- making sure that the ACD is articulated and followed
- ensuring that the person remains in control where possible.

Religious and cultural practices

In our multicultural society, it is your duty to care for people who are dying and who come from different ethnic backgrounds. Different cultures have different customs that are expected to be followed. Therefore, it is important to be aware of the religion and culture of the palliative patient. Figure 15.10 lists examples of cultural beliefs and appropriate related care prior to and after death.

FIGURE 15.10 Beliefs and care at death

BELIEF	PRIOR TO DEATH	AFTER DEATH
Buddhists believe in reincarnation – the cycle of birth, death and rebirth	The dying person may ask a monk to help them pray for a better reincarnation	Buddhists believe it is important that the body is treated with respect, but there are no essential rites for disposal of the body
Catholics believe that there is eternal life	The Catholic priest offers the Sacrament of the Anointing of the Sick or confession	The priest may comfort the family and help them make the funeral arrangements
Mormons commonly believe that death is the separation of the soul from the body	The ward bishop is called to offer support to the dying person and their family	The ward bishop comforts the family and helps them prepare the funeral arrangements
Greek Orthodox believe in eternal life	An Orthodox priest is often called to offer prayers, counselling, confession and Holy Communion	The family stay with their relative after death. The priest says the first prayer and a candle is lit. This is repeated for 40 days
Hindus believe in reincarnation. When a person dies their soul merely moves from one body to the next	Family and a Hindu priest may come to pray and sing hymns and holy chants	It may be upsetting to the family if a non-Hindu person touches the body after death. Family can wash, anoint and dress the body
Jews believe that when they die there is existence after death	A rabbi may be called to say the confessional prayer (Vidui) and affirmation of faith (Shema)	Ritual washing and dressing of the body are performed. If non-Jewish people have to handle the body, gloves are worn. All lines, catheters etc. should be left in situ
Muslims believe that life is never-ending and death is another stage when the soul is released from the body	When death is imminent, most face Mecca, the Muslim holy city. Prayers are recited from the Qur'an at the bedside	The body is washed and wrapped in a shroud for burial as soon as possible, preferably within 24 hours, and the body should face in the direction of Mecca
When an Indigenous person dies, their spirit goes back to the Dreaming Ancestors in the land	Large gatherings at the hospital may take place as it is believed that this prepares the person for the next stage of their journey	The name of the deceased person is not spoken out loud; it is believed that it will help make sure the spirit can move onto the next journey without interference

Adapted from: Palliative Care Victoria (2013). Death & Dying – Religious & Cultural Considerations. Retrieved 19 October 2019 from https://w6p3u3w8.stackpathcdn.com/wp-content/uploads/2015/11/Death-Dying-Religious-Cultural-Conderations.pdf

Culturally appropriate care for Aboriginal and Torres Strait Islander peoples

Engaging with relevant organisations and personnel in the planning, provision and monitoring of palliative care is fundamental to providing culturally safe palliative care to Aboriginal and Torres Strait Islander peoples. This ensures that culturally relevant requirements are addressed and the preferences of the person and their family are considered.

Research cultural considerations for providing end-of-life care or access the Australian Indigenous HealthInfoNet website (**http://www.healthinfonet.ecu.edu.au/related-issues/ palliative-care**) to answer the following questions:

1   How can Aboriginal liaison officers or Aboriginal health workers assist with a palliative approach in hospital and community settings?

2   Why is it important to acknowledge kinship, traditional healers and bush medicines for some individuals?

3   After a person has passed, what cultural practices should be approached with respect and continued support?

15.11 ACTIVITY

Recognise, support and report signs of deterioration or imminent death

Physical death is a progressive process, during which there are some signs that usually indicate that the death is imminent. Not all of the following changes occur and they may not appear in any particular order as the body shuts down during the dying process. Recognising that a person is deteriorating and that death is imminent is an important part of caring for that person.

Signs of impending death

Signs of impending death include the following:

- increased anxiety, restlessness and confusion, then the person becomes less responsive
- shallow and irregular (Cheyne-Stokes respirations) breathing where the person's breathing patterns become progressively irregular and shallower followed by periods of strong, deep breathing. This pattern continues until breathing ceases
- noisy (stertorous) breathing if the person is unable to cough up secretions
- speech becomes increasingly difficult, confused or unintelligible and finally impossible
- pulse becomes rapid and weak
- extremities become cold and circulation slows with the development of cyanosis
- skin may become pale, cool, clammy and mottled as death approaches
- the person may involuntarily void or defecate
- the eyes stare and appear glazed
- the patient loses consciousness.

Cheyne-Stokes respirations
Abnormal pattern of breathing, where there are periods of apnoea (no breathing) followed by periods of tachypnoea (fast breathing).

Signs of clinical death

Signs of clinical death include the following:

- the pupils do not respond to light and are permanently dilated
- the jaw may drop

- the eyes may remain open
- there is no pulse or respiration
- the body becomes cold
- blood pools with purple discolouration in the lowest areas of the body
- after two to four hours the body becomes rigid (rigor mortis)
- fluids may leak from natural body openings, particularly if decomposition is allowed to occur.

Care after death

There are considerations regarding care and preparation of the body after someone dies. Required procedures are often included in an organisation's procedure manual as well as your state/territory's Department of Health regulations. After death, a Medical Certificate of Cause of Death ('death certificate') is completed by a medical practitioner. In the event of accidental death or the cause of death being unknown, the coroner must be notified, and the body not touched until the coroner gives permission.

Care should be taken when attending to the person who has died. They are entitled in death to be treated with the same dignity and respect as any living person. It is an emotional time for families and significant others and they all require special care during this period. After a person dies it is important to give the family the time that they need with the body. Some family members might like to stay with their loved one, while others might like to be involved with washing the body. Every death and every family is individual; therefore, it is important to talk to the family and make them feel they are in a safe space to be with their loved one. It is important to respect cultural considerations or requests whenever possible.

In general, unless culture or a coroner does not permit it, a body is prepared by washing the person, removing tubes and jewellery, and then placing them in a non-porous bag. Use gloves as the body may continue to be infectious after death. The name of the deceased is written on the outside covering according to organisational policy. At all times, the deceased person is accorded the same dignity as if that person was still alive; for example, with doors closed and the body being handled gently.

Standard infection control and work health and safety guidelines should always be followed while handling and preparing a body. The body of a deceased person confirmed or suspected to have a viral respiratory disease (for example, COVID-19) should be placed in a leak-proof body bag or double bagged according to the state/territory Department of Health regulations. Precautions while handling a body include the following:

- Avoid unnecessary manipulation of the body that may expel air from the lungs.
- Wear appropriate PPE while handling the body, at all times.
- Practise hand hygiene before and after contact with the body.

If the family of the deceased person are not present, and if they wish to visit, the deceased person can be viewed in the hospital mortuary or holding bay or alternative facility. Check with hospital policy regarding where deceased individuals can be viewed.

Autopsy

In some situations, a medical examination is undertaken after death (a post-mortem or autopsy). A coronial examination is performed if the medical practitioner is unable to ascertain the cause of death or if the person died in unusual circumstances. An autopsy can be performed regardless of the family's wishes. A non-coronial autopsy is done to offer information to the medical profession on the deceased person's condition and can only be performed with the family's consent.

The immediate family may also choose to consent to an autopsy but limit the extent of the examination. They can also decide whether or not organs or samples taken from the body may be kept for further study. Once the post-mortem is complete, the body can be collected by the family's chosen funeral director before it is buried or cremated.

Loss and grief

Loss can be actual, perceived or permanent, and it occurs when someone or something can no longer be seen, heard, known, felt or experienced. Grief is the natural response to loss. It includes a range of physical, mental, emotional and spiritual responses.

Each person will grieve and recover in their own way, with normal grief reactions being:

- emotional – anxiety, fear, sadness, anger and guilt
- mental – disbelief, confusion, preoccupation and hallucinations
- physical – breathlessness, lack of energy, dry mouth, and tightness in chest and throat.

Factors that may influence the experience of loss and grief include:

- length and closeness of the person's relationship with the deceased person
- nature and quality of the person's death
- availability of a supportive environment
- knowledge and confidence about how to discuss death and dying
- the stage of the individual's growth and development
- cultural and spiritual beliefs.

It is important to remember that everyone reacts differently, and everyone's coping method is unique. The grieving period may range from months to years, with each person requiring time to make sense of what has happened.

> **Grief reactions**
> A wide array of emotions including sadness, shock, anger, guilt and depression that an individual might feel after experiencing loss.

Stages of grief

Five stages of grief were first proposed by Elisabeth Kübler-Ross in her 1969 book *On Death and Dying*. By recognising the stages that a grieving person may go through, you are better able to understand and offer support to the person. The five stages of grief and loss proposed by Kübler-Ross are outlined in Figure 15.11.

Coping with loss is a personal experience, and while nobody can understand all the emotions that the person is going through, they can offer support and comfort through the process (see Figure 15.12).

Manage grief reactions

The healthcare team need an empathetic and understanding approach and to use their listening skills to allow the family and carers to express their emotions. Strategies to assist the family and carers include:

- be accessible
- listen and respond to concerns
- do not judge
- accommodate the individual's needs; e.g., pets, music, exercise and reminiscence
- validate and support time out

FIGURE 15.11 Kübler-Ross's five stages of grief and loss

STAGE	DESCRIPTION
1 Denial and isolation	The first reaction to learning about the terminal illness, loss or death is to deny the reality of the situation. 'This can't be happening' is a normal reaction to rationalise the emotions and is a defence mechanism against the shock of the diagnosis
2 Anger	Reality sets in and the emotions are redirected and expressed as anger The anger may be directed at objects, strangers or loved ones
3 Bargaining	The normal reaction to feelings of helplessness and vulnerability is often a need to regain control: 'If only we had sought medical attention sooner …' Some people attempt to make a deal with God or a higher power in an attempt to postpone the inevitable
4 Depression	Sadness and regret are the main emotions This can be a preparation to separate ourselves and prepare to say goodbye
5 Acceptance	This phase is marked by withdrawal and calm and may not be reached if death is sudden and unexpected or if the person never sees beyond anger or denial People who are grieving do not necessarily go through the stages in the same order or experience all of them

Source: Kübler-Ross, E. (1969). *On Death and Dying* (2014 reprint edition). New York: Scribner.

FIGURE 15.12 A person experiencing grief

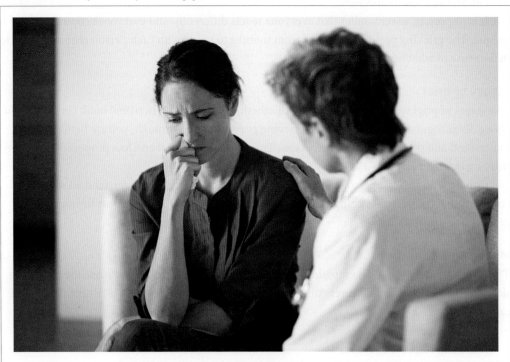

Source: iStock.com/kupicoo

- support and encourage loved ones' participation in care if requested
- acknowledge and support difficult decisions
- accommodate cultural and religious customs
- refer to services that can assist individuals to deal with issues; e.g., clergy and grief counsellors.

Remember that body language can send messages of calmness and reassurance. Eye contact indicates care about what the person is saying and that we want to support them. You can contribute by sharing information and working as a team, or informing the RN or supervisor if unsure how to communicate or how to manage reactions.

Stages of grief

Identify the stages of grief from the examples in the following table, then compare your answers with those of others in your class:

EXAMPLE	STAGE OF GRIEF
I promise to do everything I can to make this world better for the rest of my life.	
This isn't right! I don't deserve this!	
Why me? This is so unfair!	
Well, everybody dies some day.	
I will never drink again if you just bring him back.	
I don't want to see anyone.	
I'm ready for whatever comes.	
I'll just pretend it isn't there and it'll go away.	
I don't care any more.	

15.12 ACTIVITY

6 MANAGE OWN EMOTIONAL RESPONSES AND ETHICAL ISSUES

Dealing with death and dying can be challenging for members of the healthcare team. It can add considerably to workplace stress and therefore must be managed effectively. It is important that systems are in place to facilitate access to peer support, mentoring and referral. Healthcare workers should be supported to develop skills in self-care and reflective learning, and if ethical issues arise, they should be raised with the appropriate person for discussion and management according to organisation policies and procedures.

Follow organisation policies and procedures to manage own emotional responses and ethical issues

Members of the healthcare team will form individual relationships with palliative patients and their families, and it is normal to grieve when someone dies. Sometimes it is a relief to see the end of the person's suffering. However, when there has been a long relationship with the person, the grief reaction can be intense.

Pastoral care worker
A person who works within an holistic approach to health to help individuals respond to spiritual and emotional needs.

Most organisations which give care to people at the end of their lives have some form of staff counsellor, pastoral care worker, or psychologist experienced in grief counselling who can offer guidance when a difficult situation arises. Employee Assistance Programs (EAPs) are also available where the organisation supports confidential counselling services for employees. Discuss your concerns with your supervisor or RN who can give you more information, support or referral to an alternative person if required.

ACTIVITY 15.13

Support services

As well as accessing support from colleagues, healthcare organisations can provide support for employees who are experiencing grief or are having difficulty with ethical issues.

Answer the following questions regarding support services:

1 What signs and symptoms would indicate that your colleague is experiencing grief reactions?

2 Identify the support services in the organisation where you work or are undertaking work experience.

3 What professional services are available if a person needs additional support outside the workplace?

Identify, reflect and discuss your own emotional responses to death, and raise ethical issues with an appropriate person

Everyone affected by death grieves in their own way, and care workers who have been close to a deceased person can become quite distressed by their death. There may also be ethical issues that make you feel uncomfortable about the way in which the person died. Communicating your own emotional responses and raising ethical issues is an important way to deal with these feelings and concerns.

Ethical issues

Ethical and moral apprehensions occur with many end-of-life decisions. Confusion regarding sedative medications, euthanasia, withholding treatments such as 'do not resuscitate' and not providing nutrition and hydration can cause concerns for you, and the person's family and carers. Ethical, cultural, religious and moral factors are involved in these decisions and there are also worries about legal implications. As an HSA, it is important to raise your concerns with the RN or supervisor.

Withhold or withdraw treatment

Palliative care is aimed at supporting people at the end of their life. This may include withholding or withdrawing treatment, which is not considered to be euthanasia or voluntary assisted dying. Euthanasia is a deliberate act or omission, undertaken with the intention of ending a person's life. Voluntary assisted dying (VAD) laws have been passed in all of Australia's states, with those laws now applicable in Victoria and Western Australia, and to commence in 2023 in Tasmania, South Australia, New South Wales and Queensland. These laws identify self-administration, where the person takes the medication themselves, and practitioner administration, where the person is given the medication by a doctor (or in some Australian states, a nurse practitioner or registered nurse). This is sometimes called voluntary euthanasia as it is a voluntary choice and the person must be competent to make the decision.

Advance care directives may include discussions regarding 'not to perform CPR' and should be clearly documented to avoid confusion if the need to act on the decision arises. Lawful care of the terminally ill, such as withholding or withdrawing futile treatment, never involves an intention to end a person's life.

Palliative sedation

Palliative sedation is regarded as the use of sedation to reduce consciousness, relieving one or more unmanageable symptoms of pain and distress. It is important to emphasise that palliative sedation does not have the intent to directly hasten or end life but to provide comfort for the palliative patient.

Autonomy

Every person has the right to make decisions regarding their care. Part of your role is to advocate for a competent person's right to decide their own course of action, whether it is something that you feel is appropriate or not. If the person is well informed as to the consequences of their actions, they must be allowed to exercise their autonomy to do so.

Provide nutrition and hydration

Ethical issues arise when the person can no longer take nutrition or hydration because of their terminal state. Some people choose to request not to receive artificial nutrition or hydration at the end of their life, such as in an ACD. Some family members insist on trying to continue to feed their loved one even when it is no longer safe to do so. Individuals who are dying do not feel hunger or thirst and the resultant dry mouth can be made comfortable with ice chips and lip moisturiser. This should be explained to the family members to reassure them if they are concerned about nutrition and hydration in the dying individual.

Identify and initiate self-care strategies including bereavement care to address the impact of responses on self

Many areas of health care can be stressful and the emotional nature of working closely with people at the end their lives can be challenging. Stress and bereavement can result from emotional exhaustion and the inability to cope with the physical burden of caring for a palliative patient.

This can cause:

* absenteeism from work
* feelings of dissatisfaction and unhappiness
* physical and emotional symptoms such as tiredness, headaches, irritability, weight loss and sleep disturbances.

Developing self-awareness is an important step in self-care. It assists you to identify your strengths and weaknesses as well as to understand why you react the way you do in certain situations. Self-awareness can assist you to manage your emotions and prevent stress, and by actioning self-care strategies, resilience can be achieved. You can then monitor your own levels of distress and identify

Bereavement

The emotional reactions experienced after a significant loss, such as death.

and deal with potential unpleasant reactions. Building self-care into daily routines can help to avoid the build-up of stress and avoid burning out. Self-care strategies can include:

- identifying ways to leave the job behind for balance between home and work life
- doing regular exercise or relaxation activities
- enjoying time with friends and/or family
- maintaining a balanced diet
- debriefing after difficult events (see Figure 15.13)
- seeking a mentor who can provide support
- accessing supportive services, including counselling
- being proactive in raising and addressing concerns
- focusing on teamwork and a positive workplace culture
- acknowledging your grief and recognising that it is a normal reaction to the experience of loss.

FIGURE 15.13 A debriefing session

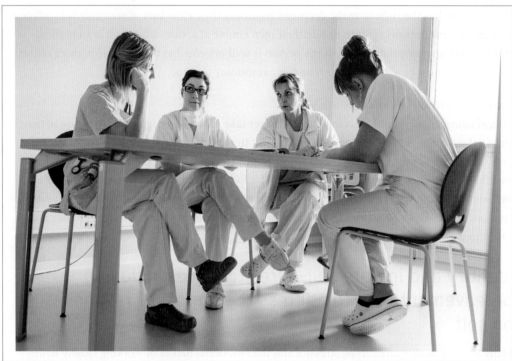

Source: Alamy Stock Photo/MBI

ACTIVITY 15.14

Developing self-awareness

Answer the following questions in relation to your work:

1. How do I feel during and after I finish work?
2. How well do I balance my work and personal life?
3. How has work impacted on my relationships (i.e., family, friends)?
4. What am I learning in my work role?
5. How have my faith and spirituality changed?
6. Reflect on your answers and consider strategies that can support you in building resilience.

SUMMARY

This chapter has described how to apply the principles and aims of a palliative approach when supporting people, while respecting their preferences for quality-of-life choices. Communication with the person, their family and carers plays a significant part in this support, as does upholding their spiritual and cultural beliefs.

This chapter emphasised that by encouraging advance care planning and open discussion about decisions for dying and death, the person can end their life with dignity and comfort. By responding appropriately to signs of pain and other symptoms and following end-of-life care strategies, the holistic needs of the person at the end of their life can be achieved.

The last part of the chapter highlighted the importance of managing your own emotional responses and discussing ethical concerns. By recognising the stress or grief that you may experience in a palliative environment and talking to your supervisors about ethical issues, you can receive support and clarification for your own, and your patient's, wellbeing.

APPLY YOUR KNOWLEDGE

Grief after death

David became a widower when his beloved wife of 59 years, Hannah, died after suffering a massive stroke in hospital. Her death was sudden and David found his coping skills were challenged. David's initial feelings were of shock and confusion and this was exacerbated because he was not there when Hannah died.

1   Elisabeth Kübler-Ross described stages of grief. What stages may David be going through in this early period?

As the healthcare worker who had been looking after Hannah, I knew that it was important not to rush David and to let him know that he did not have to talk if he didn't want to.

2   What strategies can the healthcare worker use to assist David in his initial grief reactions?

I wanted to put my arms around David but was aware of professional boundaries, so I stayed with him until his family arrived. They requested their Jewish beliefs be followed and wanted to assist with the preparation of Hannah.

3   How is the body prepared prior to being taken from the ward area?

4   What are Jewish beliefs regarding death and why is it important to support the family's religious and cultural beliefs when providing care after death?

I found David's grief stressful for my own emotional wellbeing as it reminded me of my grandparents, who I could not imagine being apart. I reflected that they would feel that part of them was missing. I discussed this with my colleagues after Hannah was taken from the ward area.

5   Using the knowledge you learnt in Chapter 1, 'Participate in workplace health and safety', what physical and psychological effects could the healthcare workers' own emotional reactions have on their ability to perform their role?

6   What self-care strategies can be used to enable healthcare workers to manage their emotional responses effectively?

7   Understanding the scope of your role is essential to performing it effectively within the healthcare team. What was the scope of the HSA's involvement in the care for David and Hannah?

◄ REFLECTING ON THE INDUSTRY INSIGHT ➕

1 How does the atmosphere of palliative day care help to alleviate clients' fears and worries?
   a The atmosphere replicates a hospital environment.
   b They can share their fears and anxieties with experienced palliative day care staff.
   c Clients can stay 24 hours in the care facility.
   d The facility can provide all medical and surgical treatments required.

2 The volunteer in the scenario provided gentle massage for the clients. Massage therapy in palliative care patients should do which of the following?
   a Promote comfort and relaxation.
   b Focus on deep tissue massage only.
   c Only be used with psychological interventions.
   d Aim to relieve pain associated with life-limiting illness.

3 What communication skills were highlighted to form a therapeutic relationship with the palliative clients?
   a Closed questions, active listening.
   b Reminiscence, reiteration.
   c Feedback, providing opinions.
   d Open questions, clarifying concerns.

SELF-CHECK QUESTIONS

1 What is your understanding of a palliative approach and how is it different to a curative approach?
2 What is the purpose of the National Palliative Care Strategy and what is the new *Palliative Care 2030* strategy's focus for palliative care?
3 How can a healthcare worker use a non-judgemental approach to encourage the palliative patient to express their needs?
4 If a person has no directive and does not have decision-making capacity, how is their treatment determined?
5 What are the functions of an enduring power of attorney?
6 What is the function of hospice care?
7 How can a healthcare worker ensure that dignity of death is maintained?
8 What are the reasons for an autopsy to be performed on the deceased?
9 What are the strategies that can assist family members to cope with grief?
10 What are your definitions of the following key words and terms that have been used in this chapter?

KEY WORD OR TERM	YOUR DEFINITION
Palliative care	
Terminal care	
Enduring guardianship	
Pastoral care worker	
Quality of life	
Advance care directive	
Bereavement	
Grief reactions	
Do not resuscitate order	
Power of attorney	

QUESTIONS FOR DISCUSSION

1   Discuss how a person's definition of quality of life may be similar or different as their illness progresses.
2   Discuss your duty of care as an HSA when working in a palliative care environment.
3   Discuss the potential barriers that may hinder discussions between healthcare workers and individuals about their distress at end of life.
4   Palliative sedation is considered to be a last resort once all other measures have been exhausted. Discuss how the lines between palliative sedation and euthanasia can be blurred.
5   Discuss the resources that are available within the community to help bereaved caregivers.

EXTENSION ACTIVITY

Caring for a person at the end of life

Edith is 86 years old and suffered a stroke a year ago. She remains weak and has right-sided weakness and difficulty swallowing (dysphagia). Her husband Harold has been caring for her at home, but over the last month her condition has deteriorated. They have no children and have been married for 65 years. The home nurse has assessed Edith and noted that she had a temperature of 38.5 degrees Celsius and consolidation in her lungs.

Edith is admitted to hospital with pneumonia. During her admission, the healthcare team discuss Edith's care plan, and Harold produces a copy of Edith's advance care directive that states that she does not want lifesaving measures, including resuscitation or nutritional support. Harold also has power of attorney for her health care.

Edith becomes more disorientated over the next two weeks. She is unable to swallow the pureed foods without choking and her weakness has progressed to the point where she cannot weight-bear. Edith is transferred to the palliative care unit and continues to deteriorate. She develops a dry mouth and becomes difficult to arouse. Pain relief is given to Edith on a regular basis, and her skin integrity is a priority as she is not mobilising.

Harold tells the nurse that he feels helpless and does not know how to make Edith comfortable. He confides to the nurse that he feels that 'she may get better now that she is receiving good care'.

The healthcare team inform Harold that Edith's condition will not improve and describe the changes that are taking place now and what will happen with further deterioration. Over the next week, Edith begins to sleep more, becomes less responsive, and her eyes remain shut. Harold asks for the chaplain as their faith has helped them throughout their lives.

Edith's life is nearing its end and Harold stays at her bedside. One morning Edith's extremities are cyanotic and her breathing irregular. The chaplain arrives and within a short time, Edith stops breathing. The doctor pronounces death and allows Harold to spend time with his wife. After Harold leaves, the healthcare team debrief and spend time talking with one another about the experience of helping Edith and Harold through the dying process.

Answer the following questions.

1 Form groups and document a nursing care plan that addresses:
   a oral hygiene for Edith
   b skin integrity and pressure injury management
   c pain management and restlessness.
2 What is the protocol for documenting Edith's advance care directive?
3 What stage of grief is demonstrated by Harold's statement?
4 How can the healthcare worker encourage Harold to talk more about his feelings?
5 Practise with a colleague one-on-one the communication techniques that you would use when encouraging Harold to talk about his feelings.
6 Why is it important for Edith and Harold to have spiritual support at end of life?
7 Why is it important for the healthcare team to express their emotions and debrief after the death of a patient?

REFERENCES

Australian Commission on Safety and Quality in Healthcare (ACSQH) (2016). Australian Charter of Health Care Rights. Retrieved 2 November 2016 from https://www.safetyandquality.gov.au/national-priorities/charter-of-healthcare-rights/

Australian Department of Health (2018). National Palliative Care Strategy 2018. Retrieved 6 May 2019 from https://www.health.gov.au/sites/default/files/national-palliative-care-strategy-2018.pdf

CareSearch (2017). Non-pharmacological approaches. Retrieved 12 November 2016 from https://www. caresearch.com.au/caresearch/tabid/751/Default.aspx

Kübler-Ross, E. (1969). *On Death and Dying* (2014 reprint edition). New York, NY: Scribner.

Palliative Care Australia (2018). *Palliative Care 2030 — working towards the future of quality palliative care for all*. Canberra: PCA. Retrieved 16 March 2022 from https://palliativecare.org.au/wp-content/uploads/dlm_uploads/2019/02/Palliative-Care-2030-public.pdf

Segal, J. & Robinson, L. (2019). Hospice and palliative care: Helpguide. Retrieved 2 November 2016 from http://www.helpguide.org/articles/caregiving/hospice-and-palliative-care.htm

South Australia Health (2020). Management of deceased during a pandemic sub-plan. Retrieved 17 March 2022 from https://www.sahealth.sa.gov.au/wps/wcm/connect/public+content/sa+health+internet/resources/management+of+deceased+during+a+pandemic+sub+plan

Victorian Department of Health. Australian Charter of Healthcare Rights. Retrieved 18 October 2022 from https://www.health.vic.gov.au/participation-and-communication/australian-charter-of-healthcare-rights

World Health Assembly (2014). *Strengthening of palliative care as a component of comprehensive care throughout the life course*. Geneva: WHA.

MAINTAIN A HIGH STANDARD OF SERVICE

Learning objectives

By the end of this chapter, you should be able to:

1   establish and maintain an appropriate relationship with people accessing services
2   act in a respectful manner at all times
3   evaluate your own work to maintain a high standard of service.

Introduction

This chapter outlines the skills and knowledge required to deliver and maintain a high standard of service in a range of community services and health contexts where direct support services are provided.

For a health services assistant (HSA), providing a high level of patient care and standard of service is a priority. This aligns to the National Safety and Quality Health Service (NSQHS) Standards which aim to improve the quality of health service provision. The services provided may be patient care, delivering timely information or organising ongoing care. The effectiveness of your work will largely depend on your communication skills, which will enable therapeutic relationships with your patients. Important communication skills addressed in this chapter as well as other chapters include how you establish rapport and respond to your patients' concerns and needs, and the actions to resolve conflict and complaints. This also requires that you act in a respectful manner at all times by maintaining confidentiality, demonstrating courtesy and providing any required assistance with behaviours of concern.

This chapter also highlights the importance of evaluating your own work performance to achieve a high standard of service. Seeking advice and reflecting will ensure that continuous improvements can be made to your service delivery.

INDUSTRY INSIGHTS 💬➕

Working in a COVID Screening Clinic

I've been working in the COVID screening clinic in our regional town for the last six months. This role is very interesting as I assist the COVID-19 Clinic Team in delivering high-quality care to clients.

I work under the direction of a registered nurse (RN) to register the clients who present for swabbing and collect their details. I also direct them to the swabbing areas and issue them with an information flyer after they have had their swab, and input their screening forms into the online database. My role also includes ensuring swabs taken are secured in a receptacle for delivery to the relevant microbiology laboratory. When the clinic is not busy, I order supplies to ensure that we have enough PPE and swabbing equipment at all times.

There is a strong focus on infection control in this role, which complies with the National Safety and Quality Health Service (NSQHS) Standard number 3 (Preventing and Controlling Healthcare-Associated Infection). We make sure that all chairs and tables are wiped down between clients; we wear PPE, including masks and gowns; and we make sure that the clients are also wearing masks (NSW Health, 2022).

I have to be respectful at all times and I try to build a rapport with the clients. This can be difficult when we are wearing masks; however, I have found that a cheery voice and eye contact works wonders. Some of the clients are very scared of having a swab in their nose so we have to build a positive relationship to gain their trust and allay their fears.

Our team has regular training and education activities regarding COVID, infection control and the various vaccinations available, so I have learnt a lot during my time at the clinic. We also have performance reviews in order to continuously improve the level and quality of service for both the clients and ourselves.

1 ESTABLISH AND MAINTAIN AN APPROPRIATE RELATIONSHIP WITH PEOPLE ACCESSING SERVICE

The NSQHS Standards were developed by the Australian Commission on Safety and Quality in Health Care in collaboration with the Australian Government, states and territories, the private sector, clinical experts, patients and carers. The primary aims of the NSQHS Standards are to protect the public from harm and to improve the quality of health service provision (Australian Commission on Safety and Quality in Healthcare, 2021).

The eight NSQHS Standards are:

1 Clinical governance
2 Partnering with consumers
3 Preventing and controlling infections
4 Medication safety
5 Comprehensive care
6 Communicating for safety
7 Blood management
8 Recognising and responding to acute deterioration.

The intention of Standard number two, Partnering with Consumers, is to provide health services that are responsive to patients and other significant people close to them, which may include carers and their families. The Standard requires that patient needs are given priority in terms of the design, implementation and review of their care plan. Health teams, which include HSAs, should work in partnership with patients by enabling them to provide input into actions that relate to quality assurance and continuous improvement. The intention of Standard two is to therefore provide a framework for active partnership with patients in the delivery of healthcare services.

National Safety and Quality Health Service (NSQHS) Standards
National standards regarding the consistent level of care people can expect from health service providers.

You should aspire to a high standard of service as required by the National Safety and Quality Health Service (NSQHS) Standards. This includes establishing rapport with patients to respond to their needs. In doing so, their care plan is given priority in terms of its design, implementation and review.

Establishing rapport and appropriate service

Rapport
A close relationship allowing a good understanding for effective communication.

As an HSA, you will spend a significant amount of time with patients and carers. As such it is important to develop and maintain relationships by building rapport. This means a close relationship with effective communication and an understanding of feelings. This will enable you to better understand the physical, social and emotional issues of the persons in your care and assist you to provide appropriate services to meet their needs.

At your first contact with the patient you should show care and compassion by your words and by your body language. Appropriate body language includes facing the person and making good eye contact, and having a relaxed posture and a pleasant smile. Do not get distracted or point at your patient and avoid inappropriate gestures like rolling your eyes or turning your back on the patient.

Using appropriate body language is the beginning of building rapport, which can be formal or informal. Formal rapport can include providing factual and objective information to patients, carers or colleagues about healthcare needs. You need to remain professional and provide clear communication. Informal rapport can include providing casual conversation about general topics including current affairs, hobbies or what happened on the weekend. Remember not to become too familiar or culturally incorrect.

SCENARIO

Formal and informal rapport

As the HSA on the morning shift you are looking after Mrs Beasley. When taking her observations you note that there are abnormalities. You use formal rapport to report your observations to the nurse in charge: 'Mrs Beasley in bed nine has a temperature reading of 38.8 this morning and is complaining of a headache.'

Later, as the HSA working in the short stay clinic, you are helping to admit a 23-year-old Muslim woman, Ms Abbas, who is having a knee arthroscopy. You use informal rapport to build a relationship with this patient: 'Hi Ms Abbas. I'm Helen, your nurse for the shift, and I will be looking after you this morning. I noticed the beautiful fabric and style of your hijab. Did you make it yourself?'

1   Reflect on these responses and suggest alternative communications that could build informal rapport with your patients.

Building rapport

Describe informal conversations you can have to build rapport with the following patients:

1   an eight-year-old child who has been admitted with tonsillitis

2   an 84-year-old woman who has been admitted with a fractured femur

3   a 32-year-old male with limited English who has been admitted with abdominal
     pain for investigation.

As you continue to provide support and develop rapport with your patients, consider these additional strategies:

- Show respect and use the name by which they choose to be addressed.
- Speak to the patient directly and not through another person who may be there at the time.
- Speak clearly and introduce yourself when you come into the ward.
- Create empathy with their feelings and be tolerant of any problems or patient issues by not showing any annoyance or frustration.
- Use active listening and explanation to keep them informed.
- Act in the patient's best interests by maintaining their safety and security and assisting them to reach their healthcare goals as determined by the nursing care plan.
- Maintain a professional approach at all times. This means working within your scope of practice and respecting the patient's privacy and dignity.
- Remember your ethical boundaries by using touch appropriately and gaining consent prior, having a respectful and courteous attitude, not giving away your personal details to a patient, and not entering into personal relationships that are not appropriate for the setting.
- Respect the patient's culture by adhering to any cultural requirements as identified in their care plan. You should refer to Chapter 6, 'Work with diverse people', where appreciating diversity is discussed in detail.

Maintaining a professional approach

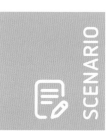

How would you respond to maintain your professional boundaries in each of the following scenarios?

1   A patient's family offer to buy you some jewellery as a gift for looking after their daughter.

2   A patient makes racist remarks about one of your co-workers and asks your opinion.

3   A patient asks you for some money so that they can catch a taxi on discharge.

4   A patient sees that you are upset and gives you a hug.

5   A patient asks you to massage their shoulders as they are aching after completing exercises.

   In these scenarios, the HSA should respond in a manner that does not offend the therapeutic relationship. Uphold your professional conduct and ethics and ensure your behaviour is in line with these as well as being within your scope of practice and organisational policies.

Establishing rapport by using appropriate body language and by being open and friendly is also important for your other contacts in the healthcare setting, including team members, visitors and allied health teams. This could include:

- doctors
- social workers

- allied health professionals
- interpreters
- spiritual advisers.

Your role is to adhere to your scope of practice and delegated responsibilities as determined by your team leader, and to support the safety and quality procedures underlying the NSQHS Standards.

Effective communication skills for quality service

Establishing a good working relationship with patients for care that is responsive to their needs will require effective communication skills. Review Chapter 4, 'Communicate and work in health and community services', where effective communication is covered in greater detail. Effective communication is more than just speaking and listening. It also covers non-verbal cues such as facial expressions, eye contact, gestures, touch and posture. Maintaining a high standard of service should embrace all aspects of your communication skills in order to establish and maintain empathy and achieve outcomes.

Key aspects of effective communication include the following:

- *Verbal communication:* You should choose words carefully for clarity and speak clearly and with sincerity. The tone of your voice should be friendly and you should pause to allow the patient time to consider a response.
- *Non-verbal communication:* Your body language should reinforce your spoken message and your rapport with the patient. Your non-verbal communication, through your body language, shows your true attitude and your genuine concern.
- *Active and reflective listening skills:* This provides feedback to the patient that you are listening. Focus on what has been said and respond appropriately with words that continue the conversation. Seek clarification and question when needed.

When communicating with patients you should:

- listen actively and allow adequate time for the patient to communicate with you
- always speak directly to the patient rather than through a third person
- check for understanding of what you have said by asking open-ended questions where the person can provide an extended reply, rather than questions requiring a 'yes' or 'no' answer; e.g., 'Tell me what the pain feels like in your arm' rather than 'Do you have pain in your arm?'
- rephrase information, using different words, if the patient appears not to have understood. You should ask questions that you know patients can easily answer; e.g., 'You need to fast from midnight for your operation tomorrow' can be rephrased as 'You cannot eat or drink anything from midnight in preparation for your operation tomorrow'.
- be positive in your words and your body language.

Trust between yourself and the patient is the foundation of a good working relationship. Trust then creates respect, where you can work with the patient to respond to their needs.

Access interpreter services

Interpreter
A person who interprets speech orally or into sign language.

When working with patients from differing cultures whose first language is not English, you may need to access interpreter services. An interpreter translates verbal communication from one language to another and acts as aide where language barriers exist.

If you are unsure about a person's ability to understand and discuss their concerns, it is always recommended you ask 'What language do you prefer to speak?' or 'Do you need an interpreter?'

Engaging an interpreter is recommended if the patient:

- demonstrates no understanding of English when asked basic questions and is unable to have an everyday conversation; e.g., the person cannot respond in English when asked their name, address or date of birth
- is only able to respond in English in a limited way, or uses English that is difficult for you to understand; e.g., the person is able to understand and uses simple greetings but little more
- relies on family or friends to communicate on their behalf
- prefers to communicate in another language
- is able to communicate in English but is in a stressful or unfamiliar environment
- uses Auslan as their primary language.

Types of interpreting

Face-to-face interpreting occurs when an interpreter attends in person. This allows the interpreter to observe body language as well as hear the spoken words. This type of interpreting is best used in long and complex interviews (see Figure 16.1).

FIGURE 16.1 Interpreter service

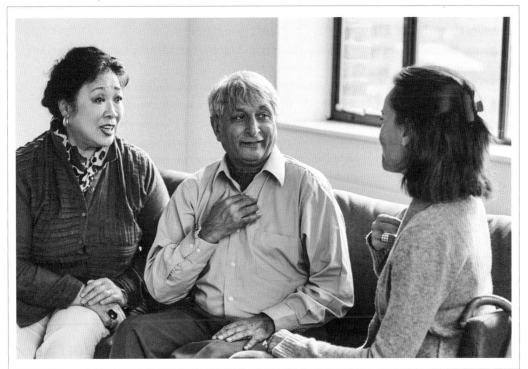

Source: iStock.com/Dean Mitchell

Telephone interpreting connects the interpreter to the person through the phone. It is widely used in regional or remote areas where access to a face-to-face interpreter is not possible and also in emergency situations to avoid delays.

Videoconferencing is an alternative where face-to-face interpreting is not available or appropriate. This is also useful for persons who have difficulty hearing or require social distancing. It also reduces miscommunication errors that may occur over the telephone (WA Health, 2017).

Interpreters are used when communication barriers exist. Figure 16.2 outlines the benefits of using a professional interpreter in healthcare settings.

FIGURE 16.2 Benefits of professional interpreters

DO ✓	DON'T ×
• Engage interpreters and translators accredited by the National Accreditation Authority for Translators and Interpreters (NAATI) at the professional level	• Use relatives or friends as interpreters • Use bilingual staff to interpret even though they may not be involved emotionally
WHY?	
• Interpreting is a professional skill • Healthcare interpreters are bilingual • Their language and interpreting skills have been tested • Interpreters are trained in medical terminology • Interpreters operate under a strict code of professional ethics which ensures that their services are impartial and confidential • Interpreters attend a number of professional development courses related to interpreting in the healthcare field	• Information transfer cannot be guaranteed • It could be a breach of duty of care which could result in legal action • Relatives or friends may not skilled in medical terminology • It breaches confidentiality and there is no guarantee of impartiality or professional conduct • It places a burden on the translator, who may be exposed to sensitive information

Aboriginal and Torres Strait Islander patients and carers

For Aboriginal and Torres Strait Islander patients and carers, consider the cultural differences (WA Health, 2017):

- 'Direct eye contact can be intimidating and be considered rude or aggressive.'
- 'A female consumer and/or carer will usually prefer a female interpreter.'
- Ask the patient's group before booking an interpreter as relationships between some Aboriginal people may determine certain behaviours.
- It is important that you tell the prospective interpreter the name of the patient so that difficult situations do not occur.

ACTIVITY 16.2

Interpreting services

Most state and territory governments will provide guidance on working with interpreters.

1 Look online to find out the interpreter polices that apply in your state or territory.

2 Find out what services are offered and their availability.

Answers will vary according to the site chosen.

Identify concerns and needs, and respond and report

As an HSA, you should attempt to identify any patient concerns. These concerns may directly relate to their care plan or may occur at any time. Standard two of the NSQHS Standards, Partnering with Consumers, identifies that services should be responsive to the needs of patients. It is the role of the HSA to report any concerns to their supervisors. This will enable up-to-date information to be included in the care plan.

Responding to patient needs should be captured in these care plans, which have been developed by the healthcare team and which are based on medical interventions, nursing care and patient support services. The purpose of the planning process should be carefully explained to patients by the registered professionals so that their feedback and input is considered and they have consented to the treatment or care. Explanation should include:

- expected outcomes to be achieved
- required medical intervention supported by nursing care
- required resources and other services to be used.

The care planning process will depend on a patient's readiness and their ability to understand and make decisions and to participate. If a patient is unable to make decisions, to understand the process or to participate, a legal guardian should act as their advocate for their care plan.

Patient responsive care planning (see Figure 16.3) means that the patient's views on their care are included in planning and this can determine the resources and services to be provided. This is a crucial part of NSQHS Standard two, which aims for an active partnership between patients and health teams in the delivery of healthcare services. As an HSA you are a part of that partnership, so you should encourage patient input into your actions to support their care plan. This can be achieved by being patient and listening to your client's responses without interrupting them when they share their health information. Prompting by saying 'Go on' and 'Can you elaborate' may also encourage them to give more information. Your reporting is also an important aspect of monitoring so that care plans are reviewed on an ongoing basis and with clear processes for responding to patient concerns and needs, and to document what has been learnt.

FIGURE 16.3 Patient responsive care planning

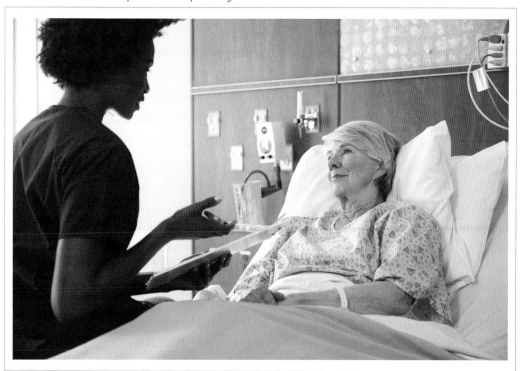

Source: Shutterstock.com / Monkey Business Images

ACTIVITY
16.3

Identifying concerns

Comment on the following statements with suggested responses to provide appropriate patient care:

1 You are admitting a patient who provides one-word answers to your questions. How would you encourage the patient to provide more information?

2 Marty has dementia and is unable to make decisions or understand the processes involving his care plan. How would you include his preferences in care planning?

3 Your patient, who is from Turkey and speaks very poor English, has been admitted into hospital for an operation. She is accompanied by her niece who speaks very good English and has agreed to be her interpreter. How would you respond?

In each of these scenarios, the HSA should report to their supervisor if they are unsure and require guidance or if the situation is outside their scope of practice.

Conflict resolution and referral to appropriate personnel

Conflict is addressed in detail in Chapter 4, 'Communicate and work in health and community services'. You should resolve conflicts directly, where an outcome can be achieved, or you may refer the conflict to your team leader for its resolution if you are unsure how to do so.

Resolving conflicts directly requires an open and collaborative communication style with strategies including the following:
- Agree on the ground rules before discussions take place.
- Allow each person time and space to tell their side of the story, from their perspective.
- Respect differences in attitudes, values and behaviours.
- Help the individuals collaborate for resolutions.
- Highlight the commonalities that can be agreed upon.
  Use the following communication techniques when resolving conflicts:
- Use active and reflective listening.
- Do not interrupt or judge.
- Remain calm, with an open posture.
- Maintain eye contact.
- Use open-ended questions and paraphrasing.
- Discuss the issue, not the individual.

Best conflict strategies

The conflict strategy of collaborating relies on problem-solving, where a mutual solution to the conflict is found by both parties cooperating in an attempt to resolve the issue. This is the best result as it allows for teamwork and maintains healthy relationships. Other strategies include compromising by both parties to resolve conflicts quickly, which is a useful strategy when the conflict is mild. A competing style of conflict management is best when decisive action is needed and someone needs to take charge to direct others to undertake specific tasks.

Avoiding the conflict allows both parties to cool down; however, a resolution must be reached before the conflict escalates. Refer to Chapter 4, 'Communicate and work in health and community services', for more information.

As an HSA, your role in conflict situations is to keep the patient safe, avoid escalation and report to your supervisor. Some conflicts are minor and can be dealt with directly; for example, interpersonal misunderstandings between colleagues. Other conflicts require input from your supervisor; for example, when the safety or emotional state of the patient is at risk.

Dealing with conflict

Complete the table by writing 'yes' in the 'Directly' column if you would deal with the conflict directly, or under 'Supervisor referral' if you would take that action, or both.

16.4 ACTIVITY

SITUATION	DIRECTLY	SUPERVISOR REFERRAL
A family member is angry with you over a medication change		
A nurse shouts at you for not documenting a patient's observations even though you did not take them		
You overhear a doctor making derogatory remarks about a patient on the ward		
You witness a doctor failing to wash her hands between patient interactions		
You have requested the weekend off; however, the roster indicates that you are on shift for Saturday and Sunday		
You see another nurse abusing a patient by shoving them into their bed		

Manage and seek advice to resolve complaints in line with organisation policy

Complaints about health service providers can be made on the basis of failing to provide satisfactory care, lack of information, lack of dignity or respect, negligence or time delays. Complaints are expressions of dissatisfaction or concerns about issues. They can be made in person, by email or survey, or by letter.

NSQHS Standard one, 'Clinical Governance', requires acute care facilities to have a complaints procedure in place to respond to complaints from patients in line with organisation policy and procedures, and to enhance their services. It is a requirement for government funding and a legal obligation under the NSQHS Standards that healthcare organisations inform their patients of the complaint procedures.

The first step when a complaint is to be made should be for the patient or family to approach the health provider to discuss their concerns. State/territory health guidelines adopt a consumer-focused approach to complaints. If staff have the authorisation to resolve complaints at first contact, escalation can be avoided and complaints can be resolved directly and quickly. Remember that all complaints should be taken seriously, even if they appear trivial.

Dealing with complaints internally

As an HSA, you will work closely with patients and you might hear complaints from them personally. Not all complaints are put in writing and even written complaints can be handled internally without the need for external involvement.

Complaints that are made to you by a patient, carer or family member may relate to an overall criticism of the care facility or could be a criticism of the personal services that you provide. Complaints may also be made about other staff members and these should be referred to your supervisor.

When receiving a complaint, it is important to do the following:

- Use active listening to the person making the complaint.
- Be non-judgemental and empathetic.
- Acknowledge their complaint and listen for understanding.
- Let them know that steps will be taken to investigate and resolve their concerns.
- Respond in a positive and helpful manner and remain calm.
- If it is a matter that can be dealt with in your delegated role, outline how you will deal with the concerns or issues that have been raised and if necessary seek advice from your team leader.

Remember, when in doubt as to whether you can resolve the complaint, ask your supervisor. Often, relevant information can be given by a superior who better understands the concerns. However, if things can be done immediately to resolve the complaint, do it straight away.

ACTIVITY 16.5

Dealing with complaints

How would you respond to each of the following scenarios?

1   Your patient is complaining about the noise in the room.
2   Your patient complains about the light from the cardiac monitor at the next bed. He is finding it difficult to sleep.
3   Your patient complains that another nurse was rude to them.

Dealing with complaints externally

You should refer any patient complaint to your supervisor for action unless it is minor and you can easily resolve it yourself; for example, adjusting pillows for comfort, re-warming a meal, or providing an extra blanket for warmth. Major complaints are those regarding the safety and security of patients and should be referred to your supervisor.

If a patient is dissatisfied with how their complaint was handled internally, they can raise their concerns with the Health Care Complaints Commission or the health department in their state or territory. This will assist in the advocacy of their complaint by:

- helping to make their concerns known to the facility
- protecting their right of access to their health information
- enabling conciliation between the patient and the provider of the health service
- assisting in the resolution of the complaint
- assessing and clarifying problems in the way health services are provided
- using information obtained to recommend improvements to services.

Supervisors can provide information to patients regarding the contact details for lodging complaints externally. If you are working in aged care, there are quality standards for residential homes. Quality standard number 6, 'Feedback and complaints', requires an organisation to have a system to resolve complaints. If a client has a concern or complaint that has not been able to be resolved by the service provider, they can contact the Aged Care Quality and Safety Commission. More information can be sourced from **https://www. agedcarequality.gov.au/providers/standards**

Complaints management

ACTIVITY 16.6

1   Match the description of the complaint to the category ('major' or 'minor') in the following table. Again, note that major complaints should be referred to your supervisor for resolution.

COMPLAINT	CATEGORY
A patient complains about a meal being too hot	
A patient complains that they cannot sleep because the room is too cold	
A patient complains that the purse in her bedside locker has been taken	
A relative complains that her mother has worsening pressure sores and that she has being left lying in a urine-soaked bed	
A patient is given the wrong medication, which has an adverse effect	
A patient complains that another patient has punched and verbally abused him	
A patient complains that the sound of the TV from the next bed is too loud	

2   Consider how you would resolve the minor complaints.

2   ACT IN A RESPECTFUL MANNER AT ALL TIMES

Respect means having regard for someone's feelings, wishes or rights. Showing respect demonstrates that you are professional and that you have empathy for a client's situation. Your responsibility is to show respect for cultural and other aspects of diversity and respect a client's confidentiality and privacy at all times. This includes an awareness of correct words, gestures and body language when dealing with those from differing cultures. You should show courtesy and provide any required assistance with behaviours of concern which includes using appropriate techniques to manage and minimise aggression.

Demonstrate respect for individual differences

You will work as an HSA with various age groups, ranging from infants to older persons. You may also have patients with language, hearing, visual, physical and intellectual disabilities where these differences will require an adjustment to the care which you provide. You should respect and show empathy for all patients, irrespective of these differences, and if required adapt the care provided so that these differences do not present a barrier to the services given.

Respect should be shown by your active and positive support and can be demonstrated by:

- introducing yourself and being friendly
- not being discriminatory
- showing support and encouragement
- treating patients with dignity
- listening and being non-judgemental.

This respect should also be extended to work colleagues and other members of health teams who have extensive knowledge that will support the care of your patients. You should also show respect for individual differences with your patients, who will have different values based on their culture and diversity. These can include:

- age and generational differences
- ethnicity
- gender, including transgender and intersex
- religious and spiritual beliefs
- sexual orientation and identity.

Culture and other aspects of diversity are outlined in considerable detail in Chapter 6, 'Work with diverse people', and you should refer to this chapter for more information. Individual differences present particular sensitivities that health teams should take into account when working with patients and their families (see Figure 16.4).

FIGURE 16.4 Respecting cultural differences

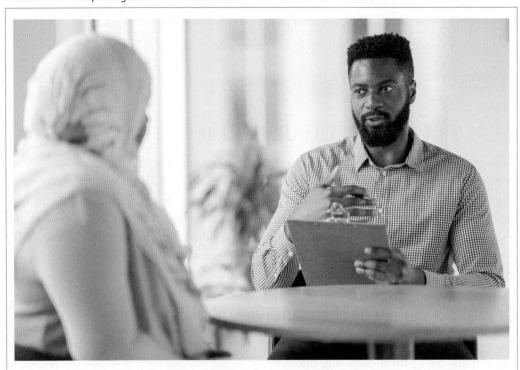

Source: iStock.com/FatCamera

Wolper Jewish Hospital

Wolper Jewish Hospital is the only not-for-profit Jewish hospital in Australia. The hospital provides rehabilitation, medical and palliative care of the highest quality to the general community within a framework of Jewish culture and religious and dietary requirements.

Transcultural care considerations include the following:

- All food is prepared with the advice of the consultant dietitian and is strictly kosher. Shabbat and all Jewish festivals are celebrated with traditional foods and special events.
- In keeping with Jewish customs, the palliative care service 'offers a warm, empathetic and reassuring environment that allows patients to maintain their dignity in an atmosphere of traditional values'.
- On Saturday there is only one rehabilitation session and Sunday is a rest day.
- 'Jewish law states that terminally ill people should remain active and productive members of society for as long as possible. Wolper provides patients with the opportunity to do this by celebrating all Jewish festivals and holidays, and providing places where patients can celebrate with family and friends while they are able.'
- 'Rabbis from a number of different synagogues visit the hospital regularly offering religious counsel, advice and assistance. Patients are able to request that their own rabbi or minister of any other religion visit them.'
- Wolper Jewish Hospital provides testing for a range of genetic disorders that occur more frequently in individuals of Eastern European (Ashkenazi) Jewish ancestry.

Wolper Jewish Hospital, 2018

Discuss how this example demonstrates respect for diversity and its importance in terms of respecting differences.

Respect and maintain confidentiality and privacy

Patients have the right to expect that their personal information will stay private and secure. The right to ensure confidentiality and privacy is outlined in Commonwealth, state and territory laws. The *Privacy Act 1988* protects each individual's personal information and ensures that such personal information is used responsibly and not for anything other than what it was obtained for; for example, it cannot be given to third parties without consent. Health records should not be disclosed to someone else, and this includes ensuring not being overheard while speaking on the phone in public places, and only discussing information with appropriate professionals.

Health records are a specific but necessary type of personal information and take several forms in acute care, including documenting a patient's:

- physical, mental and psychological health, including disabilities
- interventions received, including medications and their effectiveness
- genetic predisposition relating to aspects of health.

Refer to Chapter 10, 'Provide non-client contact support in an acute care environment', which outlines the confidentiality and privacy of healthcare information in more detail.

Healthcare privacy and consent

Health privacy is covered under Commonwealth, state and territory laws. Conduct an online search using the term 'health privacy' and then follow the links relevant to your state or territory. Answer the following questions regarding privacy and consent:

1   How are records protected in your state/territory?

2   Define implied consent.

3   Define voluntary consent.

Demonstrate courtesy in all personal interactions

You should demonstrate courtesy in all interpersonal interactions, which includes those with patients, carers, families and other visitors to your healthcare facility. The intention of NSQHS Standard two, Partnering with Consumers, is to provide health services that are responsive to patients and other significant people close to the patient. How you respond should be based on courtesy, which means being polite and well mannered, and showing genuine care and consideration for your patients.

Demonstrating courtesy involves appropriate relationship-building and effective communication. This means that you should be supportive and non-judgemental, with a desire to observe and listen to what a patient has to say. It also includes respecting different interests and views.

Assist care of individuals with behaviours of concern

Behaviours of concern are broadly based and cover unacceptable actions by patients which create harm to other people and/or themselves. Review Chapter 12, 'Respond effectively to behaviours of concern', which highlights in more detail how to respond and care for individuals with these behaviours, which include:

*   anxiety
*   aggression
*   confusion or cognitive impairment
*   intoxication
*   intrusive behaviour
*   manipulation
*   self-destructive behaviour
*   wandering.

You should identify and report any behaviours of concern to your team leader in accordance with your workplace procedures and provide any assistance required in terms of your delegated responsibilities. You should also be conscious of the patient's physical and mental health status and any prescribed medication in terms of behaviours of concern and the consequent impact.

Chapter 12 also identifies possible causes, triggers, and support strategies to control these behaviours. The behaviour support plan should be subject to monitoring strategies on an ongoing basis. Behaviours of concern are a form of communication and health workers need to work out what the behaviour indicates about possible reasons for it.

Causes of behaviours of concern

You should be conscious of the patient's physical and mental health status and any prescribed medication in terms of behaviours of concern and the consequent impact.

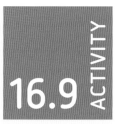

- When Peter has a migraine he becomes very angry with other people.
- Gloria has dementia and is found pacing in another patient's room.
- Sophie has a number of allergic reactions. She is continually scratching her skin, which annoys other patients and is causing a worsening of her eczema.

1 What strategies could you use to reduce these behaviours of concern?
2 Think of other health issues that may result in behaviours of concern.

Aggression management techniques

Aggression can be defined as having feelings of anger that can result in both physical and psychological harm to yourself or others. It can be verbal or physical and may cause physical or emotional issues for others as well as the patients themselves, especially if it is not handled properly. With aggressive patients you should attempt to recognise what the aggression is telling you and determine how you should calm the patient. You should be aware that the aggression may be triggered by a number of psychological causes, which could include:

- fear
- feeling frustrated
- poor self-esteem
- confusion
- dementia.

Medical causes can include infection, constipation, medication, pain or dehydration. Aggression can be displayed by physical signs including:

- heavy breathing
- pacing or agitation
- clenched fists
- flushed face
- yelling or screaming
- abusive remarks.

Responses to aggression

Review Chapter 12, 'Respond effectively to behaviours of concern', which highlights the ABC model when developing responses:

- Antecedents – factors that occurred before the behaviour
- Behaviour – what the behaviour was
- Consequence – what happened after the behaviour.

Identifying the ABCs can help in developing strategies to reduce antecedents and modify consequences.

You should show that you are in control of the situation by applying the following strategies when dealing with an aggressive patient:

- Remain calm and professional and avoid being defensive.
- Show empathy by actively listening and by reflecting on what is being said or demonstrated; e.g., 'I can see that you are irritated. Can you tell me what is causing your irritation?'

- Speak softly and use positive body language to reinforce your genuine concern.
- Keep distance between yourself and the person – do not crowd them.
- Do not argue.
- Try to establish their concerns and explore possible solutions to their anger, which will turn the dialogue from negative to positive. This is based on recognising the triggers of the aggression and moving towards an outcome which will remove the need for the aggression; e.g., 'It seems like this long wait is really frustrating you. Is there anything we can do to help?'

If a patient becomes physically aggressive and is a danger to themselves and others, then prioritise your safety. Do not attempt to handle the situation alone but rather call for help.

ACTIVITY 16.10

Strategies for aggression

Gillian, the new HSA, notified her supervisor about Anthony, who reached out and grabbed her inappropriately when she helped him out of his wheelchair. There have been other complaints about Anthony, who has an acquired brain injury after a car accident, and he has already been given a warning about this behaviour.

The acute care facility applied its risk control policies and procedures, with extra supervision and monitoring required. Actions and strategies involving Anthony's behaviour of concern resulted in a behaviour support plan for him, in consultation with his guardian and case worker, to prevent similar incidents from reoccurring. The facility provided extra training to all healthcare staff so that they all dealt consistently with Anthony's issues.

Two workers were to be used to assist Anthony with transfer, and staff were asked to speak softly and use positive body language before performing care on Anthony.

1 What additional strategies could be used for Anthony?

2 Why is it important to report and review these types of incidents?

3 EVALUATE YOUR OWN WORK TO MAINTAIN A HIGH STANDARD OF SERVICE

Regardless of your role, it is your responsibility to assist with the health and wellbeing of your patients. This means evaluating your own work for continuous improvement. Chapter 7, 'Organise personal work priorities and development', described conducting a SWOT analysis to identify strengths, weaknesses, opportunities and threats, and the importance of personal learning and professional development to improve performance. You should also seek feedback and assistance from your team leader and co-workers and be prepared to adjust your own work performance to continually improve and maintain a high standard of service for patients.

Monitor and evaluate effectiveness of interpersonal interactions

Reflection is an ideal way for you to evaluate your work performance, as long as it is done critically. This means the self-analysis of strengths and weaknesses. It will allow you to consider new goals and work on areas that need improvement.

The effectiveness of your interpersonal interactions with patients and other team members is important in terms of your emotional intelligence, which means how you understand, use and manage your emotions in positive ways to assist others. You should consider the following factors in terms of monitoring the effectiveness of your interpersonal interactions by using your emotional intelligence to ensure best-service outcomes for patients:

- Have an open mind regarding other people's perspectives.
- Stay calm and do not respond emotionally to difficult or frustrating situations.
- Allow your intuition and not your emotions to determine your interactions with other people.
- Think before you act rather than act on impulse.
- Empathise with patient wants, needs and views on expected standards of care.
- Use effective communication and social skills to resolve conflict and to build and maintain good relationships.

Self-analysis or reflection but without consideration of what others see in your performance may lead to incorrect conclusions on how to improve your skills. Seek feedback from your work colleagues and supervisors to find out what worked well and what needs improvement. Your emotional intelligence can also play a part here by reflecting on your emotions to evaluate success in interpersonal interactions. This can be done by:

- analysing the effect of your actions on your patients by 'putting yourself in their shoes'
- taking responsibility for your actions and being prepared to acknowledge fault and to correct any errors in judgement
- valuing the work of the healthcare team and striving towards its success, as opposed to seeking to achieve your own individual goals
- seeking credit for the work of the team as opposed to your own achievements
- analysing your own performance on an ongoing basis and seeking feedback from your team leader, team members and patients to achieve best-service outcomes.

Emotional intelligence

Truthfully respond to the following statements regarding your emotions:

1   I can recognise my emotions easily.
2   I find it easy to listen to patients.
3   I know what I am good at and what weaknesses to work on.
4   I have strategies to calm myself down when angry or frustrated.
5   I enjoy working in a team.
6   I tend to forget about frustrations easily.
7   I do not get stressed about conflict situations.
8   I enjoy my work.

If you answered 'yes' to most of these questions, you have some degree of emotional intelligence. If not, you will need to work on your self-awareness regarding those statements about which you gave a negative response.

Seeking advice

Seeking and receiving advice from your team leader, other team members and appropriate other sources is essential for improvement. Your team leaders are experienced and can provide motivation, support and guidance to allow you to carry out your role effectively.

Remember that it is better to ask for advice than to not ask. You will not be seen as incompetent but rather it will help you to improve your work performance. When seeking advice:

- be specific about what you require
- be positive and professional
- be timely and do not delay, as this may compromise the health of the patient
- ask for clarification if you do not understand
- incorporate the advice in future work for continuous improvement.

Review Chapter 7, 'Organise personal work priorities and development', which discusses monitoring your own work performance through self-assessment. It also outlines the importance of feedback, mentoring and performance appraisal to enhance performance. The following are suggestions on seeking and receiving advice and assistance to enhance performance:

- Your own self-assessment of performance needs to be considered alongside feedback received in terms of what worked well and what did not work so well.
- Use a 360-degree survey or similar tool which uses a questionnaire where you seek feedback from your team leader, colleagues and someone who reports to you. That said, as an HSA you would not have persons reporting to you.
- Seek feedback from patients through asking questions based on the services that you have provided in terms of their needs.
- Embrace any formal or informal mentoring schemes where a more experienced worker will assist you to learn on the job and perhaps to help in your long-term career development.
- Performance appraisal should be used to gain knowledge for continuous improvement.

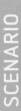

SCENARIO

Seeking advice to enhance performance

When you need help and don't ask for it, you can become more stressed and will continue with poor performance. By asking for assistance early on and being direct in your request, you can reduce unnecessary worry.

Beverly, the HSA, has been working in the general ward of a regional hospital for the last six months. Recently, the ward introduced a newer version of blood glucose monitoring machines. Beverly had used the old ones before but was unsure of the way in which the new ones were calibrated. When asking her supervisor, the following suggestions could be used:

- 'I am unsure of the way the new glucometers are calibrated. It would really help me if you could arrange for someone to show me how to do this task.'
- 'I have read the instruction manual but am still unsure if I am doing the correct calibration on the new glucometers. Could you watch me when you have time to make sure I am doing it correctly?'

1 How has Beverly been specific in her requests for assistance?
2 How has Beverly shown positive and professional communication in her request?
3 Consider additional suggestions for this request.

Adjust your own work to incorporate advice

You should adjust your work performance to incorporate any advice to improve the standard of support that you provide to your work team in servicing patient needs. The NSQHS Standards emphasise continuous improvement, which are defined as a 'systematic, ongoing effort to raise an organisation's performance as measured against a set of standards or indicators'. Continuous improvement relates to individuals and teams and should aim for small incremental changes to performance to produce significant improvements over time. Continuous improvement can be represented by the Plan, Do, Study, Act (PDSA) cycle (see Figure 16.5).

FIGURE 16.5 The Plan, Do, Study, Act (PDSA) cycle

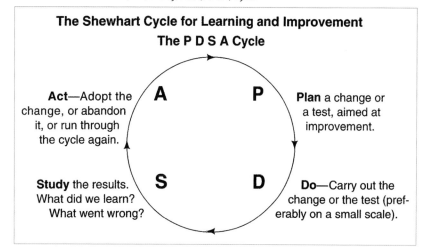

Source: Deming (2018). © 2018 Massachusetts Institute of Technology, by permission of The MIT Press.

Continuous improvement
Ongoing efforts to improve performance or processes.

This cycle assesses a change by planning to test the change (Plan), carrying out the change (Do), observing the consequences (Study) and determining what can be done for improvement (Act). Adjustments to your work based on advice to improve standards of support and service can in turn be based on your response to the following aspects of the PDSA continuous improvement cycle:

- **Plan** adjustments to your work performance:
  - Identify performance issues to be addressed.
  - Plan actions to address issues.
  - Decide how actions will occur and by when.
  - Decide how changes will be measured on your work performance.
  - Be clear on outcomes being sought in terms of improved standards of support and efforts to improve patient services.
- **Do** by implementing the required adjustments to your work performance:
  - Put the improved performance plan into practice.
  - Consult with your mentor and/or team leader on progress.
  - Seek feedback on the effectiveness of adjustments you have made on performance.
  - Identify any problems that may affect the outcomes being sought.
- **Study** by analysing the effectiveness of changed performance:
  - Evaluate all feedback received on adjustments to performance.
  - Discuss feedback with your mentor and/or team leader.
  - Decide whether adjustments to your work have resulted in improvements.
  - Analyse the doing stage to decide whether there is still scope for further improvement.
- **Act** and move onto the next stage of continuous improvement:
  - Make any further adjustments to work performance based on consideration of the Plan, Do, Study, Act stages.
  - Continue with actions that worked and work on areas that still require improvement.
  - Repeat the Plan, Do, Study, Act cycle for new action plans for further adjustments to your own work as an HSA.

Deming (2018). © 2018 Massachusetts Institute of Technology, by permission of The MIT Press.

Evaluating your work

1 Identify an aspect of your performance as an HSA which requires continuous improvement for a high standard of services.

2 Outline how you will use the Plan, Do, Study, Act (PDSA) cycle to adjust your work performance.

SUMMARY

This chapter examined the importance of maintaining a high standard of patient service with reference to the National Safety and Quality Health Service (NSQHS) Standards, which apply to your role and responsibilities as an HSA in an acute care setting. The first part of the chapter examined the importance of establishing and maintaining appropriate relationships with people who access health services. This requires effective communication and interpersonal skills including building rapport and utilising interpreter services when required. Other aspects of maintaining a high standard of service that were outlined include conflict resolution and dealing with complaints and resolving concerns.

Acting with respect for patients was further illustrated by referring to cultural and other aspects of diversity and dealing with behaviours of concern. Strategies for these behaviours were highlighted by the ABC model to manage and minimise aggression.

The last part of the chapter described how an evaluation of your own work performance can result in continuous improvement. This evaluation was gained through using emotional intelligence and seeking advice. The Plan, Do, Study, Act cycle was illustrated as a way of ensuring that a high standard of work performance and patient service is achieved.

APPLY YOUR KNOWLEDGE

Home and community care

Elaine, an HSA, has recently been given a new client as part of her role as a home care assistant. Richard, an 84-year-old widower and Vietnam War veteran, lived alone. He had diabetes and emphysema, which made mobilising difficult. Elaine's role was to assist Richard with showering, check his morning blood glucose level, and make sure he took his prescribed medications.

Since it was her first visit, Elaine knew the importance of building rapport with Richard. She chatted with him informally and found out that his son and daughter lived interstate and that he had a few ex-army friends in the local area, but found socialising difficult due to his limited mobility.

1 Why is it important for the HSA to establish rapport with Richard?

When Elaine was assisting Richard in the shower, she noticed that one of his toes was quite red and inflamed. As part of her role she recorded this in his notes and reported it to the home care registered nurse. This resulted in a doctor undertaking a home visit the next day. The doctor prescribed oral antibiotics to Richard and a medicated cream and Elaine was asked to monitor the site for any changes.

2 Using the knowledge you gained from Chapter 4, 'Communicate and work in health and community services', explain how Elaine followed communication protocols to enable high-quality care and service to Richard.

Elaine checked Richard's toe every day for two weeks and reported to the home care RN on its improved condition. During this time, Richard opened up to Elaine and spoke about his depression since losing his wife and how he would love to catch up with his old army mates. Elaine listened and responded to Richard's concerns by communicating this to the home care service. The service organised for the local community bus to transport Richard every Friday to the RSL so that he could socialise with his mates.

3   Why is it important to identify Richard's concerns and apply patient responsive care planning?

After a month, the home care service reviewed Elaine's performance with her client. They were very happy with her work and gave Elaine the opportunity to provide feedback as well. She continued to care for Richard and looked forward to chatting with him every morning and caring for him in his home environment.

4   Why is it important for Elaine to seek advice and reflect on her own work performance?

5   Understanding the scope of your role as an HSA is essential to performing your role effectively within the healthcare team. How did Elaine demonstrate an understanding of the scope of her role in supporting Richard?

◄ REFLECTING ON THE INDUSTRY INSIGHT 💬

1   The HSA mentioned a strong focus on infection control, including wiping down chairs and tables between clients and wearing PPE. How does this align to the NSQHS Standards?
   a   Demonstrates quality by ensuring that staff are cleaning the environment regularly.
   b   Aligns to standard two to ensure clients are involved in quality health care.
   c   Aligns to standard three on preventing and controlling infections.
   d   Demonstrates safety by ensuring a dust-free and tidy environment.

2   How did the HSA try to build rapport with clients when wearing a mask?
   a   Taking off the mask to communicate.
   b   Using positive body language including eye contact and a cheery voice.
   c   Asking personal questions during the interaction.
   d   Allaying their fears by joking about the swabbing procedure.

3   Performance reviews were undertaken at the COVID clinic and were necessary because they:
   a   Were compulsory sessions for all healthcare workers.
   b   Highlighted how cost savings could be made for the clinic.
   c   Allowed staff to air grievances to each other.
   d   Improved the level and quality of service for the clients.

SELF-CHECK QUESTIONS

1   Identify the NSQHS Standards which apply to acute care and other health services throughout Australia.

2   Explain the difference between formal and informal rapport.

3   Explain why it is important to use professional interpreters when required for patients.

4   Describe the communication techniques that can be used when resolving conflicts.

5   Outline how complaints procedures relate to the NSQHS Standards.

6   Explain how the *Privacy Act 1988* protects individuals' personal information.

7   Explain the ABC model when developing a response to patient aggression.

8   What factors should be taken into consideration when seeking advice from your supervisor or work colleagues?

9   Describe the PDSA cycle for continuous improvement.

10 What are your definitions of the following key words and terms that have been used in this chapter?

KEY WORD AND TERM	YOUR DEFINITION
National Safety and Quality Health Service (NSQHS) Standards	
Rapport	
Interpreter services	
Patient responsive care planning	
Continuous improvement	
Behaviours of concern	
Aggression	
Courtesy	
Emotional intelligence	
360-degree survey tool	

QUESTIONS FOR DISCUSSION

1   'The introduction of the National Safety and Quality Health Service (NSQHS) Standards with the patient as the prime focus of activity ensures that required services are appropriate and serve patient interests.' (Australian Commission on Safety and Quality in Healthcare, 2021) Describe how the NSQHS Standards provide the standards of care consumers can expect from health service organisations.

2   You have been appointed as a mentor to a new HSA who has experienced a conflict with a work colleague about coming back late from the morning tea break. Explain how you would advise this person prior to resolving the conflict situation.

3   Discuss why cultural differences may hinder establishing a rapport with patients.

4   Discuss how performance appraisal can provide for continuous improvement.

5   Discuss how the NSQHS Standard number six, Communicating for Safety, can be applied to maintaining a high standard of service for clients.

EXTENSION ACTIVITY

National Safety and Quality Health Service (NSQHS) Standards

The NSQHS Standards apply to acute care and other health services throughout Australia. These health services measure performance on eight standards and aim for consistency, with continuous improvement based around high standards of performance.

1   Go online for resources to implement the NSQHS Standards and download the accreditation workbook (**https://www.safetyandquality.gov.au/sites/default/files/migrated/National-Safety-and-Quality-Health-Service-Standards-Accreditation-Workbook.pdf**)

2   Find the section on Partnering with Consumers (Standard two) and refer to CRITERION: Partnering with patients in their own care: Action 2.3 – Healthcare rights.

3   Refer to either a hospital or community health service where you may be employed or completing your clinical placement, and after interviewing a supervisor and/or other healthcare worker, consider the extent to which the organisation adheres to actions, reflective questions and examples of evidence currently in use.

    Answers will vary according to workplace.

REFERENCES

Australian College of Nursing (2020). Maintaining professional boundaries. Retrieved 26 February 2022 from https://www.acn.edu.au/wp-content/uploads/career-hub-resources-maintaining-professional-boundaries.pdf

Australian Commission on Safety and Quality in Healthcare (2019). Person-centred care. Retrieved 30 December 2021 from https://www.safetyandquality.gov.au/our-work/partnering-consumers/person-centred-care

Australian Commission on Safety and Quality in Healthcare (2021). The NSQHS Standards. Retrieved 9 July 2022 from National Safety and Quality Health Service Standards, 2nd edn.

Australian Government (2021). The *Privacy Act*, Rights and Responsibilities. Retrieved 31 December 2021 from https://www.oaic.gov.au/privacy/the-privacy-act/rights-and-responsibilities

Deming, W. Edwards (2018). Foreword by Kevin Edwards Cahill, *The New Economics for Industry, Government, Education*, third edition, PDSA cycle - figure 13, and 211 word excerpt from Chapter 6. © 2018 Massachusetts Institute of Technology, by permission of The MIT Press.

Department of Health and Human Services, Victorian Government (2020). Language services policy and guidelines. Retrieved 23 December 2021 from https://www.dhhs.vic.gov.au/publications/language-services-policy-and-guidelines

International Journal of Nursing Studies (2018). The impact of emotional intelligence in health care professionals on caring behaviour towards patients in clinical and long-term care settings, 80, 106–17. Retrieved 30 December 2021 from https://www.sciencedirect.com/science/article/abs/pii/S002074891 8300166#:~:text=Patient%20outcomes%20can%20be%20improved,and%20empathy%20towards%20 their%20patients.&text=Emotional%20intelligence%20is%20positively%20associated,%2C%20job%20 satisfaction%2C%20and%20caring

NSW Health (2017). Interpreters – standard procedures for working with health care interpreters. Retrieved 23 December 2021 from https://www1.health.nsw.gov.au/pds/ActivePDSDocuments/PD2017_044.pdf

NSW Health (2020). Complaints management guidelines. Retrieved 29 December 2021 from https://www1.health. nsw.gov.au/pds/ActivePDSDocuments/GL2020_008.pdf

NSW Health (2022). Policy directive: Standard operating procedure for administration of COVID-19 vaccines in NSW vaccination clinics. Retrieved 25 October 2022 from https://www1.health.nsw.gov.au/pds/ ActivePDSDocuments/PD2022_040.pdf

Royal Australian College of General Practitioners (2021). *Putting prevention into practice: Guidelines for the implementation of prevention in the general practice setting*, 3rd edn. Retrieved 31 December 2021 from https://www.racgp.org.au/getattachment/2ba9e40f-fe33-44bf-8967-8bf6f18a1c1a/Putting-prevention-into-practice-Guidelines-for-the-implementation-of-prevention-in-the-general-practice-setting.aspx

WA Health (2017). WA health system language services policy guidelines. Retrieved 30 December 2021 from https://ww2.health.wa.gov.au/-/media/Files/Corporate/Policy-Frameworks/Communications/Policy/ WA-Health-System-Language-Services-Policy/Supporting/WA-Health-System-Language-Services-Policy-Guidelines.pdf

Wolper Jewish Hospital (2018). Wolper Jewish Hospital. Retrieved 27 December 2021 from https://wolper.com.au/ services/palliative-care

ASSIST WITH AN ALLIED HEALTH PROGRAM

Learning objectives

By the end of this chapter, you should be able to:

1 provide relevant information to clients
2 prepare for therapy sessions
3 provide assistance with therapy sessions
4 use therapy equipment correctly and safely
5 provide feedback on appropriate therapy information to supervising allied health professionals
6 assist in the design and construction of simple therapy materials and equipment
7 complete required administrative duties
8 work with a primary healthcare approach.

Introduction

This chapter outlines the skills and knowledge required to provide basic assistance to an allied health professional. For a health services assistant (HSA) who is working in an allied health context or as an allied health assistant, this includes providing assistance to professionals such as occupational therapists, physiotherapists, podiatrists and speech therapists. The assistant will work under the regular (direct, indirect or remote) supervision of an allied health professional to provide assistance for clients by preparing them for therapy sessions, providing information and confirming plans, following supervisor instructions and treatment plans, reinforcing therapy goals and using equipment safely and correctly.

Administrative duties are part of this role, including documenting client progress and the exchange of information between allied health teams and healthcare organisations. There is an emphasis on all the allied health professional roles as well as the limitations of the assistant in supporting them with their treatments.

This chapter highlights the promotion of health through a primary healthcare approach with added emphasis on prevention of disease, the involvement of other services, and supporting therapeutic interventions using an evidence-based practice approach.

Working in a physiotherapy clinic

I work under the supervision of a team of physiotherapists in a large rehabilitation clinic. Their expertise is a great source of knowledge for me and I am learning so much about the benefits of exercise for recovery and good health.

My supervisor has given me a copy of Mr Quade's therapy plan. Mr Quade had a heart attack four weeks ago and I have been asked to assist him with his cardiac exercise program. His program consists of exercises including walking, stretching and strength training and is personalised for his needs, as well as education and psychological support.

Since his heart attack, Mr Quade has gradually been increasing his walking on the treadmill and is up to 30 minutes a day before he needs rest. My role is to check the equipment and make sure Mr Quade warms up before the session so that his body is prepared for exercise. This also reduces the incidence of soreness afterwards. I also monitor and encourage Mr Quade during his sessions and record his progress. At the end of each session, the physiotherapist checks in on him and answers his queries and I book him in for further appointments.

Mr Quade is also receiving dietary advice and tells me that he is confident that with the healthy lifestyle changes including exercise, weight reduction, stress-relieving strategies and correct nutrition, he will strengthen his heart and live a long and healthy life.

1 PROVIDE RELEVANT INFORMATION TO CLIENTS

In order to provide relevant information to clients, you must have knowledge of the allied health services that are available and the roles of the professionals that provide these services. As an assistant to the allied health teams. you will be working across a variety of settings including rehabilitation, aged care, acute care, community care, disability and home care. The clients – both young and old – will have a range of health issues, so you must maintain confidentiality of information at all times and understand your role in the delivery of relevant information under the supervision of the allied health professionals.

Adhere to confidentiality policies

Confidentiality has been discussed in detail in Chapter 4, 'Communicate and work in health and community services'. Clients will expect that all personal information, including medical history, is not disclosed to anyone except in an emergency situation. The *Privacy Act 1988* states that all personal information is to be used responsibly and with the client's consent. The clients or their guardians should be able to know what information has been collected and how it will be used.

When discussing a client's information with supervisors or other allied health teams, always ensure that privacy is maintained and that permission has been granted. Remember to maintain privacy by:

- not discussing client matters in a public area
- keeping files secure and not accessible to the general public
- logging off computers after documenting client notes
- not leaving files open to expose confidential client details.

Confidentiality with a psychologist

At the beginning of her treatment, Sophia was given paperwork detailing the privacy policy at the psychology clinic. This explained how the information shared in the therapy sessions would be kept private. It also outlined when confidentiality may be broken – in situations when clients could cause serious harm to themselves or others.

The psychologist explained the policy to Sophia and she understood and signed the paperwork. As an assistant I was aware that this information could not be shared with anyone else and that this confidentiality allowed Sophia to feel safe in a therapeutic space.

1   Look up 'health professionals and confidentiality' in the SA law handbook on the web (**https://lawhandbook.sa.gov.au**) and list any other exceptions to breaking confidentiality.

2   Does a parent or guardian need to be present in counselling sessions if the client is under 18? Look up each state and territory's age of automatic confidentiality.

Provide basic accurate information to clients

> Allied health professionals work with people to identify and assess issues and provide treatment and to support acquisition of skills, recovery and reablement.
>
> AHPA, 2022a

Allied health professionals deliver diagnostic and therapeutic services to people and work across multidisciplinary teams (see Figure 17.1).

Allied healthcare settings

Allied health professionals provide services to maintain function of clients across a variety of workplaces. The allied health teams, including the assistants, work collaboratively with other health providers, including doctors, pharmacists and nurses, in the following settings:

Acute care

Within the public sector, particularly in the acute care setting, allied health practitioners tend to work in discipline departments with a senior of their discipline. Allied health services in acute hospital settings commonly include occupational therapists, physiotherapists, social workers, dietitians and speech pathologists. Their roles are to maximise independence and to support the client and their family through to discharge planning.

Residential aged care

Allied health professionals are an integral part of the aged care sector. As people get older they become more likely to experience ill health, including much higher rates of chronic disease and injuries resulting from falls. These elderly people can benefit from allied health programs including exercise programs, fall-prevention programs, diversional therapy programs and a variety of leisure activities and nutrition support. Allied health professionals can offer these services independently or work as part of a multidisciplinary aged care team to ensure that the aged person has the full range of treatments to manage their needs.

FIGURE 17.1 Types of allied health professionals

Allied health professional	Role description
Occupational therapist	Promote health by assisting persons to participate in everyday life, such as through personal care, feeding, household management, return to work and leisure activities
Podiatrist	Assist clients with lower limb and foot problems including bone and joint disorders, diabetes, corns and bunions, and circulatory disorders
Speech pathologist	Works with clients to treat communication disorders that are not limited to stroke, brain injuries, dementia and intellectual disabilities. Also treats persons experiencing difficulties with swallowing
Physio-therapist	Treats clients with sports injuries and musculoskeletal conditions as well as chronic health conditions such as diabetes, obesity, osteoarthritis and stroke
Dietitian	Assists clients in managing nutrition when they are affected by health conditions such as diabetes, obesity, allergies and gastrointestinal disorders
Prosthetist	Provides splints/braces or prosthetics to increase mobility and independence for persons who have limb amputations or limitations in mobility
Psychologist	Helps people change the way they think, feel, behave and react. They assist clients with behavioural issues, addictions, learning difficulties, trauma and mental health issues, as well as providing strategies to gain peak performance
Audiologist	Assesses and prescribes devices such as hearing aids for clients with hearing loss. Works with allied health teams to provide rehabilitation for clients with balance disorders
Exercise physiologist	Provides exercise interventions to restore persons to optimal functioning. They can assist with weight loss, mobility issues, chronic health issues and pain
Pharmacist	Dispenses prescription medications to patients and offers expertise in the safe use of the prescriptions. They can also provide immunisations and conduct health screening

Home care

The services of the allied health teams can be extended to home care to enable older persons or those living with a disability to live independently in the community. Disabilities can include cerebral palsy, spinal cord injury, developmental disorders and brain injuries. Services can include rehabilitative care, healthy ageing strategies and organising modifications to the home to minimise hazards. Many of these services are funded through the National Disability Insurance Scheme (NDIS), Commonwealth home support programs and home care packages.

Rehabilitation facilities

Rehabilitation plays an important part in the recovery process for clients who have had surgical repair of injury. Allied health professionals provide essential services to achieve optimal functioning in these settings. Rehabilitation facilities may be attached to hospitals or be independent facilities. They can offer day programs for those who are well enough and independent enough to come in from home or provide inpatient services that are personalised to the client's goals. These can be in the form of group sessions or individual sessions.

Rehabilitation
Restoring someone to health through training and therapy.

Specialist clinics

Within the private sector, physiotherapists, podiatrists, chiropractors, osteopaths and psychologists are the disciplines that provide the most common allied health services. Larger allied practices may also be co-located with medical practices and other health disciplines.

Allied health frameworks

The allied health workforce in Australia is either regulated by the national body, the Australian Health Practitioner Regulation Agency (AHPRA), or self-regulated, which means that each professional body is responsible for certification of qualifications. Examples of the regulated and self-regulated workforce are shown in Figure 17.2.

FIGURE 17.2 Regulated and self-regulated allied health workforce

REGULATED	SELF-REGULATED
Chinese medicine practitioners	Art therapists
Chiropractors	Audiologists
Medical radiation practitioners	Dietitians
Occupational therapists	Exercise physiologists
Optometrists	Speech pathologists
Osteopaths	Music therapists
Pharmacists	Orthoptists
Physiotherapists	Prosthetists
Podiatrists	Social workers
Psychologists	Sonographers

Allied health assistant responsibilities

For allied health assistants, each state/territory in Australia has its own frameworks and scopes of practice in its health workforces. This includes limitations on the role of an allied health assistant. Assistants do not order treatment or assess clients, nor do they make clinical decisions or prepare treatment plans. The job description for each specialised allied health role may have additional limitations on practice, so it is important to understand the limits and responsibilities of your role.

The scope of practice needs to be in line with the requirements of the service. It should be determined by the relevant staff making decisions relating to service needs in the allied health department. Remember that at all times the allied health assistant must work under the supervision of healthcare professionals. These professionals have responsibilities regarding the allied health assistant, which are to:

- remain responsible for the delivery of therapy provided by an allied health assistant
- educate, delegate, supervise and evaluate work done by allied health assistants
- have an understanding of the scope of practice for the allied health assistant workforce
- provide professional development opportunities as required.

ACTIVITY 17.2

Allied health professionals

Allied Health Professionals Australia (AHPA) is the peak national organisation for allied health professions. Look up **https://ahpa.com.au/allied-health-professions/** and then describe the following allied health roles:

ALLIED HEALTH PROFESSIONAL	ROLE DESCRIPTION
Art therapist	
Chiropractor	
Orthoptist	
Music therapist	
Osteopath	
Radiographer	
Chinese medicine practitioner	

---

2 PREPARE FOR THERAPY SESSIONS

As an assistant to an allied health professional, you may need to prepare for therapy sessions. You will be working under the instruction of your supervisor so it is important to have a clear understanding of what is required for the sessions. Additional information from relevant sources including medical records, treatment plans and organisation policies can assist with this preparation. You must also check resources and equipment for suitability and safety as well as communicating with the client to ensure that they are prepared for the session.

Confirm and discuss therapy and treatment plans and programs

Working with allied health teams means that you must have an understanding of the treatment plans in order to assist with therapy. The treatment plan outlines the therapy sessions or treatment sessions that your client will need to undertake to promote rehabilitation or recovery. Your supervising allied health professional will need to give you clear instructions either verbally or in written form and you must ask for clarification if unsure of any of their directions.

The allied health professional will determine the therapy session or treatment plan based on:

- initial referral
- understanding of medical history, supporting tests and investigations
- examination of the client
- interpretation of findings
- client goals and abilities.

Treatment plan

An outline of a patient's therapeutic treatment.

Therapy session

A therapy session involves a series of sessions with the client and allied health professional working towards a goal (see Figure 17.3). This can involve an assessment followed by a series of exercises, group meetings or individual sessions.

FIGURE 17.3 Speech pathologist undertaking therapy session with a client with dysphagia

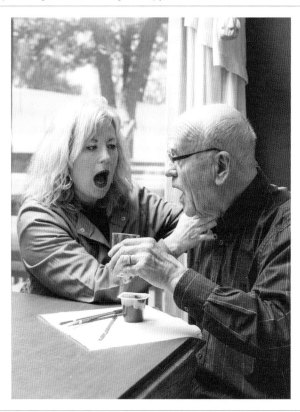

Source: iStock.com/wanderluster

SCENARIO

Therapy sessions for client with dysphagia

Madeline has dysphagia as a result of a stroke and has been referred to a speech pathologist for therapy sessions. The initial assessment session involved the speech pathologist taking a comprehensive history, including asking her about her nutritional intake and difficulties in swallowing and then going through a series of therapy exercises for her to perform at home. My role as an allied health assistant was to prepare Madeline for the therapy session by making her comfortable and ensuring that she had the correct equipment for the exercises.

Madeline's therapy sessions were aimed at increasing the strength of her chewing and swallowing muscles, so that she could maintain adequate nutrition and hydration. Madeline practised the therapy exercises to ensure she understood the correct technique. Her treatment plan for the therapy sessions included:

- **Exercise 1:** Swallow your saliva while you squeeze your mouth and neck muscles very hard. Repeat 5 times each and complete exercise 3 times a day.
- **Exercise 2:** Lie on your back without a pillow. Lift your chin to look at your feet whilst keeping your shoulders on the bed. Repeat 20 times and complete exercise 5 times a day.
- **Exercise 3:** Place a straw in your mouth and suck on it to pick up a piece of paper. Keep the suction strong enough to carry the piece of paper over to a cup and then release. Repeat with 5 pieces of paper and increase distance as your strength increases.

Madeline had no adverse effects after the practice exercises and was given a comprehensive list of additional exercises to perform once discharged and a referral for follow-up in four weeks. I clarified that Madeline understood the plan and informed her that she could contact the speech pathologist if she had any further queries.

1   Research dysphagia on the internet and describe the potential complications of this problem.
2   Why is it important for the speech pathologist to take a comprehensive history prior to initiating therapy exercises?

Treatment session

This can include a treatment or procedure to rectify an illness or injury (see Figure 17.4) with a follow-up consultation.

FIGURE 17.4 Fibreglass cast treatment for a fractured wrist

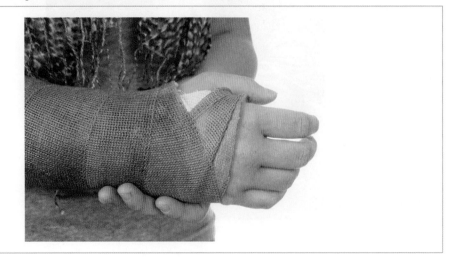

Source: iStock.com/DawnPoland

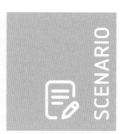

Treatment session for fractured arm

Colin has a fractured wrist as a result of a fall whilst playing tennis. He has been assessed in the emergency department and referred to the fracture clinic for casting.

Treatment at the fracture clinic involved placing a tubular stockinette over the forearm, then applying padding and wet fibreglass casting tape. The tape was then moulded to Colin's arm while it was still wet.

As an allied health assistant in the fracture clinic, I prepared the equipment and supported Colin throughout the procedure. After the cast was applied, Colin experienced heat which was a normal feeling as the cast was setting. The importance of not getting the padding wet and reporting any pain, numbness, tingling, odour or swelling was emphasised to Colin by the doctor. When the cast was set, I gave Colin a pamphlet on cast care and arranged his follow-up appointment, which included physiotherapy support. Colin was told it would take 6–12 weeks for full recovery and he assured us that he would care for the cast as advised so that he could get back to tennis as soon as possible.

1 Why is it important for Colin to notify the doctor if he experiences pain, swelling and numbness?
2 Why would it be important for Colin to have physiotherapy support after fracturing his wrist?

Obtain information from relevant sources

Many of your clients may be under the treatment of a multidisciplinary team. This combined approach enables the best decisions to be made regarding the most appropriate treatment for each client. This team can consist of doctors, nurses and various allied health professionals. It is important for you as the assistant to these professionals to understand each team member's role and to communicate effectively so that you are aware of the tasks required from each discipline. Other relevant sources of information can be obtained from the client and family, the facility, or from organisational policies and procedures.

Relevant information can be sourced from:
- medical records – identify past medical history and social and emotional status, which can provide useful information on ongoing treatment planning
- X-rays or test results – identify injuries, infections and abnormal blood levels to enable the healthcare team to manage the treatment for each client appropriately
- treatment plans – identify current treatments for illness and injury so that the entire healthcare team is aware of the client's history
- community contacts – can provide information to assist the client on discharge and through rehabilitation if required. This will enable the healthcare team to determine the best recovery/rehabilitation strategy for individual clients
- equipment usage manuals – can provide information on use, troubleshooting and maintenance so that the HSA can assist the client to use the equipment effectively.

The client

The client can be a useful source of information and may describe changes to their condition since the last session. This can include improvements or deterioration in their health status or difficulties in performing the required exercises or treatments. When obtaining information about a client, you must ensure that they consent and understand why the information is being collected and how it will be treated. When gaining consent you should also consider the surroundings and take steps to make the client feel comfortable. This may be done by taking them to a private room or lowering your voice.

The facility

Clinical pathways
Standardised, evidence-based multidisciplinary plans that identify an appropriate order of clinical interventions and timeframes for common disorders.

Your supervisor will give you relevant information regarding assisting in the therapy sessions for the clients. This may include brochures from the facility which have take-home information for client exercises. Providers can also use clinical pathways for selected disorders and their treatments. These documents outline a standard, evidence-based multidisciplinary management plan that identifies the clinical care, timeframes and expected outcomes for a client group. These roadmaps improve the quality of care by reducing variation and maximise the outcomes for clients.

ACTIVITY 17.3

Clinical pathway for Achilles tendon repair

Review the following clinical pathway for a client's rehabilitation post Achilles tendon repair and answer the questions below:

APPOINTMENTS	REHABILITATION 1–2 TIMES PER WEEK
Goals of rehabilitation	• Wound healing • Weight-bearing as tolerated using boot and crutches • After 8 weeks progress to full weight-bearing and discharge crutches
Precautions	• 0-degree plantar flexion • Watch for signs of wound infection • Sleep in boot
Exercise	• Ankle range-of-motion exercises • Upper extremity circuit training • 2–5 cm heel lifts • Straight leg raises • Isometric exercises of uninvolved muscles

1 Why is it important for the allied health assistant to have a knowledge of precautions in this clinical pathway?

2 What are isometric exercises?

3 How can the family benefit from post-operative information following this surgical procedure?

Check resource and equipment suitability and working order and minimise environmental hazards

Before any therapy session, you will need to ensure that the required equipment is in good working order. This includes checking for defects and cleanliness, and making sure batteries are charged and that no equipment is missing parts. When equipment is identified as faulty it needs to be removed for repair by appropriate persons. If equipment is on loan it will need to be returned to the supplier. Some health and government departments fund or subsidise devices and equipment depending on the clients, so it is important to determine if the client is eligible for funded support; for example, from the Department of Veterans' Affairs. Procedures for the management of equipment repairs may vary between work locations and it is recommended you review the appropriate local procedure at your facility.

Adaptive equipment and aids

Depending on the type of therapy session there will be a variety of equipment that can be used. This adaptive equipment is classified as any device or tool that can help with an activity or task when the person has trouble performing these routines. The equipment makes life easier for the person and helps them to maintain their independence. Your supervisor will advise on what is required.

Adaptive equipment
Any device or tool used to assist with completing activities of daily living.

Examples of adaptive equipment and aids include:

- *mobility equipment:* walking frames, crutches, lifters, wheelchairs, swivel seats
- *visual aids:* screen readers, Braille displays
- *personal care aids:* shower chairs, raised toilet seats, commodes, hand-held showerhead, rails, reaching devices
- *dressing aids:* sock aids, shoehorns, Velcro, elastic shoelaces
- *eating equipment:* plate guards, extra-grip cutlery, cups with lids or two handles, non-slip bowls and plates, jar openers (see Figure 17.5)
- *supportive equipment:* slings, splints, braces, wedges, cushions, rails, hearing aids, grabbers, non-slip mats, ramps.

FIGURE 17.5 Adaptive feeding equipment

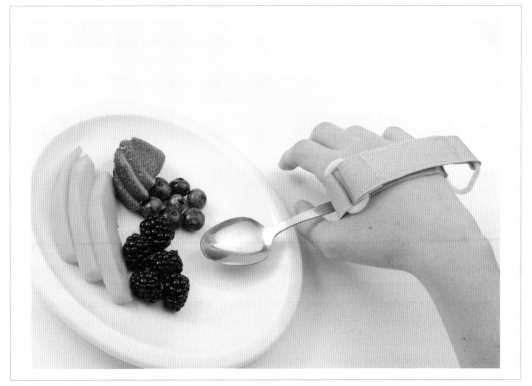

Source: Science Photo Library/Science Source

ACTIVITY
17.4

Checking hearing aids

Audiologists are trained to test hearing in those suffering from hearing loss and can prescribe hearing aids in various sizes or shapes to augment hearing.

An allied health worker can assist the client with care of their hearing aid so that they have reliable and better hearing.

TYPE OF HEARING AID	CLEANING RECOMMENDATIONS
Behind the ear hearing aid	• Remove debris with a dry cloth • Clean earmould daily by soaking in warm, soapy water • Clear tubing with water and allow to dry overnight • Remove batteries and clean battery compartment nightly
In the ear hearing aid	• Clean and clear away wax with brush provided by healthcare professional • Use hook or wax pick to clear holes • Wipe with clean, dry cloth • Remove batteries and clean battery compartment nightly

1 Why is it important to avoid wipes with chemicals or alcohol when cleaning hearing aids?

2 What should be done if the client's earmould develops an odour?

Prepare the client for therapy

Preparing the client under the direction of the supervising allied health professional is essential for a positive result with therapy. All the information you give to the client should be clear and easily understood and you should confirm their understanding at each stage of the message. Use questioning, paraphrasing and reflective listening to make sure that they understand. Chapter 4, 'Communicate and work in health and community services', outlines this in more detail.

As an allied health worker, you need to be aware that there are often psychological effects from a client's injury or disease, so there may be emotional reactions that can impact on preparation. Changed body image or being dependent on another person can have a significant impact on a person's wellbeing. This can also impact financial stability and future goals and plans, and present as:

• anger

• anxiety

• loss of control

• depression

• frustration.

You will need to use your interpersonal communication skills so that you can identify and best prepare the client for their sessions. This includes active listening, empathy, and the assistance of other team members if required; for example, a psychologist or social worker. When the client is emotionally prepared, they are more likely to undertake the session in a positive way. Consider the following:

• Have you introduced yourself and your role?

• Has consent been obtained for the therapy session?

• Has the client been informed about the procedure?

- Is the client wearing appropriate clothing for the session?
- Are they in pain – do they need medication?
- Is there any pre-existing condition that must be considered prior to therapy?
- What equipment is required for this session?
- How much assistance will be required for the client?

Importance of preparation

Think about a time when you had to prepare someone for a new activity or task and answer the following questions:

1   What communication strategies did you use to make the person feel at ease with you and listen to you?

2   What body language and signs would you look out for in a person who was feeling anxious?

3   What techniques could be used to alleviate frustration in a person who was being instructed on a task and was finding it difficult?

17.5 ACTIVITY

3   PROVIDE ASSISTANCE WITH THERAPY SESSION

When providing assistance with therapy sessions, it is important to have a good knowledge of the client's individualised treatment plans, goals and limitations of therapy. This involves an understanding of their condition and emotional status, so that therapy tasks and programs can be undertaken successfully and with the appropriate precautions. Your role will be to assist each client to achieve their goals through clear explanation, reinforcement and encouragement (see Figure 17.6).

FIGURE 17.6 Assisting with a therapy task

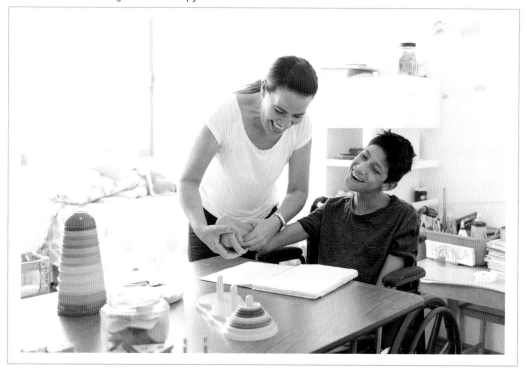

Source: iStock.com/ferrantraite

When working under the supervision of an allied health professional, you should always seek clarification and feedback if you are unsure of the instructions. You should also take appropriate actions to ensure the comfort, safety and privacy of the client, including reporting incidents.

Assist with therapy tasks and maintain general therapy precautions

A basic knowledge of anatomy and physiology gives the allied health assistant an understanding of how to assist with treatment plans and therapies and to take precautions. Chapter 3, 'Recognise healthy body systems', outlines this in more detail.

When assisting with a therapy session, you will need to consider the readiness of the client. This includes consent and a full explanation of the procedure. You will also need to understand their condition so that precautions can be taken.

Conditions requiring precautions

Respiratory disorders

Asthma, COPD and pneumonia may result in shortness of breath and limited ability to perform exercises. Clients are advised to bring their regular medications (for example, bronchodilators) prior to therapy sessions. It is important to remember to have a chair nearby if the client experiences fatigue and a sputum mug nearby if they have increasing mucous secretions. Report any signs of blood or discolouration in sputum and ask your supervisor to inform you of the best exercise position for the client when assisting with therapy sessions.

Circulatory disorders

Peripheral vascular disease, angina or swelling of limbs could cause limitations in participation in therapy sessions. Client confidence may be impacted, so it is important to observe for pain, discolouration or numbness of extremities and anxiety. These should be reported to your supervisor and the therapy session should be ceased.

Nervous system disorders

Stroke, vertigo, speech and swallowing disorders, brain injury and spinal cord injury will impact a client's ability to feel, move and participate in therapy sessions. However, the benefits of treatment can improve function considerably, and in particular strength, balance, mobility and quality of life. Report any signs of pain or dizziness and have a chair ready for the client to rest. Report coughing or choking when the client is eating or drinking and provide napkins if they bring up any food or fluids.

Musculoskeletal disorders

Joint replacements, amputations, bone and joint disorders and muscle weakness can impact mobilisation. It is important to encourage your clients as progress can be slow. The psychological effects of limitations can cause depression in your clients, so it is important to motivate, use therapeutic communication and create a supportive environment. Some clients may have an instruction plan from their surgeon regarding positioning and weight-bearing. A physiotherapist, prosthetist (see Figure 17.7) or podiatrist can use this plan to help inform decisions on therapy and to instruct the client in the required exercises or treatments.

FIGURE 17.7 Prosthetist assisting a client

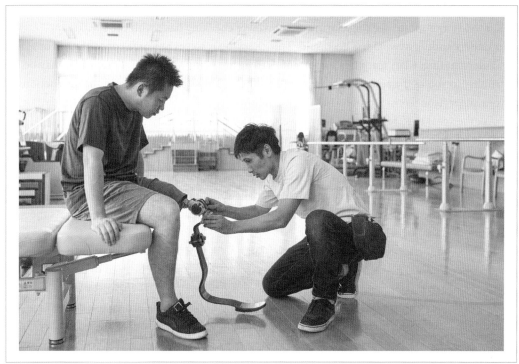

Source: Alamy Stock Photo/Aflo Co., Ltd.

Prosthetic prescription

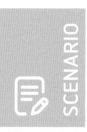

Alex is a recent amputee and is attending his first prosthetic fitting and alignment session. In previous sessions, Alex and the prosthetist decided on the type of device to be made as well as the socket design. During this fitting and alignment session, the natural position of the stump is determined as Alex stands up with a frame. Then the leg prosthesis is aligned while Alex places weight on the prosthesis. This enables the specialist to make the necessary height and angle adjustments for Alex's profile.

My role during this session was to make sure that the frame was at the correct height and in safe working order. I made sure Alex was comfortable and I ensured that he was near the bed when he first placed weight on his new prosthetic leg just in case he felt dizzy. I also looked out for any emotional distress or pain he was experiencing.

Alex's wife was a great support and she provided much-needed encouragement to Alex during the session. An occupational therapist was also organised to see if any rails or other modifications were needed at Alex's home and to work on a plan for him to return to work.

1　Why is it important for Alex to be fully informed and able to ask any questions prior to the session being undertaken?

2　How would a prosthetist, psychologist, occupational therapist and physiotherapist work together to support clients with amputations?

Seek clarification and feedback

When we communicate, seeking clarification involves checking back with the speaker on your understanding of what has been said. This checking resolves any areas of confusion or misunderstanding. Clarification is important as there are many aspects of therapy that may be unfamiliar to you as the assistant, and you need to be sure that you understand the instructions of your supervisor. Considerations include the following:

- Ask the speaker to repeat what they have said if you are unsure.
- State what you understand the speaker has said.
- Ask for examples if appropriate.

For example: 'Thanks for giving me the instructions on how to calibrate the treadmill. I'm not quite clear on a few things and I want to make sure I understand. If I heard you correctly, I need to press the hold and incline buttons until the display reads 'calibration', then press the start button. Is that right?'

It is also important for the allied health assistant to ask for feedback to improve their work practices and develop new skills. Feedback comes from others and can be used to describe positive or negative comments about your actions or behaviour.

For example: 'Can you tell me how I went today when I helped Mr Brown use the resistance bands? I have only done this a few times before and want to know if I was doing it correctly.'

Feedback
Helpful information or criticism given to improve performance.

Positive feedback

This is communication that recognises your strengths or successes. It enhances your morale and encourages good work practices.

For example: 'Thanks for putting in the extra effort to work late and finish off the filing for the clients today. Our team really appreciates your efforts and values you as a team member. You are always so positive and this helps to motivate us and makes the clinic a great place to work.'

Negative feedback

This communication points out what a person is doing poorly or what behaviours and habits are causing problems. It can be difficult to listen to if it is poorly delivered. When giving negative feedback, it is important to frame it in a constructive way so that improvements can be made. To assist in this:

- deliver feedback carefully and respectfully and consider the person's emotional state
- help the person find ways to avoid making the mistake again and provide suggestions for improvement
- be honest and sincere and let them know you are there to help them.

For example: 'Yesterday when you were speaking to Mr Barrow I noticed that you became exasperated and raised your voice at him. I know that he can be difficult at times but he is quite stressed about his rehabilitation. Next time it would be a good idea to take a minute to sit with him, acknowledge his concerns and spend time listening to him. I'm sure this will alleviate his concerns.'

Positive or negative feedback

17.6 ACTIVITY

1   Identify each of the following statements as an example of either positive or negative feedback:

STATEMENT	POSITIVE OR NEGATIVE FEEDBACK
You haven't done the 10 a.m. observations on Mrs Smith. You're making us all look bad	
I'm happy with the way that you helped your colleague with the showers this morning	
Your attitude in the meeting made it look like you didn't want to be there	
I would ask you to do an extra shift but your work ethic leaves a lot to be desired	
Thanks for staying with Mrs McGrath today. She seemed quite upset but your calming voice eased her anxiety	

2   Consider the negative feedback examples and think about how each sentence could be reworded to make it constructive feedback.

Ensuring comfort, safety and privacy of client

An important part of treating a client is to ensure they feel safe and comfortable and that their privacy is respected. A visit to an allied health clinic can involve being handled, put in uncomfortable positions and undergoing procedures that may result in pain. Person-centred care as discussed in Chapter 13, 'Work with people with mental health issues', outlines that the provision of privacy, dignity and safety empowers a person and encourages them to develop an understanding of what they want and need.

In an allied health context, this means:

- providing physical comfort; e.g., pillows, splints, pain relief
- providing emotional support by alleviating fears or anxieties
- respecting the client's values and preferences
- providing environmental privacy; e.g., screens, making sure the client is covered
- providing information, communication and education while adhering to privacy principles
- adhering to safety principles with all equipment
- showing cultural safety by being sensitive to the person's cultural values and beliefs.

Explain therapy goals to clients and support goal achievement

Allied health professions create treatment plans that outline the approach and interventions used to achieve a certain goal. Goals are established during therapy sessions and they should be general and specific. The allied health assistant should receive appropriate instructions from their supervisor and use reinforcement, clear explanation and clarification to support and motivate the clients in meeting these goals.

General goals

These are the long-term goals that summarise the purpose of the therapy or treatment. Chapter 7, 'Organise personal work priorities and development', describes goals as needing to be specific, measurable, actionable, realistic and time-based (SMART). Long-term or general goals are set to help people understand what they can expect from rehabilitation and where they can expect to be in several months. Regardless of the goal, the final outcome depends on the person's motivation and the support and coaching given by the therapy teams.

Examples of general therapy goals include:

- to improve mobility
- to maximise hearing
- to regain the ability to complete ADLs
- to restore speech to an understandable level
- to maintain adequate nutrition.

Specific goals

These short-term interventions help to achieve the general goals. Clients attending therapy sessions are encouraged to achieve the short-term goals, with the allied team monitoring the progress. The goals may need to be changed if people progress more slowly or quickly than expected. If a client can achieve the goals earlier than expected, then the targets can be stretched as long as there is no excessive discomfort. Conversely, if the client experiences discomfort in trying to reach the goals, they can be reduced. Examples include:

- increase range of motion in shoulder by 80 per cent
- walk 20 metres independently on a level surface
- safely drink single-cup sips of thin liquids without aspiration within two weeks.

ACTIVITY 17.7

Therapy teams and goals

Complete the following table by matching the allied health professional listed here with the specific goals: occupational therapist, physiotherapist, prosthetist, speech pathologist, dietitian, psychologist, audiologist.

SPECIFIC GOALS	ALLIED HEALTH PROFESSIONAL
To lose 1–2 kg a fortnight over the next three months	
To shower independently using a shower chair within two weeks	
To swallow pureed food without regurgitation over the next week	
To walk the length of the parallel bars three times without assistance using your new artificial leg	
To correctly insert and remove an in-the-ear hearing aid three times as measured by observation	
To use the Headspace app every week for the next three months to promote mindfulness	
To perform five × sit-to-stand exercises with minimal assistance over a 15-minute period	

Maslow's hierarchy of needs

Goal-setting is important for rehabilitation because it can provide the patient with motivation. Maslow's hierarchy of needs connects people's needs to motivation. This hierarchy states that physiological and safety and security needs must be satisfied first before the higher-level needs of self-esteem and self-actualisation can be met (to review in more detail, see Figure 12.1).

In supporting and coaching clients to achieve goals, the allied health worker should always consider the client's physiological needs first. This may mean relieving pain, providing nutrition and ensuring comfort before attempting to support a client in reaching their higher-level goals.

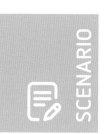

Applying Maslow's hierarchy in helping a stroke patient

Kassem has suffered a mild stroke and has resultant left-sided weakness and dysphasia. In developing a rehabilitation plan, the allied health team consider his initial needs before progressing to therapy for independence over time.

Basic physiological needs

Ensure Kassem is pain-free and has adequate nutritional support. Assist with feeding and elimination.

Security and safety

Assist Kassem with mobility and hygiene and falls prevention.

Social and emotional

Allow Kassem's family to visit whilst he is in hospital and encourage their participation in his care. Be sensitive to Kassem's cultural and spiritual needs.

Self-esteem

Encourage Kassem's progress with rehabilitation by allowing him to perform as much self-care as possible. Encourage independence by rewarding progress.

Self-actualisation

Acknowledge accomplishments so that Kassem is able to plan ahead and cope with stressful situations.

Manage and report accidents and incidents

Any risks, hazards or incidents that occur in the workplace will need to be documented and reported to your supervisor. You will need to be familiar with the policies and procedures in your facility and with any incident reporting systems used. Refer to Chapter 1, 'Participate in workplace health and safety', where accidents and incidents are covered in detail.

Remember, when filling out incident reports:

* complete time, date and place
* include the name of the client involved and the witness to the incident
* detail the incident – where and when it occurred
* describe the incident, what was being performed and if any treatment was provided

As with all reporting requirements, be clear, concise, objective and accurate, as these reports are legal documents.

4 USE THERAPY EQUIPMENT CORRECTLY AND SAFELY

Allied health professionals use a wide range of equipment and resources. A sound understanding of each piece of equipment and its purpose is required as well as their safety aspects and limitations. A manufacturer's instructions can provide some of this knowledge, as can your facility with training opportunities. It is important to follow the work health and safety guidelines for each piece of equipment and to adhere to manual handling and infection control precautions. Refer to Chapter 1, 'Participate in workplace health and safety', for more information.

Use equipment according to manufacturer and supervisor instructions

Manufacturing instructions are provided for your safety and to inform you of how to use the equipment. These instructions may guide the user in assembly of the equipment and include troubleshooting questions and answers. Safety guidelines may also be included in the instructions; for example, maximum weight-bearing loads. It is important to use the equipment as per the instructions or the product warranty may be voided.

Examples of equipment that may require instructions include:
- hoists and lifters
- wheelchairs
- stationary bikes
- rowing machines
- treadmills
- dynamometers
- tilt tables (see Figure 17.8)
- ultrasounds
- electronic therapy.

Considerations when using equipment correctly and safely include the following:
- Maintain equipment in a good state of repair and proper working order.
- Use equipment only for the operations for which it is appropriate.
- Make sure that you check all items of equipment before use.
- Ensure that safety guards or brakes are applied before using equipment on clients.
- Where equipment is found to be unsafe or broken, it must be taken out of service and sent for repair or replaced as required.
- The organisation must keep records of maintenance checks, testing and servicing.
- Make sure that instructions are kept so that all staff have access if required.
- Attend information and training sessions whenever any new equipment is purchased for use.

Follow work health and safety (WHS) guidelines for equipment

When working in an allied health context, it is essential that you understand the guidelines for manual handling and infection control for particular pieces of equipment, and how this relates to your role in assisting the physiotherapist, occupational therapist or other allied health

FIGURE 17.8 A tilt table

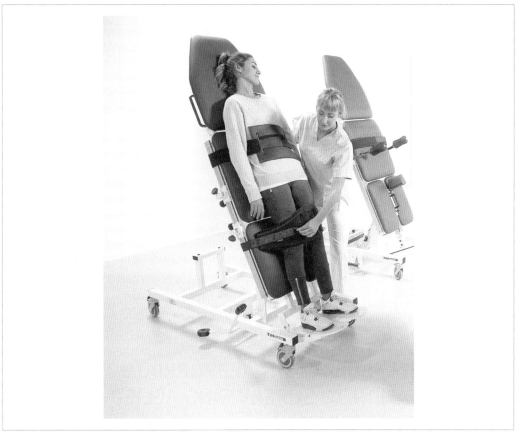

Source: Rehab Technology, www.rehabtechnology.com.au

professionals to deliver and monitor therapy programs. You will need to speak with your supervisor to receive the appropriate skills training required for your area of work.

Manual handling precautions may include:

- selecting the appropriate equipment for the procedure
- checking equipment for faults, damage and cleanliness
- checking the weight limits on equipment against the client's weight
- planning before the move, including removing obstructions
- requesting assistance if necessary.

Standard infection control precautions may include:

- appropriate hand washing – before and after patient contact
- immunisation – it is your responsibility to be up to date
- use of personal protective equipment – gloves, masks and protective eyewear if required
- cleaning equipment and workspaces
- following cough etiquette.

While delivering any therapy programs in your role, you may meet clients who are infective or suspected of being infective. It is important that you are aware of and follow infection control procedures at all times. Refer to Chapter 2, 'Comply with infection prevention and control policies and procedures'.

Occupational therapy equipment for Frank

Frank has had a total hip replacement following a fall at home. He has been discharged to a rehabilitation clinic and has been referred to an occupational therapist who will identify if any aids or adaptive equipment are required in his home.

As an allied health assistant, I was able to visit Frank's home with the occupational therapist and help assess the environment for hazards and determine what adaptive aids were needed. On inspection, Frank required:

- rails in the bathroom and a shower chair
- raised toilet seat
- non-slip mats in the bathroom
- reacher, to pick up items from the floor
- sock aids to help him put on his socks
- walker.

While in the rehabilitation hospital, Frank practised using these aids so that he was capable on return to home. My role was to assist Frank with his practice and refer any queries to the supervisor.

1   Why is it important to have a raised toilet seat after a hip replacement?
2   What manual handling precautions should you be aware of when assisting Frank in the shower?

5   PROVIDE FEEDBACK ON APPROPRIATE THERAPY INFORMATION TO SUPERVISING ALLIED HEALTH PROFESSIONAL

Feedback in an allied health context means providing information about a client's reactions to a session, how they performed a task or how they recovered after a treatment. This is then used as a basis for improvement. When providing feedback on a therapy session, remember to:

- be specific
- be timely
- focus on the behaviour not the person.

Client feedback provides valuable information about the service offered. This will give the allied health team an insight into what worked well and what did not, and where improvements can be made.

Feedback can be formal or informal. Formal feedback can be given by patients through surveys or by staff in performance development plans. Informal feedback is often given verbally; for example, 'I noticed you made Mr Roper and his wife feel very comfortable while you explained the hearing test to them today, and your explanation was very clear. They were looking a bit overwhelmed but when you gave them the brochure about hearing aids, they seemed a bit more relieved. I'll check if they have any further questions for you before they leave.'

Pass on significant information

It is important to pass on significant information to your supervisor after a therapy session. This includes the progress of the session and if any difficulties were faced by the client during the session. Additional feedback that should be given includes:

- Was there a deviation from an activity or prescribed task?
- Did they complete the session?
- What was their emotional status during the session? For example, were they motivated or uninterested?
- Were there any incidents during the session?

As an assistant to an allied health professional, you should ensure the safety of the clients by observing for any reactions or adverse effects of their treatments. Reactions or adverse effects to observe and report in your clients include:

- pain
- tightness in chest
- breathing difficulties
- pallor
- sweating
- difficulty breathing or wheezing
- dizziness
- irregular heart rate
- nausea.

Exercise physiology for chronic pain

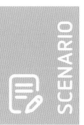

Jamal has had chronic back pain which has lasted for more than three months following a fall down the stairs at his workplace. He has had medical treatment but the pain persists. He has been referred to an exercise physiologist.

The physiologist took a detailed assessment and developed a carefully programmed exercise plan to address Jamal's symptoms. This included a review of his body mechanics, posture, and his sleeping and work habits.

As an assistant to the exercise physiologist, my role was to prepare and clean the equipment that Jamal was going to use and provide any assistance to the exercise physiologist during the session. The session involved Jamal performing stretching and flexibility exercises on a mat, aerobic exercises on a treadmill and core strengthening tasks. He was also given education on meditation and lifestyle modifications.

1   What adverse effects should be reported while Jamal is doing his exercises?
2   What safety aspects would be shown to Jamal for the treadmill?

Document information

When working with allied health professionals, you may be required to complete documentation regarding the therapy sessions given to clients. this may include:

- meeting notes
- telephone conversations
- progress notes
- information provided to clients
- follow-up or referral notes.

Documentation is covered in Chapter 10, 'Provide non-client contact support in an acute care environment', which highlights that documentation must be accurate, factual and signed by yourself as well as with a countersignature, according to organisational requirements. The chapter also provides information on how to correct errors in documentation.

The importance of documenting client's progress is that:

* it provides a record of continuity and evaluation of care
* information can be passed on to the entire healthcare team
* evaluation of care can be determined
* it informs research and statistics
* it helps in the development of a treatment plan
* it can be used as a teaching tool.

Depending on your workplace, most health service districts will have their own policy on documentation in client files. Some organisations use the SOAP method for documenting in clients' notes:

* **S** – Subjective information on what client reports
* **O** – Objective information on what you see
* **A** – Assessment of client
* **P** – Plan

Here is an example of SOAP reporting:

* S – Cameron reported that he was managing well with the cardiac menu plan as prescribed by the dietitian but deviated on a few occasions
* O – Client appeared short of breath
* A – Blood pressure 155/95, weight gain 0.2 kg from last week
* P – Dietitian consulted to reinforce diet plan and set short-term goal to reduce weight by 0.1 kg per fortnight. For follow-up referral to psychologist to work on behavioural changes.

You may also need to learn what acceptable abbreviations can be used for each allied health team.

6   ASSIST IN THE DESIGN AND CONSTRUCTION OF SIMPLE THERAPY MATERIALS AND EQUIPMENT

For many assistive devices and therapy equipment, it is essential to have training in their use and regular follow-up on their continued appropriateness. Your role includes identifying any gaps in these resources, which can be identified by yourself or the client, and then working with the allied health professional to develop solutions. This may include modification or updating materials for the individual's needs to allow them to progress through their treatment plans.

Assist identification of gaps in therapy material resources and develop solutions

Each client will have differing needs and abilities. Therapy materials and equipment are more likely to meet these needs if the individual involved can assist with the design, identifying gaps and modifying if required. The client needs to know how to use the therapy material or equipment and the goals for its use in order to identify any gaps.

Some therapy materials can cause adverse reactions in the client, and the allied health worker should be aware of these signs and consider solutions as appropriate. This can include:

- reactions to materials in therapy devices (e.g., slings, bands), which can cause redness, rash or swelling. Consideration of alternative materials needs to be made
- pressure areas causing redness and ulceration at bony prominences. The device may need to be replaced or additional padding may need to be inserted
- skin injuries for older persons who have fragile skin. Check for sharp edges and insert padding where appropriate.

Update therapy materials and construct aids and adaptations

Every client has different needs and any aids should take into account the client's abilities and lifestyle. Therapy materials and aids should therefore be adapted to suit the individual. Equipment may need to be updated or modified from time to time and this should always be done under the guidance of your supervisor.

It is essential that you have a good knowledge of the assistive device and any measurements that may be required to make adjustments. This can be obtained from the product information manual in your workplace or as instructed by your supervising health professional.

Mobility aids

Assistive devices for mobility – for example, forearm crutches or underarm crutches – can be adapted by modifying the height to the underarm and adjusting the handgrips for comfort and fit. Adding padding can also provide comfort under the arm. Walking sticks can be adjusted for the person's height. Wheelchairs are becoming more specific, with some models able to be adapted for individual needs. This includes custom-made seating to support and control posture, handles on wheels to assist with rotation and adjustable footplate heights. Check with your supervising allied health professional or information manual for this information.

Devices for ADLs

Assistive devices for activities of daily living can support the client in their hygiene, mobility and nutritional needs and can be adapted to suit each individual. Examples include the following:

- Over-the-toilet frames can be adjusted for height (see Figure 17.9).
- Hoists and lifters have slings appropriate for an individual's weight and size.
- Bath boards can be adjusted so that they are firm and secure, with some being more heavy-duty for client weight considerations.
- Shower chairs can have fixed or swing-back armrests for the particular needs of clients.

Supportive devices

Splints come in various sizes and can be custom-made – they can include foam inserts for client comfort and to relieve pressure. Hearing and vision assistive software is available to assist people who have hearing or vision disabilities so that they can participate in a range of activities. Adaptations can include larger buttons on phones or computers, screen magnification (see Figure 17.10) or adjustments to amplification.

FIGURE 17.9 An over-toilet frame

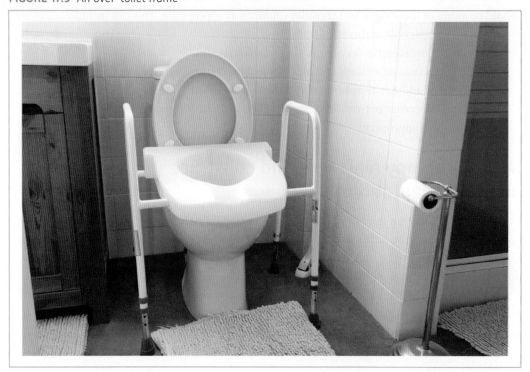

Source: Alamy Stock Photo/Ronnie McMillan

FIGURE 17.10 A screen magnifier

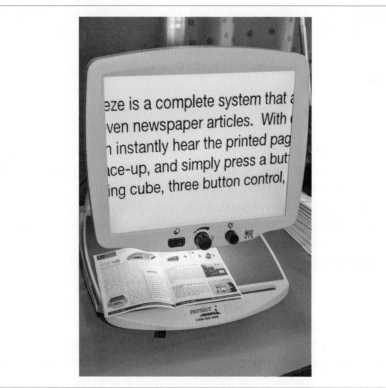

Source: Alamy Stock Photo/Jeffrey Isaac Greenberg 7+

Low vision adaptations

SCENARIO

Salina was diagnosed with macular degeneration, which has caused her to have blurred vision and reduced central vision in both eyes. She was referred to the orthoptist for assessment and provision of aids to manage her daily living tasks.

On assessment of her home, the following adaptations were made:

- tactile bump dots placed on microwave, stove and clothes washer
- big-button telephone
- additional lights
- shelf liners opposite in colour to crockery
- optical magnifier for reading
- adapting computer software by increasing size of text, changing contrast and using the narrator function.

1 What are the additional roles of an orthoptist?
2 Along with home adaptations, what additional support and services may Salina need with her low vision?

7 COMPLETE REQUIRED ADMINISTRATIVE DUTIES

Working as an assistant to the allied health team means more than providing client support and care. Maintaining data and stock, filing, and booking appointments as well as other administrative duties help to maximise clinical efficiency (see Figure 17.11). Supporting the allied health professionals through assisting with the coordination of programs and maintaining client records ensures that optimal care can be given in both the hospital and community settings.

Maintain statistics

The collection, recording and reporting of client activity data is a key strategy in supporting the performance monitoring, program measurement, and service planning and funding for allied health providers.

Knowledge of statistics helps allied health professionals evaluate research that assesses the efficacy of treatments, which benefits patient care. Statistics can measure performance and whether it has been successful or not. This establishes benchmarks or standards of service and allows for quality improvements to be made. Statistics also inform research by identifying trends that can be further explored.

Working in an allied health assistant context, you may undertake administrative duties that include the collection of statistics and data, such as:

- names, date of birth and gender of clients
- cultural/English-speaking status
- referral and admission information
- treatment plans.

It is important to remember privacy and confidentiality policies when dealing with personal information. The knowledge gained through statistics supports evidence-based practice by applying the most up-to date-evidence for patient care. This is discussed later in this chapter.

Statistics
Collection, analysis and interpretation of data.

FIGURE 17.11 Example of a hospital medical stock-ordering form

PURCHASE ORDER FORM

CUSTOMER INFORMATION

SOLD TO

Organisation: _____

Attention: _____

Street: _____

City: _____ State: _____ Postcode: _____

Phone: _____ Fax: _____

Email: _____

SHIP TO

Organisation: _____

Attention: _____

Street: _____

City: _____ State: _____ Postcode: _____

Phone: _____ Fax: _____

PAYMENT INFORMATION

PAYMENT TYPE

☐ Cheque enclosed for: $_____

☐ Bill us "Net 30 Days"

☐ Pay by credit card

CREDIT CARD INFORMATION

☐ Visa   ☐ MasterCard   ☐ AMEX

Card #: _____ Exp. Date: _____

Name on Card: _____

Signature: _____

ORDER INFORMATION

Model	QTY	Product	Colour	Size	Unit price	Total price

CONFIRMATION

☐ This confirms a phone order

    Name of Salesperson: _____

☐ I have ordered before

☐ Notify me before delivery *(may incur additional charges)*

    Phone: _____

AUTHORISATION

Name: _____ Title: _____

Signature: _____ Date: _____

PO #: _____

Maintain stock levels

You may be required to maintain an inventory of stock and report any items of equipment that require attention. Management of the stock includes identifying low levels of stock and ordering, as well as maintenance and cleaning. All equipment should be labelled with safe working loads which identify the weight limits for their use, as well as being tested and tagged. Warranties should be stored in a safe place if needed for replacement.

Ordering stock includes identifying the preferred suppliers and determining minimum and maximum orders. Stock should be rotated on shelves so that stock with the oldest expiry date is used first. It is also important to consider storage space and not to overfill shelves. Completing inventories of stock allows you to have the right amount of stock at the right time. This can be done manually with a stock book or with a computerised stock control system, depending on the size of the facility in which you work.

Book in clients for appointments

Booking clients for appointments is a common task in any healthcare service (see Figure 17.12). Efficient scheduling has a significant impact on the client's delivery of care and keeps wait times to a minimum as well as maintaining client satisfaction. Considerations when booking clients for appointments include:

- implementing patient self-scheduling – many practices now have the ability to offer real-time patient scheduling any time and from anywhere with internet access
- prioritising appointments – some clients may need the highest level of care and others can be managed by a brief appointment
- utilising an appointment reminder software system – this can improve upon the number of on-time arrivals and kept appointments
- ensuring clients are aware of what they need to bring in or wear to each appointment
- creating waiting lists to cover last-minute cancellations.

FIGURE 17.12 Booking an appointment

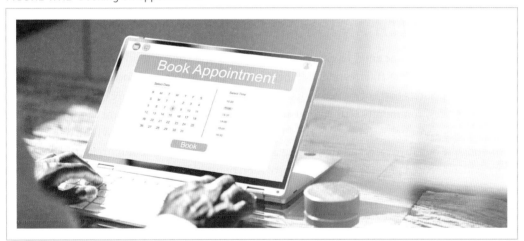

Source: Alamy Stock Photo / Andriy Popov

The types of information that you will need when booking appointments include:

- name of person
- contact information
- phone number
- appointment date and time

- first or follow-up appointment (first appointments generally take more time and may require the client to complete additional paperwork)
- treating allied health professional if in a multidisciplinary clinic
- interpreter if required
- parking availability at the facility or if transport needs to be organised; e.g., community transport
- clothing requirements for session if client needs to undertake activities
- scheduled fees for treatment and claiming information.

ACTIVITY 17.8

Client bookings

Answer 'true' or 'false' for the following statements:

STATEMENT	TRUE/FALSE
Not all appointments are the same	
Send reminders on the day of the appointments	
Schedule time between appointments in case of delays	
Waiting lists are unnecessary when scheduling properly	
Delays in appointments affect the smooth running of the clinic	
Cancellation policies should be printed clearly in the reception room	
Fees are to be collected when clients book their appointment	
Bilingual receptionists can be used as interpreters	

8 WORK WITH A PRIMARY HEALTHCARE APPROACH

Primary health care

Entry level to the health system and, usually, a person's first encounter with the health system.

Primary health care is the entry level to the health system and covers health promotion, early intervention, prevention and treatment. It includes physical, mental and social wellbeing and is usually the person's first encounter with the healthcare system. Services are delivered in general practices, community settings and allied health practices. The assistant can work with a primary healthcare approach by supporting the client in the planning and provision of services, promoting preventative care, and supporting access and equity. It is also important to reflect using evidence-based practice in your own provision of healthcare services.

Support and facilitate the involvement of the client and the community in the planning and provision of services

Supporting the client in the community and at home can reduce the need for the person to require acute care in a hospital setting. By providing services according to the instruction of allied health professionals, the client can receive early management of health conditions and receive earlier interventions for their needs.

Community services

Community services can provide allied support for health promotion, assessment, intervention and treatment in the home or in community health centres. Each of the multidisciplinary teams can deliver a comprehensive range of services in both metropolitan and rural settings. Services for Australian Rural and Remote Allied Health (SARRAH) is the nationally recognised body representing rural and remote allied health professionals. They particularly manage chronic disease and those with complex care needs. Other community services include Indigenous outreach workers, rural doctor networks, telehealth, and primary health networks.

Primary health networks

These are independent organisations that coordinate primary health care in regions and align it with local needs and expectations. Their goals are to improve access and effectiveness of health services for people, particularly those at risk of poor health outcomes. Allied health services are an integral component of the services provided.

Promote good health and a preventative approach to maintaining health as part of own work role

Health promotion and disease prevention looks at screening and maintenance to prevent future illness and treatment. By identifying and preventing potential problems, improved healthcare outcomes can be made. The allied health worker can play an important role in this strategy and in particular with chronic disease. Allied health workers have specialist expertise in working with persons to improve their health and wellbeing and avoid disease complications. Examples of chronic disease include:

- osteoarthritis
- type 2 diabetes
- mental illness
- asthma
- renal disease
- cardiovascular disease
- multiple sclerosis.

Treatments can include self-management skills, screening for prevention, exercises to optimise function and mobility, splints to reduce pain, dietary advice, counselling, group therapy (see Figure 17.13) and stress management.

The allied health teams use a holistic approach to care in that they consider the multidimensional aspects of the person when planning their care. This includes physical, mental, social and spiritual aspects.

FIGURE 17.13 Group therapy session

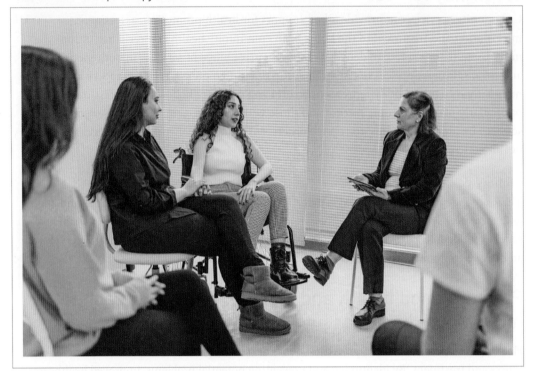

Source: iStock.com/Phynart Studio

Art therapy for mental health issues

Claudia has been diagnosed with depression. The GP at the aged care facility has recommended art therapy as an alternative treatment as Claudia has mentioned that she loves doing art, finding it comforting.

This type of therapy uses a non-judgemental approach that allows the client to detail their moods as art and then the art therapist can discuss the person's feelings. It is a method that can calm a mood through art and creativity.

Claudia attends a group session and her paintings show boats in stormy weather, which is indicative of her current emotional state. In discussions with the art therapist, Claudia is able to express her feelings of sadness, and over the course of these group sessions she is able to continue to paint her emotions and also to speak about her feelings. With the help of the therapist, Claudia is able to develop strategies to manage her depression.

1　How is art therapy a preventative health measure?

2　What alternative therapies or strategies could be used to assist persons with feelings of sadness, grief, depression or insecurity?

Recognise importance of access and equity in provision of health services

Making health services available to everyone in Australia means access to the right care at the right time while overcoming potential health barriers, such as geography, culture or socioeconomic situations, so that equity is maintained. These barriers or determinants of health are the non-medical factors that affect the health of individuals and their communities. Knowledge of the determinants and support of access and equity is an important focus for the allied health worker.

Access and equity
Providing services to all and treating them fairly.

Determinants of health

Housing

Safe, affordable and secure housing is associated with better health, which in turn impacts on people's participation in work, education and the community. Living in insecure housing can lead to decreased health, which can be seen in persons with low incomes.

Education

Education enables people to achieve employment, have an income, live in adequate housing and make informed healthcare choices. An individual's education level affects not only their own health but that of their family and community.

Nutrition

People who don't have access to healthy foods are less likely to have good nutrition. That raises their risk of health conditions like heart disease, diabetes and obesity and can lower life expectancy.

Individual characteristics

Genetics plays a part in determining lifespan, healthiness and the likelihood of developing certain illnesses. Personal behaviour and coping skills also determine health, with smoking, drinking and drug use affecting health, as well as how we deal with life's stresses and challenges.

Health equity and access

> Health equity is defined as the absence of unfair and avoidable or remediable differences in health among population groups defined socially, economically, demographically or geographically.
>
> WHO, 2022

In Australia, healthcare facilities and services provide some degree of equity to the population; however, some groups, including Aboriginal and Torres Strait Islanders, those affected by chronic mental illness and those in insecure low-paid employment, still experience health inequality.

People living in remote and very remote areas generally also have poorer access to health services than people in regional areas and major cities. They may need to travel long distances to attend health services and these populations rely more on general practitioners (GPs) to provide healthcare services, due to less availability of local specialist services (Australian Government Department of Health, 2016).

The Australian Government has developed the National Preventive Health Strategy, which outlines the overarching, long-term approach to health promotion and equity in Australia over the coming decade (see Figure 17.14). Its aim is to improve the health and wellbeing of all Australians through investment in prevention and prioritising disadvantaged populations.

FIGURE 17.14 National Preventive Health Strategy 2021–2030

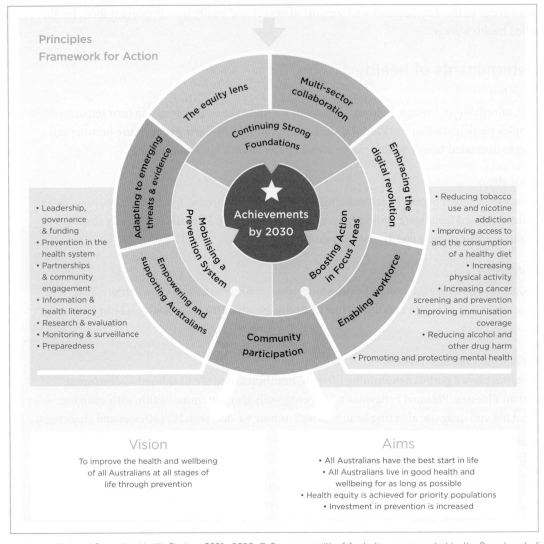

Source: National Preventive Health Strategy 2021–2030, © Commonwealth of Australia as represented by the Department of Health 2021, p. 8. Licensed under Creative Commons Attribution 4.0 International Public License. © Commonwealth of Australia (Department of Health) 2021.

ACTIVITY 17.9

Aboriginal diabetes education in South Australia

The South Australian Aboriginal Chronic Disease Consortium has developed a series of video resources featuring members of rural and remote Aboriginal communities, to capture diabetes stories that highlight challenges and successes in managing diabetes and diabetes risks and complications.

The videos feature health professionals, including allied health workers, and provide explanations about the disease and its management in language that is appropriate for Aboriginal people with diabetes.

Visit **https://www.community.healthconnections.com.au** and navigate to 'Aboriginal Diabetes Education Video Resources' to watch Aboriginal and Torres Strait Islander people share their diabetes stories.

1   Why is it important to use Aboriginal and Torres Strait Islander community members to share their diabetes stories?

Reflect evidence-based practice in own provision of healthcare services

Evidence-based practice (EBP) means using the 'best available evidence' to underpin clinical decision-making and provide the best possible outcomes for clients (see Figure 17.15). This problem-solving approach encourages the healthcare worker to provide individualised and comprehensive care. It helps you to build your own knowledge and improve your practices.

As an assistant to allied health professionals, you'll understand that health care depends on correct decisions. In your role, you can reflect on evidence-based practice to:

- evaluate and implement the most current, clinically relevant care based on research
- draw on your clinical expertise with what has worked and what has not
- consider the preferences of your clients.

You will be working under the guidance of your supervising allied health professional, which provides you with an opportunity to ask questions, research evidence and evaluate the care that has been prescribed for the clients.

The benefits of evidence-based practice include the following:

- As the preferences of the patient are taken into consideration, an advantage of evidence-based practice is that the needs of the patients are prioritised.
- As each nursing action is backed up by research, there is no need to engage in activities that are not proven.
- Research-backed evidence ensures your practices are current and relevant, and this builds your confidence as a healthcare worker.

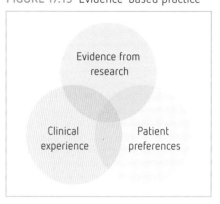

FIGURE 17.15 Evidence-based practice

Evidence from research

Clinical experience

Patient preferences

Evidence-based practice for nutrition

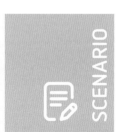

SCENARIO

Dietitians use evidence-based practice when providing information to clients for their nutritional wellbeing.

Valerie has heart disease and type 2 diabetes and has been referred to the dietitian for nutritional advice. She is significantly overweight and has high blood pressure. The dietitian takes a full medical history as well as asking Valerie what foods she consumes on a regular basis. These foods include:

- sugar-sweetened beverages
- fast food
- frozen meals
- snacks, including chips and cakes.

An evidence-based diet plan is developed for Valerie which includes:

- eating wholefoods and avoiding processed foods.
- a wide variety of vegetables and fruits
- limiting full-fat dairy products.
- eating a few portions of oily fish per week
- healthful fats, such as olive oil and avocados
- nuts, seeds and legumes.

Valerie is also referred to an exercise physiologist to design an appropriate strength and cardio program for her, based on her preferences, abilities and home environment. The exercise physiologist will also provide goal-setting techniques to motivate Valerie in achieving her outcomes.

1 How could the allied health assistant use evidence-based practice to support Valerie in her nutritional choices?

2 Why is it important for the exercise physiologist to set goals in order to motivate Valerie to maintain correct nutritional choices?

3 What are two example goals that would be specific for Valerie?

SUMMARY

The allied health sector is very diverse, with each professional working to assess conditions and provide treatment to enable recovery and/or reablement. This chapter identified this diverse workforce and outlined the roles and responsibilities of both the allied health professionals as well as the allied health assistants. The assistive roles include preparation of the client for therapy by providing relevant information and providing assistance with therapy sessions, while giving feedback to the supervising professionals.

The importance of using therapy equipment safely was highlighted as well as the adaptations that can be made to suit the individual's needs. This chapter also examined the administrative roles that allied health workers undertake, such as maintaining data and stock, filing, and booking appointments, which all help to maximise clinical efficiency.

The last part of the chapter identified that healthcare workers play a central role in providing essential services that promote health and prevent disease to individuals and communities based on the primary healthcare approach. Using evidence-based practice and reflection ensures that the quality of health care for the population is maintained.

APPLY YOUR KNOWLEDGE

The multidisciplinary approach

Justin has had motor neurone disease for the last 18 months. This disease causes destruction of motor neurons and results in the muscles not receiving signals from the brain, so they begin to waste. The disease also causes muscle stiffness and overactive reflexes. Justin has begun to have trouble speaking clearly and the weakness in his legs and arms has progressed. This has made him feel depressed as he finds it difficult to help out at home.

Justin's GP has referred him to an allied health team consisting of a physiotherapist, speech pathologist, psychologist and occupational therapist to assist him with his health and wellbeing.

1 Describe the roles of these allied health professionals.

Allied health assistants work under the supervision of these healthcare professionals, who are responsible for the delivery of therapy provided by the assistant. The physiotherapist prescribes splints to prevent contractures in Justin's arms and designs a treatment plan to maintain Justin's mobility. The allied health assistant is assigned to assist Justin with this plan by supporting him with passive exercises.

2   How does the allied health assistant ensure that they have full understanding of the treatment plan and therapy?

3   Using the knowledge you learnt in Chapter 3, 'Recognise healthy body systems', how can the allied health assistant perform passive exercises with Justin?

The occupational therapist undertakes a home visit to determine how Justin performs everyday activities and asks him what he finds difficult. She develops a plan to assist Justin which includes adaptive equipment for his personal care needs.

4   What assistive personal care devices would benefit Justin, who has weakness in his hands and legs?

During Justin's clinic session, the speech pathologist works with him to develop a plan for his slurred and slow speech. The speech pathologist listens to him as he goes through the exercises, and the allied health assistant stays with him as he continues with the exercise plan. This includes speaking more slowly, pausing to take breaths between words and sentences, and over-emphasising words and breaking them into distinct syllables. The allied health assistant reports back to the speech pathologist and records Justin's progress in the notes using the SOAP method of documentation.

5   What is the SOAP method and why is it important to document Justin's progress?

Justin is aware that he will require more and more help with all aspects of day-to-day living as the disease progresses. He and his family are confident that the allied health professionals will continue to support him and that they will tailor their plans to provide increasing assistance as it is needed.

6   Justin had a variety of treatment plans with each of the multidisciplinary team members. What was the scope of the allied health assistant's involvement in these treatment plans?

◀ REFLECTING ON THE INDUSTRY INSIGHT

1   Mr Quade's cardiac exercise program has been personalised for his needs and includes:
    a   Visits to the psychiatrist and physiotherapist.
    b   Stretching and education for his family.
    c   Education and strength training.
    d   Running to improve his endurance.

2   Why is it important for Mr Quade to warm up prior to his exercise session?
    a   To decrease pain associated with limited blood flow to the heart.
    b   To reduce the incidence of soreness or injury post-exercise.
    c   To reduce his body temperature so that he does not perspire during exercise.
    d   To maximise his endurance when increasing the pace of the session.

3   Healthy lifestyle choices recommended for Mr Quade include:
    a   Eating more saturated fats and starting a new sport.
    b   Increasing exercise, sleeping well and fasting.
    c   Drinking more water, stretching and eating more meat.
    d   Exercise, weight reduction and correct nutrition.

SELF-CHECK QUESTIONS

1   In your own words, describe the role of allied health professionals.
2   List the limitations in scope of practice for allied health assistants.
3   Explain how treatment plans assist with therapy for clients.
4   Explain the difference between a treatment session and a therapy session.
5   Outline how the client can be a useful source of information when reviewing therapy plans.
6   Explain why it is important to understand the physical and emotional limitations of the client before assisting with therapy sessions.
7   Explain the difference between general and specific goals when planning sessions for the client.
8   Why is it important to adapt therapy aids and equipment to suit the individual?
9   How can health promotion and disease prevention minimise future illness and maintain the client's wellbeing?
10 What are your definitions of the following key words and terms that have been used in this chapter?

KEY WORD AND TERM	YOUR DEFINITION
Rehabilitation	
Scope of practice	
Clinical pathway	
Clarification	
Feedback	
Adaptive equipment	
Statistics	
Primary health care	
Equity and access	
Evidence-based practice	

QUESTIONS FOR DISCUSSION

1   Discuss the non-client sources used to obtain health information on a client.
2   Discuss why it is important to explain goals to a client prior to undertaking therapy sessions.
3   Discuss the adaptive devices used to support ADLs that an occupational therapist could prescribe for a client who has had a stroke with resultant right-sided weakness.
4   Discuss the importance of statistics to health care and research.
5   Discuss the importance of access and equity in the provision of health services.

EXTENSION ACTIVITY

Radiographer assistant roles and responsibilities

Radiographer assistants support a radiographer in obtaining X-ray or other medical images of patients. Other duties and responsibilities include ensuring imaging machines are functioning properly, interacting with patients and performing administrative tasks. Completing a Certificate III in Allied Health Assistance and undertaking a training course in medical imaging will enable you to qualify for this role.

As a newly qualified allied health assistant, Lucas has learnt how to safely check and clean the medical imaging equipment and modify the equipment for patient comfort. His additional roles include patient bookings and maintaining records.

Lucas finds that many patients experience anxiety during the imaging process, particularly during CT and MRI scans where the procedure is done in a confined space. Explaining the imaging procedures and putting the patients at ease is something that he is becoming skilled in, although sometimes a sedative is required to help patients relax during the procedure.

Additional preparation includes checking that the patient has removed all jewellery and that they do not have a pacemaker or implanted device. Lucas instructs the patients to lie still during the procedure and lets them know that they may have to hold their breath at some stages of the scanning process. He also lets them know that the machine makes a noise and the scan may take up to 30 minutes.

When the scan results are not positive and patients require further surgery, therapeutic communication is a priority as well as referrals to both medical and additional allied health professionals.

1   How can Lucas develop a therapeutic relationship with his clients at admission?
2   What comfort adaptations could Lucas use when the patient is lying on a scanning table?
3   Explain why it is important for patients to remove metal objects before CT scans and describe the types of metal objects that need to be removed.
4   What additional allied health professionals could be used when scan results indicate further disease requiring surgery?
5   How can Lucas use evidence-based practice to continue with his learning journey?
6   Form two groups and discuss how medical imaging supports a health promotion and disease prevention strategy, with reference to the principles, vision and aims of the National Preventive Health Strategy 2021–2030.

REFERENCES

Allied Health Professionals Australia (AHPA) (2022a). Allied health professionals. Retrieved 31 December 2021 from https://ahpa.com.au/allied-health-professions/

Allied Health Professionals Australia (AHPA) (2022b). Rehabilitative care. Retrieved 31 December 2021 from https://ahpa.com.au/key-areas/rehabilitation/

Australian Government Department of Health (2016). National Strategic Framework for Rural and Remote Health. Retrieved 1 January 2022 from https://www1.health.gov.au/internet/main/publishing.nsf/Content/national-strategic-framework-rural-remote-health

Australian Government Department of Health (2021). What primary health networks are. Retrieved 10 January 2022 from https://www.health.gov.au/initiatives-and-programs/phn/what-phns-are

Australian Institute of Health and Welfare (2016). Primary healthcare in Australia. Retrieved 4 January 2022 from https://www.aihw.gov.au/reports/primary-health-care/primary-health-care-in-australia/contents/about-primary-health-care

Indigenous Allied Health Australia (IAHA) (2020). Indigenous allied health. Retrieved 2 January 2022 from https://www.indigenousalliedhealth.com.au

New South Wales Health Department (2018). Introduction to evidence-based practice and CIAP. Retrieved 5 January 2022 from https://www.ciap.health.nsw.gov.au/training/ebp-learning-modules/module1/evidence-based-practice-is.html

Portugal, Salvador E. (2021). Rehabilitation for speech disorders. Retrieved 5 January 2022 from https://www.msdmanuals.com/en-au/home/fundamentals/rehabilitation/rehabilitation-for-speech-disorders

Public Health Association Australia (2012). Policy-at-a-glance – Health Inequities Policy. Retrieved 5 January 2022 from https://www.phaa.net.au/documents/item/691

Queensland Health (2017). Occupational Therapy Learner Guide – Support the fitting of assistive devices. Retrieved 9 January 2022 from https://www.health.qld.gov.au/__data/assets/pdf_file/0026/650582/LG-fit-assistive-device.pdf

Services for Australian Rural and Remote Allied Health (SARRAH) (2022). Making a difference. Retrieved 10 January 2022 from https://sarrah.org.au/

St Vincent's Hospital Melbourne (2022). Occupational therapy: A guide for lower limb amputees. Retrieved 6 January 2022 from https://www.svhm.org.au/ArticleDocuments/3201/Occupational%20Therapy%20-%20A%20guide%20for%20lower%20limb%20amputees.pdf.aspx?embed=y

University of St Augustine for Health Sciences (2020). The role of evidence-based practice in nursing. Retrieved 10 January 2022 from https://www.usa.edu/blog/evidence-based-practice/

World Health Organization (WHO) (2022). Social determinants of health. Retrieved 9 January 2022 from https://www.who.int/health-topics/social-determinants-of-health#tab=tab_1

GLOSSARY

acceptable abbreviations
Abbreviations that are approved for use by each health organisation.

access and equity
Providing services to all and treating them fairly.

acronym
A word formed by the initial letters of each word in the complete phrase.

active and reflective listening
Focusing on what someone is saying to you by asking questions, paraphrasing, seeking clarification and summarising.

active exercise
Using your own muscle power to move muscles and joints in the body.

activities of daily living (ADLs)
A set of activities necessary for normal self-care. The activities are feeding, bathing, dressing, toileting, mobility and continence.

adaptive equipment
Any device or tool used to assist with completing activities of daily living.

additional precautions
Also called transmission-based precautions. Special infection control measures used when standard precautions alone may not be sufficient to prevent the transmission of infection.

advance care directive (ACD)
Sometimes called a 'living will', this is an outline of your preferences for your future care along with your beliefs, values and goals when you can no longer make these decisions yourself.

Alzheimer's disease
A physical disease of the brain with progressive damage to brain cells, which causes dementia.

anti-thrombosis (TED) stockings
Calf- or thigh-length elastic stockings that help prevent DVT and pulmonary embolism. Work by compressing the leg in a graduated fashion to increase the return of blood up the leg veins.

anxiety
Feelings and experiences that occur at times of stress. Symptoms include nervousness, fear, worry, excessive sweating, irritability, breathlessness, palpitations and racing pulse.

arrhythmia
An irregular heartbeat, ordinarily associated with a fluttering in the chest.

arteries
Thick-walled blood vessels that carry oxygenated blood from the heart to tissues and organs in the body.

assertion
Being emphatic in a calm and positive way, without being either aggressive or passive.

assistive device
Any device that is designed, made or adapted to assist a person to perform a particular task.

assumption
Something taken for granted or accepted as true without proof; a supposition.

asthma
A type of chronic airways disease with symptoms of wheezing, breathlessness and chest tightness.

atherosclerosis
Hardening and narrowing of the arteries caused by cholesterol, fat and other substances lining the arteries.

Australian Standards
Documents setting out specifications, procedures and guidelines for Australia.

autonomic nervous system
Automatic or involuntary responses of the nervous system, as in the actions of smooth muscles, cardiac muscles and glands.

autonomy
Having control and choice over one's life.

bacteria
Microorganisms capable of causing disease and infection.

bariatric person
A person who is obese or severely obese.

barrier nursing
Local isolation of a patient with an infectious disease to prevent the spread of the disease. The 'barrier' takes the form of gowns, caps, overshoes, gloves and masks that are donned by staff and visitors before approaching the patient and discarded before returning to the normal environment.

bereavement
The emotional reactions experienced after a significant loss, such as death.

biohazard bag
Specialist disposal bag for clinical waste.

bipolar disorder
Extremes of mood, between manic and depressive, that interfere with everyday life.

bladder scanning
Provides a 3D image of the bladder on a display screen.

blood glucose level (BGL)
Level of glucose present in the blood, the measurement of which is undertaken when a person has or is suspected to have diabetes. Normal BGL is between 4.0 and 8.0 mmol/L.

blood pH
The acidity or alkalinity of blood.

body cavities
Spaces inside the body that hold and protect internal organs.

body mechanics
The way a person moves and holds their body when they sit, stand, lift, carry and bend.

body temperature
The level of heat produced and sustained by the body, the measurement of which provides information regarding general health and possible infection. Measured with a thermometer.

brain stem
Merges with the spinal cord at the base of the brain to relay messages to other parts of the body.

capillaries
The smallest blood vessels, which connect arterioles with venules.

cardiovascular system
Refers to the heart, blood vessels and blood.

cartilage
Tough connective tissue that lines joints and gives structure to the nose, ears, larynx and other parts of the body.

centre of gravity
The point at which the entire mass of the body is assumed to be concentrated – waist/hip height.

cerebellum
The part of the brain that lies beneath the cerebrum and coordinates muscle activity and balance.

cerebrum
The part of the brain that controls thought, language, reasoning, perception and voluntary movement.

charting by exception
Where only significant findings or exceptions to the predefined standards are documented in detail.

chemical waste
Waste that is made from harmful chemicals such as solvents and mercury.

Cheyne-Stokes respirations
Abnormal pattern of breathing, where there are periods of apnoea (no breathing) followed by periods of tachypnoea (fast breathing).

clarification
A communication technique used to clear up confusion or uncertainty.

cleansing
The cleaning of surfaces or instruments with warm water and mild detergent.

clinical constraints
Clinical restrictions that need to be taken into consideration when giving care; for example, IV, IDC, drain.

clinical handover
Transfer of information, accountability and responsibility for patients from one healthcare worker to another.

clinical hand wash
A longer routine hand wash that takes a minimum of 60 seconds and is used by healthcare workers before commencing a dressing or procedure on a resident or patient, or before opening sterile equipment.

clinical pathways
Standardised, evidence-based multidisciplinary plans that identify an appropriate order of clinical interventions and timeframes for common disorders.

clinical waste
Any waste that has the potential to cause or spread disease.

communication
Sending, receiving or exchanging information.

community mental health services
Services and teams that deliver care outside of inpatient settings.

community transport personnel
People who assist community members with transportation to and from activities, health services, appointments, etc.

Community Treatment Order
Sets out the terms under which a person must accept medication and therapy, counselling, management, rehabilitation and other services while living in the community.

confidentiality
Having another's trust or confidence.

conflict of interest
A situation in which the concerns or aims of two different parties are incompatible.

contingencies
An outline of what you are going to do when something does not go to plan.

continuity of care
Where health care is provided for a person in a coordinated manner by a health team.

continuous improvement
Ongoing efforts to improve performance or processes.

COPD (chronic obstructive pulmonary disease)
A disease with symptoms of mild or severe shortness of breath. COPD includes emphysema and chronic bronchitis.

coroner's court
A court that deals with finding out the identity of the deceased person, when and where they died, how they died and the medical cause of death.

critical incident
Any situation that creates a significant risk of substantial or serious harm to the physical or mental health, safety or wellbeing of another.

cultural bias
Assumptions about other cultures or about a particular cultural group that affects related perceptions.

cultural competence
The ability of systems to provide care to patients with diverse values, beliefs and behaviours.

cultural identity
The feeling of belonging to a group.

cultural safety
'Creating a workplace where everyone can examine our own cultural identities and attitudes, and be open-minded and flexible in our attitudes towards people from cultures other than our own.' (SafeWork NSW, 2020)

culturally and linguistically diverse (CALD)
People born in a country where English is not the main spoken language.

cultures
Growing microorganisms in a nutrient medium.

curative care
Healthcare practices using medication and therapies that treat patients with the intent of curing them.

deadline
An urgent goal that is non-negotiable and has to be met by a certain time.

debriefing
Providing a summary update of a condition or situation to the affected or concerned people.

delirium
An acute confusional state that can be caused by acute illness or drug toxicity. It is often reversible.

dementia
A progressive state of confusion and deterioration of intellectual and physical ability, resulting in eventual death.

diagnosis
Identifying a disease, illness or problem.

diagnostic images
Visualisations such as X-ray, CT scans, MRI scans and ultrasounds.

diastolic
Blood pressure when the heart is relaxed and refilling with blood – the lower reading.

dignity of risk
A person's right to make their own choices and decisions, even when those decisions could put them at risk, with benefits that might include gaining greater self-esteem and independence.

discharge planning
The plan of how the client's medical requirements will be met after he or she is released from treatment.

disclosure
Revealing or uncovering information that was intended to be private.

discrimination
Treating a person or people unfairly due to their age, gender, race, religion, sexuality, marital status etc.

disinfection
The removal or elimination of pathogenic microorganisms (except spores) with the use of chemical solutions.

distraction
Used to refocus the attention of a person with dementia from a negative behaviour to a positive one.

DNR order (do not resuscitate)
A medical order to withhold cardiopulmonary resuscitation (CPR) techniques.

Doppler ultrasonography
Involves the transmission of sound waves through the skin using a Doppler machine.

duty of care
The requirement to ensure health and safety by eliminating risks.

early intervention
Responding early in the course of a mental health disorder or illness, and early in an episode of illness, to reduce the risk of escalation.

electrocardiogram (ECG)
Provides graphical record (a trace) of the heart's electrical action.

electronic medical records (EMRs)
Online medical records and forms used to standardise documentation, prevent errors and allow ease of access for all healthcare staff.

embolism
The obstruction of a blood vessel by a foreign substance or a blood clot.

emergency action plan
A plan that outlines an organisation's policies and procedures in response to an emergency situation.

empathy
The ability to understand and share the feelings of another.

empowerment
Defined by the WHO as the 'process of taking control and responsibility for actions that have the intent and potential to lead to fulfilment of capacity'.

endocrine system
The system of glands and organs that secretes hormones into the bloodstream to regulate bodily functions.

enduring guardianship
Allows you to legally appoint a decision-maker of your choice to make lifestyle and healthcare decisions should you lose the capacity to do so.

enteral tube feeding
Delivery of nutritionally complete food directly into the gut via a tube.

erythrocytes
Red blood cells.

ethnocentrism
The belief that your own cultural or ethnic group is superior to others.

experiential learning
Learning process based on 'learn by doing' and by reflecting on the experience.

feedback
Helpful information or criticism given to improve performance.

fluid balance chart
Helps to accurately record fluid intake (i.e., oral and IV) and output (i.e., urine, vomitus and drainage).

food record chart
Used to monitor and assess the nutritional intake of patients where there is concern about their nutrition. Helps to inform dietitian treatment plans.

formal learning
Structured learning programs that may be accredited in terms of a unit of competence or completion of a qualification.

fungi
Yeasts or moulds that may cause infections in the hair, nails, skin and mucous membranes.

gastrointestinal system
Responsible for the digestion and absorption of food and liquids into the blood for cell energy and function.

general waste
Domestic and recyclable waste which does not cause any concern as a biological, chemical, radioactive or physical hazard.

genotoxic or cytotoxic waste
Includes cytotoxic drugs (e.g., used in chemotherapy).

Glasgow Coma Scale (GCS)
A tool that is used to assess a person's level of consciousness. A score of 15 indicates an alert and orientated person, whereas less than 8 indicates they are comatose.

glucometer
Measures the levels of glucose in a patient's blood.

grief reactions
A wide array of emotions including sadness, shock, anger, guilt and depression that an individual might feel after experiencing loss.

grievance
A complaint because an event is believed to be incorrect or unfair.

group dynamics
The processes involved when people in a group interact.

haematoma
A collection of blood outside of blood vessels.

hazard
Anything that has the potential to harm the health or safety of a person.

health record
A chronological record of interactions, observations and actions relating to a particular patient.

hierarchy of control
A step-by-step approach to eliminating or reducing risks, with a ranking of risk controls from the highest level of protection through to the lowest and least reliable protection.

homeostasis
The ability of a system to maintain its internal equilibrium.

hospital-acquired infection
Also called nosocomial infections. An infection acquired in the healthcare facility by a patient who did not have it on admission.

human rights
The basic freedoms and protections that belong to every single human.

hybrid record
A health record comprising paper, digitised and electronic formats. A hybrid health record is created and accessed using both manual and electronic processes.

hypothyroidism
Where the thyroid gland is underactive and fails to secrete enough hormones into the bloodstream.

incident
An event or particular occurrence; for example, a falls incident.

inclusive practice
Not discriminating against people or treating them unfairly on the basis of differences when caring for them.

incontinence
Any accidental or involuntary loss of urine from the bladder or faeces from the bowel.

individual service plans
Plans that set out goals and strategies and explain the support provided by each member of the healthcare team, as well as who is responsible for what and when.

infection
Damage to tissue or cells by invading microorganisms.

infectious waste
Waste contaminated with blood and/or other body fluids.

informal learning
Incorporates applied learning in everyday situations.

informed consent
A person's voluntary decision to agree to healthcare intervention after accurate information has been given regarding choices.

integumentary system
The bodily system consisting of the skin and its associated structures, such as the hair, nails, sweat glands and sebaceous glands, all of which protect the body from damage, injury and infection.

interfacility transport
Transport from one facility to another.

interpersonal communication
Face-to-face exchange of information, feelings and meaning through verbal and non-verbal messages.

interpreter
A person who interprets speech orally or into sign language.

joints
Where two or more bones meet to allow for movement.

key performance indicator (KPI)
A measurable value that demonstrates how effectively objectives and goals are being met.

lamina flow environment
An environment that minimises the amount of dust and particles in the air by filtering and exhausting the air in one direction only.

ligaments
Fibrous connective tissue that connects bones to other bones.

lymphatic system
Specialised vessels and organs that collect and circulate excess fluid in the body; plays a part in the body's immune response.

mandatory reporting
The legal requirement to report suspected cases of child abuse and neglect.

marginalised groups
Specific groups of people who have been pushed to the lower or outer edge of society.

menopause
The period in a woman's life (typically between the ages of 45 and 50) when menstruation ceases.

mental illness
Conditions that significantly affect how a person feels, thinks, behaves and interacts with others.

mentoring
Assisting an individual in terms of achieving their work goals with the use of a more experienced person.

microorganism
Any living microscopic entity, including bacteria and viruses.

multiculturalism
Incorporating ideas, beliefs or people from many different countries and cultural backgrounds.

musculoskeletal system
The bones, joints, cartilage, ligaments and connective tissue that support the body and help you move.

near miss
An accident that is just barely avoided; for example, almost receiving a needlestick injury.

National Safety and Quality Health Service (NSQHS) Standards
National standards regarding the consistent level of care people can expect from health service providers.

nervous system
Receives and interprets stimuli (via neurons) to control and coordinate activities in the body.

non-verbal communication
All the messages in a conversation that are not expressed in words.

nursing history
Data collected about a client's physical, cognitive, social and emotional history.

olfactory cells
Passes along smell sensations to the brain.

organelles
A number of organised or specialised structures within a living cell.

orientation
A person's ability to identify their position in the environment relative to known landmarks (i.e., knowing where they are and where they are going).

ostomy appliance
Used when a patient has an artificial opening in the colon or ileum due to disease or surgery to the digestive tract.

palliative care
Care that improves the quality of life of a person and their family through the prevention and relief of suffering by assessment and treatment of pain and other problems – physical, psychosocial and spiritual.

parasites
Microorganisms that survive and thrive on others while contributing nothing to the host cell. Protozoa and helminths are types of parasites.

passive exercise
Exercise performed with the assistance of a person who moves your muscles and joints through their range of motion.

pastoral care worker
A person who works within an holistic approach to health to help individuals respond to spiritual and emotional needs.

pathogens
Microorganisms that produce disease.

pathological waste
Waste that includes human tissue, organs or fluids.

patient history
Information gained by asking specific questions, either of the patient or significant others.

pelvic floor exercises
Isometric exercises to strengthen the muscles around your bladder, bottom, and vagina or penis.

performance appraisal
A review of your job performance with feedback on further growth and development.

peristalsis
Involuntary constriction and relaxation of the muscles of the intestine or another canal.

person-centred approach
Caring holistically for the person, which includes their preferences, needs and values, and those of their carers.

person conducting a business or undertaking (PCBU)
Individuals, businesses or organisations that are conducting business.

personal protective equipment (PPE)
Clothing and equipment designed to be a barrier between the worker and the hazard.

pharmaceutical waste
Unused, expired or leftover medication that is no longer needed.

point of care solution
A device that is used where direct patient care is delivered.

policy directive
An official or authoritative instruction.

post-traumatic stress disorder (PTSD)
A disorder that develops in some people who have seen or lived through a shocking, frightening or dangerous event. Main symptoms are re-experiencing the trauma (memories, nightmares or flashbacks), avoiding reminders of the trauma, and negative thoughts and mood.

power of attorney
Gives an assigned third party the power to make decisions on a person's behalf regarding managing assets and financial affairs in the event that they are unable to do so when the need arises.

prefix
A one- or two-syllable word part placed before a word to modify or alter its meaning.

protocols
The set of rules that explain the correct conduct and procedures to be followed in formal situations.

protozoa
Single-celled parasites causing infections such as gastroenteritis after ingestion of infected food or water.

proxemics
The space that people feel is necessary to maintain between themselves and others.

pressure injury
Also known as a pressure ulcer, pressure sore, bed sore or decubitus ulcer; they are a risk for anyone who is immobile. Unrelieved pressure damages underying tissue by decreasing circulation. Categorised from Stage I to Stage IV.

primary health care
Entry level to the health system and, usually, a person's first encounter with the health system.

pulse
A wave of distension of an artery following the contraction of the heart.

pulse oximeter
Measures heart rate (as bpm) and oxygen saturation (as SpO2) in the blood.

quality of life
Includes a person's physical, social, psychological and spiritual needs and can only be determined by each individual.

range of motion
The measurement of movement around a specific joint or body part.

rapport
A close relationship allowing a good understanding for effective communication.

reality orientation
Attempts to orientate the person with the present using reminders of the time (clocks), the day (calendars) and current surroundings (signage).

recovery-orientated practice
Sets of capabilities that support people to recognise and take responsibility for their own recovery and wellbeing and to define their goals, wishes and aspirations.

reflection
Mirroring the feeling or tone of someone's message so that the person can better understand their own thoughts and feelings.

rehabilitation
Restoring someone to health through training and therapy.

respiration
The process of inhalation (breathing in) and exhalation (breathing out) to exchange oxygen and carbon dioxide. When measuring, observe the rate, rhythm, volume and symmetry.

residual risk
The risk of loss or harm remaining even after all controls have been implemented.

reminiscence
Using written, pictorial or oral life histories to enhance the psychological wellbeing of a person with cognitive impairment.

respiratory system
The organs involved in breathing with the exchange of oxygen and carbon dioxide.

restrictive practice
An intervention that restricts the rights or freedom of movement of an individual.

rickettsiae
Microorganisms that can only survive within living tissue and are spread by lice, fleas and ticks, causing infections such as typhus.

risk
The possibility that a hazard will actually cause harm.

risk assessment
Analysis of the potential risks that may be involved in an activity.

risk control
A hazard management process aimed at identifying risks and eliminating or reducing the likelihood of injury.

risk management
The culture, processes and structures that are directed towards realising potential opportunities while managing adverse effects.

root word
Usually indicates the involved body part and refers to the main body of the word.

routine hand wash
Lasts between 40 and 60 seconds and is used to remove visible soil and transient microorganisms.

scope of practice
Procedures, actions and processes that a healthcare worker is permitted to undertake.

self-assessment
Reflecting on the quality of the work you have done, including strengths and weaknesses.

sharp
Any equipment that contains a needle, scalpel or blade.

skin integrity
Skin that is whole, intact and undamaged.

social media
Websites and other online means of communication that are used by large groups of people to share information and to develop social and professional contacts.

somatic nervous system
Carries motor and sensory information to skin, sense organs and skeletal muscles.

specimen collection
The process of obtaining tissue or fluids for analysis; for example, urine for urinalysis, faeces for occult blood testing, or sputum for testing for pathogens.

sphincter
A circular muscle that constricts a passage or closes a natural orifice. When relaxed, a sphincter allows materials to pass through the opening.

spinal cord
Carries motor and sensory messages to and from the brain.

spores
Cells produced by bacteria and fungi that can develop into new bacteria or fungi.

standard precautions
Basic level of infection control that reduces the spread of possible infection.

statistics
Collection, analysis and interpretation of data.

stereotype
A generalised idea or image about a person or thing that is often oversimplified and offensive.

sterilisation
The complete removal of and destruction of all microorganisms (including spores) from equipment by either steam, chemicals or gamma irradiation.

stigma
A mark or label that sets a person apart. It can create negative attitudes and prejudice.

stretch target
A target that cannot be achieved by small improvements and requires extending oneself.

suffix
A one- or two-syllable word part attached to the end of a word to modify or alter its meaning.

surgical hand wash
Completed prior to surgery or an invasive procedure, and takes between two to five minutes. The hands and forearms are scrubbed as well as areas under nails.

SWOT analysis
A strategic planning technique used to help a person or organisation identify strengths, weaknesses, opportunities and threats.

synovial fluid
Thick liquid located between joints to provide lubrication.

systolic
Blood pressure when the heart is contracting – the upper reading.

tendons
Connective tissue that connects muscle to bone.

therapeutic relationship
In nursing, a relationship between the healthcare person and the patient that improves physical, social and emotional wellbeing.

transcultural strategies of care
Care that acknowledges an individual's culture, values, beliefs and practices.

transducer gel
Water-based conductive medium that is used in ultrasound, ECG and scanning therapies.

treatment plan
An outline of a patient's therapeutic treatment.

Universal Declaration of Human Rights
The internationally agreed declaration stating that all people everywhere have the same human rights that no-one can take away from them.

urinalysis
Tests the urine for the presence of various substances.

urinary catheter
Drains urine from the bladder into a drainage bag.

urinary system
Produces, stores and eliminates fluid waste (urine) from the body.

validation therapy
A communication technique that focuses on the individual's emotions, rather than reality. Its primary goal is to try to see the world from the individual's point of view.

vasodilation
Dilation or widening of a blood vessel.

veins
Thin-walled blood vessels that carry deoxygenated blood to the heart from tissues and organs in the body.

viruses
Microorganisms that multiply only within the living cells of a host. Examples include the common cold, chicken pox and HIV.

Waterlow or Braden pressure ulcer assessment tool
A screening tool that provides predictive information about the risk of developing a pressure sore.

weighing scales
Used to determine the patient's weight; can include chair scales or standing scales.

work health and safety induction
An overview of the general WHS obligations, policies and procedures of your organisation.

work role boundaries
The clear definition of a healthcare worker's duties, rights and limitations.

INDEX